Essentials of
CRITICAL CARE MEDICINE
for the Physician

Essentials of
CRITICAL CARE MEDICINE
for the Physician

Jamshed Sunavala
MD FCCP FICP FISE (Hon)
Director
Department of Critical Care and Emergency Services
Jaslok Hospital and Research Centre, Mumbai, India
Consultant Intensivist
Breach Candy Hospital & Research Centre and
B D Petit Parsee General Hospital
Mumbai, India

Foreword
Farokh E Udwadia

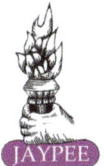

JAYPEE BROTHERS MEDICAL PUBLISHERS
The Health Sciences Publisher
New Delhi | London

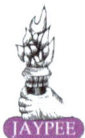 **Jaypee Brothers Medical Publishers (P) Ltd**

Headquarters

Jaypee Brothers Medical Publishers (P) Ltd
EMCA House, 23/23-B
Ansari Road, Daryaganj
New Delhi 110 002, India
Landline: +91-11-23272143, +91-11-23272703
+91-11-23282021, +91-11-23245672
Email: jaypee@jaypeebrothers.com

Corporate Office

Jaypee Brothers Medical Publishers (P) Ltd
4838/24, Ansari Road, Daryaganj
New Delhi 110 002, India
Phone: +91-11-43574357
Fax: +91-11-43574314
Email: jaypee@jaypeebrothers.com

Overseas Office

JP Medical Ltd
83 Victoria Street, London
SW1H 0HW (UK)
Phone: +44 20 3170 8910
Fax: +44 (0)20 3008 6180
Email: info@jpmedpub.com

Website: www.jaypeebrothers.com
Website: www.jaypeedigital.com

© 2022, Jaypee Brothers Medical Publishers

The views and opinions expressed in this book are solely those of the original contributor(s)/author(s) and do not necessarily represent those of editor(s) of the book.

All rights reserved. No part of this publication may be reproduced, stored or transmitted in any form or by any means, electronic, mechanical, photocopying, recording or otherwise, without the prior permission in writing of the publishers.

All brand names and product names used in this book are trade names, service marks, trademarks or registered trademarks of their respective owners. The publisher is not associated with any product or vendor mentioned in this book.

Medical knowledge and practice change constantly. This book is designed to provide accurate, authoritative information about the subject matter in question. However, readers are advised to check the most current information available on procedures included and check information from the manufacturer of each product to be administered, to verify the recommended dose, formula, method and duration of administration, adverse effects and contraindications. It is the responsibility of the practitioner to take all appropriate safety precautions. Neither the publisher nor the author(s)/editor(s) assume any liability for any injury and/or damage to persons or property arising from or related to use of material in this book.

This book is sold on the understanding that the publisher is not engaged in providing professional medical services. If such advice or services are required, the services of a competent medical professional should be sought.

Every effort has been made where necessary to contact holders of copyright to obtain permission to reproduce copyright material. If any have been inadvertently overlooked, the publisher will be pleased to make the necessary arrangements at the first opportunity. The **CD/DVD-ROM** (if any) provided in the sealed envelope with this book is complimentary and free of cost. **Not meant for sale**.

Inquiries for bulk sales may be solicited at: jaypee@jaypeebrothers.com

Essentials of Critical Care Medicine for the Physician

First Edition: 2022

ISBN: 978-93-5465-478-7

Dedicated to

Goolu, Anahita, Ayesha and Nergish

AND

All the selfless frontline workers who battled the COVID-19 pandemic.

*"Any (Human) death diminishes me,
because I am involved in mankind"*

— *John Donne*

Guest Contributors

Aabha Nagral MD
Hepatologist and Gastroenterologist
Apollo Hospitals, Navi Mumbai and
Jaslok Hospital and Medical
Research Centre
Mumbai, Maharashtra, India

Amey Sonavane
DNB (Medicine) DNB (Gastroenterology)
Hepatologist and Gastroenterologist
Apollo Hospitals
Navi Mumbai, Maharashtra, India

Ayesha Sunavala
DNB (Med) FNB(Infectious Diseases)
Consultant, Infectious Disease
P D Hinduja Hospital
Mumbai, Maharashtra, India

Azad Marazban Irani
MBBS DNB (Medicine) DNB (Neurology)
Junior Consultant
Jaslok Hospital and Research Centre
Mumbai, Maharashtra, India

Bhupendra V Gandhi MBBS
Certified Diplomate
American Board of Internal
Medicine and American Board
of Nephrology
Mentor, Department of Nephrology
and Renal Transplant
Sir H N Reliance Foundation
Hospital and Breach Candy Hospital
Mumbai, Maharashtra, India

Bomi B Ichaporia MD DM(Card)
Consultant Cardiologist
Breach Candy Hospital
Mumbai, Maharashtra, India

Camilla Rodrigues MD
Consultant Microbiologist
P D Hinduja Hospital and Medical
Research Centre
Mumbai, Maharashtra, India

Dipsha Kriplani Suvarna
MD FHO FCH
Clinical Associate
Hematology and Hemato-oncology
Breach Candy Hospital
Mumbai, Maharashtra, India

Fali Poncha MD DM
Consultant Neurologist
Jaslok Hospital and Research Centre
Mumbai, Maharashtra, India

Joanne Mascarenhas
DNB (Medicine) EDIC IDCCM
Consultant Intensivist
Breach Candy Hospital Trust
Mumbai, Maharashtra, India

Karuna Tiwari MD
Consultant Microbiologist
Dr Lal Path Labs
Mumbai, Maharashtra, India

Kunal Thakkar MD DM
Consultant Endocrinologist
Sterling Ram Krishna Speciality Hospital
Gandhidham, Gujarat, India

Nalini S Shah MD DM
Emeritus Professor
Department of Endocrinology
Seth G S Medical College and
KEM Hospital
Mumbai, Maharashtra, India

Nitin Burkule MD DM DNB FACC FASE
Director
Department of Cardiology
Jupiter Hospital
Thane, Maharashtra, India

Rajeev Soman MD FIDSA
Consultant Infectious
Diseases Physician
Jupiter Hospital
Pune, Maharashtra, India

Guest Contributors

Rakshita Eashwernath MD
Fellow in Infectious Diseases
Jupiter Hospital
Pune, Maharashtra, India

Ram E Rajagopalan
MBBS AB (Internal Medicine) AB (Critical Care)
Professor and Head of Clinical Services
Sri Ramachandra Medical Centre and
Sri Ramachandra Institute of Higher
Education and Research, Porur
Chennai, Tamil Nadu, India

Rishit Harbada
MBBS MD (Medicine) DNB (Medicine)
MRCP(London) DNB(Nephrology) ESE
(Nephrology)
Clinical Associate Nephrology
Department of Nephrology and Renal Transplant
Sir H N Reliance Foundation Hospital
Mumbai, Maharashtra, India

Sarosh M Katrak MD DM FRCP (Edin)
Emeritus Professor
Department of Neurology
GMC and Sir J J Group of
Hospitals, Mumbai
Director Emeritus
Department of Neurology
Jaslok Hospital & Research Centre
Mumbai, Maharashtra, India

Shruti Tandan Pardasani
MD FNB (Critical Care Medicine)
Consultant Intensivist
Jaslok Hospital and Research Centre
and Bhatia Hospital
Mumbai, Maharashtra, India

Vibhor Pardasani MD DM
Assistant Professor
Department of Neurology
Bombay Hospital Institute of
Medical Sciences
Mumbai, Maharashtra, India

Foreword

It gives me great pleasure to write a foreword to this book on Critical Care Medicine by Dr Jamshed Sunavala, a colleague with whom I have been associated for several decades. Dr Sunavala together with a number of other specialist colleagues have written on several important problems encountered in Intensive Care. The book consists of seven sections, each section being devoted to a particular aspect of critical care, there being altogether thirty-five chapters in this book.

The chapter on Acute Respiratory Failure incorporates basic respiratory physiology. Unfortunately, even today, many consultants as also intensivists have not given this aspect of respiratory care due consideration.

Every single chapter has been well-written, each being informative and instructive. The material in each chapter has been brought quite up-to-date. This is due to the fact that several consultants, each a specialist or super-specialist in his or her field has made valuable contributions.

I found the chapter on the Use of Antibiotics in the ICU written by Dr Ayesha Sunavala as also the chapters on Coma and Pitfalls in the Diagnosis of Brain Death written by Dr Sarosh Katrak particularly commendable. The case studies of Critical Care Infections by Dr Rajeev Soman and Rakshita Eashwernath are both interesting and informative.

The great importance of adequate nutrition in critically ill patients is not sufficiently realized. Dr Jamshed Sunavala's chapter on Nutritional Support is of critical value.

With all the advances in critical care, with all the sophisticated gadgetry at one's disposal it should not be forgotten that the knowledge and practice of basic good medicine which unquestionably involves taking a good history and performing a meticulous clinical examination, remains the bed-rock of critical care medicine.

I would recommend this book as a very good compendium to all critical care units in our country.

Farokh E Udwadia
MD FRCP (London) FRCP (Edinburgh) Master FCCP Hon DSc
Emeritus Professor of Medicine
Grant Medical College and JJ Group of Hospitals, Mumbai
Consultant Physician and Director of Critical Care Unit
Breach Candy Hospital, Mumbai
Consultant Physician, BD Petit Parsee General Hospital, Mumbai

Preface

One might call it 'audacity' to write a book, where a plethora of excellent books on the subject, are available on the stand. Therefore, I do not intend to add another exhaustive textbook on critical care medicine and definitely not a voluminous reference book; for such a venture you require multiple contributors or yourself be a prolific writer. *This book is aimed to target a specific readership and will be invaluable to:*

- *Consulting physicians in medicine and allied subjects* whose clinical practice includes caring for patients in the ICU and who need to understand the current 'best practice' standards in critical care medicine. In our own, and also many other countries, 'open' and 'hybrid' ICUs are prevalent and well-accepted, which allow admission rights to primary consultants. This may raise an issue of 'expertise' because a nonintensivist physician may not be thoroughly acquainted with the nuances involved in certain aspects of critical care medicine. Further, nonintensivist physicians though not required to do intricate monitoring and therapeutic procedures, should have adequate knowledge of their clinical application and procedural complications.
- *Residents in training for post-graduation in medicine or allied subjects* who seek a painless introduction to critical care medicine before their mandatory posting in the ICU. The book would also help those who have more than a passing interest in the entirety of critical care medicine and go beyond their assigned obligations towards routine patient care.
- *Young intensivists* who are beginning their ICU training. For them this book would be an excellent introduction to the fundamentals of the subject and a valuable guide for translating evidence into practice.

Well then, how is this book different from the rest? For one, it is brief but factual and adequate for the readership towards whom it is directed. Secondly, the book was written to make the science and art of critical care medicine accessible and understandable without going into pages of minute details which are more useful to a full time intensivist. Further, those chapters covered adequately in standard textbooks of medicine are not included here, in which case the book would have been much too long and encyclopedic and lost its purpose. Rather, the subject material included has been selected for its value to practising physicians hence those specific problems which are best handled by the intensivist are covered in this book, thereby broadening the physician's perspective, intrinsic to critical care. Chapters have been selectively chosen and divided within sections appropriate to the clinical approach of the subject (e.g. shock, supports, organ dysfunction, monitoring etc.), unlike other standard textbooks. Also, they are more or less independent as a result of which, they need not be read in a prescribed sequence. Further, in an attempt to avoid repetition and to make the book readable and short, certain important topics such as fluid resuscitation, shock (classification) and coagulation in brief, have been incorporated within the appropriate chapters. Basic principles of resuscitation and emergency procedures are an essential part of critical care training best learnt "hands-on" at the bedside. In every textbook the treatment of cardiac arrest, both Basic and Advanced Life Support, is consistent and follows the American Heart Association Guidelines which need no repetition in this book. Lastly, much emphasis has been placed to maintain clarity and simplicity so that those without any background or training in critical care medicine can easily comprehend the message. A precise knowledge of general medicine from reading standard textbooks of medicine (e.g. Harrison or Cecil), is an integral part of the practice of critical care medicine, without which the intensivist remains nothing more than a procedural technician.

Jamshed Sunavala

Acknowledgments

This book would remain incomplete without the contribution from my colleagues who readily agreed to write some of the chapters relevant to their expertise. I am genuinely grateful to all of them, as I believe that they have captured the essence of critical care medicine in their particular subject, which I hope will be useful to all who read this book. I am thankful to Dr Dhruva Chaudhry and Dr Nimish Shah who took time off from their busy schedule to vet some of the chapters relevant to their specialty and for their suggestions and Ms Parmi Gala (Clinical Pharmacologist) for help in compiling appendix I.

My sincere thanks to Dr Farokh E Udwadia who graciously consented to write the foreword to this book. His immeasurable contribution in pioneering critical care medicine in our country cannot be overlooked and that he has personally gone through almost all the chapters, was most encouraging.

I am grateful to Mr Neeraj Chawan whose conscientious efforts in typing the manuscript during the pandemic helped in the timely completion of the book.

I am thankful to Dr Ruby Kharas for proof reading the manuscript. I am greatly indebted to Mr Freddy Nagarvala for designing the front and the back cover of the book. A special thanks to Dr Pheroza Godrej for her help in obtaining permission for the copy of the painting from the Tate Gallery, London. Finally, my sincere thanks to the management of Jaypee Brothers Medical Publishers at New Delhi and Mumbai for publishing this book and particularly Mr Sameer S Mulla (Business Manager-Channel Sales) and Ms Nikita Chauhan (Senior Development Editor) for the assistance and support throughout the making of this book.

Contents

SECTION 1: HISTORY

1. Critical Care Medicine Over the Years 3
   Jamshed Sunavala

SECTION 2: RESUSCITATION

2. Airway Management 19
   Jamshed Sunavala

3. Postcardiac Arrest Care after Return of Spontaneous
   Circulation 26
   Jamshed Sunavala

SECTION 3: ORGAN DYSFUNCTION

4. Acute Respiratory Failure 35
   Jamshed Sunavala

5. Acute Respiratory Distress Syndrome 56
   Jamshed Sunavala

6. Intensive Care Management of Acute Heart Failure and
   Cardiogenic Shock 69
   Ram E Rajagopalan

7. Acute Kidney Injury in the ICU and Renal Replacement
   Therapies..84
   Bhupendra V Gandhi, Rishit Harbada

8. Coma in the ICU: A Clinical Approach 104
   Sarosh M Katrak

9. Stroke for Physicians and Intensivists...................................... 113
   Fali Poncha, Azad Marazban Irani, Vibhor Pardasani

10. Acute Liver Failure.. 126
    Amey Sonavane, Aabha Nagral

SECTION 4: INFECTION

11. Sepsis and its Sequelae 141
    Jamshed Sunavala

12. Antimicrobial Therapy in the Intensive Care Unit 155
    Ayesha Sunavala

13. Optimal Usage of the Microbiology Laboratory in the ICU .. 179
    Karuna Tiwari, Camilla Rodrigues

14. Invasive Fungal Infections in the ICU: Diagnosis and
    Management 193
    Rajeev Soman, Rakshita Eashwernath

15. Ventilator-associated Pneumonia 206
    Joanne Mascarenhas

16. Case Studies in ICU Infections 213
    Rajeev Soman, Rakshita Eashwernath

SECTION 5: SUPPORTS

17. Indications of Mechanical Ventilation 231
    Jamshed Sunavala

18. Basics of Mechanical Ventilation 235
    Jamshed Sunavala

19. Advanced Modes of Mechanical Ventilator 245
    Joanne Mascarenhas

20. Weaning from Mechanical Ventilator 252
    Jamshed Sunavala

21. Extracorporeal Membrane Oxygenator 261
    Jamshed Sunavala

22. Mechanical Circulatory Supports 265
    Jamshed Sunavala

23. Approach to Nutritional Support 273
    Jamshed Sunavala

SECTION 6: MONITORING

24. Hemodynamic Monitoring 299
    Jamshed Sunavala

25. Arterial Blood Gases and Acid-base Abnormalities 322
    Jamshed Sunavala

26. Echocardiography in Critical Care 341
    Nitin Burkule, Bomi B Ichaporia

SECTION 7: PROBLEM ORIENTED TOPICS

27. Postoperative Atrial Fibrillation 363
    Jamshed Sunavala

28. An Approach to Acute Abdomen 374
    Shruti Tandan Pardasani

29. Endocrine Emergencies 379
    Nalini S Shah, Kunal Thakkar

30. Management of Exacerbation of Chronic
    Obstructive Pulmonary Disease 403
    Joanne Mascarenhas, Jamshed Sunavala

31. Approach to a Patient with Hyponatremia 411
    Bhupendra V Gandhi, Rishit Harbada

32. Intensive Care Unit-acquired Weakness 425
    Vibhor Pardasani

33. Seizures in the Intensive Care Unit 430
    Vibhor Pardasani

34. Medical Management of Post-traumatic Hemorrhage
    and Coagulopathy... 437
    Jamshed Sunavala, Dipsha Kriplani Suvarna

35. Pitfalls in the Diagnosis of Brain Death 449
    Sarosh M Katrak

Appendices

Appendix I: Antibiotic Formulary Used in Critically-ill Patients 455
Appendix II: Important Scorings Used in Critical Care Patients 464
Appendix III: Inotropes Used in ICU...467
Appendix IV: Mnemonics 468

Index 473

SECTION 1

History

○ **Critical Care Medicine Over the Years**
  Jamshed Sunavala

CHAPTER 1

Critical Care Medicine Over the Years

Jamshed Sunavala

■ INTRODUCTION

Medical history is vague about the exact time when critical care medicine as we understand today, began. However, the practice of caring for critically ill patients is not a new concept and does not differ greatly from the past. From the time of Hippocrates to Galen to Florence Nightingale and to the present times, the watch words have remained the same—vigil, speed, support, and compassion. These four pillars that constitute the spirit of critical care were also practiced by good old physicians and family friends—*Luke Fildes* painting of the country doctor says it all **(Fig. 1)**.

In the further discourse, I have no intention to elaborate on the history of medicine—there are better books available on the subject. My main objective is to firstly acknowledge the men and women whose contributions over the years have made it possible for the standards of critical care accessible today and secondly, to understand the many limitations and inadequacies in our present approach to critical care medicine.

■ HIPPOCRATES

The physician from the island of Kos revealed for posterity the face of impending death—"The Hippocratic Facies". He also observed the respiration

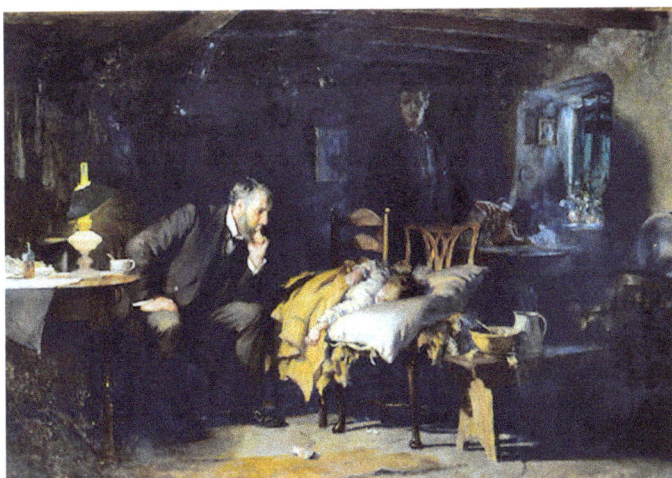

Fig. 1:. The Doctor, exhibited in 1891, Sir Luke Fildes. Presented by Sir Henry Tate, 1894.
Photo: Courtesy Tate

of a patient with high fever, akin to that of a *"man recollecting himself whilst breathing large and deep"*—here possibly he was describing a case of severe sepsis in respiratory failure. Much before *John Cheyne* and *William Stokes* (both Scotsmen) were historically linked together to describe *"Cheyne-Stokes breathing"*, the notable gasp from a failing respiratory center was already described by Hippocrates as vividly as we see today—*"gasping irregular breathing which would cease quarter of a minute and restart, first slow then heavy and fast and cease again".* He also commended all physicians caring for the critically ill, who conducted the treatment better than others. The present day intensivists seem to have taken him too seriously and are appalled by the mention of "open intensive care units (ICUs)".

■ AFTER HIPPOCRATES

Indeed there is a long line of pioneers in the medical field following Hippocrates without whom we may have required another century or probably more, to be able to achieve today's modern science of critical care medicine. *Celsus* provided us with the signs of inflammation—"calor, rubor, tumor, dolor". Anatomy was relatively nonexistent till the 16th century and the coming of *Andreas Vesalius* and his artistic anatomic atlas. June of 1543 saw two cherished works of the European Renaissance, one—"On the Revolutions of the Heavenly Spheres" a monumental work by Nicolaus Copernicus, and the other—"De Humani Corporis Fabrica Libri Septem" by Andreas Vesalius on the fabric of the human body. This masterpiece by Vesalius was illustrated by no other than Titian and his school of artist in the city of Padua. Till this time and for the previous 14 years, the gospel of Galen was considered the Bible of Medicine. Vesalius adored Galen, but he soon found discrepancies with Galen's manuscripts showing the anatomy of the human body which were at odds with his findings. He initially refused to believe this and he even entertained the theory that the anatomy of the human body had changed over the years, but when Galen's shortcoming became glaringly obvious, he realized that the great God of medicine had erred. It was Vesalius again in 1555 who first described the possibility of inserting a tube or a reed in an opening made in the trachea and blowing into it and thereby inflating the lungs. However, it was Paracelsus (1493-1541) who first demonstrated a type of assisted ventilation through a tube inserted in the patient's mouth. Interestingly, Vesalius who was wrongly accused by his enemies, was sent on a pilgrimage to the Holy Land as punishment for dissecting a Spanish Nobleman who they claimed, stirred on application of the scalpel and some went as far as to blame him for dissecting the body on a beating heart. During this voyage he was shipwrecked and died of hunger on the Greek Island of Zante (Zakynthos).

Robert Koch and *Louis Pasteur* dispelled *Pettenkofer's* belief of "miasma" or vapors being responsible for disease and were the first to identify the microbial agents as cause of infectious diseases. *Florence Nightingale* introduced a triage system for the critically ill wounded soldiers of the Crimean war. *Drinker's Iron Lung and Fleming, Florey, and Chain's* discovery of penicillin, the double helix of *Watson and Crick* and many others with their discoveries were the first to sow the seeds of what we reap today. However, the unbelievable advances in technology in the field of critical care medicine and progress in the last 60 years cannot be denied. The first attempt at using a positive pressure ventilator was during the polio epidemic in Europe in the early fifties. This period is probably the beginning of the modern concept of an ICU as we understand today.

▪ POLIO EPIDEMIC OF COPENHAGEN

The polio epidemic struck Copenhagen in 1952. *Bjorn Ibsen*, an anesthetist, was consulted because the negative pressure iron lung was not helping the victims, though theoretically the bellows function of the iron lung, pushing air in and out, should have sufficed for the polio-afflicted patients who suffered from type II respiratory failure. Ibsen, to his surprise, observed increased blood levels of CO_2 reflecting persistent uncorrected respiratory acidosis despite being ventilated on the iron lung and obliviously concluded that the patients were inadequately ventilated and oxygenated. He improved the system by introducing positive pressure intermittently (through a tracheostomy), and in synchrony with the negative pressure phase provided by the iron lung. His crude, but effective method of providing the positive pressure intermittently [intermittent positive pressure (IPP)] was by introducing a Bennett's positive pressure valve in line with the continuous positive pressure applied from the other end. This supplemented positive pressure worked and substantially improved survival. Later the improved version of this contraption/device was also helpful in patients with primary type I respiratory failure with intractable hypoxemia by keeping the collapsed alveoli open, and this was the earliest mode of recruitment attempted and the rest is history. I believe that this period of the early 50s was the beginning and the first step to the multidisciplinary ICU of today.

▪ THE TWO VITAL INTERVENTIONS THAT MADE THE DIFFERENCE

Respiratory Support

Respiratory, hemodynamic, nutritional management, and nursing are the four supports on which all critically ill patients depend on during the life-threatening phase of their illness. However, the first two have made a stronger impact as major supports in improving outcomes. After *Ibsen's* innovation of the IPP ventilator, more refined volume-cycled ventilators were developed by the mid-50s—these included the *Bang* and *Engstrom* ventilators, soon followed by *Bennett MA-IB*. With time, more sophisticated ventilators entered the market with various modes mainly used for lung recruitment and weaning. The most vital and universally used mode is the concept of positive end-expiratory pressure (PEEP) which followed the observation of *Furman* that when the exhalation limb of the circuit from the tracheostomy was inserted under

1-4 cm of water, it provided expiratory resistance and improved oxygenation by opening the collapsed alveoli and increasing the functional residual capacity (FRC). PEEP is today a standard mode used in most patients and has proved enormously successful in ventilating patients with ARDS. *Barach's* study describing the use of positive pressure respiration for treatment of pulmonary edema preceded *Ibsen* and was published in the Annals of Internal Medicine in 1938, however the emphasis was on providing positive pressure without intubation, as ventilation was not the prime concern. Two other historical landmark papers, which completely revolutionized the future of mechanical ventilation, were *Ashbaugh, Bigelow, and Petty's* publication on acute respiratory distress syndrome (ARDS) in Lancet 1967 and later the ARDS Network Study in New England Journal of Medicine (NEJM) 2000, stressing on the use of low tidal volumes in ARDS. It is remarkable that this (lung protection strategy), is the only mode that has shown significant survival benefit.

Hemodynamic Support

William Harvey's "De Motu Cordis" published in 1628, detailed the circulation of blood and he can rightly be called the father of hemodynamics. However, the complete pathway for circulation was identified half a century later by *Marcello Malpighi,* also famous for his discovery of capillaries connecting veins to arteries. The English clergyman *Stephen Hales* crude 4 feet glass tube inserted into the artery of a horse in 1733 was of course too cumbersome for our modern ICUs, but thankfully the Austrian physician *Karl Samuel Ritter von Basch* designed the first portable sphygmomanometer in 1881. He claimed haughtily that cutting open a patient's artery would no longer be required, but had he lived a century longer, he would have been quite disappointed to note that we puncture open radial arteries a bit too enthusiastically in our ICUs today. Till the turn of the 19th century, one could measure only systolic blood pressure and it was only in 1905 that *Nikolai Korotkoff* was able to measure diastolic pressure by identification of certain sounds, now known as Korotkoff sounds.

The modern concept of hemodynamics as we understand today can be credited to *John Womsley* (1907-1958) and *Donald McDonald* (1917-1973). McDonald's thesis on "Blood Flow in Arteries" has since been a standard work in the field of hemodynamics. The Nobel prize in medicine for performing the first right heart catheterization in a human went to *Werner Theodor Otto Forssmann* who inserted a urethral catheter in his own basilic vein and advanced it into the right heart, when he was only a 25-year old surgical resident. He was dismissed from the hospital for his reckless act in attempting such a suicidal experiment and disrespecting the reputation of his department. We are not certain as to which department took umbrage, whether it was cardiology or urology. Later *Drs Andre Cournard* and *Dickinson Richards* innovated new catheters which could be advanced into the pulmonary arteries and they joined Forssmann in receiving the Nobel Prize in 1964. However, it was not until *Jeremy Swan* and *William Ganz* invented the balloon floating pulmonary artery catheter (PAC) for measurement of right-sided pressures that opened the possibility of bedside hemodynamic monitoring. Unfortunately, this catheter gained instant notoriety after the moratorium decreed by no other than *Dr Roger Bone* at the end of the last century. Today intensivists who rail against the use of Swan-Ganz catheters should remember that "any tool can be a weapon in the wrong hands". Fluid resuscitation now followed the adage that "cardiac filling pressure is not fluid responsiveness"; dynamic values of stroke volume variation (SVV) and pulse volume variation (PVV) are now considered appropriate, and just measuring pulmonary wedge pressure as an index of left ventricular filling pressure may not always reflect the improvement in the cardiac output to volume challenge. To understand this subject, it would be well to refer to a landmark paper in *Clinics in Chest Medicine,* 2003 on hemodynamic monitoring by *Michael Pinsky*.

Methods of supporting patients with severe cardiogenic shock or refractory cardiac failure have made considerable strides in the last two or three decades with newer inotropes, but more significantly due to better understanding and application of both inotropes and vasopressors already in use. Introduction of intra-aortic balloon pumps (IABPs) and newer ventricular assist devices such as the Impella device have contributed immensely for bridging patients to interventions, surgery, or even to conceivable recovery. Adding extracorporeal membrane oxygenation (ECMO) to the Impella (ECPELLA) can help patients with cardiac and respiratory failure with refractory hypoxia.

GENESIS OF TODAY'S INTENSIVE CARE UNITS

The concept of close monitoring of the critically ill was first conceived by *Florence Nightingale* during the Crimean War in the 1850s. She was also possibly the first to arrange and separate the sick according to the severity of their illness, keeping the ones who required close monitoring nearest to the nursing station, a concept that we call "Triage" today. In 1923, *Walter Dandy* opened a separate three-bedded unit for critical postneurosurgical patients at the Johns Hopkins Hospital in Baltimore, USA. By the 1930s, many such postoperative recovery rooms for close monitoring and observation, mushroomed during the Second World War and special shock units to provide the best resuscitation facilities, were setup on the fronts. 1958 saw the first modern prototype of a multidisciplinary ICU at Baltimore City Hospital, USA, under *Dr Peter Safar* and soon hospitals all over USA and Europe adopted the same plan for their ICUs.

In India, most of the hospitals till the early 70s were designed to look after critical cardiac patients and called them intensive cardiac units. They exclusively looked after the patients with coronary artery disease and their main purpose was to closely monitor arrhythmias requiring immediate cardioversion or pacing, and in the event of an arrest, to resuscitate. But there was little facility available to support over time, patients with organ failure.

Quoting Dr FE Udwadia's introductory lines from the preface of his Textbook of Critical Care Medicine, "....... these units, though centralized were designed and equipped chiefly to offer intensive care to patients with acute myocardial infarction. Mechanical ventilation was primitive; its use being mostly restricted to token gesture of graces offered to a patient about to depart from the world".

The concept of advanced respiratory and hemodynamic support developed post availability of good positive pressure ventilators together with facilities to monitor hemodynamics at the bedside along with the availability of Swan-Ganz catheters.

However, our main challenges in India today are the lack of ICU beds, poor patient-to-nurse ratios, lack of excellent training facilities, and affordable treatment.

Battle of the Bugs

Bacteria have lived and owned the world billions of years before us and perhaps we live here only because they allow us to, but definitely we could not survive without them. The ones in our gut help to fight foreign microbes, which could otherwise make us sick. They divide and breed but once every million divisions they may mutate and the mutant bacteria may have an added advantage of being resistant to antibiotics. Antibiotic resistance can of course occur in many ways, mainly because of overuse and abuse and consequently we are faced with the dreadful dilemma of multidrug resistance (MDR) and pandrug resistance (PDR). Drug resistance, with no new and effective antibiotics in sight, has become the greatest predicament we face in our ICUs today.

Increasing population of elderly patients in our ICUs with diseases and drugs, which suppress their immune system, are at the biggest risk of developing serious infections. In most cases our immune system fights back, but not before unleashing a cytokine storm from a dysregulated host response to infection, which leads to life-threatening organ failure. Sepsis was defined in 1992 by *Roger Bone* and colleagues as a systemic inflammatory response syndrome (SIRS) but now the latest definition of 2016, Sepsis-3, is all about organ dysfunction.

■ ERA OF ORGAN TRANSPLANT AND IMMUNOSUPPRESSANTS

The earliest attempts in human transplant were done in India almost a thousand years ago; of course, what described were not organ transplants but autotransplant of flaps. The first attempt at human-to-human kidney transplant was done by Dr Yu Yu Yuronoy in 1936 which failed in the early postoperative period due to rejection. However, the credit to the first successful kidney transplant goes to Dr Murray and his team from Boston in 1954 and it was performed between identical twins. On the other hand, it was not till late 60s that several successful liver transplants were done where all patients received immunosuppression with azathioprine and cortisone though none survived beyond 23 days.

It was not until the discovery of cyclosporine, refinement of surgical techniques and donor supports that both kidney and liver transplant were no more considered experimental but seriously offered as therapy. By the early 1990s the introduction of tacrolimus, which has a greater potency than cyclosporine, paved a way for longer survival. Further, advance in organ procurement and preservation and newer immunosuppressants following the calcineurin era has made organ transplant (especially kidney and liver) a routine surgical procedure today with a high success rate.

The increasing organ transplant program and the large gamut of immunosuppressants in use have created an enormous burden on the ICU. The intensivist today has to deal with early and in-hospital post-transplant complications and they need to be conversant with the drugs and their various side effects ranging from hematological complications following the use of azathioprine, mycophenolate, sirolimus, and antibodies (monoclonal and polyclonal antibodies). Cyclosporine has side effects on the kidney and heart whereas tacrolimus in addition to the side effect on the kidney also has central nervous system (CNS) toxicity. The newer class of immunosuppressants such as belatacept is relatively safe but a few cases of post-transplant CNS problems such as an increased risk of multifocal leukoencephalopathy and post-transplant lymphoproliferative disorder have been described with its use. To further compound the work of the already stressed ICU staff is the use of steroids causing new-onset diabetes mellitus with uncontrolled high sugar levels. Patients on immunosuppressants also present in the ICU with perplexing problems, especially fever of unknown etiology and most of these medications have unique interactions with the commonly prescribed adjunct agents such as antibiotics, antifungals, antihypertensives, and antidepressants. Despite progress, the future of transplant holds a lingering fear of alarming zoonotic transmitted infections such as the Ebola virus, etc., with the ongoing experimental trials of xenotransplantation.

It was not until 1980 that a lung transplant with an acceptable outcome was achieved by Joel Cooper and Colleagues. However, the overall survival rate even today is approximately 50% at 5 years. Despite major advances, complications of post lung transplant are not uncommon. Bronchial stenosis at the anatomic site and unexplained noncardiogenic pulmonary edema within 72 hours following transplant and wide spectrum of infections are the main complications that the intensivist may have to deal with in the first or second week post-transplant. The first cardiac transplant was successfully performed by Christiaan Barnard in 1967. Now heart transplant has become a standard surgery for treating patients with advanced and refractory heart failure. In the majority of patients, the immediate postoperative course would be similar to post bypass surgery requiring ventilatory support and management of possible arrhythmias. Rejection and problems of immunosuppression are usually experienced later. However, the intensivist should be on guard to deal with immediate surgery-related infections and well versed with management of advanced support such as IABP and temporary left ventricular assist device (LVAD).

■ EVIDENCE-BASED MEDICINE

As doctors, most of us must have read *AJ Cronin's* "The Citadel" written in 1937, which became the moving spirit behind the foundation of the National Health Service (NHS) in Great Britain. The man behind the main theme of the novel was Dr Mason, whose management of patients was based not only on his skill as a doctor with independent thinking but also on uncompromised and sound ethical principles. I am not sure how well he would have fared in today's time where he would have to abandon his lateral thinking and diagnostic skills developed through experience, and now compelled to restrain his personal views and act in accordance with the evidence of others, strictly adhering to protocols and bound by technology.

Very often evidence was based on a single trial and discarded by another to become invalidated. This has been revealed by retrospectively reviewing, a vast body of literature published in the last 30–40 years from which we have learnt that single-centered randomized controlled trials (RCTs) have failed often by not being replicated in larger multicentered RCTs. A typical example is the strongly advocated early goal-directed therapy (EGDT) *of River's* published in NEJM in 2000, a single-centered RCT confirming a survival benefit that was not substantiated in later studies. This shows that guidelines will change with newer and better controlled trials hence a single study from one center should not cloud one's judgment.

Evidence, besides providing useful guidelines, has also given us insight into certain aspects of bedside care that were considered perfunctory. For instance, early intubation is beneficial for critically ill patients; also, head elevation to 30° and improved oral hygiene decreased incidence of ventilator-associated pneumonia (VAP). It was helpful, among many others, in formulating guidelines such as the surviving sepsis campaign and septic bundles and glycemic control protocol. Probably the greatest benefit evidence-based medicine (EBM) revealed was the importance of teamwork for more efficient ICU functioning.

■ END-OF-LIFE CARE FOR THE TERMINALLY ILL

In general, the patient population admitted to ICUs today is older than they were 40 years ago. This means greater morbidity for obvious reasons and many elderly patients with comorbidities succumb to a critical illness. A few, pull on, with the help of cardiopulmonary support till they are labeled terminally ill with little hope of complete recovery and many have no meaningful existence even after a protracted recovery period. The other group of patients, young or old, are those who have survived a successful resuscitation but with a very dismal outcome. Less than a quarter survive to discharge and of these only a handful have a meaningful recovery. Hence, it behoves that the treating doctor to deal with both the patient and the family with responsibility and utmost sensitivity, but sooner or later the sensitive issue of do not resuscitate (DNR) will be brought up.

Before considering DNR, repeated counseling of the family members is essential and discussions should include an honest picture of the patient's functional status and prognosis of future outcome. Relatives' preferences should be carefully understood and sympathetically considered, before pronouncing views regarding futile resuscitation. The counseling doctor has to be well aware that often our ability to prognosticate the outcome may not be perfect. Hence, using phrases such as "meaningful existence, morality issues, and dignity in death", may often carry a certain degree of arbitrariness and should be used carefully, sensing the poignancy of the moment, even though the family has accepted the inevitable. Further, avoid using a self-fulfilling prophecy to coerce the patient into accepting DNR.

With organ transplants on the rise, the modern ICUs have to contend with the ethics of certifying brain death for organ donation. *Mollaret and Goulon* in 1959 were the first to describe death based on the loss of function of the brain. Guidelines for determination of brain death have been framed by multiple scientific committees, to instruct clinicians to accurately examine patients, to avoid risk of diagnostic error and legal implications. It is important to remember not to callously disregard the last hope of living, which every family desires, so be thoughtful before pronouncing "futile resuscitation".

Four centuries ago, Francis Beacon defended the art of reasoning by general and liberal education of all humanities and advised not to lose our perspective only in the worship of science. This promoted a wise judgment of ends to accompany the scientific improvement of means. His words seem more applicable to our times, with an increasing population of the terminally ill, taxing our reasoning and judgment.

■ CORONAVIRUS DISEASE-2019 PANDEMIC: THE INDIAN SCENARIO

The ongoing pandemic of coronavirus disease-2019 (COVID-19) infection has created a serious impact on the future of our understanding of viral infections. It has opened a new perspective on the physiological and immunological aberrations, responsible for the varied clinical manifestations and complications that has thrown light on the therapeutic implications of the drugs and interventions used. The intensivists particularly have struggled to improve outcomes of the critically ill and many new challenges and predicaments have been an eye opener.

The COVID-19 pandemic spread worldwide in 2020 and continued to rage even through 2021. The pandemic was caused by the severe acute respiratory syndrome coronavirus-2 (SARS-CoV-2) and was first reported in December 2019 from the Wuhan provenience of China from where it originated, but the first case reported in India was on 30th January 2020. At the time of writing this book (May 2021) India was in the midst of a second wave of COVID-19 pandemic and by now has had the second largest number of confirmed cases (after the United States), with 26 million reported cases and over 3 lacs deaths. This second wave advanced with enormous casualties which was far more devastating than the first wave in September 2020 and the experts predicted a catastrophic rise of COVID-19 infection with a mounting death rate by the end of this surge. The magnitude of the second wave left India totally unprepared with shortage of hospital beds, oxygen, ventilator, vaccines, and drugs, moreso in the rural areas. Multiple factors were proposed for this unprecedented surge, including a rampant disregard to personal protection by the public. People let lose their guard, soon following the first wave with the incidence of COVID showing a dramatic decline in comparison to other countries. This self-assured hubris among the public and the government, led to complacency resulting in relaxation of preventive control measures.

In consistency with current chapter, it is relevant to discuss those serious cases requiring ICU care. Critically ill patients of COVID presented with a myriad complications, which are otherwise seen rarely in one disease. Patients during the onset of the pandemic throughout the first wave presented in the ICU with a clinical picture suggestive of ARDS and likewise the management guidelines were prototyped to correction of refractory hypoxia and prevention of alveolar capillary leak. However, with time many features of respiratory affliction following COVID were at odds with that of ARDS as known to us. Firstly, many patients tolerated oxygen desaturation (even below 90%) without displaying any signs of respiratory distress. Secondly, during the very acute phase there was no evidence of refractory hypoxia as most cases of severe oxygen desaturation (well below 90%) were corrected with nasal oxygen delivery of 2-4 L/min and this was out of line with the very definition of ARDS. With time, majority (over 95%) of these patients recovered but of which only few required ventilator support and here too most responded to noninvasive ventilation (NIV) or high-flow nasal oxygen (HFNO). Though ground glass appearance on the chest CT was common with ARDS, the distinctive appearance of peripheral pneumonia hinted in favor of COVID. The confidence of managing hypoxia without ventilatory support conveniently favored home management in mild-to-moderate cases, especially during the second wave, when there was an acute shortage of hospital beds.

The few with refractory hypoxia went from NIV to intubation and mechanical ventilation and had high mortality rates and even with the best of ICU care, almost over 60% did not make it to recovery. ECMO was the last resort for refractory hypoxia and though the outcome was very poor, it was offered to the younger population mainly on compassionate grounds. The only therapies that showed benefit in serious cases of COVID were:
- Oxygen with or without mechanical ventilation
- Prone positioning

- Steroids—dexamethasone 6–8 mg per day or methylprednisolone 40 mg twice a day to be used judiciously
- Anticoagulants—low-molecular-weight heparin (LMWH) or oral anticoagulants (apixaban 2.5 mg twice a day)
- Interleukin-β (IL-β) inhibitor tocilizumab available in the market as "Actemra".

Timing of giving the above medications was of paramount importance—too early may be ineffective or even harmful at times and too late was like offering the last ministrations to the dying. Steroids for instance was a case in point. Tocilizumab used in patients without ruling out underlying bacterial or fungal infection can lead to life-threatening septic shock. At the same time, it should be cautiously used and timed before patient becomes terminally ill with a full-fledged cytokine storm and on ventilator/inotropic support.

Thromboembolic complications emerged as an important issue in patients with COVID-19 infection. They were due to a procoagulant pattern and very likely related to an endothelial thromboinflammatory syndrome and the common complications emerging from this syndrome were pulmonary embolism and cerebrovascular accidents. Hence, appropriate use of anticoagulants was advocated with worsening of symptoms even at times prior to hospitalization.

Since the first wave much has happened and by the time second phase reached its peak many unusual complications were recorded. Though acute respiratory failure with refractory hypoxia was the leading cause of death other unexpected fatal complications were recorded. These included:

- *Cardiac failure*: Here uncertainty remains whether the virus was directly causing myocarditis or the cardiac damage was secondary to the severity of the illness.
- *Secondary infections*: Bacterial and bloodstream infections were commonly seen. However, fungal infection of the lung such as aspergillosis and mucormycosis were not that uncommon in the sickest of the patients.
- Acute liver injury and liver failure occurred rarely but was very sudden with a high mortality. It was not certain whether this was a result of direct harm from the virus or other antecedent causes.
- Acute kidney injury (AKI) seemed to be a common complication secondary to the hemodynamic and respiratory compromise in the severely ill cases. Most of them recovered from AKI with improvement in their respiratory and cardiac function but some of the cases did require hemodialysis.
- Disseminated intravascular coagulation (DIC) leading to undue clotting or bleeding occurred mainly in the critically ill patients or during a cytokine storm or associated with severe sepsis.
- Pneumomediastinum and pneumothorax as complications were seen in the critically ill patients with COVID infection and not necessarily in ventilated patients. The worse sequelae to this were bronchopleural

fistula, which could lead to a protracted stay in the ICU and very often a poor outcome.

The second wave of COVID-19 showed progressive worsening in most parts of India taking a high toll on life and economy. Lockdown periods had been extended in most parts of India, though in certain regions such as Mumbai, some evidence of plateauing was emergerging by July 2021. Lately the use of monoclonal antibody cocktail (casirivimab + imdevimab) which mirrors human antibodies was found to be useful in thwarting the infection in the early phase of the disease. Its use is mainly restricted to mild-to-moderate high-risk symptomatic patients (before the requirement of supplemental oxygen) where it was found to be most effective.

Perspective and Conclusion

I would like to end this chapter by stressing on the human aspects of critical care which seems to be lost in the midst of advanced technology, invasive therapies, slow erosion of clinical medicine and the influence of the corporate health care structure today. In the near future, I fear that ICUs may become a brutal place for patients, relatives and the care givers. For the patient it might mean dehumanization of the individual, relatives will be considered mere customers in the waiting room and the patients families will be constantly under stress of escalating cost with unpredictability of prognostication. Doctors and nurses may lose their clinical acumen and remain vulnerable despite the availability of high-tech imaging, integrated monitoring systems and the limitations of the many lifesaving machines.

Modern technology may be considered as a triumph for medicine but at a staggering cost, if it prolongs lives only to confront us to a new form of misery. Thus medicine may turn into a meaningless exercise, once it is realized that therapy meant to heal has only bought more time to be ill. The future raises the daunting possibility of an industrial or a corporate model evoking image of an 'assembly line' management of health care. For this not to happen we need to answer the all important question – "Whether a world without disease is possible". If not, then the medical profession has to hone their skills and change current prospectives that will allow the doctors to preserve and augment their clinical acumen, judgment and humanity.

How do we put all these problems in place so that it can be managed in a more civilized manner? At the outset, we need to recognize that we are slowly dehumanizing the intensive care unit. Better communication skills should be the essence of critical care training in order to assuage a stressful encounter for patients and relatives in and out of the ICU. Technology should be used as an aid and not a replacement for clinical skills and judgment. It is imperative to understand that doctors and nurses are mere humans and they too have personal fear of death, conflicting religious and personal convictions, untoward experiences with patients, constantly battle with feeling of remorse, guilt and peer pressure. All these can result in a "Burn-out" syndrome.

Thus critical care is a blend of vigil, speed, skill, compassion and care balanced and supported by the use of five senses - without which all technology is virtually useless.

■ SUGGESTED READING

1. Acute Respiratory Distress Syndrome Network, Brower RG, Matthay MA, Morris A, Schoenfeld D, Thompson BT, et al. Ventilation with lower tidal volumes as compared with traditional tidal volumes for acute lung injury and the acute respiratory distress syndrome. N Engl J Med. 2000;342(18):1301-8.
2. Al-Aby Z, Xie Y, Bowe B. High-dimensional characterization of post-acute sequelae of COVID-19. Nature. 2021;594:259-64.
3. Ashbaugh DG, Bigelow DB, Petty TL, Levine BE. Acute respiratory distress in adults. Lancet. 1967;290(7511):31-23.
4. Friedman M, Friedland GW. Medicine's 10 Greatest Discoveries. New Haven: Yale University Press; 1998.
5. Funk DJ, Parrillo JE, Kumar A. Sepsis and septic shock: a history. Crit Care Clin. 2009;25(1):83-101.
6. González-Crussi F. A Short History of Medicine. New York: Modern Library; 2008.
7. Gordon R. The Alarming history of Medicine: Amusing Anecdotes from Hippocrates to Heart Transplants. New York: St. Martin's Press; 1993.
8. Ibsen B. The anaesthetist's viewpoint on the treatment of respiratory complications in poliomyelitis during the epidemic in Copenhagen, 1952. Proc R Soc Med. 1954;47(1):72-4.
9. Linden PK. History of solid organ transplant and organ donation. Crit Care Clin. 2009;25(1):165-84.
10. Lyons AS, Petrucelli RJ. Medicine—An Illustrated History. New York: Abradale Press; 1997.
11. O Malley CD. Andreas Vesalius of Brussels. California: University of California Press; 1964.
12. Patone M, Thomas K, Hatch R, Tan PS, Coupland C, Liao W, et al. Mortality and critical care unit admission associated with SARS-CoV-2 lineage B.1.1.7 in England. Lancet Infect Dis. 2021;S1473-3099(21)00318-2.
13. Pinsky MR. Hemodynamic monitoring in the intensive care unit. Clin Chest Med. 2003;24(4):549-60.
14. Sherman IW. The Power of Plagues. Washington DC: ASM Press; 2006.
15. Swan HJC, Ganz W, Forrester J, Marcus H, Diamond G, Chonette D. Catheterization of the heart in man with use of a flow-directed balloon-tipped catheter. N Engl J Med. 1970;283:447-51.
16. Udwadia FE. Man and Medicine: History. Oxford: Oxford University Press; 2000.
17. Wijdicks EFM, Rabinstein AA. The family conference: end-of-life guidelines at work for comatose patients. Neurology. 2007;68(14):1092-4.
18. Wijdicks EFM. Brain Death, 2nd edition. New York: Oxford University Press; 2011.

SECTION 2

Resuscitation

- **Airway Management**
  Jamshed Sunavala

- **Postcardiac Arrest Care after Return of Spontaneous Circulation**
  Jamshed Sunavala

CHAPTER 2

Airway Management

Jamshed Sunavala

■ ANATOMY AND FUNCTION OF THE AIRWAYS

Management of the airway remains a crucial part of resuscitation and support in critically ill patients. A thorough knowledge of the anatomy and function of the airway is mandatory for all physicians and nurses involved in the respiratory care of such patients. The atmospheric air on its way to the lungs for purpose of gas exchange, needs to pass through the nose, down the oral cavity, the upper airways, trachea, the main bronchial branches and finally to the small airways, before it reaches the alveoli for gas exchange. During this journey through the nasal passage, the inspired air is filtered, humidified and warmed, the latter two processes continue in the pharynx and the tracheobronchial tree. This is the reason why external sources of humidification are to be incorporated whilst on mechanical ventilation (MV) with artificial airway. Unrequired particles in the air >10 µm are trapped by hair in the nasal mucosa, and smaller particles reaching the mucosa of the bronchus, cause reflex irritation and are coughed out, away from the lungs, with the help of "cilia" which line the respiratory tract from the nose to the bronchioles, only sparing the vocal cords. However, particles <2 µm in diameter may reach the alveoli, where they are ingested by the macrophages. The larynx prevents food and other foreign bodies from being aspirated into the trachea, by reflex closure of the glottis during swallowing. In elderly or unconscious patients or in patients with poor gag reflex due to lower cranial nerve palsy, there is a high risk of pulmonary aspiration. This needs to be anticipated in all such patients hence oral feeds should be avoided and alternative routes for enteral feeding should be used.

Assessing adequacy of airways forms an important aspect of airway management and it includes checking for protective reflexes (gag reflex) as mentioned earlier and patency of the airways to ensure a smooth flow of O_2, regardless of the delivery system (nasal prongs or face masks). Lastly, a protected patent airway with a good O_2 delivery system would be useless, without an adequate respiratory drive in a spontaneously breathing patient. This can be clinically assessed most times, though an objective assessment with pulse oximeter or arterial blood gases can give a good idea of a patient's ventilatory efforts. If the underlying factors for the poor respiratory drive cannot be addressed or corrected promptly due to oversedation or other causes of type II respiratory failure, positive pressure ventilatory support may become mandatory.

AIM OF AIRWAY MANAGEMENT

It is primarily to establish a patent and secure airway for adequate ventilation. It should also be able to deliver inspired oxygen by noninvasive methods or by MV, noninvasively, it can be administered by a nasal cannula or a face mask. The main disadvantage of the nasal cannula is that it cannot deliver >30% of O_2; on the other hand, face masks can deliver higher concentrations of O_2. A simple face mask has vents that allows dissipation of humidity and heat, it also allows room air to enter the mask and hence cannot deliver O_2 concentration in excess of 50% at the most even on very high-flow rates. However the same mask with a reservoir bag attached to it (partial rebreathing or nonrebreathing masks) can deliver inspired O_2 concentrations up to 60–80%. Venturi masks have a device that can entrain a known proportion of ambient air when a set concentration of 100% O_2 is allowed to pass through a venturi device, thereby enabling a delivery of a near exact concentration of inspired O_2, which could range between 25 and 35%.

Securing a Patent Airway

It may be achieved initially by simple manoeuvres such as right positioning and clearing the airway of any extraneous materials such as thick saliva, food, blood, broken teeth, or dentures by suctioning or using a finger wrapped in gauze, to wipe clear any larger solid particles in an unconscious patient. *Triple airway manoeuvre* involves "head tilt" to extend the neck, "jaw thrust" by pulling the mandible forward and mouth opening which is often beneficial in obtunded patients. However, this manoeuvre is contraindicated in trauma patients with spine as instability. Here immobilization of the spine is mandatory before performing any manoeuvre.

To keep the airway open for prolonged periods, artificial airways are available which can be introduced between the tongue and the posterior pharyngeal wall, and one such commonly used airway is the oropharyngeal airway (OPA). However, this is only a temporary measure to keep the airway patent and will have to be replaced by a more permanent intervention such as the endotracheal tube (ET) intubation. However, some advanced artificial airways are available as a bridge before introducing the ET, in patients with difficult intubation. These adjuncts are known as "supraglottic airways (SGAs)", like the laryngeal mask airway (LMA) **(Fig. 1)**, which is a mask mounted on a tube, which can be placed blindly in the lower pharynx overlying the glottis, with an inflatable cuff which seals the inlet, allowing manual ventilation through an Ambu bag or ventilator. LMA is used most commonly in emergency resuscitations during prehospital transport by paramedics or doctors in cases of difficult intubation. LMAs come in various sizes, usually size 3 for females and size 4 for males**.** Now many newer and improved SGA devices are available, which are easier to insert and have better oropharyngeal seal, therefore less risk of aspiration.

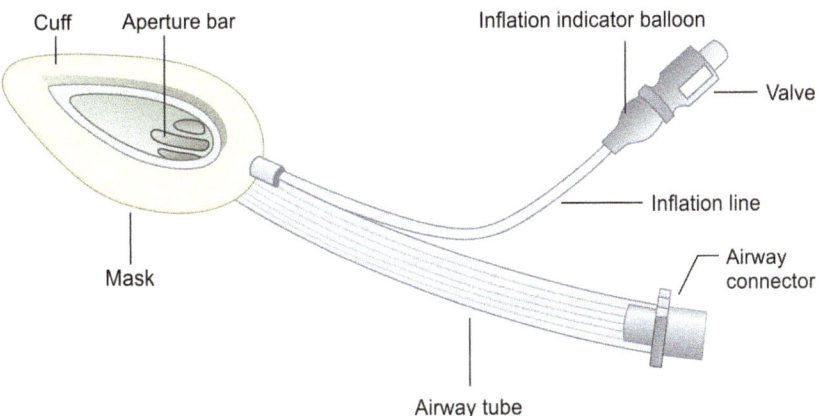

Fig. 1: Laryngeal mask airway (LMA).

Endotracheal Intubation

It is of course the most effective and secured method of providing a semi-permanent airway, especially for delivering a positive-pressure ventilation, with the minimum risk of aspiration. Its invasiveness is a major deterrent in many situations, where a judgment call has to be made between noninvasive ventilation (NIV) and intubation to provide MV. Techniques of intubation require practice and skill for which every internist should be trained, particularly for using the orotracheal intubation route, which is the most widely used technique using direct laryngoscopy. In semi-conscious patients who may gag on the laryngoscope, one may have to use sedatives to minimize or abolish the protective laryngeal/pharyngeal reflexes. Commonly, sedatives such as midazolam or induction agents like propofol or opioids (fentanyl) are used. However, the intensivist has to be extremely well trained to quickly intubate such patients, to prevent occurrence of life-threatening hypoxia or when difficult intubation is anticipated, then it would be best to take the help of an anesthetist.

■ DIFFICULT AIRWAY

It is a serious situation by itself and when one anticipates this, the clinician in-charge should assign an experienced individual and if required, call upon an anesthetist, familiar with the algorithmic steps well described in the latest guidelines (e.g., American Society of Anesthesiologists) for management of difficult airways. Usual conditions associated with difficult airways are listed in **Box 1**.

Unanticipated difficult airway is a serious situation, especially in the hands of an inexperienced individual. It is thus mandatory that the intensive care unit (ICU) protocol ensures that all intubations need to be done by well-trained personnel. All trained individuals should be familiar with alternative airway devices and techniques as patients with unanticipated difficult airway

> **BOX 1** Conditions associated with difficult intubation.
> - Mouth bleeding
> - Foreign body
> - Small mouth
> - Large tongue
> - Acromegaly
> - Facial muscle spasm
> - Facial burns
> - Tetanus
> - Cervical spine trauma or surgery
> - Short neck
> - Neck stiffness
> - Obesity
> - Inability to reach base of epiglottis with laryngoscope blade

may provide very little breathing time for both (themselves and the doctors), before becoming seriously hypoxic and hemodynamically unstable. Here restoration by 100% oxygen needs to be delivered immediately by mask or by using an SGA device as a bridge to invasive ventilation via a cricothyrotomy or minitracheostomy.

It is important for the intensivist to be familiar with manoeuvres, techniques, and various appliances available to negotiate difficult airways. Preoxygenation with 100% O_2 delivered through Ambu bag and mask or NIV can reduce hypoxemia and facilitate intubation by relaxing the mouth and muscles of the upper airways. Further, preoxygenation helps to overcome the unduly prolonged apnea time. Malleable stylets placed inside the ET can help to easily direct the ET through a poorly visualized glottis, different sizes and shapes of laryngoscopic blades and fiberoptic intubation can be very useful, if readily available. A Frova intubating stylet can be used to tide over a difficult scenario since it has a ventilating port.

Once the ET is inserted, its position in the trachea should be immediately confirmed by auscultating for equal air entry in both lungs, failure to recognize tube misplacement in one bronchus or the other, below the carina, can cause collapse of the opposite unventilated lung. Very often during emergencies, ET may be misplaced in the esophagus and may be difficult to confirm in a patient with severe respiratory distress and at times, one hears transmitted breath sounds from the esophagus, over the lung fields.

■ CANNOT INTUBATE–CANNOT VENTILATE

It is the worst possible situation for a critically ill patient requiring urgent respiratory support as well as for the intensivist who finds himself in this helpless situation. Fortunately, it is not a common scenario but when it occurs it is best for all intensivists to follow a protocol, which should begin, by calling for appropriate help, instead of struggling to force an ET in a patient who may have anatomic or physiological restrictions to intubation. Intubation with

LMA may be used as a bridge to attempt ventilation. However, surgical intervention by tracheostomy should be initiated, as fast as possible, by doing a minitracheostomy or calling for surgical help.

In cannot intubate–cannot ventilate situations, one will have to resort to a surgical tracheostomy, or a less invasive needle cricothyrotomy or subcutaneous tracheostomy. Hence, all intensivists should be well trained in these procedures. *Needle cricothyrotomy* is done in an absolute emergency, as it enables to maintain satisfactory oxygenation for a short period. However, it does not create a definitive airway and will be inadequate for CO_2 to escape through the needle-sized cannula. Here a 14 gauge "intravenous (IV) cannula over a needle," attached to a syringe, is pierced through the cricothyroid membrane by continuously applying negative pressure, until there is a give and air enters the syringe, at which point, one has to slide the cannula off the needle, into the trachea.

A *surgical cricothyrotomy* is a more permanent procedure, whereby, after injecting a local anesthetic, an incision of 1–1.5 cm is made over the cricothyroid membrane incising the superficial fascia and subcutaneous fat. Then one proceeds to divide the membrane (with blunt forceps or the handle of the scalpel), through which is inserted a cuffed tracheostomy tube between the thyroid and cricoid cartilages. Presently, many commercial prepacked kits are readily available such as the "Portex® Mini-Trach®" kit marketed by Smiths Medical Products, where a small-sized cannula can be inserted through the cricothyroid membrane with the help of a scalpel and an introducer. A Mini-Trach® kit with Seldinger technique is available, which accurately and safely guides the cannula with minimal risk of bleeding or creating surgical emphysema, from misplacement due to misalignment of tissue.

All the above procedures are useful in dire emergency following a failed ET intubation but for a more permanent airway, planned tracheostomy should be done where the trachea is opened, between the second and third tracheal rings or one space higher. *Tracheostomy* is indicated in cases where a patent airway is required for long-term periods, as it provides better access for suctioning and maintaining a good tracheobronchial toilet. Further, it may enable easier and possibly a faster weaning from the ventilator, as it creates a reduced anatomic dead space. However, tracheostomy should be avoided or deferred if there is local inflammation over the operating area and also when excessive bleeding is anticipated in patients with coagulation abnormalities. Timing of tracheostomy is left, to the judgment of the physician or intensivist managing the patient and though there is no fixed consensus, most favor doing a tracheostomy by 1–2 weeks of ET placement or even earlier, in patients anticipated to need a longer period of artificial airway. Conventionally, surgical tracheostomy is best performed by a surgeon, as risk of bleeding, misplacement and surgical emphysema are higher **(Table 1)**. However, *percutaneous tracheostomy* using commercially available kits like the "Mini-Trach®", can be performed by a

TABLE 1 Complications of tracheostomy.

During the procedure	Postprocedure	Late complications
• Bleeding • Creating a false tract • Pneumothorax • Pneumomediastinum • Hypoxia (if patient is not oxygenated through endotracheal tube during the procedure) • Injury to posterior wall and oropharynx	• Self extubation • Bleeding • Infection	• Infection • Tracheal stenosis • Tracheoesophageal fistula • Tracheomalacia

TABLE 2 Airway management summary.

Aim	• To establish a patent and secure airway for adequate ventilation
Simple manoeuvres to clear the airways	• Clearing the airways of extraneous material, food, salvia, dentures, etc., by suctioning or finger swipe • Positioning and triple airway manoeuvres • Immobilization of unstable cervical spine
Oxygen delivery system	• Nasal prongs and simple mask • Venturi mask and mask with reservoir bag • Partial rebreathing and nonrebreathing masks with reservoir bag
Airways for clear ventilation	• Oropharyngeal airways • Nasopharyngeal airways • Esophageal obturator airways (EOA) • Laryngeal mask airways
Airways for mechanical ventilation	• Endotracheal tube • Tracheostomy tube
Rapid sequence intubation	• Prepare and position the patient. Set the instrument tray with laryngoscope with different sized blades. Check the light on laryngoscope. Preoxygenate the patient • Apply carotid pressure. Rapid administration of induction agent. Direct laryngoscopic-guided intubation • Verification of correct tube placement
Difficult airways	• Difficult mask ventilation (jaw advancement, beard, obesity, age > 60 years, edentulous, and sleep apnea) • Difficult intubation (see Box 1)
Choice of pharmacological adjuncts	• Hypnotics • Propofol • Midazolam • Etomidate • Ketamine • Neuromuscular blocking agents

trained intensivist. To, summarise, airway management involves maintenance of a clear airway, appropriate device for O_2 delivery, invasive and noninvasive means of ventilator support and management of difficult intubation **(Table 2)**.

■ SUGGESTED READING

1. Andriolo BN, Andriolo RB, Saconato H, Atallah AN, Valente O. Early versus late tracheostomy for critically ill patients. Cochrane Database Syst Rev. 2015;(1):CD007271.
2. Apfelbaum JL, HagbergCa, Caplan RA, Blitt CD, Connis RT, Nickinovich DG, et al. Practice guidelines for management of the difficult airway: an updated report by the American Society of Anesthesiologists Task Force on Management of the Difficult Airway. Anesthesiology. 2013;118(2):251-70.
3. Engels PT, Bagshaw SM, Meier M, Brindley PG. Tracheostomy: from insertion to decannulation. Can J Surg. 2009;52(5):427-33.
4. Frerk C, Mitchell VS, McNarry AF, Mendonca C, Bhagrath R, Patel A, et al. Difficult Airway Society 2015 guidelines for management of unanticipated difficult intubation in adults. Br J Anaesth. 2015;115(6):827-48.
5. Joffe AM, Deem S. Airway management. In: Tobin MJ (Ed). Principles and Practice of Mechanical Ventilation, 3rd edition. New York: McGraw-Hill Companies; 2013.
6. Kallstrom TJ, American Association for Respiratory Care (AARC). AARC clinical practice guidelines: oxygen therapy for adults in acute care facility. Respir Care. 20002;47(6):717-20.
7. Maxwell BG, Ganaway T, Lighthall GK. Percutaneous tracheostomy at the bedside: 13 tips for improving safety and success. J Intensive Care Med. 2014;29(2):110-5.

CHAPTER 3

Postcardiac Arrest Care after Return of Spontaneous Circulation

Jamshed Sunavala

■ INTRODUCTION

Return of spontaneous circulation (ROSC) is defined as return of normal or near normal pulse and rhythm following cardiac resuscitation and the immediate goal is to initiate hemodynamic and respiratory stabilization. This implies that resuscitation will need to continue following ROSC and is termed as postcardiac arrest care (PCAC). Simultaneously, it is important to establish the cause or trigger for the cardiac arrest and this should be incorporated as a part of PCAC.

■ CHECK LIST

Immediately after ROSC a rapid check list to identify correctable causes and comorbidities should be commenced in order to avoid recurrence of arrest, serious arrhythmias or hemodynamic compromise. I have used a mnemonic "POSTATTACK" to quickly identify the common underlying conditions which can serve to promptly identify the correctable triggers **(Table 1)**. These include clinical, laboratory and bedside tests, to establish a diagnosis within minutes following ROSC.

TABLE 1 Clinical, laboratory and bedside tests, to identify correctable causes and comorbidities which could result in recurrence of cardiac arrest and help to stabilize the patient.

P—Rule out tension **P**neumothorax (post resuscitation complication)	
O—**O**xygen-persistent hypoxia (requiring immediate intubation and mechanical ventilation)	Can be immediately diagnosed on clinical examination
S—**S**troke/decreased sensorium (requiring further respiratory support)	
T—Hypo**T**ension (requiring volume or vasopressors)	
A—**A**cidosis (ABG)	
T—Coronary **T**hrombosis (ECG)	Tests for confirmation at bed side
T—Pericardial **T**amponade (2D echo)	
A—**A**ortic tear (X-ray chest and 2D echo)	
C—**C**ongestive cardiac failure (X-ray chest)	
K—Hypo**K**alemia (serum electrolytes)	

(ABG: arterial blood gas; ECG: electrocardiogram)

■ STABILIZATION POST-RETURN OF SPONTANEOUS CIRCULATION (BOX 1)

Cardiac arrest results in an abrupt cessation of blood circulation to the brain, heart, and other vital organs. Survival, both short and long term, would depend on prompt cardiopulmonary resuscitation (CPR) and ROSC. However, hypoxic brain injury with resultant neurological deficit, remains a major problem and the impact of the injury is worsened because of the double hit—with the initial injury, occurring during cardiac arrest, followed by further injury during immediate reperfusion and in the next 48–72 hours after ROSC. Neurological injury could range from mild deficits to severe compromise in the level of consciousness. To limit brain injury during CPR, an uninterrupted cardiac compression, airways management and 100% oxygen is strongly recommended **(Box 2)**. The American Heart Association (AHA) guidelines for CPR are now universally practiced and certification from this association for both basic and advanced life support should be mandatory, for all residents working in major hospitals.

After ROSC, the optimum levels of oxygen and carbon dioxide over and above other interventions need to be maintained **(Box 2)**. Though it is uncertain as to the exact levels of oxygen and carbon dioxide required to avoid further brain injury, there is enough evidence to suggest that extreme hyperoxia and hypocapnia are potentially harmful and may result in poor neurological outcomes. In order to circumvent this uncertainty it is best to titrate fraction of inspired oxygen (FiO_2) to a minimum, necessary to achieve oxygen saturation (SpO_2) of 94%. The role of carbon dioxide and end-tidal carbon dioxide ($EtCO_2$) monitoring is still uncertain. However, extreme hypocapnia following hyperventilation is shown to be detrimental to neurological recovery, whereas moderate hypercapnia may have a beneficial effect as a vasodilator, by increasing blood flow to the brain. To this effect monitoring of $EtCO_2$ may be useful in maintaining normal or slightly higher levels of partial pressure of carbon dioxide ($PaCO_2$).

BOX 1 Stabilization after ROSC—outcome associated with O_2, CO_2, and BP optimization.

Oxygenation:
- Recommended—lowest FiO_2 to maintain SpO_2 of 94%
- To avoid hyperoxia
- Emerging evidence suggests that very high PaO_2 values in the first 24 hours may be detrimental

Carbon dioxide:
- Recommended to maintain $PaCO_2$ between 35 and 40 mm Hg
- Hypocarbia due to hyperventilation has shown poor neurological outcomes

Mean arterial pressure (MAP):
- Maintaining higher MAP of 90 mm Hg to 100 mm Hg has shown better neurological outcomes than maintaining MAP of 60–70 mm Hg

(BP: blood pressure; FiO_2: fraction of inspired oxygen; $PaCO_2$: partial pressure of carbon dioxide; PaO_2: partial pressure of oxygen; ROSC: return of spontaneous circulation)

> **BOX 2** Essential interventions and therapies to be considered after cardiac arrest.
>
> *During CPR:*
> - Uninterrupted good quality cardiac compression (as per the AHA guidelines for CPR)
> - Defibrillation for VF/VT
> - For pulseless electrical activity (PEA)
>   - IV epinephrine and continue CPR—if shockable rhythms appears → defibrillate
> - O_2 delivery and ventilation
>   - Studies have shown that maintaining higher O_2 levels during prolonged CPR have improved neurological outcomes
>
> *After return of spontaneous circulation (ROSC):*
> - Checklist **(Table 1)**
> - Stabilization **(Box 1)**
> - Therapeutic hypothermia **(Box 3)**
> - Triage for percutaneous coronary intervention (PCI)
> - Predicting neurological recovery **(Box 4)**
>
> (AHA: American Heart Association; CPR: cardiopulmonary resuscitation; IV: intravenous; VF/VT: ventricular fibrillation/ventricular tachycardia)

The AHA guidelines have recommended maintaining of a systolic pressure of 90 mm Hg initially by volume challenge, followed by vasopressor and inotropes as required. Other reversible causes will of course need to be addressed at the earliest. The COMACARE multicenter Scandinavian pilot study of 120 out-of-hospital cardiac arrest (OHCA) patients with witnessed ventricular fibrillation (VF) was designed to compare high or low normal levels of partial pressure of oxygen (PaO_2) (75–110 vs. 150–190 mm Hg), $PaCO_2$ (34–35 vs. 44–45 mm Hg) and mean arterial pressure (MAP) (60–70 vs. 80–100 mm Hg) for 36 hours, after intensive care unit (ICU) admission. This novel study used a neurofilament light (NFL) as a biomarker to predict postcardiac arrest outcome. The study concluded that targeting higher MAP of 80–100 mm Hg was associated with less likelihood of hypoxic brain damage, however, no significant difference was seen between groups targeting low-normal or high-normal PaO_2 or $PaCO_2$. Optimizing oxygenation, carbon dioxide and blood pressure levels are essential parts of resuscitation but these have shown limited therapeutic value, in order to improve secondary brain injury in the first 72 hours of ROSC. Temperature control by inducing therapeutic hypothermia (TH) in the first 24 hours has shown a slightly more favorable response in improving neurological outcomes.

■ THERAPEUTIC HYPOTHERMIA (BOX 3)

Decrease in the cerebral metabolic rate following TH was believed to be the main mechanism of action in providing brain protection. However, recent studies have suggested that a combination of possible mechanisms could be responsible in avoiding neurological injury. Recent studies have shown that mild-to-moderate hypothermia after cardiac arrest has beneficial effects

> **BOX 3** Therapeutic hypothermia—management.
>
> *Indications*:
> Patients with decreased sensorium who cannot be aroused
> *Contraindications*:
> Serious bleeding, pre-existing temperature below 34°C, and cryoglobulinemia
> *Aim*:
> - To begin immediately after ROSC
> - To induce hypothermia to 34°C
> - To maintain hypothermia between 34°C and 36°C (latest studies have shown no difference in outcomes on maintaining temperature between 34°C and 36°C)
>
> *Method*:
> - *Induction:* Ice cold (4°C) infusion of normal saline to a core body temperature of 34°C
> - *Maintenance:* To maintain core temperature preferably to 34°C, however up to 36°C is acceptable
> - *Cooling:* By using endovascular cooling or surface cooling or using both simultaneously
>
> *Monitoring*:
> Intracerebral temperatures are best measured by pulmonary artery catheter or tympanic thermometer. However in practice, core (rectal or lower esophageal) temperatures are measured
> *Complications*:
> Shivering, bleeding, bradycardia, hypotension, hypokalemia, and infection
>
> (ROSC: return of spontaneous circulation)

on the brain with good neurological outcomes. Temperatures of 33–36°C, 28–32°C, and below 28°C are usually referred to as mild, moderate and deep hypothermia, respectively.

Earlier studies, such as the multicentered European trial [New England Journal of Medicine (NEJM) 2002] and the one by Bernard et al. (NEJM 2002), showed a favorable neurological outcome following TH after OHCA associated with VF or pulseless ventricular tachycardia (VT). This prompted the Liaison Committee on Resuscitation to recommend TH for such patients. However, with emerging evidence, TH is now considered appropriate for any patient who remains unresponsive following ROSC, regardless of the location [OHCA or in-hospital cardiac arrest (IHCA)] or the underlying rhythm. The only major contraindications are serious bleeding, preexisting hypothermia of below 34°C or cryoglobulinemia. There are various ways of inducing TH, though endovascular cooling is the most favorable method. Surface cooling may fail to achieve and maintain target TH.

At times both surface and endovascular cooling may be necessary to maintain the desired temperature. Endovascular cooling is done immediately after ROSC by infusing large volumes (30 mL/kg) of ice cold (4°C) of normal saline intravenously after insertion of a central venous catheter. The infusion should be rapid and given in aliquot of 500 mL at 10 minutes intervals to induce hypothermia up to 34°C. However, there are two practical problems that we have encountered: (1) giving 500 mL of saline usually takes longer and it loses its required temperature of 4°C rapidly, hence we give 100 mL subdivisions of the aliquot and (2) achieving TH of 34°C rapidly during induction, is manageable but it is quite difficult to sustain the temperature despite both endovascular and surface cooling. Hence we have accepted 36°C for maintenance, which has shown favorable outcomes in recent studies. Shivering is a common problem during induction which can increase body temperature, hence it is preferable to simultaneously run an intravenous (IV) midazolam infusion. However, management of refractory shivering will need neuromuscular blocking agents. Other complications of TH include bradycardia, hypotension, hypokalemia, and bleeding. Bradycardia is common during TH and is associated with good neurological outcome and should be preferably left alone if there is no hemodynamic compromise. Hypokalemia should be corrected cautiously to avoid hyperkalemia. Nonconvulsive status epilepticus has been reported, hence a continuous electroencephalogram (EEG) recording, is recommended during the induction period of TH. Clotting factors and platelet depletion or dysfunction may cause bleeding in patients on TH after cardiac arrest and concurrent acidosis may further impair coagulation. The changes in the routine coagulation tests are difficult to assess as laboratories adjust the temperature of all samples to a standard 37°C. Hence doing thromboelastography (TEG) in this setting, would rightly detect the dynamic changes in blood coagulation during resuscitation and be useful to guide transfusion therapy. Tight glycemic control is mandatory during TH as hyperglycemia induced by hypothermia is associated with poor neurological outcome. The list of usual complications related to TH is given in **Box 3**.

■ TRIAGE FOR PERCUTANEOUS CORONARY INTERVENTION

Majority of patients after cardiac arrest and particularly those occurring out of hospital (OHCA) would have succumbed to acute coronary syndrome and if no other obvious cause was ascertained, this group of patients could benefit with percutaneous coronary intervention (PCI). Survivors of cardiac arrest with postrecovery electrocardiogram (ECG) showing ST-segment elevation myocardial infarction (STEMI) have a particularly good prognosis from the neurological point of view. PCI is contraindicated for patients with major complications such as bleeding. Comatose patients on continuous TH need not be excluded. The final decision would depend on the clinician's judgment where age, signs predicting poor neurological recovery, presence of other comorbidities and the relatives' consent would have to be seriously considered.

■ OUTCOMES

One of the largest and multicentered studies reviewing the outcome after cardiac arrest is the European Registry of Cardiac Arrest (EuReCa) published in 2016 and which included 10,672 patients from 27 European countries with OHCA. This study reported a considerable variation in incidence and outcome after OHCA, with an incidence ranging from 19 to 104 per 100,000 people per year and an overall survival to discharge of 10.3%. Another study reported by Weisfeldt et al. in NEJM in 2011 observed that the majority of the survivors had an initial rhythm of VF or pulseless VT. Interestingly, studies have shown that bystander witnessed OHCA (in public places) showed a significantly higher survival at discharge compared to OHCA occurring at home, and over the years this disparity increased with improving survival rates for patients with bystander witnessed cardiac arrest at public places. This was more evident in a Danish study by Wissenberg et al. in the Journal of the American Medical Association (JAMA) 2013, and was probably contributed by the Danish national drive to train increasing number of bystanders in CPR (beginning at school level). Though outcomes documented increasing survival rates in the West, a similar trend was not observed following OHCA in Asia except in Japan, where "All Japan Registry" (2005-2014) identified an increase in survival as well as improved neurological outcomes. Probably the initiative of CPR training among adults and at school level, improved the bystander witnessed neurologically favorable survival rates from 9.8% to 20.6% (Kitamura et al. Circulation, 2012).

Survival alone would be retroproductive if there is a poor neurological outcome. Hence, the term "survival with neurologically favorable" or "survival with poor outcome" is more appropriate. The main purpose of improving survival following CPR and ROSC is to offer a meaningful life on hospital discharge. A Cerebral performance category (CPC) scale of 1 to 2 or modified Rankin Scale (mRS) of 0 to 3 is generally acceptable as a good neurological outcome **(Box 4)**. Current studies for IHCA patients have also shown short- and long-term increase in survival with favorable outcomes, especially in those with underlying rhythms of VF or pulseless VT.

BOX 4 Predicting neurological outcomes at discharge.

Cerebral Performance Category (CPC) scale:
1. Conscious and alert
2. Conscious and alert but with moderate disability
3. Conscious with severe disability
4. Comatose or persistent vegetative state
5. Brain dead

Modified Rankin Scale (mRS):
0. No symptoms
1. Some symptoms with usual activities possible
2. Slight disability—unable to do all previous activities, but independent
3. Moderate disability—requiring some help but able to walk without help
4. Severe disability—bed ridden and incontinent
5. Dead

CONCLUSION

Survival after cardiac arrest with reasonably good neurological recovery depends on the following:
- *Timely CPR*: This is best expected form a bystander, well trained in CPR in OHCA, which presently is unlikely in our country.
- Immediate resuscitation with a prompt-coded response in IHCA patients who have VF or pulseless VT as initial rhythms and with effective response to defibrillation by automated external defibrillator (AED).
- Uninterrupted good quality cardiac compression during CPR.
- Relatively younger group of patients with least comorbidities.
- Patients of OHCA or IHCA who have underlying STEMI and are eligible for PCI. These patients usually have VF or pulseless VT. Note: STEMI can be ascertained only after the recovery of cardiac rhythm.
- Prompt interventions as in **Box 2** after ROSC may help.

It is important to understand that all the above are perceptions and may only benefit a small percentage of patients to survive and achieve a normal neurological recovery.

SUGGESTED READING

1. Batista LM, Lima F, Januzzi JL, Donahue V, Snydeman C, Greer DM. Feasibility and safety of combined percutaneous coronary intervention and therapeutic hypothermia following cardiac arrest. Resuscitation. 2010;81(4):398-403.
2. Drebek T, Patrick K. Is there a role of therapeutic hypothermia in critical care? In: Deutschmann CS, Neligon PJ (Eds). Evidence-based Practice of Critical Care, 3rd edition. Amsterdam, Netherlands: Elsevier; 2020.
3. Gough CJR, Nolan JP. Outcome of cardiopulmonary resuscitation. In: Vincent JL (Ed). Annual Update in Intensive Care and Emergency Medicine 2017. Heidelberg, Germany: Springer; 2017.
4. Holzer M. Targeted temperature management for comatose survivors of cardiac arrest. N Engl J Med. 2010;363(10):1256-64.
5. Hosmane VR, Mustafa NG, Reddy VK, Reese CL 4th, DiSabatino A, Kolm P, et al. Survival and neurological recovery in patients with STEMI resuscitated from cardiac arrest. J Am Coll Cardiol. 2009;53(5):409-15.
6. Merchant RM, Topjian AA, Panchal AR, Cheng A, Aziz K, Berg KM, et al. Part 1: Executive Summary: 2020 American Heart Association Guidelines for Cardiopulmonary Resuscitation and Emergency Cardiovascular Care. Circulation. 2020;142:S337-57.
7. Wihersaari L, Ashton NJ, Reinikainen M, Jakkula P, Pettilä V, Hästbacka J, et al. Neurofilament light as an outcome predictor after cardiac arrest: post hoc analysis of the COMACARE trial. Intensive Care Med. 2021;47:39-48.

SECTION 3

Organ Dysfunction

- **Acute Respiratory Failure**
  Jamshed Sunavala

- **Acute Respiratory Distress Syndrome**
  Jamshed Sunavala

- **Intensive Care Management of Acute Heart Failure and Cardiogenic Shock**
  Ram E Rajagopalan

- **Acute Kidney Injury in the ICU and Renal Replacement Therapies**
  Bhupendra V Gandhi, Rishit Harbada

- **Coma in the ICU: A Clinical Approach**
  Sarosh M Katrak

- **Stroke for Physicians and Intensivists**
  Fali Poncha, Azad Marazban Irani, Vibhor Pardasani

- **Acute Liver Failure**
  Amey Sonavane, Aabha Nagral

CHAPTER 4

Acute Respiratory Failure

Jamshed Sunavala

■ DEFINITION

Acute respiratory failure (ARF) is a state of a severely reduced partial pressure of arterial oxygen (PaO_2) below 60 mm Hg or an elevated partial pressure of carbon dioxide ($PaCO_2$) above 50 mm Hg caused by an acute failure of lung function.

The term "acute on chronic respiratory failure" can apply to a combination of ventilatory and oxygenation failure, as in chronic obstructive pulmonary disease (COPD). These group of patients though suffering from chronic failure may be leading a relatively normal life, but can present with sudden respiratory distress and acute failure when beset by complications such as lower respiratory tract infections. Acute respiratory distress syndrome (ARDS) on the other hand, always manifests as an acute presentation of severe hypoxemic respiratory failure.

■ CLASSIFICATION OF RESPIRATORY FAILURE (TABLE 1)

Respiratory failure can be classified according to the:
- Physiological abnormality in gas exchange
- Anatomical site of the derangement
- Disease etiology

Physiological Abnormality

Type I: Hypoxemic Respiratory Failure

Here the main gas exchange abnormality is a severe fall in PaO_2 (<60 mm Hg) and $PaCO_2$ in most instances is also low, as it is washed out due to hyperventilation.

Type II: Hypercapnic Respiratory Failure

Here the failure is mainly due to alveolar hypoventilation and the main gas exchange abnormality is an elevated $PaCO_2$ (>50 mm Hg). The PaO_2 is mildly reduced corresponding to the degree of hypoventilation, but never below 60 mm Hg. For PaO_2 to fall below 60 mm Hg there would be near absent ventilation or respiratory arrest.

Combined respiratory failure: Acute exacerbation of COPD or Asthma COPD Overlap Syndrome (ACOS) with tight bronchospasm is one of the conditions

TABLE 1	Classification of respiratory failure.		
Physiological (abnormality)	**Anatomical site**	**Disease etiology**	
Type I: Hypoxemic respiratory failure • $PaO_2 < 60$ mm Hg—main gas exchange abnormality • $PaCO_2$—usually reduced due to hyperventilation • V/Q < 1	• Alveoli • Lower airways	ARDS, severe pneumonia, ILD with supra-added infection, pulmonary edema, atelectasis, and pulmonary embolism	
Type II: Hypercapnic respiratory failure • $PaCO_2 > 50$ mm Hg—main gas exchange abnormality • PaO_2—mildly reduced, appropriate to the $PaCO_2$ level • V/Q = 1 (normal)	• Central neurological • Spinal cord, peripheral nerves, and neuromuscular • Upper airways • Chest wall	• Sedative drug overdose, medullary lesions, brain trauma, CVA, metabolic encephalopathy, septic encephalopathy, and meningitis • Cervical cord injury, poliomyelitis, Guillain–Barré syndrome, myasthenia gravis, myopathies, and critical care neuropathy • Upper airways obstruction • Flail chest, pleural effusion, and increased intra-abdominal pressure	
Combined respiratory failure—hypercapnic and hypoxic • $PaCO_2 > 50$ mm Hg • $PaO_2 < 60$ mm Hg	Airways	Acute exacerbation of COPD	

(ARDS: acute respiratory distress syndrome; COPD: chronic obstructive pulmonary disease; CVA: cerebrovascular accident; ILD: interstitial lung disease; PaO_2: partial pressure of arterial oxygen; $PaCO_2$: partial pressure of carbon dioxide; V/Q: ventilation to perfusion ratio)

where patient may have both hypoxic and hypercapnic respiratory failure and I prefer to classify them separately as "combined type of respiratory failure"(**Table 1**). Interestingly, a few studies have shown that the inhibitory effect of acute respiratory acidosis on muscle contractility can decrease respiratory muscle endurance. This may be one of the reasons for the sudden deterioration that we see in patients with severe COPD, fostering a sharp rise of $PaCO_2$ from the already elevated levels.

The other condition where we may encounter a combined failure is in case of severe refractory hypoxemic failure, where the PaO_2 falls as the shunt fraction increases progressively. Initially the $PaCO_2$ remains constant but starts rising, at times even up to 50 mm Hg or more, when the shunt fraction exceeds 50%.

Anatomical Site of Derangement

Respiratory failure can occur due to a disease or abnormality afflicting any of the anatomical sites involving the central and peripheral nervous system, the chest wall, the airways, and the lung parenchyma. Usually all causes involving the respiratory center, spinal cord, peripheral nerves, muscles, and thoracic cage affect the bellows movement of the lung, leading to hypoventilation and type II ventilatory failure, whereas type I hypoxic respiratory failure occurs if the lower airways and mainly the alveoli, which are the main site of gas exchange, are involved.

Disease Etiology

Common diseases responsible for respiratory failure are listed in **Table 1**.

■ GAS EXCHANGE IN RESPIRATORY FAILURE

pO_2–pCO_2 Relation in Acute Respiratory Failure (Fig. 1)

- The graph in **Figure 1** is plotted with partial pressure of oxygen (pO_2) and partial pressure of carbon dioxide (pCO_2) on the horizontal and vertical axis, respectively.
- The straight line AB represents a normal V/Q and runs from point B to point A through point N, where B extends to meet the ambient O_2 at sea level (150 mm Hg). N is the meeting point of normal PaO_2 and $PaCO_2$.

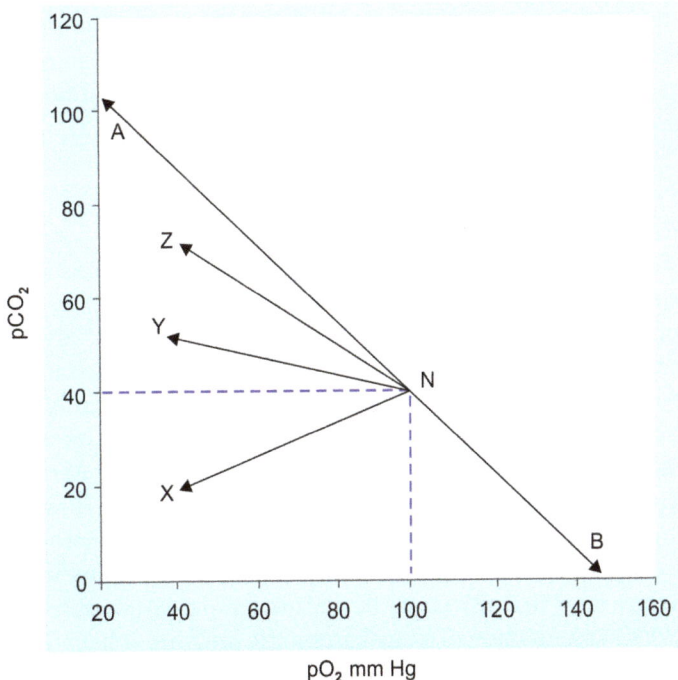

Fig. 1: Gas exchange in acute respiratory failure.

TABLE 2: Respiratory and nonrespiratory causes of hypoxemia.	
Respiratory causes	**Nonrespiratory causes**

• Decreased P_AO_2
  – Alveolar hypoventilation as in type II hypercapnic respiratory failure
• Decreased transport of oxygen from alveoli to pulmonary capillaries
  – Diffusion impairment (ILD)
  – V/Q mismatch
	• Decreased PiO_2
	  – Low barometric pressure at high altitude
	• Decreased FiO_2
	  – Anesthetic accident (very rare)
	  – Right-to-left intracardiac shunt

(FiO_2: fraction of inspired oxygen; ILD: interstitial lung disease; P_AO_2: partial pressure of alveolar oxygen; PiO_2: partial pressure of inspired oxygen; V/Q: ventilation to perfusion ratio)	

- Gas exchange for *hypercapnic type II respiratory failure* is always towards the direction of N → A, reflecting a high $PaCO_2$, and a mild fall in PaO_2 commensurate with the $PaCO_2$ levels.
- Patients with *hypoxic type I respiratory failure* with low V/Q or shunt effect will move in the direction of N → X, where both PaO_2 and $PaCO_2$ values are low, the latter being a result of hyperventilation.
- With severe protracted hypoxia remaining uncorrected, the gas exchange values will shift in the direction of Y showing a rise in $PaCO_2$. This happens over time because of decreasing respiratory effort following muscle fatigue.
- Patients with COPD who may have a mixed picture of both hypoxia and hypercapnia move towards N → Z. However, these patients are dependent on hypoxic respiratory drive and can abruptly become markedly hypercapnic if the respiratory drive is cutoff by administration of high oxygen concentrations or excessive sedation resulting in CO_2 narcosis.

Approach to Hypoxemia

Hypoxemia in general can be due to respiratory causes and nonrespiratory causes **(Table 2)**. Respiratory causes are secondary to a low partial pressure of alveolar oxygen (P_AO_2) as in type II respiratory failure, as described earlier, or due to an impairment of oxygen transfer from the alveoli to the pulmonary capillaries but with a normal P_AO_2, as in type I respiratory failure. The underlying physiological aberration in the latter is primarily a result of ventilation to perfusion ratio (V/Q) mismatch or a diffusion defect **(Fig. 2)**. Diffusion impairment is commonly seen in patients with interstitial lung disease (ILD) but they rarely present with a low PaO_2 at rest. However, if the transit time of the pulmonary circulation is shortened, as with increase in heart rate after exercise, the PaO_2 will fall significantly. The nonrespiratory causes of a low PaO_2 are rare **(Table 2)**. It may be due to a low partial pressure of inspired oxygen (PiO_2) as a function of a low barometric pressure at high altitudes, or to a right-to-left intracardiac shunt or a decrease in fraction of inspired oxygen (FiO_2). Decrease in FiO_2, however, occurs very rarely, following an anesthetic

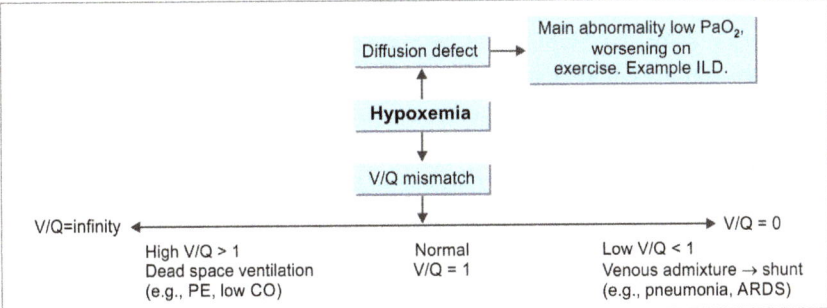

Fig. 2: Physiological causes of hypoxemia. (ARDS: acute respiratory distress syndrome; CO: cardiac output; ILD: interstitial lung disease; PaO₂: partial pressure of arterial oxygen; PE: pulmonary embolism; V/Q: ventilation to perfusion ratio)

accident from an improper installation of oxygen lines. Note that the FiO_2 is not affected by altitude; hence oxygen delivery (DO_2) at high flow rates helps in mountain sickness.

pO₂ Cascade

- *Partial pressure of oxygen in the atmosphere* ($PatmO_2$) is a product of the barometric pressure (P_B) and the fraction of O_2 concentration in the air (FiO_2).

  Patm would be $P_B \times FiO_2$
  i.e., Patm (at sea level) = 760 × 0.21 = 159 mm Hg (rounded to 160 mm Hg)

- PiO_2 is the partial pressure of oxygen in the inspired air humidified in the nasopharynx. This is saturated with water vapor hence it dilutes the alveolar gases by a dilutional factor.

  $$PiO_2 = FiO_2 (P_B - P_{H_2O});$$ where P_{H_2O} is the water vapor pressure
  PiO_2 (at sea level) = 0.21 (760 – 47) = 150 mm Hg

- *Partial pressure of O_2 in the alveoli* (P_AO_2) is the partial pressure of O_2 when it reaches the alveoli, where it drops further to a level as calculated by "*alveolar gas equation*"

  $$P_AO_2 = PiO_2 - \frac{PaCO_2}{R}$$

  where R is the respiratory quotient, R = 0.8 or (1.2 as a numerator)

  $$P_AO_2 = FiO_2 (P_B - P_{H_2O}) - 1.2 (PaCO_2)$$
  P_AO_2 (at sea level) = 0.21 (760 – 47) – 1.2 (40)
  = 102 mm Hg

- *Alveolar-arterial oxygen gradient P(A-a)O₂:* Though the PaO_2 from arterial blood gas (ABG) is useful to establish the type of respiratory failure, PaO_2 alone is insufficient to gauge the adequacy of oxygen transfer without reference to P_AO_2. Adequacy of oxygen transfer is determined by knowing the $P(A-a)O_2$.

$P(A-a)O_2$ is 7–17 mm Hg in normal healthy adults at room air, but varies with extremes of age. Hypoxemia with a normal $P(A-a)O_2$ suggests a type II ventilatory failure whereas an increased gradient confirms a lung parenchymal disease (type I failure). $P(A-a)O_2$ is an essential calculation in clinical practice because PaO_2 alone has a wide range of normality and is a function of three variables—ventilation, FiO_2, and respiratory quotient (R). Calculating $P(A-a)O_2$ can help to unravel subtle impairments of gas exchange which are otherwise not clinically apparent.

Consider the following possibilities where $P(A-a)O_2$ will be helpful:

- As already mentioned earlier, it distinguishes between hypoxemia due to hypoventilation secondary to central or neuromuscular causes, from that of diseases involving the lower airways and alveoli affecting the oxygen transfer.
- Symptomatic mountain climbers at high altitudes cannot be clinically differentiated to having a mild mountain sickness from a more serious event such as high-altitude pulmonary edema (HAPE) by PaO_2 alone. Low PaO_2 at high altitudes is an expected physiological measure of low barometric pressure and may be of little help, hence determining an increased alveolar-arterial gradient would be more conclusive of HAPE.
- A breathless young woman presenting in the emergency medical services (EMS) with a clear chest on auscultation, normal X-ray chest, a low $PaCO_2$ of 25 mm Hg (due to hyperventilation) and PaO_2 of 85 mm Hg and oxygen saturation (SaO_2) of 96% should not be dismissed as a case of anxiety or panic attack. Her calculated $P(A-a)O_2$ was markedly increased to 35 mm Hg and later she was diagnosed as having pulmonary embolism (PE).
- Take an example of a patient with COPD and high fever transferred to the wards from the EMS. He was reported to be hyperventilating and was fully conscious in the EMS where he was receiving 2 L/min of oxygen by nasal prongs and no sedation was given; but on transfer to the ward he was semiconscious and markedly hypoventilating. His PaO_2 and $PaCO_2$ done in the EMS were 150 mm Hg and 60 mm Hg, respectively. At 2 L/min of oxygen flow rate by nasal prongs, one would expect an FiO_2 of approximately 0.28, hence calculated P_AO_2 should be:

$$P_AO_2 = FiO_2 (Patm - P_{H_2O}) - 1.2 (PaCO_2)$$
$$= 0.28 (760 - 47) - 1.2 (60)$$
$$= 128 \text{ mm Hg}$$
$$P_AO_2 - PaO_2 = 128 - 150 = -22 \text{ mm Hg}$$

This is not possible as PaO_2 can never by higher than P_AO_2; hence the patient must have received a much higher concentration of oxygen than 28%. Estimating FiO_2 based on flow rates from face mask or nasal prongs is not reliable. The increased FiO_2 probably suppressed the patient's respiratory drive and was responsible for his poor sensorium and the sharp rise in $PaCO_2$.

- a/APO_2 Ratio

P(A-a)O$_2$ is influenced by changing FiO$_2$ whereas arterial-alveolar pO$_2$ ratio (a/APO$_2$) remains relatively unaffected by FiO$_2$. Hence by using P(A-a)O$_2$, it is not possible to assess the patient's course of gas exchange accurately, more so, in patients with respiratory failure where alveolar-arterial gradients are very high needing an increasing FiO$_2$ anywhere from 0.4 to 1. Further, the ratio (a/APO$_2$) would be useful to monitor patients using face mask or nasal prongs where FiO$_2$ of delivered oxygen cannot be precisely measured limiting the accuracy of P(A-a)O$_2$.

Oxygen Dissociation Curve (Fig. 3)

Unlike CO$_2$ which is carried in plasma, almost all O$_2$ is bound to hemoglobin (Hb). A very small amount of oxygen (in physical solution) is carried in plasma and is in equilibrium with oxyhemoglobin and is measured as PaO$_2$. The relation between the saturated Hb and PaO$_2$ is nonlinear and well recognized as the S-shaped curve on the oxygen dissociation curve.

- The S shape of the oxyhemoglobin dissociation curve has an upper prolonged plateau **(Fig. 3)** which offers one distinct advantage that a marked drop in PaO$_2$ from 100 to 60 mm Hg does not significantly affect

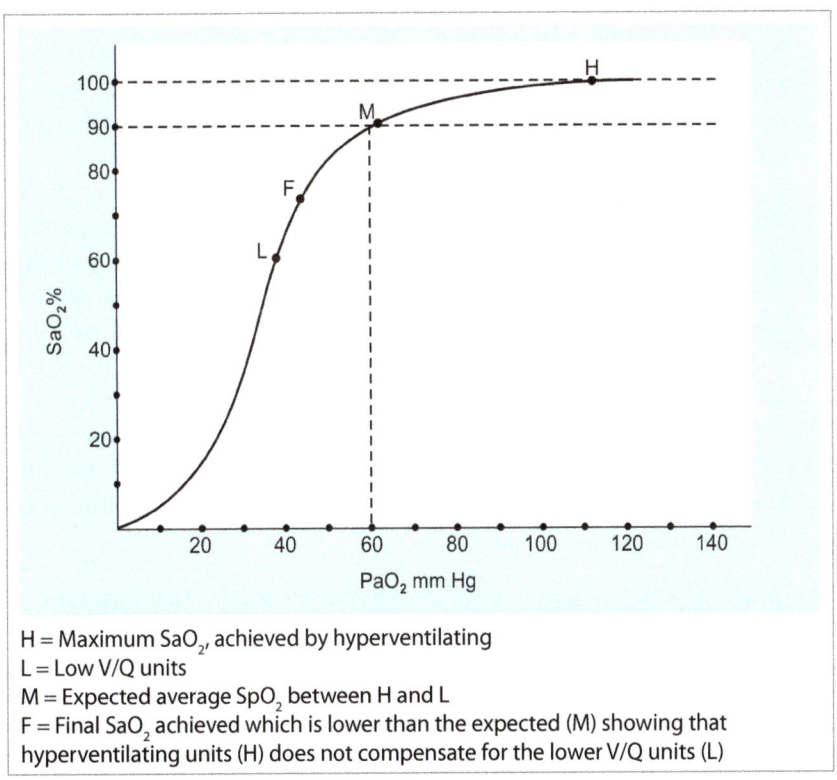

H = Maximum SaO$_2$, achieved by hyperventilating
L = Low V/Q units
M = Expected average SpO$_2$ between H and L
F = Final SaO$_2$ achieved which is lower than the expected (M) showing that hyperventilating units (H) does not compensate for the lower V/Q units (L)

Fig. 3: Oxygen dissociation curve showing poor compensation to low V/Q units by hyperventilating.

O_2 saturation. The SaO_2 and content remains high (above 90%) during mild-to-moderate hypoxemia and sharp drop in SaO_2 occurs only after the PaO_2 drops below 60 mm Hg. Hence, monitoring SaO_2 with a pulse oximeter would suffice with the knowledge that as long as SaO_2 is above 90%, the patient is reasonably well oxygenated. Further, it explains why a PaO_2 of 60 mm Hg is considered a reference point for the interpretation of type I respiratory failure.

- PO_2 in the pulmonary capillary is almost the same as the partial pressure of venous oxygen (PvO_2), which lies on the steep portion of the curve. This creates a significant gradient from P_AO_2 to capillary pO_2 alveolar-capillary gradient enabling a smooth transfer of oxygen.
- At the peripheral tissue level the capillary circulation is more acidic, because the CO_2 which is an acidic gas is greater in concentration here; hence the curve shifts to the right. The rightward shift results in reduced Hb affinity to oxygen, thereby facilitating oxygen unloading to the tissues. However at the level of pulmonary circulation, the CO_2 concentration is lower and the curve shifts to the left which favors oxygen uptake in the Hb. The overall effects of this shift of the oxygen dissociation curve helps to maintain good tissue oxygenation.
- A question commonly raised is whether low V/Q units can be compensated by high V/Q units through hyperventilation. Yes, $PaCO_2$ can be compensated but not PaO_2. Hence, in patients who are hypoxemic due to V/Q imbalance cannot be compensated to a normal V/Q by hyperventilating, whereas high $PaCO_2$ is more than compensated even to lower than normal values. The answer lies in the difference between the CO_2 and O_2 dissociation curves **(Fig. 4)**. The linear curvature allows the high pCO_2 to fall appropriately in response to hyperventilation. However, this is not the case with the "S"-shaped oxygen dissociation curve which determines the final PaO_2 levels in the pulmonary capillaries derived from high, normal, and low V/Q units. The final PaO_2 level is not an average of the partial pressures of oxygen, but is the average of the unequal aliquots of SaO_2 and content in pulmonary capillaries. The high and normal V/Q units all lie on the flat portion of the curve with little difference in their saturation or content and hence cannot compensate for the low oxygen content lying on the steep downslope **(Fig. 3)**.

▇ APPROACH TO DIAGNOSIS OF ACUTE RESPIRATORY FAILURE

Clinical Diagnosis

Dyspnea is the predominant symptom of ARF. Though exertional dyspnea may be present in a deconditioned or an *obese* patient, the most frequent presentation in ARF is dyspnea at rest. Dyspnea is a subjective sensation of awareness of breathing or discomfort and is usually described as increased effort to breathe, air hunger, or chest tightness. However, one need not ask

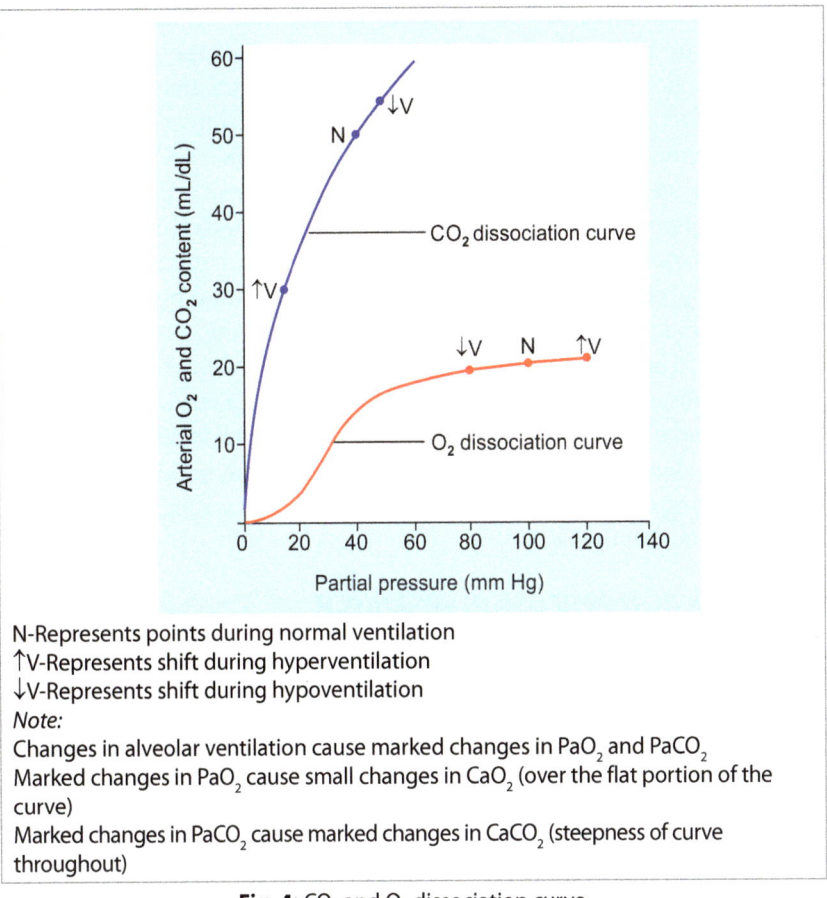

N-Represents points during normal ventilation
↑V-Represents shift during hyperventilation
↓V-Represents shift during hypoventilation
Note:
Changes in alveolar ventilation cause marked changes in PaO_2 and $PaCO_2$
Marked changes in PaO_2 cause small changes in CaO_2 (over the flat portion of the curve)
Marked changes in $PaCO_2$ cause marked changes in $CaCO_2$ (steepness of curve throughout)

Fig. 4: CO_2 and O_2 dissociation curve.

a patient of ARF to qualify or quantify dyspnea as it is so very apparent and cannot be missed. The usual auscultatory findings such as wheeze/rhonchi or rales/crackles may not be apparent in patients with severe breathlessness. There may be no breath sounds heard in patients with severe bronchospasm (Silent Chest). Similarly in patients with cardiac failure, peribronchial edema may present with a wheeze instead of expected rales/crepitations. Hypoventilating patients with decreased respiratory drive may not display signs of respiratory distress. In these patients, shallow breathing may be overlooked during a cursory examination but on counting, their respiratory rate would be rapid. In cases of severe degree of respiratory depression, the minute ventilation (V_E) may be seriously compromised because of both slow and shallow respiration.

There is no reliable clinical symptom or sign to predict either hypoxic or hypercapnic respiratory failure. Cyanosis, flapping tremors, tachycardia, bounding pulse, mental confusion, etc., were once useful to make an educated guess; but these are now replaced with the prompt and easy availability of

ABG and pulse oximetry. However, many patients in the intensive care unit (ICU) who are under observation for pneumonia, postoperative recovery, COPD, respiratory depression following sedation, brain trauma, Guillain–Barré syndrome, etc., may suddenly deteriorate. Here an astute clinician should be able to anticipate trouble irrespective of the patient's SpO_2 level or ABG findings. Hence mild-to-moderate hypoxia may present with unexplained clinical symptoms and signs such as confusion, behavioral change, irritability, restlessness, headache, diaphoresis, and decreased mental performance, which may precede respiratory failure. With worsening hypoxia, a more serious alteration in the sensorium or seizures can occur. Also unexplained bradycardia or tachycardia, hypotension or hypertension, would point towards a sudden deterioration in gas exchange and impending respiratory collapse. One common observation suggestive of hypoxemia is a feeling of excessive heat in an adequately air conditioned room, with the patient demanding further cooling or increasing the speed of the fan; this is a sign of air hunger and should not be missed.

VENTILATION/PERFUSION MISMATCH

Lung units can either be poorly ventilated but well perfused or well ventilated but poorly perfused. In other words, we have nonuniform ventilation with uniform perfusion which represents a right-to-left shunt (physiological shunt) or uniform ventilation with nonuniform perfusion representing physiological dead space **(Fig. 5)**. This mismatching of ventilation to perfusion (V/Q mismatch) is the most important determinant of hypoxemia due to a defective oxygen transfer. As V/Q of a normal healthy lung is equally balanced between ventilation and perfusion, the ratio is around 1 (though the respiratory exchange ratio "R" between ventilation and pulmonary circulation is between 0.8 and 1). However, the range of V/Q in disease states can vary anywhere from zero (low V/Q units) to infinity (dead space units) **(Fig. 2)**. Though the term V/Q mismatch embraces both the physiological shunt and physiological dead space, however, routinely for all clinical purposes it denotes a low V/Q imbalance producing a physiological shunt, because physiological dead space by itself is not a common cause of hypoxemia. Gas exchange abnormality cannot be ascertained by measurement of PaO_2 and $PaCO_2$ alone, as one would need to know the alveolar-arterial gradient $P(A-a)O_2$, as described earlier, to confirm a V/Q mismatch.

Quantifying the Shunt

Firstly let us understand the distinction between venous admixture and right-to-left physiological shunt, as both terms should not be interchangeably used. Hypoxemia can occur with low V/Q lung units of varying degrees from partially ventilated to totally unventilated alveoli. Hypoxemia from lung units with low V/Q ratios where alveolar air is less than the capillary perfusion will result in

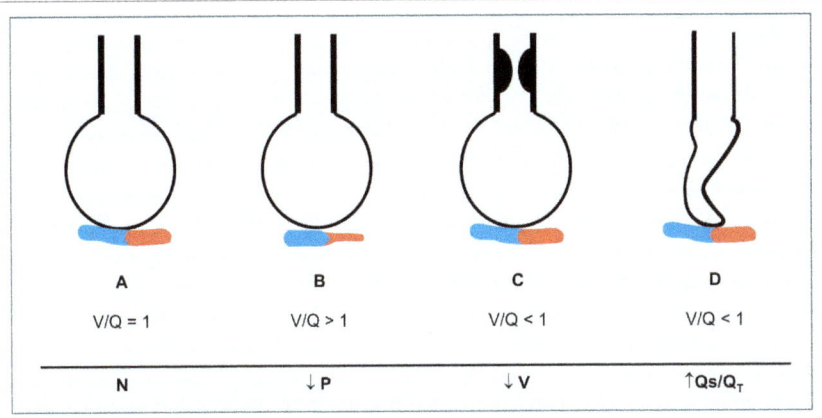

A = Normal lung (uniform ventilation and perfusion)
B = Physiological dead space effect (uniform ventilation and nonuniform perfusion)
C = V/Q mismatch (nonuniform ventilation and uniform perfusion)
D = Shunt effect due to a collapse lung unit

Fig. 5: V/Q mismatch and shunt. (N: normal; P: perfusion; Q_s/Q_T: total shunted blood flow/cardiac output; V: ventilation; V/Q: ventilation/perfusion)

venous admixture, whereas lung units where capillary blood receives no air from the totally unventilated alveoli result in a right-to-left physiological shunt **(Fig. 5)**. Treating venous admixture with 100% oxygen will correct hypoxemia and eliminate venous admixture entirely, but if some degree of hypoxemia is left uncorrected, it can be assumed that this fraction of venous admixture is due to the shunt effect. For this reason, supplemental oxygen will not significantly improve hypoxemia and the response of PaO_2 to the increasing concentration of FiO_2, will vary according to the degree of shunt fraction. If 40% or more of cardiac output is shunted there will be negligible or no response to PaO_2. Shunt is best calculated by delivering 100% O_2 (on mechanical ventilator) and using the shunt equation:

$$\frac{Q_s}{Q_T} = \frac{CcO_2 - CaO_2}{CcO_2 - CvO_2}$$

where Q_T = Total cardiac output; Qs = Total shunted blood flow
CaO_2, CvO_2, and CcO_2 are arterial, venous, and capillary O_2 contents, respectively.

Normal Qs/Q_T is 3–5% coming from the bronchial circulation and bypassing the alveoli.

The actual calculation requires pulmonary catheterization to obtain CvO_2 and assuming that on breathing 100% O_2, the CcO_2 is 100%. However, routine shunt calculation is hardly ever used at the bedside; alternatively, the *PaO_2/ FiO_2 ratio*, which gives a fairly good idea of the degree of shunting is commonly used at the bedside. For instance, a PaO_2 of 90 mm Hg will be a good PaO_2/ FiO_2 ratio >450 at sea level while breathing room air, but not so on receiving

> **BOX 1** Causes of tissue hypoxia.
> 1. Inadequate O_2 carrying capacity (CaO_2)
>   - $CaO_2 = (SaO_2 \times Hb \times 1.34) + (0.003 \times PaO_2)$
>   - If Hb = 15 g%; normal CaO_2 = 20 mL/100 mL of blood = 200 mL/L
> 2. Inadequate O_2 transport (DO_2)
>   - $DO_2 = CO \times CaO_2$
>   - If CO = 5 L/min; normal DO_2 = 5 × 200 = 1,000 mL O_2/min
> 3. Inadequate peripheral O_2 extraction
>   - Normal O_2 extraction = 25% of DO_2 = 250 mL
>
> (Hb: hemoglobin)

60% O_2 (FiO_2 = 0.6), as this would significantly decrease the PaO_2/FiO_2 ratio to 150. The main limitation of PaO_2/FiO_2 ratio occurs when using an open face mask or nasal prongs for O_2 delivery, as FiO_2 cannot be accurately estimated.

In conclusion, therefore the respiratory causes of arterial hypoxemia can be due to any disturbance along the O_2 cascade—a low PiO_2, FiO_2, or P_AO_2; a diffusion defect or a V/Q mismatch due to venous admixture, or right-to-left physiological shunt. However, one should be aware that tissue hypoxia can occur without arterial hypoxemia as a result of an inadequate oxygen carrying capacity (CaO_2), an inadequate DO_2, or an inadequate peripheral O_2 extraction (***Box 1***).

■ pCO_2 AND VENTILATION

The term ventilation, when used broadly, usually implies to a movement of air in and out of the lungs. To be more precise, we need to qualify this term to its specific function, so that there is no ambiguity in our understanding of what we are exactly implying.

Minute Ventilation

This is the total amount of air breathed in a minute and is conveniently measured on a sample of expired air. The symbol for minute ventilation is V_E, which stands for volume per unit time of expired air. Hence for measurement, V_E = respiratory rate (f) × tidal volume (V_T), and is the sum of alveolar and dead space ventilation (V_D).

Alveolar Ventilation

The correct definition of alveolar ventilation (V_A) is the volume of air that reaches the alveoli and takes part in gas exchange between the alveoli and pulmonary capillaries. The portion of alveolar gas that is not involved in gas exchange because of dead space is not considered a part of V_A.

$$\text{Hence } V_A = f \times (V_T - V_D)$$

where f = respiratory rate, V_T = tidal volume; V_D = dead space volume (physiological and anatomical).

Dead Space Ventilation

It is that portion of V_E that is not involved in gas exchange and hence is labeled as "wasted ventilation". V_D includes (1) anatomical V_D which remains in the airways and never reaches the alveoli and (2) physiological V_D that reaches the alveoli but for some reason does not take part in gas exchange. Disease complications such as low cardiac output or PE, which result in normal ventilation but under perfused by capillary blood (uniform ventilation with nonuniform perfusion), are two common causes of physiological dead space. In normal subjects with normal gas exchange, the V_D is approximately 30% of tidal volume (V_T), which is mainly the air in the airways that does not take part in gas exchange (anatomical dead space). Dead space is calculated as a ratio of dead space to tidal volume (V_D/V_T)

$$\frac{V_D}{V_T} = \frac{PaCO_2 - PeCO_2}{PaCO_2}$$

$PeCO_2$ is the expired partial pressure of CO_2

An increase in V_D/V_T above 0.5 will result in hypercapnia and the most common cause is ventilated but under perfused alveoli, as in low cardiac output states. The dead space effect in PE is usually transient due to a passing embolus; when it occurs it may manifest more as a relative hypercapnia and is evidenced by a marked disparity between V_E and $PaCO_2$, where the $PaCO_2$ will not fall in proportion to the hyperventilation. This subtle disparity in a patient with isolated dyspnea may at times be the only clinical expression of PE. At times, patients receiving high positive pressures on a mechanical ventilator may also present with dead space effect and hypercapnia because of overdistention of the alveoli resulting in nonuniform gas exchange.

■ HYPERCAPNIA

Hypercapnia is defined as a $PaCO_2$ level above 45 mm Hg; however, this rise should not be due to a compensated metabolic alkalosis. Except for the routine application during ABG analysis most physicians are not conversant with the intricacies of pCO_2 physiology. Importance of $PaCO_2$ is that it is the only gas that provides information on ventilation, oxygenation and acid base balance which cannot be over emphasized **(Fig. 6)**.

To understand the physiological basis of hypercapnia we need to appreciate the following aspects of $PaCO_2$—from its production in the body to its elimination by the lungs in a clinical setting.
- *CO_2 production:* In the body, CO_2 is the byproduct of food metabolism and needs to be continuously eliminated by the lungs. This is accomplished by virtue of the small pressure gradient existing between the mixed venous pCO_2 and alveolar pCO_2 (approximately 6 mm Hg) across the alveolar capillary membrane. CO_2 is transported in the blood largely as bicarbonates, carbamino compounds, and as a dissolved fraction in the

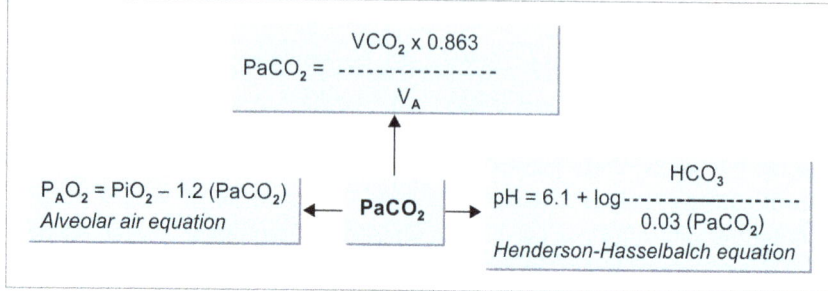

Fig. 6: Relationship of $PaCO_2$ to the three important equations of oxygenation and acid-base balance. (V_A: alveolar ventilation; PiO_2: partial pressure of inspired oxygen; VCO_2: carbon dioxide production)

plasma and this fraction of CO_2 is responsible for the measured $PaCO_2$ in the blood.

- CO_2 production (VCO_2) is a continuous process and if for whatever reason it increases (e.g., exercise) the excess load is eliminated by hyperventilation, thereby maintaining a constant normal $PaCO_2$–not resulting in hypercapnia. Hypercapnia would result only if the CO_2 excretion is impaired as in COPD or alveolar hypoventilation or development of physiological dead space. Hence, an increased CO_2 production is responsible for hypercapnia only when the lungs ability to CO_2 elimination is compromised. Interestingly but rarely, in the ICU setting VCO_2 may increase also due to a high carbohydrate meal which has a high respiratory quotient (RQ) of 1 compared to a normal RQ of 0.8.

$$RQ = \frac{VCO_2}{VO_2} = 0.8 \text{ (normal)}$$

- If such a patient on high carbohydrate diet is in the ICU on mechanical ventilator *receiving fixed V_E*, his ability to eliminate CO_2 is limited and will result in hypercapnia, and difficult weaning.
- *CO_2 elimination*: As explained earlier, $PaCO_2$ is inversely proportional to V_A and this relationship of $PaCO_2$ to ventilation is best expressed by the most important equation in respiratory medicine

$$PaCO_2 = \frac{VCO_2 \times 0.863}{V_A}$$

In this equation, VCO_2 is the CO_2 production in the body in mL/min and V_A in L/min has to be converted to mm Hg as $PaCO_2$ is expressed in mm Hg. This is achieved by the constant 0.863.

In routine clinical practice we can easily measure V_E by the use of spirometer. However, as tidal volume also includes V_D, hence V_E (V_T × respiratory rate) does not give information regarding the adequacy of gas transfer which can only be assessed by knowing the value of V_A. The only test that provides this information is $PaCO_2$, as seen from the $PaCO_2$ equation. The equation also shows that $PaCO_2$

is inversely proportional to V_A and is directly proportional to CO_2 production. Similar to the $PaCO_2$-$V_A CO_2$ relationship, there is also relationship between $P_A O_2$ and $PaCO_2$ which is well illustrated by the line AB in (**Fig. 1**). Both $P_A O_2$ and $PaCO_2$ are two independent variables balancing on either side of the scales and an increase in one is associated with a decrease in the other. In other words, hypoventilation raises the $PaCO_2$ with an associated fall in $P_A O_2$ and vice versa and this is only true for primary alveolar hypoventilation or hyperventilation. However, if there is a V/Q abnormality causing impairment of gas transfer due to disease or damage to the lung parenchyma, the relationship between PaO_2 and $PaCO_2$ will be different as shown in details in **Figure 1**. Also the extent to which the $PaCO_2$ could rise is constrained by the lowest $P_A O_2$ compatible with life and likewise, the maximum $P_A O_2$ achievable breathing room air is limited by the extent to which one can continue to hyperventilate and drop the $PaCO_2$.

- *Hypercapnia in the clinical setting*: One should recognize the fact that decreased V_A in relationship to carbon dioxide production is the fundamental reason for hypercapnia (except on directly inhaling CO_2) and this is the main physiological basis for carbon dioxide retention in clinical medicine. Hence, decrease in V_A can be caused by either inadequate V_E or increase dead space (V_D) and their causes have already been discussed earlier in the chapter.

The morbidity caused by high $PaCO_2$ levels is not due to elevated $PaCO_2$ alone but more due to its associated complications. (1) A marked fall in PaO_2 occurring from a very sharp rise in $PaCO_2$ due to hypoventilation and though supplemented oxygen can correct this but if there is any further rise in $PaCO_2$ it may create a precipitous fall in PaO_2 which could be incompatible with life if not assisted by mechanical ventilation. (2) Similarly, a rise in $PaCO_2$ will lead to a fall in pH and the resulting acidemia in critically ill patients can trigger arrhythmias and persistent pH levels below 7.25 could even be life-threatening. Therefore, a raised $PaCO_2$ should not be sole criteria to intubate and ventilate a patient but to be judged along with other clinical and laboratory parameters. Worsening of respiratory fatigue, decreased sensorium, a persistently low pH, and a refractory hypoxemia are few of the associated features that would certainly mandate ventilator support.

- *Hyperventilation is the main cause of low $PaCO_2$ levels*. However, it is important to stress that in clinical practice we see instances where $PaCO_2$ may not typically reflect the degree of hyperventilation and a disparity between the two variables may be obvious. This may happen because of an inability to hyperventilate beyond a point as in asthmatics with severe bronchospasm or in cases of respiratory muscle fatigue with increasing dead space. Here, the patient is unable to raise the V_A *and washout CO_2* despite all effort. Hence, in this scenario even a normal or near normal $PaCO_2$ is a sign of impending respiratory failure requiring ventilator support.

PULSE OXIMETRY

Pulse oximetry is a safe and noninvasive measurement of the SaO_2 but it does not measure PaO_2 which requires blood gas evaluation by arterial puncture. The basic pulse oximeter probe is usually placed on the index or middle finger or even on the big toe. The probe has two sides—the upper contains the light emitting diodes which emit monochromatic light at two wavelengths which pass through the finger and are detected by the photo detector placed on the opposite and lower side of the probe. The transmitted light passes through an amplifier which amplifies only the pulsatile waves and blocks the nonpulsatile waves selectively. This ensures that the light waves will selectively focus on the analysis of arterial blood by eliminating the nonpulsatile Hb in the veins. The two different wavelengths of the transmitting light are a reflection of the difference in deoxygenated hemoglobin (dHb) and oxygenated hemoglobin (HbO_2) concentrations in the arterial blood. The final pulse oximeter saturation is expressed in percentage by the equation:

$$SpO_2 = \frac{HbO_2}{HbO_2 + dHb} \times 100$$

The pulse oximeter levels are fairly reliable at SaO_2 levels above 70%, with minimal fluctuation from actual SaO_2 levels. Its main limitation is being a less sensitive measure of oxygenation compared to PaO_2, and this is because a significant reduction of PaO_2 (up to 60 mm Hg) results in only a minimal reduction in SaO_2 throughout the flat portion of the oxygen dissociation curve.

In carboxyhemoglobinemia and methemoglobinemia, the SaO_2 levels decrease because the oxyhemoglobin fraction decreases. However, the SpO_2 recorded on the pulse oximeter remains normal, thereby overestimating the true SaO_2. This happens because the standard pulse oximeter has only two wavelengths of light and does not detect the two variants of Hb, thus becoming an unreliable marker of SaO_2 in patients with either of these two variants.

Pulse oximeters give a near accurate reading of SaO_2 in hypotensive and anemic patients when the mean arterial pressure does not fall below 30 mm Hg and Hb remains above 3 g%, provided there is no accompanying vasoconstriction or hypoxemia. There are studies which have shown that dark skin decreases the accuracy of pulse oximeters at low levels of SaO_2, but fingernail polish showed minimal discordance between SpO_2 and SaO_2, though this did not hold true for artificial nails.

Usefulness of the pulse oximeter cannot be denied and it is a requisite for safe, noninvasive monitoring not only in ICUs, EMS, or operation theaters, but even as a part of routine monitoring of vitals by the nurses in general wards. SpO_2 can also increase the predictive value of SvO_2 or $ScVO_2$, in presence of declining cardiac output as in cardiogenic shock. The SpO_2-$ScvO_2$ gap could be a good and relatively noninvasive equation for estimating the degree of oxygen extraction and may be used as a marker for tissue hypoxia.

CAPNOMETRY

Capnometry is the measurement of CO_2 in the exhaled gas. This is measured during a single expired tidal volume with the help of an infrared CO_2 analyzer. During mechanical ventilation, the infrared CO_2 probe is attached to the airway in series with the expiratory tubing and is connected to a transducer where the photo detector can measure changes in CO_2 during each exhalation. Usually when gas exchange is normal, the end-tidal pCO_2 ($PetCO_2$) matches the $PaCO_2$. However, when the gas exchange is impaired, as in increased V_D, the $PetCO_2$ is decreased in relation to $PaCO_2$. The $PaCO_2$-$PetCO_2$ gradient is normally 3-5 mm Hg, and increased gradients are commonly associated with increase in anatomical dead space (shallow breathing) and physiological dead space (low cardiac output state, PE, COPD, or hyperinflation of the lung). Hence, a sudden increase of gradient should alert the intensivist to an inadvertent displacement of the ET tube or PE.

Capnography is also very useful for continuous noninvasive monitoring of $PaCO_2$ in operation theaters or during transport. It can also help during the weaning process as a rise or fall in $PetCO_2$ could mean increased respiratory work load or shallow breathing with muscle weakness, respectively, and in both cases it is a sign of weaning failure. However, $PetCO_2$ monitoring for weaning trial has its limitations because capnometry is possible only in a closed circuit during mechanical ventilation; however, this can be overcome by using a modified nasal cannulae available commercially. Alternatively, transcutaneous capnometers are also available.

TREATMENT

Treatment should mainly cover the two major concerns of ARF: (1) the deranged physiology of gas exchange—correcting hypoxemia and ventilatory support are most vital; and (2) specific treatment of the underlying etiology.

Correcting Hypoxemia and Ventilator Support

As discussed earlier, the "oxygen cascade" continues from the atmosphere, transferring oxygen across the lungs into the pulmonary capillaries and via the bloodstream to its final destination of oxygenating the peripheral tissues and vital organs. For this cascade to be sustainable, we need appropriate devices for delivering oxygen to the alveolar bed and innovative strategies to enable oxygen transfer through an impaired alveolar capillary membrane. Hemodynamic support may at times be required to improve the DO_2 in the bloodstream in order to reach the peripheral tissue.

Oxygen delivery devices have been adequately covered in the chapter 2 on Airways Management. However, the immediate decision to intubate or not depends on the clinical circumstances and is the quintessence of emergency management. Life-threatening or progressive organ dysfunction due to hypoxia (with or without hemodynamic compromise) and hypoxemia due to upper airways obstruction are absolute clinical emergencies that warrant immediate intubation and mechanical ventilation. In patients with hypercapnic type II respiratory failure, a selected few with adequate ventilatory effort may be observed on oxygen delivered by mask or noninvasive ventilation (NIV), but any worsening of hypoxemia, hypercapnia, or respiratory drive requires immediate intubation. NIV may also obviate the need for intubation in a subset of patients with hypoxemic respiratory failure. These include patients whose PaO_2/FiO_2 ratios are above 200 and who are clinically stable and their underlying disease is expected to respond with therapy early. For example, patients of cardiac failure and minimal pulmonary edema have a good possibility of recovering after diuresis, provided they have no other hemodynamic instability. Patients with bilateral pulmonary infiltrates do not generally respond to NIV, though one may attempt it in mild cases of ARDS ($PaO_2/FiO_2 > 200$), as discussed earlier. Absolute contraindications to NIV are mentioned in **Figure 7**.

For nonintubated patients and those not on NIV, oxygen needs to be supplemented through nasal prongs or face mask, but these may not be adequate to achieve the required PaO_2. In order to maximize the FiO_2, masks with reservoir bags are available with two different devices, the *partial rebreathing* and the *nonrebreathing masks*. The partial rebreathing devices achieve around 60–70% FiO_2 and the nonrebreathing types can approximately achieve as high as 80% FiO_2, after making allowances for the leakage from around the masks. Venturi masks with O_2 delivery via controlled flow are useful, especially in patients with COPD, where excessive oxygen supplementation may cause respiratory depression and worsening hypercapnia. Respiratory depression occurs here because the respiratory center is deprived of its hypoxic drive.

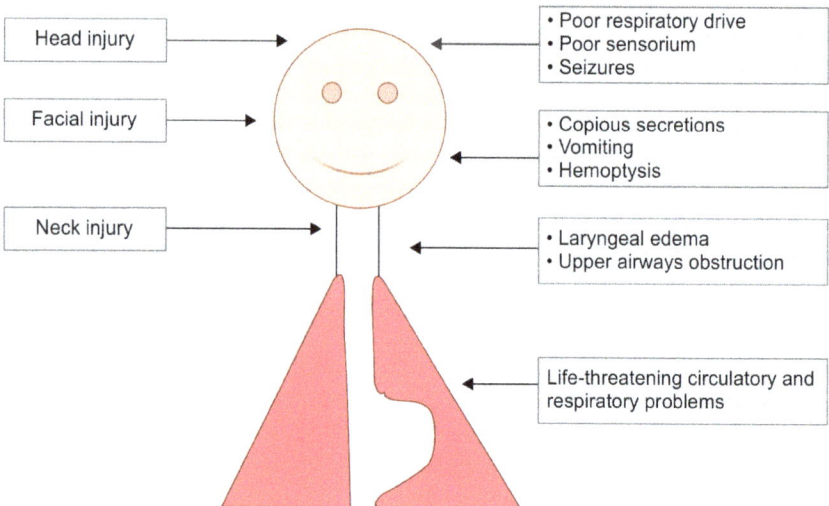

Fig. 7: Contraindications of noninvasive positive pressure ventilation (NIPPV).

One new system of noninvasive oxygen delivery is the *humidified high-flow nasal oxygen (HFNO) device by* which oxygen can be delivered through wide bore nasal prongs. In addition to providing high flow rates from 1 to 60 L/min and achieving high FiO_2, it also creates a positive pressure in the nasopharynx which acts like a positive end-expiratory pressure (PEEP) and prevents collapse of alveoli during expiration. HFNO has become a popular alternative to intubation and mechanical ventilation in selective cases of hypoxemic respiratory failure and particularly in severe cases of community-acquired pneumonia. It has also been amply proven to be effective during the recent pandemic of coronavirus disease-2019 (COVID-19).

The approximate FiO_2 delivered by various devices varies depending on the type of masks and their interface, maintaining a close fit with minimal leakage. Nasal cannula at 4 L/min can raise the FiO_2 up to 30%; higher flow rates by nasal prongs are not usually tolerated and hence, are replaced by oxygen masks. Simple masks can achieve up to 40–50% of FiO_2 at 8 L/min with an optimum interface. Partial rebreathing and nonrebreathing masks with reservoir bags can achieve anywhere from 60 to 80% FiO_2 at high flow rates of 8–10 L/min. Since some degree of leakage always occurs, as no interface is perfect hence, one cannot achieve 100% FiO_2. Whichever device is used, the aim is to maintain a PaO_2 well above 60 mm Hg or a SaO_2 of 92% or more. Patients suffering from acute coronary or cerebrovascular diseases should be maintained on a slightly higher level of oxygenation, as they are more vulnerable to the sudden changes in gas exchange.

Finally, if acceptable levels of oxygen are not achievable with noninvasive devices including NIV, intubation, and ventilator support become mandatory. Advanced modes of lung recruitment may be necessary for patients with refractory hypoxemia. In patients with ARDS, lung protection strategy mainly using low tidal volumes with permissive hypercapnia should be implemented throughout to avoid ventilator-induced lung injury (VILI). Conventionally, the clearest indication for oxygen therapy (invasive or noninvasive) is respiratory failure with a PaO_2 of <60 mm Hg. However, patients with any level of hypoxemia, and particularly those with the possibility of impending respiratory failure, or associated with other critical comorbidities, will benefit with oxygen therapy.

Treatment of the Underlying and Iatrogenic Causes

Along with the resuscitation measures for correcting hypoxemia or acidosis, the underlying cause and its management must also be attended to urgently. History may reveal an obvious cause, which when managed without delay could reduce mortality and save time of ICU stay. Patients with more serious and protracted causes of respiratory failure such as ARDS, severe pneumonia, polytrauma, and severe sepsis who have marked V/Q mismatch or refractory hypoxia will have to be managed in the ICU on mechanical ventilator using appropriate modes of lung recruitment. Patients with acute exacerbation of COPD may be tried on NIV initially, as this subset of patients with respiratory failure are difficult to manage on invasive ventilation and even more difficult to wean. However, timely intubation and ventilation is warranted if they show worsening gas exchange on NIV. Patients requiring ventilator support for longer periods have their own inherent problems like VILI, ventilator-associated pneumonia (VAP), intubation-related injuries to the trachea, and compromise of cardiac function due to raised intrathoracic pressure following PEEP.

Lastly, while patients on long-term mechanical ventilator may have many *iatrogenic complications,* the three major concerns that require separate attention are VAP, VILI, and Oxygen Toxicity. Causes and prevention of VAP and VILI are discussed separately in the chapters on "mechanical ventilation" and "strategies on mechanical ventilation in ARDS", respectively. *Oxygen toxicity* is one aspect in the management of adult patients with ARF which remains unclear, though there is compelling evidence of hyperoxic lung injury in neonates. The term *hyperoxia* is generally applied when PaO_2 levels are between 120 and 200 mm Hg, but when above 200 mm Hg, it is considered as *severe hyperoxia* and is supposed to manifest with symptoms of cough, dyspnea, pleuritic chest pain, and retrosternal discomfort. Pathological features of inflammation resembling ARDS have been postulated in some studies, but this remains uncertain.

The association of oxygen toxicity with morbidity and mortality in critically ill patients has always been difficult to prove because of the existing serious nature of the underlying disease; however, one study reported in *Crit Care Med (2017)* has shown a linear relationship between the duration of hyperoxia and mortality. Though the clinical and pathological effects of hyperoxia on the lungs are still not confirmed, there is increasing evidence to suggest an association between high levels of PaO_2 and lung damage in critically ill patients and this is possibly one of the causes of VILI. However, the exact PaO_2 level and duration at which O_2 therapy causes toxicity remains unclear. In practice, it would be wise to limit the FiO_2 below 60% once satisfactory SaO_2 levels (90–92%) are achieved.

■ SUGGESTED READING

1. American Thoracic Society. Dyspnea: mechanism assessment and management. A consensus statement. Am J Respir Crit Care Med. 1999;159(1):321-40.
2. Baydur A. Respiratory muscle strength and control of ventilation in patients with neuromuscular disease. Chest. 1991;99(2):330-8.
3. B R O'Driscoll, L S Howard, J Earis, and V Mak, on behalf of the BTS Emergency Oxygen Guideline Development Group. British Thoracic Society Guideline for oxygen use in adults in healthcare and emergency settings. BMJ Open Respir Res. 2017; 4(1): e000170.
4. Bryan TG, Whyte RP, Neligan PJ. Is oxygen toxic? In: Deutschman CS, Neligan PJ (Eds). Evidence Based Practice of Critical Care, 3rd edition. Amsterdam, Netherlands: Elsevier; 2020.
5. Duarte AG, Bidani A. Evaluating hypoxia in critically ill. J Respir Dis. 2005;26(5):209-19.

6. Gray BA, Blalock JM. Interpretation of alveolar-arterial oxygen difference in patients with hypercapnia. Am Rev Respir Dis. 1991;143(1):4-8.
7. Roussos C, Koutsoukou A. Respiratory failure. Eur Resp J Suppl. 2003;47:3s-14s.
8. Udwadia FE. Acute respiratory failure in adults. In: Udwadia FE (Ed). Principles of Critical Care, 3rd edition. New Delhi: Jaypeee Brothers Medical Publishers (P) Ltd.; 2014.
9. Udwadia FE. Respiratory monitoring in adults. In: Udwadia FE (Ed). Principles of Critical Care, 3rd edition. New Delhi: Jaypeee Brothers Medical Publishers (P) Ltd.; 2014.
10. West JB. Ventilation perfusion inequality. In: West JB (Ed). Respiratory Physiology: The Essentials, 8th edition. Baltimore: Lippincott Williams & Wilkins; 2007.

CHAPTER 5

Acute Respiratory Distress Syndrome

Jamshed Sunavala

■ DEFINITION

Since first description of acute respiratory distress syndrome (ARDS) in Lancet by Ashbaugh DG et al. in 1967, many changes have been made in its definition. However, the defining characteristics have remained the same as the initial description of an acute onset of respiratory compromise with refractory hypoxemia and tachypnea. The American-European Consensus Conference (AECC) in 1994 in its definition of ARDS laid particular stress in distinguishing between cardiogenic (hydrostatic) and noncardiogenic pulmonary edema. They advocated the use of pulmonary artery catheter (PAC) to exclude an increased left atrial pressure by measuring pulmonary capillary wedge pressure (PCWP) which should be <18 mm Hg. Further the AECC labeled this clinical entity as acute lung injury (ALI) in patients with partial pressure of arterial oxygen/fraction of inspired oxygen (PaO_2/FiO_2) ≤ 300 mm Hg and ARDS for PaO_2/FiO_2 ≤ 200 mm Hg. The new updated Berlin definition in 2011 **(Table 1)** incorporated the following changes to the AECC definition: (1) Only an objective assessment or echocardiography was necessary to exclude cardiac failure and it did not mention the use of PAC to exclude left atrial hypertension (2) The term ALI for patients with PaO_2/FiO_2 ≤ 300 mm Hg and ≥ 200 mm Hg as described in the AECC definition was now replaced by ARDS for all

TABLE 1 The Berlin definition of ARDS.

Acute respiratory failure
- Occurring within 1 week of a known clinical insult, or new or worsening respiratory symptoms
- Not explained by cardiac failure or fluid overload. May need objective assessment like two-dimensional echocardiography to rule out hydrostatic edema
- Characterized by bilateral lung opacities which are not fully explained by effusions, consolidations, or collapse

Severity of ARDS in relation to the degree of hypoxemia

Mild	Moderate	Severe
PaO_2/FiO_2 ≤ 300 mm Hg but >200 mm Hg on PEEP 5 cmH_2O	PaO_2/FiO_2 ≤ 200 mm Hg but >100 mm Hg on PEEP 5 cmH_2O	PaO_2/FiO_2 ≤ 100 mm Hg on PEEP 5 cmH_2O

(ARDS: acute respiratory distress syndrome; FiO_2: fraction of inspired oxygen; PaO_2: partial pressure of arterial oxygen; PEEP: positive end-expiratory pressure)

levels of PaO_2/FiO_2 below 300 mm Hg and patients were stratified into mild, moderate, and severe ARDS according to the PaO_2/FiO_2 ratio along with 5 cm of positive end-expiratory pressure (PEEP) to diagnose the grade of severity.

■ DIAGNOSIS

Primarily the diagnosis is based on the criteria included in the latest Berlin definition. ARDS presents with an acute onset of dyspnea with PaO_2/FiO_2 ratio of ≤300 mm Hg and the severe hypoxemia is not corrected on delivering oxygen by nasal prongs or simple mask. Partial breathing or non-rebreathing masks with high flow oxygen or noninvasive ventilation (NIV) or nasal high-flow oxygen (NHFO) may tide over mild cases of ARDS (PaO_2/FiO_2 > 200 mm Hg). However, severe cases or progressive hypoxemia will require intubation and mechanical support. Though chest X-rays may be clear in the first few hours of the onset of symptoms, these would later show bilateral patchy pulmonary infiltrates often described as "bilateral fluffy shadows". In fact, these pulmonary infiltrates soon progress to show the classic X-ray picture of ARDS, with a ground-glass appearance evenly distributed throughout both lungs without evidence of pleural effusion.

The radiological picture of permeability pulmonary edema is due to the alveolar capillary leak and is often indistinguishable from cardiogenic pulmonary edema. The history, along with signs and symptoms of an underlying cardiac disease and two-dimensional (2D) echocardiography may be useful in differentiating cardiogenic from noncardiogenic pulmonary edema. Earlier an elevated PCWP (>18 mm Hg) was used to rule out cardiogenic pulmonary edema, however, as there was growing evidence from many studies that both ARDS and cardiogenic edema with high left atrial pressures may coexist, the latest "Berlin definition" has not mentioned the use of PAC in its defining criteria but has instead stated that in suspected cases of ARDS, respiratory failure should not be fully explained by cardiac failure or fluid overload. This of course leaves a great deal of ambiguity and is not very helpful to the clinicians in making a diagnosis and this is where the definition lacks specificity.

Knowing the *predisposing conditions* and high-risk factors associated with ARDS can help towards predicting the diagnosis of ARDS. It increases the probability of ARDS when confronting a clinical and radiological picture, which overlaps with other etiologies of respiratory failure with similar lung shadows. For example, knowing the fact that 25% of all patients succumbing to smoke inhalation injury will develop ARDS leaves no ambiguity in predicting the diagnosis. Shock, sepsis, gastric aspiration and pneumonia still remain the common predisposing conditions for ARDS in the intensive care unit (ICU). **Table 2** lists the important predisposing and high-risk conditions commonly seen in the ICU. Usually the combination of these conditions not only adds to the predictability of ARDS but is also used to calculate the Lung Injury Prediction Score (LIPS). This scoring system was primarily created to help in

| TABLE 2 | Predisposing conditions for ARDS. |

Major predisposing conditions

Infection related	Noninfectious causes
• Septicemia	• Gastric aspiration
• Septic shock	• Transfusion related (TRALI)
• Pneumonia	• Pancreatitis
• Septic abdomen	• Shock (cardiogenic/hemorrhagic)
Postoperative	Post-trauma
• Major abdominal surgery	• Polytrauma
• Aortic surgery	• Multiple fractures
• Cardiac surgery	• Extensive burns
• Thoracic surgery	• Lung contusion
• Spine surgery	• Near drowning
	• Smoke inhalation

Risk modifiers
These are risk factors when combined with predisposing conditions are probably more prone to developing ARDS
- Heavy smoking
- On chemotherapy
- Alcohol abuse
- Obesity
- Hypoalbuminemia
- High APACHE II score
- On high FiO_2
- Acidosis < 7.35

(APACHE II: Acute Physiology and Chronic Health Evaluation II; ARDS: acute respiratory distress syndrome; FiO_2: fraction of inspired oxygen; TRALI: transfusion-related acute lung injury)

designing an "ARDS prevention study" which could also serve as a checklist to ensure certain preventable independent risk factors (risk modifiers) **(Table 2)**.

Bronchoalveolar Lavage

The analysis of the lavage fluid for presence of neutrophils and protein is reliable in distinguishing cardiogenic from noncardiogenic pulmonary edema. *However, it is rarely used as the procedure carries a high risk in cases of severe ARDS.* In patients with ARDS, the lavage fluid has neutrophils which are >80% of recovered cells compared to normal subjects. Similarly, lavage fluid rich in protein is evidence of ARDS and is helpful in distinguishing hydrostatic pulmonary edema from ARDS-related pulmonary edema.

■ PATHOLOGY AND PHYSIOLOGICAL CONSEQUENCES

Dysregulation of inflammation, increased alveolar capillary permeability and activation of coagulation pathways are the main pathological features of ARDS. These changes evolve progressively over the course of the disease through the three phases viz. exudative, proliferative, and fibrotic. These three phases may not necessarily occur as distinct entities over time but may coexist in different areas of the lungs at the same time, over the course of the disease.

Exudative phase is the initial response to the lung injury and begins within 24 hours of the insult. During this phase, there is activation of the innate immune system with recruitment of neutrophils, which results in the damage to the alveolar endothelium and capillary epithelium, thereby leading to the breakdown of the alveolar-capillary barrier. It is important to note that injury to both the epithelium and the endothelium is required to break the barrier, resulting in an increased alveolar-capillary permeability which allows the influx of protein-rich fluid into the interstitium and alveolar space.

The lung injury also causes surfactant dysfunction and dysfunctioning of the alveolar epithelial cells. The former leads to atelectasis and the latter causes failure of resorption of the fluid from the alveoli back into the pulmonary capillaries, both of which further augment the injury to the lung parenchyma and impair gas exchange.

Proliferative phase of ARDS may be termed as the repair phase where attempts are made to re-establish the epithelial integrity thereby reversing the fluid influx back from the alveoli to the pulmonary capillaries. This phase is also marked by the repair of the alveolar architecture while restoring the general hemostasis, slowly transiting into a continuing process of regaining the normal structure and function of the lung. However, for some unexplained reason, a few patients do not progress to a normal process of repairing and instead retrogress, to a fibrotic phase of ARDS.

In the *fibrotic phase*, profibrotic mediators like transforming growth factor-β (TGF-β) are released which lead to fibrosing alveolitis. The process of fibrosis may start shortly after injury and is associated with increased ventilator days and mortality, though a vast number of cases do recover, only after a protracted course of illness in the ICU. ARDS Network and other studies have associated the fibrotic phase of ARDS to ventilator-induced lung injury (VILI), and the fact that clinical observation of using lung protective strategies have shortened the days on ventilator, seems to give some credence to this theory. Here, the volutrauma and atelectrauma activate the inflammatory cascade, which is similar to other insults which lead to lung injury. It particularly damages the epithelial cells of the alveoli causing epithelial sloughing, formation of the hyaline membrane, and pulmonary edema.

Activation of the coagulation pathways causing inhibition of fibrinolysis leading to fibrin formation also occurs early in ARDS and is commonly reported to be present in the lung specimens during autopsy.

Physiological Consequences

The main physiological characteristics of ARDS are stiff lungs and shunting. The exudation of the proteinaceous fluid from the pulmonary capillaries causes the lung to be stiff, requiring high airway pressures to expand the lungs and achieve the required tidal volume (V_T), and this is manifest by a low compliance. A low compliance is a reduced change in lung volume per unit change in distending pressure. A marked decrease in ventilation/perfusion (V/Q) causing physiological shunting is the main cause of abnormal gas exchange in ARDS. Here the blood is shunted past the collapsed alveoli, which accounts for the hypoxemic type I respiratory failure of ARDS. In the early stages, it is the venous admixture which is responsible for the low PaO_2 and low partial pressure of arterial carbon dioxide ($PaCO_2$), the latter being due to the marked hyperventilation. However in the very late stages of unresolving ARDS, hypercapnia manifests and this is related to the increase in physiological dead space. Dead space ventilation occurs from the regions of the lung with normal ventilation but minimal or no perfusion caused by microthrombi and hypoxic vasoconstriction. The latter is also responsible for the increased pulmonary vascular resistance seen in severe cases of ARDS. For further details on V/Q imbalance and its consequences, refer to the Chapter on Acute Respiratory Failure.

■ UNDERSTANDING THE SEVERITY OF LUNG INJURY

The most common variable used to assess the severity of ALI is the PaO_2 to FiO_2 ratio (PaO_2/FiO_2), and understandably the Berlin definition of ARDS (*see* **Table 1**) has used the same criteria. According to the Berlin definition, a PaO_2/FiO_2 ratio of 200 mm Hg or less but >100 mm Hg is classified as moderately severe and a ratio of 100 or less is severe. In both cases, the patient is expected to be on a PEEP of 5 cmH_2O or more. Hence, we have to assume that the lower the PaO_2/FiO_2 ratio, greater the lung injury and thus greater lung parenchymal involvement. However, this may not be entirely true as some large studies have questioned the tenability of this assumption as they have found no clear association between the degree of hypoxia (PaO_2/FiO_2) and outcomes. Neither have they noted on CT imaging that oxygenation was dependent on the structural changes of lung parenchyma occurring across time (early, intermediate, or late ARDS), except when the lung damage was excessive and the nonaerated percentage of lung tissue was >60%. The findings of this study are important because in practice we are often faced with this disparity between the PaO_2/FiO_2 and the extent of lung involvement on high-resolution computed tomography (HRCT) image. Hence, it seems that the outcome does not always depend on the severity of hypoxia as assessed by the PaO_2/FiO_2 ratio, but more on the fraction of the nonaerated lung tissue which cannot be recruited, suggesting that CT analysis would give a more reliable assessment of overall lung severity and final outcome. However for bedside monitoring, the PaO_2/FiO_2 ratio is most convenient and a reasonably good measure of the extent of lung injury.

■ VENTILATOR-INDUCED LUNG INJURY

The aim of ventilator strategy in ARDS is to correct severe hypoxia by recruiting collapsed alveoli using what we term as *"open lung approach"* which includes use of high levels of PEEP and other recruitment maneuvers. However, there is a thin line between optimum recruitment and VILI resulting in worse outcomes.

Use of large tidal volumes of 10-14 mL/kg for ARDS patients were acceptable guidelines in the seventies and eighties. At that time, the main concerns were oxygen toxicity and barotrauma hence, avoiding high levels of PEEP and rapid reduction of FiO_2 were considered an appropriate approach in ventilator therapy for ARDS. By 1988, a study by Dreyfuss revealed that high tidal volumes of 12 mL/kg led to greater lung injury compared to patients receiving 4-6 mL/kg of V_T, and the focus shifted to *"volume overdistension"* as the primary cause of VILI in ARDS patients. This concept became widely recognized as *volutrauma* and this changed the strategy for ARDS to *low tidal volume (LTV)* ventilation of 6 mL/kg with limited inspiratory pressure. This came to be known as *lung protective strategy* and rightly so, as revealed in a large study in the New England Journal of Medicine (NEJM) in 2000, which had to be discontinued as the conventional arm (12 mL/kg) showed a significantly higher mortality compared to the LTV arm (6 mL/kg).

Interestingly, two studies in 2002 and 2005, both published in the American Journal of Respiratory Critical Care Medicine, showed that high plateau pressure (Pplat) independently predicted mortality even when V_T was held constant. Though no exact pressure was apparent, it was however accepted that Pplat should not rise above 30 cmH_2O, as that would be a reflection of excessive alveolar volume. To this day, lung protective ventilation is the only mode, which has shown decreased mortality in ARDS.

Four types of VILI have been described—barotrauma, volutrauma, atelectrauma, and biotrauma.

Barotrauma

It has been one of the earliest VILI described in ARDS patients and it is caused by air leaks from ruptured airways resulting in pneumothorax and pneumomediastinum. This was earlier suspected to be directly related to barotrauma but could also be well related to volutrauma.

Volutrauma

In ARDS, lung structure is unevenly formatted in areas of varying sizes that appear normal, poorly aerated, overinflated, and nonaerated. The aerated areas are inflamed but fully recruitable with near normal compliance and the larger these areas, the lesser the severity of ARDS. In severe ARDS, there is only a small component of these aerated areas, which consequently bear the maximum stress and strain of high inflation pressures and more so if large V_T are delivered. Studies showed that high inflation volumes rather than pressures were responsible for causing VILI. The term volutrauma and the inception of low volume ventilation were adopted following these studies.

Atelectrauma

The repetitive opening and closing of the small airways during mechanical ventilation, which is typical of ARDS, can cause damage to airway epithelium due to the excessive shearing force. The lung injury here can be reduced by using low levels of PEEP, which perhaps acts as a stent, keeping the small airways open during end-expiration.

Biotrauma

Positive pressure ventilation in ARDS may promote the release of pro-inflammatory cytokines from the lungs and cause lung injury. This could happen at accepted levels of inflation pressures which would ordinarily not be responsible for lung damage. Hence, mechanical ventilation can itself be a cause of systemic inflammatory response syndrome (SIRS) injuring the lungs. It may also injure other distant organs and the trigger mechanism here, is probably the release of intracellular mediators, which translocate into the systemic circulation through areas of increased alveolar capillary permeability as in ARDS.

■ STEPWISE APPROACH TO MECHANICAL VENTILATION IN ACUTE RESPIRATORY DISTRESS SYNDROME

Before discussing stepwise modalities of ventilation, it is imperative to understand that *lung protection ventilation (LPV)* is an uncompromised strategy which improves survival in ARDS. It should be adopted as the standard method of mechanical ventilation in all ARDS patients. LPV is designed to minimize the risk of VILI. This includes LTV ventilation at 6 mL/kg of predicted body weight, keeping the Pplat below 30 cmH_2O, and maintaining a minimum PEEP of 5 cmH_2O to prevent atelectrauma. However, LTV ventilation in ARDS patients with excessive respiratory demands may cause $PaCO_2$ to rise, but this may be permissible as long as the arterial pH does not fall below 7.25 and $PaCO_2$ does not rise beyond 70 mm Hg. This was first described by Keith Hickling in 1990 and was termed as *permissive hypercapnia*. However, it is best to avoid a persistently low pH <7.3; in which case one needs to increase the respiratory rate to a maximum of 30–35 breaths per minute. If the pH goes any lower than 7.25, keep the respiratory rate at 35 breaths per minute and try increasing the V_T by 1 mL/kg, though Pplat may exceed its target of 30 cmH_2O as a "trade-off". At this stage, serious lung recruitment strategies would be the only option and in case of an unrelenting severe respiratory acidosis, application of extracorporeal CO_2 removal ($ECCO_2$-R) is a feasible option available today.

Step 1: Assess the Severity of Acute Respiratory Distress Syndrome

Milder cases of ALI with PaO_2/FiO_2 of 200–300 mm Hg may be successfully ventilated using NIV. However, patients with marked respiratory distress and/or low PaO_2/FiO_2 below 200 mm Hg would need endotracheal (ET) intubation and ventilation. Needless delay in intubating and ventilating or pursuing with NIV despite inadequate response can lead to poor outcomes. Higher FiO_2 requirement despite high-flow nasal oxygen (HFNO) or NIV is suggestive of a greater shunt fraction and similarly, escalating $PaCO_2$ suggests respiratory muscle fatigue. In both these cases, immediate intubation and ventilator support is vital. On the other hand, if PaO_2/FiO_2 can be maintained reasonably well on NIV with stable $PaCO_2$ values, it suggests that the respiratory muscles are able to deal with the stress of reduced compliance. In which case NIV support may be continued, however, this decision rests on the clinician's judgment. With the rising popularity of NIV, there is often a needless delay in getting control of the airways which is always fraught with peril and regret. NIV is of course contraindicated in unconscious and semiconscious patients and those with poor respiratory effort. **Box 1** enumerates other conditions where NIV is contraindicated or avoided.

Step 2: Endotracheal Intubation

Most patients with ARDS present with severe respiratory distress with heavy rapid breathing and can pose difficulty during intubation. For discussion on difficult intubation, refer to the Chapter on Airway Management.

Step 3: Initial Ventilatory Settings

One does not have the opportunity to assess lung physiology amidst the bustle of resuscitation; hence, postintubation the ventilator settings are applied as per the set protocol. Briefly, the initial settings commonly applied are as shown in **Box 2**.

Step 4: Sedation

Most patients will require some degree of sedation and probably muscle relaxants to avoid ventilation asynchrony resulting from increased respiratory demand and when given in the early stages, it has shown to improve outcomes. However, prolonged periods of heavy sedation and muscle paralysis have their own adverse consequences, producing loss of respiratory muscle tone with total dependency on the mechanical ventilator, impeding early weaning

---

BOX 1 Contraindication for NIV.

- Unconscious or semiconscious patients
- Poor respiratory effort
- Uncontrolled seizures
- Life-threatening circulatory or respiratory failure
- Copious tracheal secretions
- Vomiting/hemoptysis
- Serious injuries of the face and neck
- Laryngeal edema or obstruction

(NIV: noninvasive ventilation)

> **BOX 2** On initiating mechanical ventilation in ARDS.
>
> V_T = 6–8 mL/kg
> FiO_2 = 0.7–1.0 depending on PaO_2/FiO_2
> Rate = 15–20 (increased if patient continues to fight the ventilator after sedation)
> I:E = 1:2
> PEEP = 5 cmH_2O
> Mode = VCV or PCV or ACV or PRVC
>
> (ACV: assist-controlled ventilation; ARDS: acute respiratory distress syndrome; FiO_2: fraction of inspired oxygen; I:E: inspiratory:expiratory; PaO_2: partial pressure of arterial oxygen; PCV: pressure-controlled ventilation; PEEP: positive end-expiratory pressure; VCV: volume-controlled ventilation; V_T: tidal volume, PRVC: Pressure regulated volume control)

or using spontaneous modes of ventilation. It also has a deleterious effect on gas exchange by causing upward shift of the paralyzed diaphragm, thereby resulting in further lung collapse. Sedative drugs are usually given as a loading dose followed by a continuous intravenous (IV) infusion **(Table 3)**.

Step 5: Positive End-expiratory Pressure Trials

As soon as the patient is reasonably stable after initiation of mechanical ventilation, a stepwise increase in PEEP levels should be attempted to obtain optimal lung recruitability. PEEP should be increased stepwise from 5–15 cmH_2O keeping V_T, inspiratory:expiratory (I:E) ratio, and FiO_2 constant. In normal practice, each stepwise increase is done after every 20 minutes, monitoring the peripheral oxygen saturation (SpO_2) and lung compliance (as judged by Pplat). Achieving an SpO_2 of 90% or more reflects an optimum PEEP and recruitability. Once the SpO_2 remains steady above 90%, gradually decrease the FiO_2 to 0.6, by further increasing the PEEP levels to a minimum necessary, but not above 20 cmH_2O. However, one should bear in mind that PEEP trials based on SpO_2 titration have a low sensitivity and specificity and this may not give a correct idea of recruitability in comparison to HRCT of the chest but it is still the most practical bedside method.

Step 6: Refractory Hypoxia

Most patients do not advance to a more severe form of ARDS with refractory hypoxia and they can continue on mechanical ventilator with acceptable levels of FiO_2 and without compromising the safe limits of airways pressure. However, there is subgroup of patients who need aggressive ventilator strategies as rescue therapies. These include prone positioning, inverse ratio ventilation, intermittent short recruitment trials, airway pressure release ventilation (ARVP), or in worse scenarios, ECMO may be used (Refer to Chapter on ECMO).

Most large studies in severe ARDS patients have shown that *prone positioning* consistently improved oxygenation. It is now an accepted therapy to prone patients with life-threatening refractory hypoxia. CT scans have

TABLE 3 Commonly used sedatives for patients on mechanical ventilator.

Drug	Dosage	Comments
Fentanyl	Bolus: 0.35–0.5 µg/kg Infusion: 0.7–10 µg/kg/h	Short-acting opioid No dose adjustment for renal failure Less of adverse hemodynamic effects
Remifentanil	Loading: 1.5 µg/kg Infusion: 0.5–15µg/kg/h	Ultra-short-acting opioid and effect is lost within 10 minutes of stopping infusion No dose adjustment for renal failure
Midazolam	Loading: 0.01–0.05 mg/kg Infusion: 0.02–0.1 mg/kg/h	Rapid-acting benzodiazepine Infusion to be limited to <48 hours
Lorazepam	Loading: 0.02–0.04 mg/kg (not exceeding 2 mg as bolus dose) Infusion: 0.01–0.1 mg/kg/h (not to exceed 8 mg/h)	Longer-acting benzodiazepine Propylen glycol toxicity lasts up to 6 hours in high doses (lactic acidosis and delirium)
Dexmedetomidine	Loading: 1 µg/kg over 10 minutes Infusion: 0.2–0.7 µg/kg/h	Cooperative sedation (like awakening from deep sleep and restoring back to sleep) Sedation can be continued during SBTs during weaning High loading and infusion rates can cause life-threatening bradycardia Contraindicated in patients with heart blocks or cardiac failure

(SBTs: spontaneous breathing trial)

shown more homogeneous gas distribution with opening of collapsed alveoli, mainly at the lung bases in the prone position and it also prevents or at least delays VILI. However, studies have shown that proning is beneficial mainly in the subgroup of patients with severe ARDS whose PaO_2/FiO_2 remains below 100 mm Hg. It has failed to show significant improvement in mild or moderate cases of ARDS. Ideally patients should be intermittently proned for at least 12-16 hours in a day.

Step 7: Weaning

Most patients with ARDS are difficult to wean and will take a longer time to wean, particularly if they have been on ventilator support for a protracted period. Once the lung pathology seems to be resolving and the PaO_2/FiO_2 ratio is >150 mm Hg, the clinician should consider the possibility of weaning. The best clinical assessment would be to screen the patient for pretest probability followed by a preweaning test and later attempt weaning trials. Refer to the Chapter on "Weaning from Mechanical Ventilation" for further discussion.

Many intensivists prefer to use pressure support ventilation (PSV) as part of weaning trials. Here the main advantage is the decreasing need for sedation and encouraging some degree of spontaneous breathing, with the assumption that, it may improve gas exchange because of better flow distribution and also maintain respiratory muscle tone. However, this notion is debatable and PSV cannot be tried in patients with ARDS who are not sufficiently resolved. Later in the recovery phase when the patient is more stable and not requiring sedation or muscle relaxants, it may help towards early weaning.

In *conclusion*, some patients of mild ARDS whose underlying pathology has substantially resolved can be ventilated noninvasively (NIV). However, this depends on the clinician's judgment and experience. Most patients require intubation and mechanical ventilation but they can be managed well on the usual modes of ventilation. However, a subgroup of patients with severe ARDS can have refractory hypoxia requiring aggressive strategies using advanced ventilatory modes to help recruit collapsed alveoli and improve oxygenation. Prone positioning is now found to be very helpful in improving oxygenation in patients with severe ARDS. In the process of pursuing with aggressive ventilation, there is always a danger of developing VILI, hence "LPV" remains an uncompromised strategy in all ARDS patients.

■ OTHER STRATEGIES

Steroids

A potential benefit in patients of ARDS with persistent inflammatory response has been reported in several anecdotal articles. However, the National Institute of Health (NIH)-sponsored ARDS Network evaluated the use of steroids for patients with persistent ARDS in the fibroproliferative phase and found no significant difference in outcomes between the steroid and placebo groups.

Steroid treatment in ARDS still remains controversial till more definitive studies become available. However if one is inclined to use steroids, the Society of Critical Care Medicine (SCCM) and European Society of Intesive Care Medicine (ESICM) have after reviewing literature suggested the use of methylprednisolone early in moderate-to-severe ARDS ($PaO_2/FiO_2 < 200$ mm Hg) with an appropriate dosage regimen.

Inhaled Vasodilators

Use of inhaled nitric oxide (NO) was based on the rationale that they may serve as vasodilators and help in improving pulmonary hypertension and oxygenation. Current literature does not support the role of inhaled NO in routine management of patients with ARDS, in fact, meta-analysis suggests that it may cause harm. The use of nebulized prostaglandins has showed no significant improvement in oxygenation.

Extracorporeal Membrane Oxygenation

The basic principle of extracorporeal membrane oxygenation (ECMO) is to draw deoxygenated blood and return oxygenated blood (after removal of CO_2), back into circulation. Depending on the clinical scenario, either venovenous ECMO (VV-ECMO) or venoarterial ECMO (VA-ECMO) configurations can be applied. Various other configurations are possible as per the demands made by the complexities of the clinical settings. VV-ECMO setup is primarily used for refractory hypoxia in severe ARDS and is particularly considered in patients with life-threatening but potentially reversible respiratory failure.

Ideally, VV-ECMO would be indicated if anticipated mortality approaches 75–80%, that is at a stage where $PaO_2/FiO_2 < 100$ mm Hg or FiO_2 remains $\geq 90\%$, and/or Murray score is 3–4 despite optimal care and rescue attempts for 6 hours. It may also be indicted in uncompromised hypercapnia with pH < 7.2 not corrected on mechanical ventilation with high Pplat. The Murray score is based on the severity of respiratory failure which includes four important criteria—PaO_2/FiO_2 ratio, level of PEEP, dynamic lung compliances and the number of quadrants infiltrated on chest X-ray. However, according to the Extracorporeal Life Support Organization (ELSO), ECMO may be considered at any stage where the risk of impending mortality is >50% with $PaO_2/FiO_2 \leq 150$ mm Hg or $FiO_2 > 90\%$ and Murray score of 3. Whenever rising hypercapnia and severe respiratory acidosis become a serious concern (pH < 7.2), $ECCO_2$-R may have to be used in order to selectively remove CO_2.

Most trials have not shown significant mortality benefit with ECMO; however, the Conventional ventilation or ECMO for Severe Adult Respiratory failure (CESAR) study has shown that in centers having capable facilities, ECMO has shown improved survival. Coagulation abnormality where anticoagulation is not possible, becomes the main contraindication to ECMO. Also, terminal cases of ARDS or those with major comorbidities where poor outcomes are anticipated, ECMO becomes a relative contraindication.

■ SUGGESTED READING

1. Acute Respiratory Distress Syndrome Network, Brower RG, Matthay MA, Morris A, Schoenfeld D, Thompson BT, et al. Ventilation with lower tidal volumes as compared with traditional tidal volumes for acute lung injury and the acute respiratory distress syndrome. N Engl J Med. 2000;342:1301-8.
2. ARDS Definition Task Force, Ranieri VM, Rubenfeld GD, Thompson BT, Ferguson ND, Caldwell E, et al. Acute respiratory distress syndrome: the Berlin definition. JAMA. 2012;307(23):2526-33.
3. Ashbaugh DG, Bigelow DB, Petty TL, Levine BE. Acute respiratory distress in adults. Lancet. 1967;2(7511):319-23.
4. Bellani G, Laffey JG, Pham T, Madotto F, Fan E, Brochard L, et al. Noninvasive ventilation of patients with acute respiratory distress syndrome. Insights from the LUNG SAFE Study. Am J Respir Crit Care Med. 2017;195(1):67-77.
5. Brower RG, Lanken PN, MacIntyre N, Matthay MA, Morris A, Ancukiewicz M, et al. Higher versus lower positive end-expiratory pressures in patients with the acute respiratory distress syndrome. N Engl J Med. 2004;351(4):327-36.

6. Dreyfuss D, Saumon G. Ventilator-induced lung injury: lessons from experimental studies. Am J Respir Crit Care Med. 1998;157(1):294-323.
7. Gattinoni L, Protti A, Caironi P, Carlesso E. Ventilator-induced lung injury: the anatomical and physiological framework. Crit Care Med. 2010;38(10 Suppl):S539-48.
8. Guérin C, Reignier J, Richard JC, Beuret P, Gacouin A, Boulain T, et al. Prone positioning in severe acute respiratory distress syndrome. N Engl J Med. 2013;368(23):2159-68.
9. Papazian L, Forel JM, Gacouin A, Penot-Ragon C, Perrin G, Loundou A, et al. Neuromuscular blockers in early acute respiratory distress syndrome. N Engl J Med. 2010;363(12):1107-16.
10. Pham T, Rubenfeld GD. Fifty Years of research in ARDS. The epidemiology of acute respiratory distress syndrome. a 50th birthday review. Am J Respir Crit Care Med. 2017;195(7):860-70.
11. Thompson BT, Chambers RC, Liu KD. Acute respiratory distress syndrome. N Engl J Med. 2017;377(19):1904-5.
12. Writing Group for the Alveolar Recruitment for Acute Respiratory Distress Syndrome Trial (ART) Investigators; Cavalcanti AB, Suzumura EA, Laranjeira LN, Paisani DM, Damiani LP, et al. Effect of lung recruitment and titrated positive end-expiratory pressure (PEEP) vs low PEEP on mortality in patients with acute respiratory distress syndrome: a randomized clinical trial. JAMA. 2017;318(14):1335-45.

CHAPTER 6

Intensive Care Management of Acute Heart Failure and Cardiogenic Shock

Ram E Rajagopalan

■ INTRODUCTION

Severe respiratory distress and hemodynamic instability related to acute heart failure (AHF) are common problems encountered by the general intensivist. Though a multidisciplinary effort is often necessary to identify and treat the root cause of AHF, initial symptom-directed management by the intensivist is a life-saving component of emergency care.

While chronic heart failure (CHF) is approached in a systematized manner, based on information from a multitude of randomized clinical trials, much of the care in AHF is focused on symptom relief and stabilization of vital signs and varies with different clinical presentations. Recent attempts at standardizing acute care has shifted the emphasis to a time-bound approach, similar to our tactics in handling acute coronary syndromes (ACS) and stroke, to ensure rapid initial stabilization and the mitigation of long-term compromise.

■ DEFINITION AND TIME-BOUND APPROACH

Acute heart failure is defined as a rapid onset of *new or progressively worsening signs and symptoms of heart failure.* These manifest as a spectrum of cases with varying intensities of acute *hypoxic respiratory failure* (common) and *hemodynamic compromise* (rarer), some of which are potentially life-threatening and require emergent in-hospital treatment. It is conventional to categorize the variable presentations into *"phenotypic" patterns* describing predominant presenting characteristics:

- Mild-to-moderate AHF; normal blood pressures and minimal/moderate pulmonary edema;
- Hypertensive AHF;
- Cardiogenic pulmonary edema;
- Cardiogenic shock;
- Right ventricular (RV) or high-output failure.

However, such categorization does not always identify the specific direction of the initial therapy required to stabilize the patient. A guideline promoted by the European Society of Cardiology (ESC) identifies individual clinical variations in perfusion (cold or warm) and congestion (wet or dry) obtained by bedside clinical examination to derive four broad hemodynamic profiles that allow better individualization of acute care **(Tables 1 and 2)**.

This approach, along with rapid identification and stabilization of respiratory and cardiovascular life threats, constitutes the backbone of

> **TABLE 1** Clinical definition of "hypoperfusion" (cold state) and "congestion" (wet state) used to derive the hemodynamic profiles of acute heart failure. These are simple bedside assessments.
>
> **Hypoperfusion (cold)**
> - Narrow pulse pressure
> - Symptomatic hypotension
> - Cool extremities
> - Impaired mental status
>
> **Congestion (wet)**
> - Orthopnea/PND
> - Peripheral edema
> - Distended jugular veins
> - Rales
> - Hepatojugular reflux
> - Ascites
>
> (PND: paroxysmal nocturnal dyspnea)

> **TABLE 2** Hemodynamic profiles based on clinical definitions of hypoperfusion and congestion (Table 1); initial therapy is directed by the presenting profile.
>
> | | No congestion (dry) 5% | Congestion present (wet) 95% | |
> | --- | --- | --- | --- |
> | Hypoperfusion absent (warm) | Warm-dry
Compensated failure

• Adjust oral Rx | Warm-wet

Predominant congestion

• Diuretic
• Vasodilator | Predominant hypertension

• Vasodilator
• Diuretic |
> | Hypoperfusion present (cold) | Cold-dry
Hypovolemic (diuresed) and hypoperfused

• Careful fluid challenge
• Inotropes (if hypoperfusion persists) | Cold wet

SBP < 90 mm Hg
"Cardiogenic shock"
~ 5%

• Inotropic agent
• Vasopressor (if refractory)
• Diuretic (after restored perfusion)
• Consider mechanical support | SBP > 90 mm Hg

• Vasodilator
• Diuretic
• Consider inotrope (if refractory) |
>
> (SBP: systolic blood pressure)

initial care. Identification of specifically treatable conditions and provision of multidisciplinary care is then advanced in a time-bound fashion. Finally, in the patient who has responded to acute care, a transition to long-term oral therapies ensures safe discharge **(Fig. 1)**.

■ PRECIPITATING CAUSES

About *20% of all acute episodes present de novo*, with no prior history of chronic cardiorespiratory failure, while over 75% are seen either as a sudden worsening

Chapter 6 | Intensive Care Management of Acute Heart Failure and Cardiogenic Shock

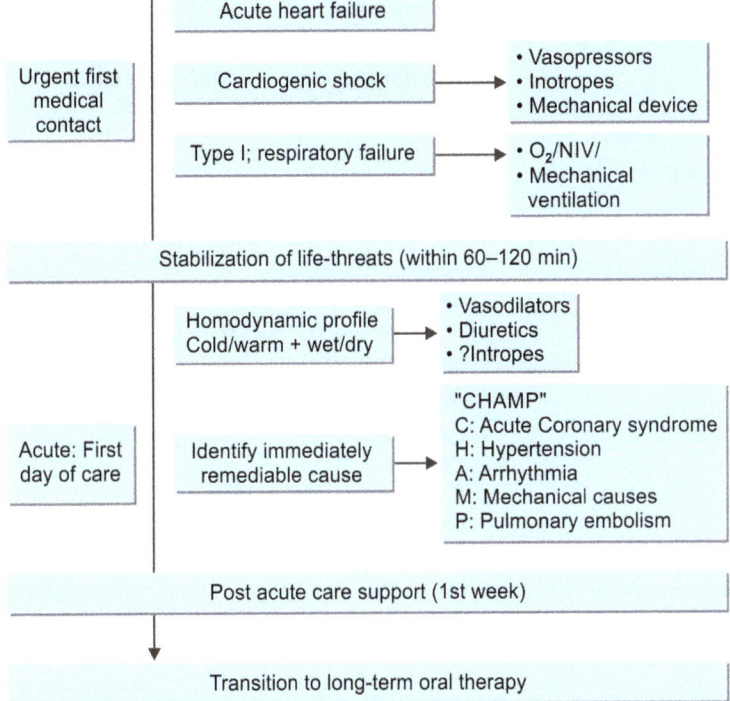

Fig. 1: A time-bound treatment approach to acute heart failure. (NIV: noninvasive ventilation)
(*Source:* Modified from the 2016 Recommendations of the European Society of Cardiology)

in patients with established CHF or a progressive deterioration of a subacute nature, reaching a threshold of severity that requires emergent treatment (acute decompensation of chronic heart failure; ADCHF).

While in most de novo cases, the precipitating cause is an ACS, a large number of cardiac and noncardiac causes can initiate acute decompensation in CHF, as summarized in **Table 3**. Identification of these causes may be of value in the stabilization of patients after initial resuscitative care.

■ THERAPEUTIC APPROACH TO ACUTE HEART FAILURE

Step 1: First Contact (Initial 60–120 Minutes after Admission) (Fig. 2)

A variety of other conditions may mimic the hemodynamic and respiratory changes that are the presenting features of AHF. Supportive care, directed at the life threats (cardiogenic shock and hypoxic respiratory failure), is the crux of initial care. Laboratory testing and imaging to confirm AHF proceeds in parallel to this initial therapy.

Hemodynamic Instability

Cardiogenic shock constitutes a minority of patients of individuals presenting with AHF, and only the most significant issues will be discussed here.

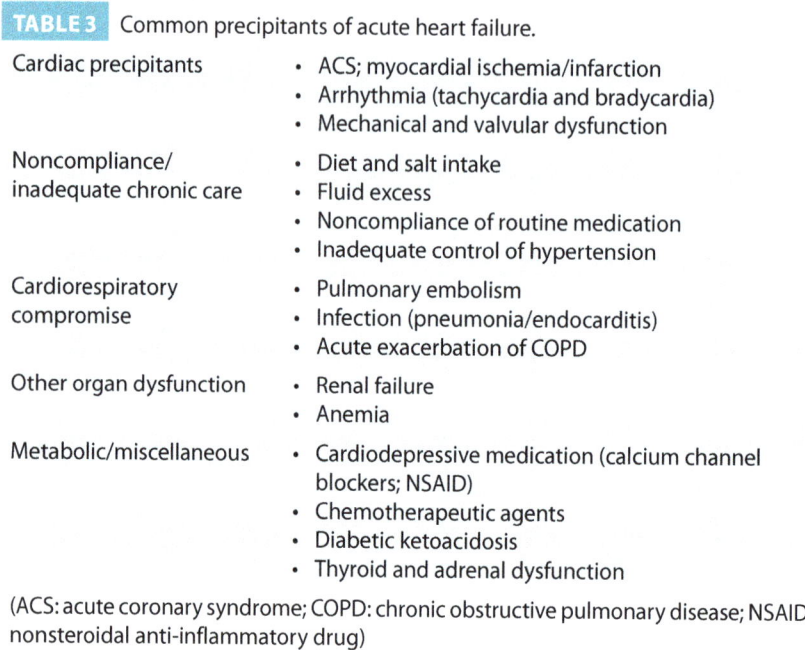

TABLE 3: Common precipitants of acute heart failure.

Cardiac precipitants	• ACS; myocardial ischemia/infarction • Arrhythmia (tachycardia and bradycardia) • Mechanical and valvular dysfunction
Noncompliance/inadequate chronic care	• Diet and salt intake • Fluid excess • Noncompliance of routine medication • Inadequate control of hypertension
Cardiorespiratory compromise	• Pulmonary embolism • Infection (pneumonia/endocarditis) • Acute exacerbation of COPD
Other organ dysfunction	• Renal failure • Anemia
Metabolic/miscellaneous	• Cardiodepressive medication (calcium channel blockers; NSAID) • Chemotherapeutic agents • Diabetic ketoacidosis • Thyroid and adrenal dysfunction

(ACS: acute coronary syndrome; COPD: chronic obstructive pulmonary disease; NSAID: nonsteroidal anti-inflammatory drug)

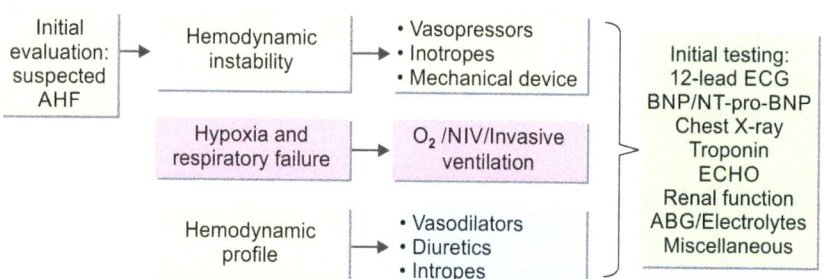

Fig. 2: Therapy and diagnosis at first contact (0–120 minutes from presentation). (ABG: arterial blood gas; AHF: acute heart failure; BNP: B-type natriuretic peptide; ECG: electrocardiogram; ECHO: echocardiogram; NIV: noninvasive ventilation; NT-pro-BNP: N-terminal pro-B-type natriuretic peptide)

Identification: It is characterized by a systolic blood pressure (SBP) <90 mm Hg along with signs of underperfusion (narrow pulse pressure, cold extremities, and organ dysfunction). Pulmonary edema is often present (cold-wet profile), though patients on chronic diuretic therapy may have minimal lung congestion or edema (cold-dry profile). A rapid differential diagnosis from other causes of shock can be attained by point-of-care (POC) ultrasonography. The existence of left ventricular failure is identified qualitatively on the two-dimensional (2D)-echocardiogram or measured by M-mode analysis of the mitral annular plane systolic excursion (MAPSE; see further). If taken together with evidence excluding volume depletion [inferior vena cava (IVC) distension/presence of

B-lines on the lung ultrasound; see further], the diagnosis of cardiogenic shock becomes very likely.

The primary goals of treatment would be to optimize the blood pressure, recognizing that an adequate arterial pressure is essential for preservation of coronary flow and for minimizing end-organ dysfunction. A wide variety of vasopressors and inotropes have been recommended for short-term use to stabilize blood pressure and improve organ perfusion, without evidence of the clear superiority of any specific agent over others. The agents include dopamine and noradrenaline (vasopressors) and dobutamine, levosimendan, and milrinone (inotropes).

- *Invasive arterial pressures* should be monitored in all patients with cardiogenic shock.
- *Stop β-blockers and vasodilators* that may be used for chronic care of the patient.
- In patients with hypotension (SBP <90 mm Hg) a *vasopressor should be initiated first*. The goal of vasopressor use is to raise systolic pressure above 90 mm Hg; higher blood pressure targets may increase the afterload in the failing heart and should be avoided. Subgroup evaluation of patients with cardiogenic shock in the SOAP (Sepsis Occurrence in Acutely Ill Patients) randomized trial implied that the risk of death increases with dopamine in comparison with noradrenaline, and the latter may be the preferred vasopressor in most cases.
- *Inotropes* may be considered as initial agents if SBP is at least >80 mm Hg or if clinical underperfusion persists after mean arterial pressure (MAP) has been raised with vasopressors. All inotropes [dobutamine, levosimendan, and phosphodiesterase (PDE) inhibitors] will vasodilate and uptitration of vasopressors may be needed to maintain adequate systolic pressures. While dobutamine is used widely, preferential use of levosimendan or PDE inhibitors may be considered if prior β-blockade is contributing to the shock state.
- All patients, especially those with de novo shock, should have an immediate *12-lead electrocardiogram (ECG)*. *Echocardiographic evaluation* would help identify significant valve pathology and other mechanical complications.
- If an acute *transmural myocardial infarction (MI)* is detected, immediate *revascularization* (catheter-based or surgical) is needed to improve hemodynamics and result in better survival. The revascularization procedure should be restricted to the culprit vessel that is responsible for the infarction and should not be a multivessel strategy.
- *Intra-aortic balloon pumps* (IABP) have not resulted in improved outcomes if inserted as a support in the perirevascularization period and should not be routinely used.
- Recent registry data imply that *percutaneous mechanical support devices* (microaxial left ventricular assist devices) are associated with poorer

outcome and increased bleeding risk when compared to IABP, despite increasing recent use.

Support of Oxygenation

Hypoxic respiratory insufficiency is common in AHF. While the administration of supplementary oxygen is logical, noninvasive ventilation (NIV) has significant value in patients with severe respiratory distress. The use of *bilevel NIV* or *continuous positive airway pressure (CPAP)* is an early consideration in the management of hypoxia and respiratory failure in this setting. Beside their value in optimizing oxygenation, their effectiveness lies in the favorable changes that they produce on the physiology of the failing heart. A reduction in ventricular preload (induced by a reduction in venous return from positive intrathoracic pressure) and a decreased afterload (mediated by reduced negative pleural pressure swings and reduced transmyocardial pressures), account for the favorable effects on the failing heart. The use of NIV and CPAP reduces mortality and the need for endotracheal intubation for invasive ventilation.

The *recommended steps* to handle hypoxic respiratory failure are summarized as:

- Continuously monitor oxygen saturation by *pulse oximetry* (SpO_2) in all patients with AHF.
- *Arterial blood gases* will additionally identify hypercarbia and acidosis and allow better estimation of the extent of shunting.
- *Administer oxygen* by an appropriate device to maintain SpO_2 > 90% and preferably not much >95%, to avoid the adverse effects of hyperoxia [partial pressure of oxygen (pO_2) > 300 torr]. There is no current evidence to show worse clinical outcomes with hyperoxia.
- *Early use of NIV/CPAP* may benefit by quicker restoration of abnormal cardiac physiology in AHF. There is no clear advantage of any one of these methods over the other.
- *Early intubation and invasive ventilation* is recommended in failure of NIV/CPAP to optimize AHF or when NIV/CPAP is contraindicated (typically after a respiratory arrest, in severe hemodynamic instability or in unconscious patients).
- *Discontinuation of ventilation* is handled differently in AHF. With improvement in oxygen needs and respiratory distress, discontinuation of the ventilator should be planned after a trial (30 minutes) on low pressure support and positive end-expiratory pressure (PEEP) (typically 7 cm H_2O each). T-piece trials will unmask heart failure and are contraindicated.
- *NIV should be initiated after extubation* in these patients who are at a high risk of reintubation because spontaneous ventilation adversely affects the loading conditions on the heart.

TABLE 4	Cardiac and noncardiac causes of elevated natriuretic peptides.
Cardiac	**Noncardiac**
• Heart failure • Acute coronary syndrome • Pulmonary embolism • Pulmonary hypertension • LVH/hypertrophic cardiomyopathy • Myocarditis • Tachyarrhythmias • Congenital and valvular heart disease • Myocarditis • Traumatic contusions/heart surgery • Cardioversion	• Age • Ischemic stroke/SAH • Renal dysfunction • Hepatic failure (cirrhosis/ascites) • COPD • Infections, pneumonia, and sepsis • Endocrine/metabolic abnormalities

(COPD: chronic obstructive pulmonary disease; LVH: left ventricular hypertrophy; SAH: subarachnoid hemorrhage)

Initial Investigations in Acute Heart Failure

Laboratory tests and diagnostic imaging are performed in this initial stage while supportive measures are being undertaken.

- *Plasma natriuretic peptide levels* [BNP, NT-proBNP, or midregional pro-atrial natriuretic peptide (MR-proANP)] are typically elevated by cardiac chamber distension and are very sensitive markers of AHF. However, a wide variety of chronic cardiorespiratory and noncardiac causes also increase these peptides **(Table 4)** and they cannot be considered as diagnostically confirmative without considering the clinical picture.
    - Very low BNP levels (<100 pg/mL) rule out AHF.
    - High BNP levels (100–500 pg/mL) are by themselves nonconfirmatory. Their diagnostic accuracy is sufficient to identify AHF only if the clinical likelihood is increased. A prior history of CHF together with any two of the following: a history of coronary artery disease (CAD), presence of pulmonary edema, pedal edema, cephalization of the pulmonary artery (PA) on chest X-ray or cardiomegaly at presentation increase the diagnostic certainty of AHF with BNP measured in this range.
    - Very high BNP values (>500 pg/mL) are probably confirmatory of AHF if the two of the above clinical criteria are present irrespective of a history of CHF.
    - The performance of BNP and NT-proBNP are similar; but cutoff values differ. NT-proBNP < 300 pg/mL rules out AHF.
    - Natriuretic peptide levels have strong prognostic implications.
- *A 12-lead ECG* must be obtained in all suspected cases of AHF.
    - Identification of ST-elevation MI warrants an immediate revascularization procedure in cardiogenic shock.
    - Non-ST changes may mandate initiation of interventional therapy if the AHF remains refractory to medical therapy.
    - Identification of arrhythmia is essential for patient stabilization.

- *Echocardiography*
    - Echocardiography is recommended immediately in all unstable patients and within 48 hours in all others to evaluate structural and functional changes.
    - *POC echocardiogram by the intensivist* (pending a formal evaluation) can direct acute therapy more effectively. Physician competence at level I (basic) is adequate to broadly assess LV function, guestimate-filling status from the respiratory variation of IVC size and to identify isolated enlargement of the right ventricle to raise suspicion of pulmonary embolism in shock patients.
    - *Qualitative assessment* of heart function can be augmented by measurement of the *mitral annular plane systolic excursion (MAPSE)* on the M-mode to allow tracking of progression over time by different clinicians **(Figs. 3A and B)**.
    - Identification of valvular dysfunction and other mechanical causes by an expert sonologist will be needed in few patients and is often deferred to a later phase. Patients with CHF also will require reevaluation for assessment of progression.
- *Chest radiograph and ultrasonography (USG) lung*
    - While classic features on a *bedside chest X-ray* must be sought (cardiomegaly, cephalization of pulmonary vasculature, Kerley B-lines, and perivascular cuffing), they are inadequate to diagnose AHF. Their specificity increases in combination with elevated levels of natriuretic peptide (see above).
    - *Lung ultrasound* at the point of care is a quick alternative to radiography. The presence of *septal B-lines* [characterized as discrete regularly-spaced vertical hyperechoic artifacts; narrow base at pleural line, extending through the screen without fading and moving synchronously

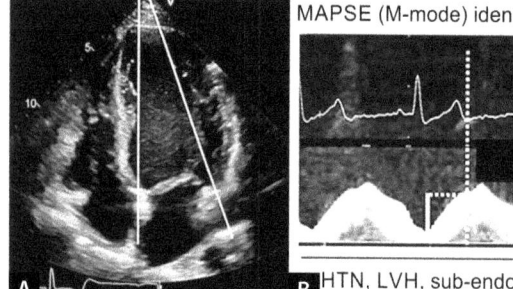

Figs. 3A and B: (A) Mitral annular plane systolic excursion (MAPSE) is evaluated by M-mode in a line from the LV apex to the mitral annulus (septal or free wall); (B) The maximum excursion of the annulus in this plane is measured. (EF: ejection fraction; HTN: hypertension; LV: left ventricle; LVH: left ventricular hypertrophy; MI: myocardial infarction)

with lung sliding **(Figs. 4A to C)**] is a sensitive and specific indicator of cardiogenic pulmonary edema. At least three such B-lines must be detected in each intercostal space and in two or more spaces on each side of the chest (diffuse involvement). However, alteration of the B-line pattern (subpleural consolidation and pleural line irregularity, inhomogeneity, areas of sparing, and an absence of lung sliding), reduce the specificity and could indicate a noncardiogenic interstitial-alveolar involvement including acute respiratory distress syndrome (ARDS).
- *Laboratory tests* must include cardiac troponins, renal function tests, thyroid functions, arterial blood gases, complete blood count, blood glucose, and electrolytes. These would help to differentiate the precipitating conditions and mimics of AHF.

Customized Support Based on Bedside Hemodynamic Profiles

Diuretics, vasodilators, and inotropes are the primary medications used in the treatment of AHF in patients not needing vasopressor therapy. Though diuretics are always administered first, the preferred sequence of *treatment should be tailored to the presenting hemodynamic profile* (*see* **Tables 1 and 2**).
- *Warm-dry profiles* indicate compensated heart failure that may require no specific alteration of therapy in patients on long-term oral medications except dose titration.
- *Warm-wet profiles* are seen in the majority of patients with AHF. Blood pressure and perfusion status may not be compromised, with some patients having significant hypertension. Congestive changes are present in these cases and often require diuresis. However, treatment is also customized based on the dominance of hypertension or congestion. If hypertension

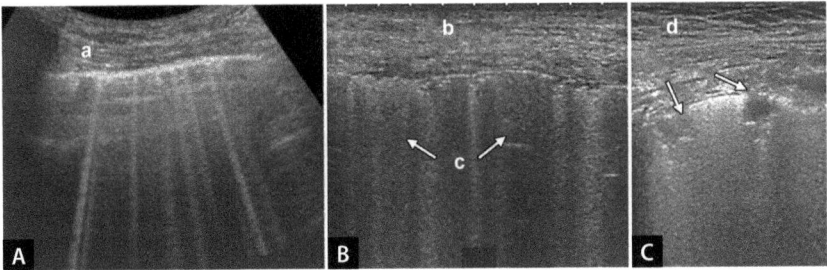

Figs. 4A to C: (A) On lung ultrasonography; typical septal B-lines of cardiogenic pulmonary edema (a) are evenly distributed narrow lines of unchanged intensity extending from a uniform pleural line which moves well with respiration. This pattern has excellent sensitivity and specificity for acute heart failure (AHF). Other patterns seen on the middle and left are noncardiogenic; (B) The uneven pleural line (b) and heterogeneous B-line distribution (c), with areas of "sparing" are usually an "inflammatory pattern" compatible with acute respiratory distress syndrome (ARDS) or other interstitial lung involvement; (C) Subpleural consolidation (d) is another feature of noncardiogenic edema. Pleural line movement is often restricted or absent in these cases.

is present, vasodilator therapy (see further), takes pre-eminence over diuretic therapy.
- *Cold-wet profiles* may present with significant hypoperfusion, but blood pressure may be either preserved or low (<90 mm Hg). The latter constitute cardiogenic shock that has been discussed earlier. If the blood pressure is preserved above 90 mm Hg vasodilator therapy is the preferred primary treatment.
- *Cold-dry profiles* are extremely rare and are often seen in patients who have been subject to long-term diuretic therapy. Careful hydration with intravenous (IV) fluid initially and use of inotropes in refractory cases are indicated.

Medications Used in the Early Phase of Treatment

Diuretics: Though traditionally considered the cornerstone of therapy for AHF, hemodynamic profiles influence their role in treatment. Since the majority of AHF presents as a warm-wet profile without severe hypertension, it remains the most common treatment in these patients. However, in hypertensive patients or individuals presenting with "cold" profiles, vasodilators acquire pre-eminence.

Mechanism: Loop diuretics, principally furosemide, are the diuretics of choice. Its effect on the renal tubular Na/K transport channels initiates a vigorous diuresis and it is traditional to attribute the "decongestive" action in CHF to the reduction in vascular volume and hence preload. However, in AHF clinical effect occurs early (15 minutes), long before the peak diuretic effect (1–2 hours). It is seen that parenteral furosemide has a strong effect on venous capacitance, which reduces preload well in advance of maximal diuresis.

Safe and effective use of loop diuretics in AHF can be achieved by:
- *Restricting the initial use of diuretics* to normotensive patients who demonstrate a "warm-wet" profile. Do not use them initially in cardiogenic shock, or in other "cold" (hypoperfused) profiles. Warm-wet patients with severe hypertension should be initiated on vasodilators before therapy with a diuretic.
- In patients who present with de novo AHF, the *dose of IV furosemide is 20–40 mg*.
- Patients on regular diuretic therapy should be given *an IV dose equivalent to their regular daily dose*.
- Bolus doses will have an ideal effect on preload and may be preferred to continuous infusions, though studies do not show a difference in efficacy.
- Patients resistant to the initial diuretic bolus should have *added vasodilator therapy*.
- *Large doses* of furosemide (typically 2.5 × the oral dose) may produce more diuresis but increase *the risk of renal injury*.
- *Combination* with a thiazide or aldosterone inhibitor may benefit poor responders.

Chapter 6 | Intensive Care Management of Acute Heart Failure and Cardiogenic Shock

- In patients with refractory pulmonary edema and increasing renal dysfunction, *ultrafiltration is not more effective* than uptitration of diuretic therapy and may increase the risk of worsening renal dysfunction.

Vasodilators: There is an increasing recognition of the role of vasodilators, especially in the warm-wet hemodynamic profile; it is even being recommended as the first-line therapy in hypertensive patients with AHF. Though there is no evidence of benefit on survival, symptomatic improvement is accelerated.

Nitroglycerin is the most common vasodilator used. *Nitroprusside* needs careful titration and invasive arterial pressure monitoring. Considering its toxicity with continued infusions, it is usually a second-line choice. Newer agents like *nesiritide* (recombinant BNP) and *ularitide* (a synthetic analog of the vasodilator urodilatin) are also effective in relieving the symptoms of AHF, though without benefits on other clinical outcomes. Recent registry data imply the absence of harm and suggestion of a nonsignificant benefit with the use of vasodilators in AHF.

Mechanism: All of these drugs benefit AHF by reducing the preload through venodilatory effects (identical to the mechanism of parenteral diuretics) and can also be titrated up to reduce afterload. Small clinical studies demonstrate their equivalence to diuretic therapy in symptom resolution. Nitroglycerine (NTG) is typically used in the following manner:

- All patients on vasodilator therapy should have a *minimum of continuous noninvasive blood pressure monitoring* (invasive arterial pressure must be used if nitroprusside is administered).
- NTG is *preferred* therapy in the *hypertensive patient with congestive signs (warm wet)* and as an adjunct to diuretic therapy in normotensive nonresponders. It is also primary therapy in *cold-wet (hypoperfused) patients with an SBP > 90 mm Hg*. It is contraindicated in cardiogenic shock (*see* **Table 2**).
- NTG is administered via a syringe pump (50 mg in 50 mL diluent; 0.6 mL/h will deliver 10 µg/min).
- Treatment with *NTG is initiated at venodilatory doses* (5-20 µg/min). As these doses may cause hypotension in the hypovolemic patient, it should be administered with caution. (Acute pulmonary edema can be precipitated by myocardial ischemia even in hypovolemic patients.)
- If hypotension develops with venodilatory doses, the medication is discontinued.
- If the blood pressure is stable or hypertension persists in a patient who remains symptomatic, *afterload reduction* can be achieved by titrating the dose up to 1-2 µg/kg/min.

Vasopressors and inotropes: The most widely used agents are *dopamine* and *noradrenaline* (vasopressors) and *dobutamine, levosimendan,* and *milrinone* (inotropes). There are no clinical trials demonstrating survival benefits with any of these agents. Beside the SOAP study showing adverse outcome with dopamine use in cardiogenic shock, registry data reveals a reduction of long-term survival with the use of these agents. The use of these vasoactive agents is therefore restricted to individuals with severe hypotension (cardiogenic shock), that contraindicates diuretics and vasodilators, or to patients with persistent hypoperfusion after such initial therapy. The inotropes often vasodilate and may cause profound hypotension when administered alone; vasopressors may be needed in addition in many cases.

- All patients requiring vasopressor and inotropic support should be ideally monitored using intra-arterial pressure measurements.
- In *cold-wet patients* with *symptomatic hypotension* (SBP < 90 mm Hg) attempt to raise pressure to the minimum threshold with vasopressor therapy. *Noradrenaline is preferred over dopamine* in these patients. Attempting to raise pressures to "normal" ranges can adversely affect afterload.
- If *symptomatic hypoperfusion remains* despite improvement of SBP or in patients with hypoperfusion but not hypotension, inotropic therapy may be considered.
- There is no preference for one specific inotrope over another, but in patients on long-term β-blockers, dobutamine may be less effective and levosimendan or milrinone may be initial choices.
- Given the *safety concerns*, inotropes should not be administered in refractory heart failure in the absence of symptomatic hypoperfusion or hypotension.

Other Medications

Morphine: Though traditionally administered for symptom relief and its benefits on hemodynamics, it also carries a significant risk of respiratory depression. Data from the Acute Decompensated Heart Failure National Registry (ADHERE) implies a greater need for intensive care unit (ICU) admission and ventilator use in AHF patients administered an opiate. Risk-adjusted mortality is also reported to be independently associated with its use. It is preferable to avoid routine use of morphine in AHF.

Digoxin: While digitalis glycosides have no direct role in the management of AHF, they remain the preferred therapy for controlling the rate in atrial fibrillation in this setting. As β-blockade may need to be avoided in hypoperfused and hypotensive patients, digoxin is an effective alternative for rate control.

Step 2: First Day (After Initial 60–120 Minutes for Stabilization) (*see* Fig. 1)

In this stage of care, after early stabilization, a multidisciplinary effort is initiated to identify and treat acutely reversible processes that will increase the probability of survival. While a large number of potentially treatable conditions can perpetuate AHF (*see* **Table 3**), only some of them need urgent attention. The CHAMP mnemonic suggested by the ESC is a reasonably comprehensive list of conditions that could provide benefit at this stage.

CHAMP

Coronary syndromes: The identification of ST-segment elevation myocardial infarction (STEMI) is essential for management of cardiogenic shock, as immediate revascularization has a positive impact on survival. Even in non-STEMI (NSTEMI), the development of heart failure is a major adverse risk warranting the need for angiography and intervention. "The American Heart Association (AHA) recommends coronary angiography in all patients with de novo AHF".

Hypertension: The modern focus on the use of vasodilators probably impacts the frequency of hypertension as a precipitant of intractable AHF. The high afterload imposed under these circumstances is significant and attempts to normalize blood pressure can result in significant benefits. Besides the traditional vasodilators, the addition of parenteral β-blockade may need to be considered, but should be balanced against its negative inotropic properties. While labetalol is widely available, its long half-life makes titration cumbersome and preference for short-acting agents like esmolol add flexibility to initial treatment.

Arrhythmia: By definition, patients with arrhythmia in AHF are unstable and require immediate cardioversion of tachyarrhythmias. However, electrical cardioversion is usually reserved for hemodynamically unstable patients or for those with poor response to initial therapy with diuretics, vasodilators, and respiratory support. Atrial fibrillation is common and rate control is preferred using β-blockers or digoxin. The ESC endorses them as first-line therapy, recommending amiodarone only as a "consideration".

Mechanical complications of ACS such as rupture of the ventricular free wall or septum, acute mitral insufficiency, endocarditis, aortic dissection, and rarely, cardiac tumors require early identification. Echocardiography (not the limited POC evaluation by the intensivist), both transthoracic and transesophageal need to be performed early to plan percutaneous or surgical intervention.

Pulmonary emboli may mimic or precipitate AHF. The gold standard for diagnosis today is the CT angiogram. Echocardiographic features of acute right heart overload may not be seen with consistency in patients with stable hemodynamics. Treatment with thrombolysis or thrombectomy, catheter based or surgical, may need to be considered.

In addition to the multidisciplinary attack on the CHAMP precipitants, the intensivist should make an attempt to identify infections as potential triggers. *Respiratory infections* may be particularly difficult to differentiate. Considerable clinical overlap of presenting characteristics and subtle differences in radiographic features make it a challenge and careful evaluation is needed to avoid overuse of antibiotics. Though procalcitonin (PCT) is often recommended to "differentiate", it is only a nonspecific marker of the severity and prognosis of inflammation. A subthreshold PCT would justify withholding of antibiotics, but higher values do not establish the diagnosis of an infection and need to be interpreted with caution.

Step 3: Postacute Care (After First 24 Hours through First Week of Hospitalization) (*see* Fig. 1)

After the initial day of therapy and cross-disciplinary interventions, the patient who has stabilized, preferably weaned off parenteral vasopressors, inotropes and vasodilators and not requiring invasive or high NIV, should transition to evidence-based therapies for chronic support of heart failure. While medications need to be customized to individual patients, the broad stepped care should include:
- Angiotensin-converting enzyme (ACE) inhibition
- Acute respiratory disease (ARD) (if ACE is contraindicated)
- Angiotensin receptor neprilysin inhibitor (ARNI); sacubitril/valsartan
- β-adrenergic blockade
- Loop diuretics
- Aldosterone antagonists
- Dietary and lifestyle recommendations.

In the stable patient, we traditionally suggest initiation of ACE inhibition to verify tolerance. The change to angiotensin-receptor blocker (ARB) or ARNI is usually left to the discretion of the long-term physician or cardiologist. We defer β-blockade until the tolerance for ACE inhibition is established, (typically in 48 hours or so), unless coronary disease raises the indication for earlier therapy. Loop diuretics at standard doses (20–40 mg furosemide) are initiated and the addition of aldosterone antagonist or thiazides is left to the long-term carers. These therapies are initiated in all de novo AHF and are changed according to the prior use in acute congestive heart failure (ACHF).

Step 4: Prognostication and Safe Discharge from the Intensive Care Unit

Data from the ADHERE registry suggests that patients admitted with AHF can be *risk stratified* on the basis of three clinical criteria:
1. Blood urea nitrogen (cutoff > 43 mg/dL);
2. Serum creatinine (cutoff > 2.75 mg/dL); and
3. SBP (cutoff < 115 mm Hg).

Presence of all three criteria at admission classifies a high-risk patient with nearly 13 times the odds of dying in hospital when compared to low-risk patients without any of these criteria.

Keeping these risks in mind, discharge from the ICU is based on a large number of parameters besides subjective improvement noted by patient. These include:
- *Stable hemodynamics*: Resting heart rate <100 bpm; stable blood pressure with no ongoing need for parenteral vasoactive agents. Tolerance of initiated long-term medications would also be ideal.
- *Improved respiratory function*: Normal breathing effort; minimal oxygen (low flow on nasal prongs) or minimal/intermittent NIV use.
- *Adequate organ perfusion* suggested at a minimum, by adequate mental function and urine output. With the exception of chronic renal disease, normalization or decline in serum creatinine levels would be objective evidence of the same.

Discharge planning from the ICU must take into consideration issues other than just care of heart failure by a cardiologist, but must, as appropriately needed, include support for renal function and the multiple comorbidities that may be highly prevalent in these patients.

Management of AHF is very much within the ambit of the general intensive care specialist and early treatment by the intensivist can provide an opportunity for subsequent multidisciplinary actions that can minimize progressive deterioration of CHF.

SUGGESTED READING

1. Al Deeb M, Barbic S, Featherstone R, Dankoff J, Barbic D. Point-of-care ultrasonography for the diagnosis of acute cardiogenic pulmonary edema in patients presenting with acute dyspnea: a systematic review and meta-analysis. Acad Emerg Med. 2014;21:843-52.
2. Čerlinskaitė K, Javanainen T, Cinotti R, Mebazaa A, Global Research on Acute Conditions Team (GREAT) Network. Acute heart failure management. Korean Circ J. 2018;48:463-80.
3. Fonarow GC, Adams KF Jr, Abraham WT, Yancy CW, Boscardin WJ; ADHERE Scientific Advisory Committee, Study Group, and Investigators. Risk stratification for in-hospital mortality in acutely decompensated heart failure: classification and regression tree analysis. JAMA. 2005;293:572-80.
4. Hu K, Liu D, Herrmann S, Niemann M, Gaudron PD, Voelker W, et al. Clinical implication of mitral annular plane systolic excursion for patients with cardiovascular disease. Eur Heart J Cardiovasc Imaging. 2013;14:205-12.
5. Mebazaa A, Motiejunaite J, Gayat E, Crespo-Leiro MG, Lund LH, Maggioni AP, et al. Long-term safety of intravenous cardiovascular agents in acute heart failure: results from the European Society of Cardiology Heart Failure Long-Term Registry. Eur J Heart Failure. 2018;20:332-41.
6. Ponikowski P, Voors AA, Anker SD, Bueno H, Cleland JGF, Coats AJS, et al. 2016 ESC Guidelines for the diagnosis and treatment of acute and chronic heart failure: The Task Force for the diagnosis and treatment of acute and chronic heart failure of the European Society of Cardiology (ESC) Developed with the special contribution of the Heart Failure Association (HFA) of the ESC. Eur Heart J. 2016;37:2129-200.
7. Strunk A, Bhalla V, Clopton P, Nowak RM, McCord J, Hollander JE, et al. Impact of the history of congestive heart failure on the utility of b-type natriuretic peptide in the emergency diagnosis of heart failure: results from the Breathing Not Properly Multinational Study. Am J Medicine. 2006;119:69.e1-11.

CHAPTER 7

Acute Kidney Injury in the ICU and Renal Replacement Therapies

Bhupendra V Gandhi, Rishit Harbada

■ INTRODUCTION

Acute Kidney injury (AKI) is one of the most common complications in critically ill patients admitted to the Intensive Care Unit. It is emerging as a major health care problem affecting millions worldwide. AKI is associated with multiple adverse clinical outcomes, increasing costs, high morbidity and mortality. AKI is a strong and independent risk factor for Chronic Kidney Disease. Hence early detection and prompt management of AKI is essential to improve outcomes.

■ DEFINITIONS

Acute kidney injury (AKI) has now replaced the older terminology of acute renal failure, in an attempt to broaden the definition and include lesser degrees of renal dysfunction, which may not necessarily result in overt kidney failure, but still cause metabolic changes without being associated with poor outcomes. AKI is thus defined as a sudden loss of renal function resulting in an inadequate excretion, with accumulation of water and metabolic waste products along with electrolyte imbalance, secondary to a direct or indirect injury to the kidneys. Serum creatinine (SCr) still remains the classical biomarker for the diagnosis in clinical practice, despite the fact that it may be less reliable in the very elderly or critically ill patients.

Currently the most accepted definition for AKI is given by the Kidney Disease: Improving Global Outcomes (KDIGO) in 2012. The KDIGO guidelines define AKI as any of the following: (1) an increase in SCr by 0.3 mg/dL within 48 hours; (2) an increase in SCr by 1.5 times from the baseline value, which is known or presumed to have occurred within the prior 7 days; or (3) urine output of <0.5 mL/kg/h for 6 hours.

■ STAGING SYSTEMS FOR ACUTE KIDNEY INJURY

The RIFLE criterion is the oldest staging system proposed for AKI. The acronym RIFLE stands for Risk, Injury, and Failure as per increasing severity, and the last two are outcome classes, i.e. Loss and End-Stage Renal Disease (ESRD). Though the RIFLE criteria correlated well with the prognosis and relative risk of death stagewise, there were some limitations. The change in SCr did not correlate with the percent decrease in glomerular filtration rate (GRF) as cited by the RIFLE criteria and further, the change in SCr also did not correlate well

TABLE 1	KDIGO AKI staging.	
Stages	Serum creatinine (SCr)	Urine output
Stage 1	1.5–1.9 times baseline OR ≥0.3 mg/dL absolute increase in SCr	Urine volume <0.5 mL/kg/h for 6–12 hours
Stage 2	SCr ≥2.0–2.9 times baseline	Urine volume <0.5 mL/kg/h for ≥12 hours
Stage 3	SCr ≥3.0 times from baseline OR Increase in SCr to ≥4.0 mg/dL OR Initiation of renal replacement therapy OR In patients <18 years, decrease in eGFR to <35 mL/min per 1.73 m^2	Urine volume <0.3 mL/kg/h for ≥24 hours OR Anuria for ≥12 hours

(AKI: acute kidney injury; eGFR: estimated glomerular filtration rate; KDIGO: Kidney Disease: Improving Global Outcomes)

with the mortality risk as predicted by the RIFLE criteria based on the decline in urine output.

Acute Kidney Injury Network (AKIN) diagnostic criteria were developed in 2007 to further standardize the diagnostic criteria and classification of AKI. However, this modified version of the RIFLE criteria with some notable changes did not significantly help to predict hospital mortality.

The KDIGO classification of AKI was proposed to be used as a guideline in 2012 as a modified version of both RIFLE and AKIN criteria **(Table 1)**. However, it excluded GFR for staging, and only SCr and urine output were used. Further, it did not stipulate that the criteria should be applied only after adequate fluid administration or after exclusion of urinary tract obstruction. Despite the potential limitations of using only urine output and SCr as the variables, the KDIGO classification has been accepted.

ETIOLOGY OF ACUTE KIDNEY INJURY

Acute kidney injury is a syndrome and its etiologies are mainly classified as kidney specific and kidney nonspecific conditions. Kidney specific causes of AKI include acute interstitial, glomerular, and vascular renal diseases. Kidney nonspecific conditions include sepsis, ischemic, toxin, and drug-induced causes, as well as prerenal azotemia and acute postrenal obstructive nephropathy. Traditionally AKI has been classified as prerenal AKI, intrinsic renal diseases, and postrenal obstructive nephropathy **(Box 1)**. Prerenal and postobstructive pathologies are consequences of extrarenal conditions and cause decrease in GFR, whereas only intrinsic renal disease represents true kidney disease. Persistence of pre/postrenal conditions will cause intrinsic renal disease.

> **BOX 1** Etiology of AKI.
>
> *Prerenal causes*
> - Intrarenal vasoconstriction (hemodynamically mediated)
> - Drugs—NSAIDs, ACE inhibitors, ARBs, and calcineurin inhibitors—cyclosporine and tacrolimus
> - Cardiorenal syndrome and hepatorenal syndrome
> - Hypercalcemia
> - Abdominal compartment syndrome
> - Systemic vasodilatation—sepsis and neurogenic shock
> - Volume depletion—renal losses due to diuretics and osmotic diuresis in ketoacidosis
>
> *Intrinsic renal causes*
> - Glomerular diseases—glomerulonephritis and rapidly progressing glomerulonephritis (RPGN)
> - Interstitial—drugs-penicillin, cephalosporin, sulfonamides, fluoroquinolones, NSAIDs, and proton pump inhibitors
> - Infections—viral, bacterial, and fungal
> - Systemic diseases—lupus and sarcoidosis
> - Tubular—ischemia and prolonged hypotension
> - Nephrotoxic—radiocontrasts, cisplatin, aminoglycosides, methotrexate, endogenous-rhabdomyolysis, tumor lysis syndrome, myeloma, and pigment nephropathy
> - Vascular—renal infarction, renal vein thrombosis, scleroderma renal crisis, malignant hypertension, and renal atheroembolic disease
>
> *Postrenal causes*
> - *Extrarenal obstruction:* Prostate hypertrophy, neurogenic blabber, retroperitoneal fibrosis, cervical bladder, and prostate cancer
> - *Intrarenal obstruction:* Stones, clots, and tumors
>
> (ACE: angiotensin-converting enzyme; AKI: acute kidney injury; ARBs: angiotensin receptor blockers; NSAIDs: nonsteroidal anti-inflammatory drugs)

Sepsis is one of the most common causes of AKI, but it is also a common complication of AKI and at times both are interrelated. In the intensive care unit (ICU) setting, serious infection, sepsis, hypotension, ischemia, and nephrotoxic drugs are the most common causes of AKI.

In large developed cities and tertiary hospitals, causes of AKI remain the same as in the developed world mostly viz. ischemia, sepsis, and drug toxicity; whereas in the remote rural areas, the causes are chiefly community acquired. Common causes in these areas include infections, diarrhea, mainly due to unsafe drinking water and poor hygiene, snake or arthropod envenomation, ingestion of natural, ayurvedic, or herbal medications mainly containing heavy metals, and poor obstetric care. Malnutrition, lack of sanitary infrastructure, poverty, uncontrolled urbanization, and deficient public health systems are frequent problems that add significantly to the disease burden in these regions. Also a large seasonal variation is seen with a spike occurring immediately during or after the rainy season. A few limited studies have shown a high frequency and early mortality in these patients, mainly due to lack of access to healthcare facilities including renal replacement therapy (RRT).

PATHOPHYSIOLOGY OF ACUTE KIDNEY INJURY

The chief pathophysiology involved in prerenal AKI is due to reduction in glomerular perfusion causing reduction in glomerular capillary pressure. This overwhelms renal autoregulation and decreases GFR causing AKI. Normally GFR is well maintained with the help of afferent arteriolar vasodilation and efferent arteriolar vasoconstriction, mediated by vasodilatory eicosanoids and angiotensin 2 (AT-2), respectively. *Volume depletion is the most common cause of prerenal AKI,* while in cases of postrenal (obstructive) AKI, obstruction of the extrarenal system at any level (renal pelvis, ureters, bladder, or urethra) will increase intratubular pressure, which opposes glomerular filtration pressure and decreases GFR.

In intrinsic renal disease, *acute tubular necrosis (ATN) is seen as a result of impaired renal perfusion, i.e., ischemic and nephrotoxic injury chiefly due to drugs or sepsis.* ATN occurs due to systemic hypotension and renal hypoperfusion affecting the renal autoregulation, causing decrease in GFR. Other mechanisms which are incompletely understood include endotoxemia leading to AKI by renal vasoconstriction, maladaptation of tubuloglomerular feedback (TGF), tubular obstruction, transtubular back leakage of the filtrate, interstitial inflammation and the release of inflammatory cytokines causing enhanced secretion of reactive oxygen species (ROS), leading to renal injury. The exact pathophysiology of intrinsic renal injury is still incompletely understood. Thus the main pathophysiologic abnormalities in ATN include intrarenal hemodynamic changes and ischemic and toxic injuries to tubular cells.

Uncomplicated ATN normally recovers within 2–3 weeks; however, multiple comorbidities or superimposed renal insults, like repeated hypotension, often alters this pattern and prolongs renal recovery. Nonrecovery of renal function after 2–3 weeks is an indication for renal biopsy.

SYSTEMIC EFFECTS OF ACUTE KIDNEY INJURY

Systemic side effects of AKI are listed in **Table 2**. However one serious side effect commonly encountered in the ICU patients is volume overload, which imperatively needs to be constantly monitored.

DIAGNOSTIC APPROACH TO PATIENTS WITH ACUTE KIDNEY INJURY

Early diagnosis and management of AKI is imperative because it is associated with improved outcomes. Diagnostic approach towards a patient of AKI is usually individualized and complete evaluation should be done including a comprehensive history, review of past medical records and complete and detailed clinical examination **(Table 3)**. The aim should be to identify preceding events including systemic events, e.g., hypotension, sepsis, or rhabdomyolysis. Other events include exposure to nephrotoxic agents or

TABLE 2 Common systemic side effects of AKI.

Neurological	Uremic encephalopathy
Cardiac	• Volume overload and pulmonary edema • Myocarditis • Myocardial depression
Liver	Hepatitis with elevated liver enzymes and coagulation abnormalities
Hematological	Bone marrow suppression and thrombocytopenia
Gastric	Uremic gastritis causing vomiting and nausea
MODS	The effects alone, or in combination, cause multiple organ dysfunction

(AKI: acute kidney injury; MODS: multiple organ dysfunction syndrome)

TABLE 3 Preceding events to be considered in the evaluation of patients with AKI.

Systemic events	• Hypotension • Sepsis • Rhabdomyolysis
Exposure to nephrotoxic agents	• Nephrotoxic drugs • Contrast
Volume contraction	• Diarrhea • Vomiting • Blood loss • Trauma • Surgery
Recent exposure to tropical diseases	• Leptospirosis • Malaria • Dengue
Poisons	• Smoke and insect envenomation • Alleged poisoning with nephrotoxic agents

(AKI: acute kidney injury)

any medications, volume contraction due to diarrhea, vomiting and surgery, exposure to tropical diseases (e.g., malaria and dengue), and exposure to rodents (e.g., leptospirosis and hantavirus) and snake or insect envenomation.

Physical examination should include complete examination with special emphasis on pulse, blood pressure, including orthostatic hypotension to check for postural drop, jugular venous pressure (JVP), skin turgor, and edema, which may guide towards the volume status of the patient. Daily intake output charting is also required. Detailed systemic examination with special emphasis on the abdomen to rule out any underlying obstructive causes including a distended bladder should be carried out. The next process should always aim to exclude prerenal and postrenal causes of AKI, as these are potentially reversible.

Knowledge of prior SCr will help in understanding the reversibility of AKI because it can be difficult to distinguish between AKI and AKI on chronic kidney disease (CKD). Patient with CKD are at an increased risk of AKI. Basic laboratory evaluation includes complete blood count (CBC), SCr, blood urea nitrogen (BUN), electrolytes, bicarbonate, and urine analysis. These tests are not only useful for the diagnosis, but also for assessment of complications, and the results of these primary tests help in further evaluation of the condition. Ratio of BUN to creatinine in healthy individuals is 10-15:1 (when both are expressed in mg/dL). It may be >20:1 in prerenal AKI due to disproportionate elevation in urea reabsorption due to elevated serum vasopressin levels. However, upper gastrointestinal tract bleeding, systemic corticosteroid administration, sepsis, and increased protein intake can also raise BUN levels.

In AKI, urinary volume plays a very important role, as it directly correlates with the residual GFR. Oliguria (urine output < 500 mL per day) is associated with worst outcomes in critical care settings. If a patient has anuria (urine output < 50 mL in 24 hours), then bilateral obstructive uropathy, bilateral renal vein thrombosis, bilateral renal arterial occlusion, renal cortical necrosis, antiglomerular basement membrane (GBM) disease, or hemolytic uremic syndrome (HUS), i.e., thrombotic microangiopathy, need to be ruled out.

Urinalysis/urine microscopy is a validated tool for diagnosis and prognosis in hospitalized patients with AKI and should be done whenever possible. Ideally a fresh urine sample should be centrifuged and should be examined for cells, casts, or any crystals. Hyaline casts are seen in prerenal AKI, while muddy brown, granular casts, and renal tubular epithelial cells are seen in ATN. Broad waxy casts may point towards CKD. Urine analysis and microscopy itself gives a vast clue to various diagnosis including glomerulonephritis (GN), interstitial nephritis, etc., and hence urinalysis remains an invaluable tool in the diagnosis of kidney diseases.

Other tests may be used in appropriate settings like C3 and C4 (complement levels) usually in cases of GN. Low levels are seen in postinfectious GN, lupus nephritis, and membranoproliferative glomerulonephritis (MPGN), whereas normal levels are seen in antineutrophil cytoplasmic antibody (ANCA)-associated vasculitis. Other tests such as lactate dehydrogenase (LDH), peripheral smear for schistiocytes, antinuclear antibody (ANA), and ANCA may be ordered in the appropriate clinical setting.

Imaging tests also help in the evaluation of patients with AKI—ultrasound helps to diagnose obstruction, polycystic kidneys, and number and size of kidneys. Doppler studies help in knowing the status of arteries and veins but are observer variable. CT scan can be useful to differentiate calculi; pyelonephritis and noncontrast magnetic resonance imaging (MRI) can be used to assess arteries and veins.

Kidney biopsy is not done routinely. It is done only in a few selected cases in which prerenal and postrenal AKI have been excluded or treated, and the causes of intrinsic renal AKI like GN, interstitial nephritis, vasculitis, etc., need to be ruled out after 2-3 weeks of nonresolution of ATN.

In a clinical setting, a clinician is commonly faced with the two most common diagnoses, i.e., prerenal AKI and ATN. Sometimes, differentiating prerenal AKI

TABLE 4 Clinical and laboratory parameters differentiating prerenal AKI and ATN.

	Prerenal AKI	**ATN**
History	History of vomiting, diarrhea, blood loss, or hypotension	History of sepsis, fever, drug, or nephrotoxin exposure
Clinical presentation	Dry skin, orthostatic hypotension, tachycardia, and signs of volume depletion	No specific signs or symptoms
Laboratory features		
Urine output	Mainly responsive to volume and removal of offending factor	Usually oliguria
Serum BUN/creatinine ratio	>20	<20
Urine sodium	<20 mmol/L	>20 mmol/L
Urine osmolality	>500 mmol/kg	<350 mmol/kg
Fractional excretion of sodium (FENa)	Mostly <1	>1
Sediment	Hyaline casts	Muddy brown granular casts
Novel biomarkers	None	Cystatin C, NGAL, and KIM-1

(AKI: acute kidney injury; ATN: acute tubular necrosis)

from ATN in hospitalized patients may be a difficult task, when both the effective arterial blood volume (EABV) and the time and course of AKI are not known. Some clues listed below, may help to differentiate between the two **(Table 4)**.

These are common differentiating factors between prerenal AKI and ATN. Fractional excretion of sodium, also called FENa, is commonly used to assess tubular function. FENa is the ratio of urine serum concentrations of sodium to urine serum concentrations of creatinine.

$$\text{FENa} = \frac{\text{Urine sodium} \times \text{Serum creatinine}}{\text{Serum sodium} \times \text{Urine creatinine}} \times 100$$

The basic concept in FENa is that urinary sodium is absorbed by renal tubular cells in prerenal injury as they are intact, while it is not absorbed by the damaged tubular cells in ATN. Hence, a FENa below 1 is consistent with prerenal injury, while >1% is consistent with ATN. However this has many exceptions in ATN, it can be <1% in cases of sepsis, radiocontrast, hemoglobinuria, and cirrhosis. While in prerenal AKI, it can be above 1% in patients with underlying CKD, and in those on diuretics, intravenous (IV) fluid resuscitation, etc.

The fractional excretion of uric acid (FEUA) is developed on lines similar to FENa. FEUA < 35 is seen in prerenal causes, while >35% is seen in ATN. None of these tests are totally sensitive, but application of multiple parameters helps to differentiate ATN from prerenal AKI, and use of multiple tests increases the sensitivity and specificity.

Novel Biomarkers in Diagnosing Acute Kidney Injury

Even today, the most used biomarker to assess renal function is creatinine. Creatinine is chiefly an assessment of renal function but not an indicator of renal parenchymal injury. SCr varies with a lot of variables such as age, sex, race, muscle mass, hydration, and medications. Also, rise in SCr is not seen until around 50% of renal function is lost. Further, it does not rise immediately in AKI, and there is a significant lag time of around 8–48 hours between AKI and loss of function as measured by creatinine. Due to this fallacy in SCr, there is a major risk of missing a therapeutic opportunity in the lag time. The main aim of these novel biomarkers is to provide an opportunity to intervene in this lag window to help in reducing the morbidity and mortality in AKI.

Various biomarkers for diagnosing AKI include cystatin C, neutrophil gelatinase-associated lipocalin (NGAL), kidney injury molecule-1 (KIM-1), interleukin-18, and N-acetyl-β-D-glucosaminidase (NAG), to name a few. The chief pathophysiology associated with accumulation of these biomarkers is inflammation and injury, as postulated from animal studies. These biomarkers accumulate in the plasma and urine of patients with AKI and represent different pathophysiological events such as tubular epithelial synthesis (NGAL, KIM-1, IL-18, and NAG), impaired proximal tubular reabsorption (cystatin C and NGAL), or increased secretion due to inflammation or sepsis.

Biomarkers are available for evaluation of functional change and cellular damage, early diagnosis, risk assessment, and prognosis of AKI patients. Novel serum and urine biomarkers with potential as early indicators of AKI may allow for improved prognostication and insight into the specific cause of AKI.

■ MANAGEMENT

Prevention and early diagnosis of AKI are of primary importance and should be the main goal. Once AKI has been detected, efforts should be made to attenuate the effects of injury and treat its consequences. No specific treatment is available for AKI. The first step in its management is its prevention, by doing a risk assessment. Multiple risk calculators are available online and few are validated for use to calculate risk for contrast-induced AKI and also in the ICU. The aim should be to identify and if possible, reverse the risk factors. The most important risk factor is CKD; hence, a baseline kidney function including SCr should be identified whenever possible. Newer serum and urinary biomarkers play a very important role in early diagnosis of AKI.

Nondialytic Management of Acute Kidney Injury

Volume resuscitation forms a very important initial strategy in all patients of AKI. It is commonly indicated in patients with sepsis, hypotension, and

> **BOX 2** Four basic phases of fluid therapy.
> 1. *Rescue:* Immediate fluid therapy to correct hypotension and hypovolemia (500 mL bolus within 15–20 minutes)
> 2. *Optimization:* Adjustment of fluid amount, type and rate following fluid challenge to achieve adequate tissue perfusion
> 3. *Stabilization*: A maintenance therapy preferably equal or a slightly negative balance for adequate hemodynamic support
> 4. *De-escalation*: Minimize fluid therapy as to maintain balance with the urine output

hypovolemia. Optimizing volume status helps in achieving adequate perfusion, as well as maintains the hemodynamics and cardiac output. It also helps to ensure renal perfusion and avoid further kidney injury. Adequate fluid resuscitation has proven to be an effective strategy in preventing as well as improving outcomes in AKI.

Fluid resuscitation is guided by nonspecific and nonsensitive markers such as heart rate, blood pressure, central venous pressure, and urine output. Newer methods like point-of-care ultrasound (POCUS) of inferior vena cava (IVC) collapsibility at end of expiration act as a good surrogate marker of fluid status. Rescue, optimization, stabilization, and de-escalation form the four basic phases of fluid therapy **(Box 2)**. KDIGO AKI guidelines suggest that crystalloids should be used instead of colloids like hydroxyethyl starch and albumin for volume expansion in patients with risk of AKI. Albumin can be used when substantial amounts of crystalloids are needed to maintain adequate mean arterial pressure (MAP), especially in patients with sepsis. Fluid overload is dangerous as it results in cardiopulmonary complications, delayed wound healing, accelerated kidney injury, and increased mortality. Fluid overload is associated with increased mortality as well as delayed recovery in patients with AKI; hence optimization of fluid balance is of utmost importance. *Loops diuretics are used commonly. They help in managing volume, but it should be borne in mind that they do not contribute to renal recovery, decreasing dialysis sessions, or mortality.* However, furosemide can be used to predict the risk of stage 3 of AKI and need for RRT. In early AKI, urine output after a furosemide stress test (FST) can be used to predict the need for RRT. Patients for FST should be hemodynamically stable and euvolemic. *Furosemide is injected intravenously in a dose of 1–1.5 mg/kg, and urine output is measured for 2 hours thereafter. A 2-hour urine output of 200 mL or less has been shown to have the best sensitivity and specificity to predict development of stage 3 AKI and requirement of RRT.* To minimize the risk of hypovolemia, urine output may be replaced with IV fluids. Other treatment modalities such as nesiritide, fenoldopam, or statins have been tried in various studies, but KDIGO does not currently recommend their use for treating AKI.

Vasopressors are recommended in AKI after adequate volume resuscitation is achieved to maintain MAP above 65 mm Hg. Ideally, norepinephrine is the vasopressor of choice, but vasopressin is equally effective. Dobutamine should be used in cases of myocardial dysfunction or in presence of ongoing signs of hypoperfusion. Optimal range for MAP in cases of sepsis is not well defined; however, most studies say it should be individualized depending on the age, presence of hypertension, peripheral vascular disease, or kidney disease. *A study by Asfar et al. showed maintaining MAP in the range of 80–85 mm Hg was more effective in reducing AKI and RRT, but increased the chances of atrial fibrillation.*

Multiple other pharmacotherapies, including N-acetyl cysteine, vasoactive agents like dopamine, and fenoldopam (pure dopamine type-1 receptor agonist) have been used in various studies but are not recommended presently as scientific evidence to justify their use is still lacking. The use of nephrotoxic drugs should be guided based on the GFR and presence of other comorbidities, after adjusting the dose and regularly monitoring renal function. However, combinations of multiple nephrotoxic drugs should be avoided.

One of the newer promising therapies for AKI is multipotent stem cells (MSCs). They have immune-modulatory and anti-inflammatory properties which are said to be helpful in sepsis, myocardial ischemia, and AKI. A phase I clinical trial has been conducted to test the safety and efficacy of MSCs in patients at high risk for AKI.

Dialytic Therapy in Treatment of Acute Kidney Injury

Use of RRT has revolutionized the care of patients with AKI and helped in reducing mortality to some extent. In 1946, Wilhem Kolf performed the first successful dialysis of a patient with AKI. Use of RRT over time has definitely shown to improve outcomes and helped in reducing mortality in patients with AKI. No single modality of RRT has shown to be superior over the other. The initiation of RRT in patients with AKI helps in preventing uremia and immediate death from the adverse complications of renal failure. The management of patients AKI is supportive, with RRT indicated in patients with severe AKI. Acute renal replacement therapy (ARRT) use in the ICU has it owns challenges as the aim is to improve the metabolic, biochemical parameters, and achieve fluid balance in hemodynamically unstable patients.

Multiple modalities of RRT are available. These include intermittent hemodialysis (IHD); continuous renal replacement therapies (CRRTs); and peritoneal dialysis (PD) and hybrid therapies, also known as prolonged intermittent renal replacement therapies (PIRRTs), a nomenclature endorsed by the Acute Dialysis Quality Initiative (ADQI), such as sustained low-efficiency dialysis (SLED) and extended-duration dialysis (EDD). PIRRT is a hybrid treatment that provides RRT for an extended period of time (i.e., 6–18 hours), but is intermittent (at least three times per week). PIRRT includes both convective (i.e., hemofiltration) and diffusive [i.e., hemodialysis (HD)] therapies, depending on the method of solute removal. No clear cut guidelines or studies exist about the best modality (continuous vs. intermittent), the optimal time for starting (early vs. late initiation), and the dose of dialysis to be delivered to patients.

Accepted urgent indications for RRT in patients with AKI generally include:
- Fluid overload refractory to diuretics
- Severe hyperkalemia (plasma potassium concentration >6.5 mEq/L) or rapidly rising potassium levels refractory to medical treatment
- Signs of uremia, such as pericarditis, encephalopathy, or an otherwise unexplained decline in mentation, uremic bleeding
- Severe metabolic acidosis refractory to medical therapy (pH <7.1)
- Drug, poisons, and certain dialyzable alcohol intoxications.

A unique point about ICU patients with AKI requiring RRT is that multiple indications coexist in these patients simultaneously. Other than these urgent indications of ARRT, volume and solute control, and drug and nutrition delivery are other renal support indications of AKI as given in the modified KDIGO AKI guidelines 2012.

Timing of Initiation of Renal Replacement Therapy

Again no consensus is available for the timing of initiation of RRT. Some studies say RRT should be initiated electively in patients with AKI, prior to the development of severe electrolyte disturbances and volume overload despite aggressive attempts at diuresis, particularly if they have increasing oxygen requirements. However, the results are ambiguous as the definition of early versus late RRT was heterogeneous in all these studies.

In the absence of clinically significant uremic symptoms or specific indications, the optimal timing of RRT initiation is controversial, particularly if the BUN is <110 mg/dL. In the absence of these conditions, generally dialysis is avoided as long as possible, on the lines similar for patients with CKD stage 5. However, RRT is often delayed in patients who may recover on their own, as well-known risks associated with the RRT include arrhythmias, hypotension, membrane bioincompatibility, and complications due to vascular access and anticoagulation. RRT may compromise recovery of renal function, and thus increase the progression of CKD.

Three major randomized control trials (RCTs) viz. ELAIN, AKIKI, and IDEAL-ICU, have not provided any consistent evidence for early initiation of RRT. The KDIGO guidelines state that RRT should be initiated emergently when life-threatening changes in fluid, electrolyte, and acid-base balance exist, but also suggest that among patients who do not have life-threatening indications, the clinician should consider the broader clinical context, the presence of conditions that can be modified with RRT, and trends of laboratory tests, rather than using any specific BUN or creatinine threshold, when making the decision to initiate RRT.

The current understanding of the literature reveals that initiation of early RRT in critically ill patients with AKI did not show any mortality benefit when

> **BOX 3** Factors while considering RRT.
>
> *Necessity of RRT*
> - Associated other organ dysfunction
> - Underlying comorbidities
> - Likelihood of recovery of renal function without the need of RRT
>
> *Risks of RRT*
> - Hemodynamic instability
> - Vascular access
> - Risks of infection
> - Immobilization
> - Clearance of trace elements/drugs/vitamins
>
> *Other factors*
> - Patient and family wishes
> - Healthcare costs
> - Availability of trained nursing staff/dialysis technicians and machines
> - Overall goals of care
>
> (RRT: renal replacement therapy)

compared to a standard initiation strategy. More ongoing RCTs and studies will provide more scientific data and may pave the way towards deciding whether early or late initiation of RRT is recommended.

Modality of Renal Replacement Therapy

Current data and studies do not support the superiority of any particular mode of RRT in patients with AKI. The ADQI consensus states that the modality should be guided by clinical practice, local resources, including staff, their training and experience and financial costs. The choice of the modality should be made available by balancing these issues. However, in selected patients, other factors may prevail and should be kept in mind **(Box 3)**.

The ideal RRT modality should be rapid, inexpensive, and easy to use with simple monitoring. It should mimic the physiology of the native organ, ensuring adequate blood purification, good solute and toxin clearance, favor nutrition administration, have minimum or no complications, should be hemodynamically tolerable and thus favor organ recovery. However, currently no ideal RRT modality is available. Various modalities currently available differ in the mode of delivery, clinical tolerability, and efficiency **(Table 5)**.

Continuous renal replacement therapy: CRRT represents a family of modalities that provides continuous support for severely ill patients with AKI. These include continuous hemofiltration (CHF), continuous hemodialysis (CHD), and continuous hemodiafiltration (CHDF) and slow continuous ultrafiltration (SCUF). Commonly used modalities are:
- *Continuous venovenous hemofiltration (CVVH):* CVVH uses hydrostatic pressure to induce the filtration of plasma water across the hemofilter membrane. Solutes are removed entirely by convection. Dialysate fluid

TABLE 5 Comparison between various RRT modalities.

	Intermittent hemodialysis (IHD)	Sustained low-efficiency dialysis (SLED)	Continuous renal replacement therapy (CRRT)	Peritoneal dialysis (PD)
Clearance	Diffusion	Largely diffusion (convection added in SLED-f)	Diffusion and convection	Diffusion and osmotic ultrafiltration
Blood flow (Qb)	250–300 mL/minute	150–200 mL/minute	100–150 mL/minute	• NA • Usually peritoneal blood flow is 50–100 mL/min
Dialysate flow	300–800 mL/minute	300 mL/minute	1,000–3,000 mL/hour	1,000–2,000 mL/hour
Ultrafiltration rate	500–750 mL/hour	• 100–300 mL/hour • Can be increased as tolerated	• 100–300 mL/hour • Can be increased as tolerated	Unpredictable
Duration	4 hours	• 6–10 hours • Can be used up to 24 hours (c-SLED)	Continuous	Continuous
Advantages	• Rapid removal of low-molecular-weight substances/toxins • Due to intermittent nature provides time window for diagnostic and therapeutic procedures • Lower costs, less expertise and no need for a separate machine, less exposure to anticoagulation hence less risks of bleeding	• Better hemodynamic stability • Lower costs, less expertise and no need for a separate machine, less exposure to anticoagulation hence less risks of bleeding • Due to intermittent nature provides time window for diagnostic and therapeutic procedures	• Continuous removal of toxins, most near physiological • Better in hemodynamically unstable patients with more stable fluid control • Better to provide nutrition • Some removal of middle-molecular-weight substances possible • Can be coupled with other extracorporeal devices like ECMO	• Technically simple • Better hemodynamic stability • No need for vascular access and anticoagulation • Less costly

Contd...

Contd...

	Intermittent hemodialysis (IHD)	Sustained low-efficiency dialysis (SLED)	Continuous renal replacement therapy (CRRT)	Peritoneal dialysis (PD)
Disadvantages	• Rapid fluid removal leading to hypotension and hemodynamic instability • Dialysis disequilibrium • Needs RO water treatment plant • Not possible to combine with other organ support systems like ECMO	Slower solute removal	• Slower solute and toxin clearance • Needs prolonged anticoagulation • Expensive and needs separate apparatus and trained staff • Needs dedicated separate filters and fluid bags • Being continuous does not provide window for diagnostic or therapeutic purposes	• Slower solute and toxin removal • No control over fluid (UF) removal • Increased chances of infections, peritonitis, hyperglycemia, and protein loss • Impairs ventilation • Stand-alone therapy and cannot be combined with other extracorporeal therapies
Clinical indications	• Hemodynamically stable patients poisoning with a dialyzable toxin • Rapid ultrafiltration (UF) removal (isolated UF)	• Hemodynamically unstable patients on inotropes • Less resource settings	Hemodynamically unstable patients chiefly indicated in liver disease, or increased intracranial pressure or cerebral edema as indicated by KDIGO	• Hemodynamically unstable patients having difficult vascular access, coagulopathy and increased intracranial tension • Children with AKI especially <10 kg

(AKI: acute kidney injury; ECMO: extracorporeal membrane oxygenation; KDIGO: Kidney Disease: Improving Global Outcomes; RO: reverse osmosis)

is not used. Small and middle molecular weight molecules (i.e., <5,000 Daltons) such as urea and electrolytes are removed in roughly the same concentration as that of plasma. There is therefore no change in the plasma concentrations of these solutes by hemofiltration. However, the administration of substitution fluid lowers by dilution, the plasma concentrations of solutes such as urea and creatinine that are not present in the substitution fluid.

- *Continuous venovenous hemodialysis (CVVHD)*: CVVHD primarily removes solute by diffusion. Dialysate fluid is used. As in IHD, dialysate fluid is run countercurrent to the direction of blood flow at a rate of 1-2 L/hour. In CVVHD, ultrafiltration (UF) is limited to the rate at which net fluid removal is desired, and no IV fluid replacement is required.
- *Continuous venovenous hemodiafiltration (CVVHDF)*: CVVHDF combines diffusion with convection. CVVHDF requires infusions of both replacement fluid and dialysis fluid. Similar to CVVH, the UF volume is variable, and replacement fluid must be given to maintain euvolemia. The amount of replacement fluid that is given is determined by the net volume removal that is desired.
- *Slow continuous ultrafiltration*: SCUF is used to treat isolated fluid overload. SCUF is not useful in patients who are uremic or hyperkalemic, because solute removal is minimal. SCUF can safely remove up to 8 L of fluid per day. Neither replacement fluid nor dialysate fluid is used.

Although superior clearance of middle- and larger-molecular-weight molecules is associated with convective therapies (hemofiltration) compared with diffusive therapies (HD), there are no studies clearly showing improved clinical outcomes compared with the type of solute transport. No specific CRRT modality has been shown to provide better outcomes.

All modalities for CRRT used today utilize venovenous circuits with blood flow through the dialyzer/hemofilter driven by an extracorporeal blood pump. All require placement of a dual-lumen IV HD catheter. Arteriovenous modalities, in which blood flow was driven by the gradient between the MAP and venous pressure, are no longer used because of risks associated with the need for arterial access (embolization and bleeding). The only advantage to arteriovenous modalities was that they did not require a blood pump.

Prolonged Intermittent Renal Replacement Therapy

It includes sustained low-efficiency (daily) dialysis (SLEDD), sustained low-efficiency (daily) diafiltration (SLEDD-f), extended daily dialysis (EDD), slow continuous dialysis (SCD), go slow dialysis, and accelerated venovenous hemofiltration (AVVH) or hemodiafiltration. The indication for PIRRT is dialysis-requiring AKI in a patient who is too hemodynamically unstable to tolerate standard IHD.

Dialysis machine and hemodialyzer: PIRRT can be performed on most machines that are used for standard IHD. Machines used for PIRRT should have the capability to run at low blood and dialysate flow rates. Some machines are designed specifically for PIRRT and have specific capabilities for solute removal by convection, diffusion, or both.

For CRRT, the hemofilter is a high-permeability, high-flux biocompatible membranes used for all modalities of CRRT. The typical membrane materials used are polyacrylonitrile (AN69), polyarylethersulfone (PAES), and polyethersulfone (PES). There are no data suggesting that one type of membrane is better than the others. Theoretically, because of their negative charge, polyacrylonitrile membranes may allow more adsorption and removal of middle-molecular-weight solutes, such as cytokines. However, no difference in outcomes has been demonstrated.

Vascular access: A nontunneled or tunneled dialysis catheter in a central vein is the preferred access for PIRRT, even among ESRD patients who have an arteriovenous fistula (AVF) or graft.

Session length: PIRRT should be performed at least three times per week to provide an adequate dialysis dose. The time per session ranges from 6 to 18 hours but is typically approximately 8 hours. The time per individual session is often determined after assessing the patient response to the initial UF rate (fluid removal per hour). CRRT is performed as a continuous modality over 48–72 hours or even longer.

Anticoagulation: Anticoagulation is recommended to prevent clotting of the extracorporeal system. However, some clinicians choose to not use anticoagulation in all patients, at least initially. Better clinical outcomes have not been shown with anticoagulation versus no anticoagulation in PIRRT. Methods of anticoagulation include systemic unfractionated heparin and regional citrate anticoagulation (RCA).

Dose of Renal Replacement Therapy

Kt/V is a measure of the volume of plasma cleared of urea during an HD session (time) = Kt divided by the volume of distribution of urea. However, it is difficult and tedious to calculate the Kt/V and newer methods like online clearance monitoring (OCM) calculated directly by the HD machine are used in IHD or SLED. *Comparison between various RRT modalities is given in* **Table 5**.

One of the key factors in deciding on the RRT modality is whether the AKI is a part of single organ dysfunction or multiorgan dysfunction [multiple organ failure (MOF)]. AKI without MOF is less complex, and the same RRT techniques used for the treatment of CKD such as IHD, PIRRT, or PD may be used, while the AKI associated with MOF is a complex condition and requires more flexible and physiological RRT like CRRT.

Both the KDIGO (2012) and the ADQI guidelines suggest CRRT rather than IHD in hemodynamic unstable patients, AKI with MOF receiving multiple extracorporeal supports like extracorporeal membrane oxygenation (ECMO), plasma exchange, adsorbent sorbent therapies like cytoSorb for sepsis, and in patients where metabolic fluctuations are poorly tolerated like in cases with acute brain injury, brain edema, or liver failure. Theoretically, CRRT offers slower fluid removal and better fluid balance, avoids large fluid and solute shifts, uses more biocompatible membranes, allows nutrition without restriction and is better adapted to the needs of critically ill patients.

Disadvantages include the longer immobilization affecting diagnostic and therapeutic procedures, more need for anticoagulation, hypothermia, and increased costs.

The PIRRT techniques like SLED are preferred in situations where mobilization and rehabilitation of patients is required and fluid and metabolic fluctuations are well tolerated. Also it is used widely for logistical and cost reasons. Few studies have shown better hemodynamic tolerability, better MAP, and less hypotension in CRRT than in SLED, but a Cochrane review failed to show it. Lack of trained staff, limited availability, and increased costs limit the use of CRRT in developing countries like India.

Extracorporeal Blood Purification beyond Acute Kidney Injury in Sepsis and Organ Support System

Continuous renal replacement therapy helps to restore immune homeostasis by altering or removing the inflammatory mediators of AKI. It is achieved by adsorption of inflammatory mediators onto the surface of the hemofilter. However, it may cause the removal of both anti-inflammatory as well as proinflammatory cytokines. Hemoperfusion therapy using various blood purification techniques such as oXiris, CytoSorb, high cutoff (HCO) membranes, and high effluent flow rate have been combined with CRRT for cytokine removal in septic patients. Current scientific evidence does not support their routine use and larger RCTs are required to prove any renal or mortality benefits.

In ICUs, critically ill patients with acute respiratory distress syndrome (ARDS), fulminant hepatic failure, and cardiogenic shock develop AKI. Few studies have shown that RRT, especially CRRT, may have a supportive role in their management along with other extracorporeal organ support devices such as ECMO and ventricular assist devices. Trials such as UNLOAD trial and CARRESS-HF have showed that they help in UF removal, especially in heart failure cases refractory to medical therapy and are even recommended by the American College of Cardiology (ACC). Similarly in ARDS and fulminant hepatic failure, they are used to reduce hypervolemia and extravascular lung volume. Molecular adsorbent recirculating system (MARS) also called albumin/liver dialysis, fractionated plasma separation and adsorption (FPSA-Prometheus), and CRRT are modalities used as a bridge therapy to liver transplant. All these modalities are in the experimental stage and there is no robust evidence currently present to suggest that these modalities reduce morbidity and mortality.

Discontinuation of Renal Replacement Therapy

Renal replacement therapy is usually continued until the patient manifests evidence of recovery of kidney function. Most often, recovery is assessed based on empirical data. In oliguric patients, the primary manifestation of recovery of kidney function is an increase in urine output; however, this finding may not be apparent in patients who are nonoliguric. Recovery of kidney function may also be manifested by a progressive decline in SCr concentrations after initial attainment of stable values despite a constant dose of renal support. More objective assessment of recovery of kidney function can be obtained by measurement of creatinine clearance. As an example, in the Acute Renal Failure Trial Network (ATN) study, creatinine clearance was assessed on 6-hour timed urine collections obtained when the urine output exceeded 30 mL/hour. In the ATN study, renal support was discontinued when the measured creatinine clearance exceeded 20 mL/min and was left to the discretion of the providers when in the range of 12-20 mL/min.

Complications of Renal Replacement Therapy

Hypotension, abnormalities in serum electrolytes like hypokalemia, hypophosphatemia and hypocalcemia, alkalosis, albumin and amino acid losses, hypothermia, infection, and bleeding are all well-recognized complications of RRT. Others complications include arrhythmias, membrane bioincompatibility, complications due to vascular access, and subtherapeutic antibiotic concentrations. The clinician should be aware of these complications while using the various RRT modalities and appropriate corrective measures should be carried out early in the course of treatment.

CONCLUSION

Acute kidney injury is one of the most common clinical syndromes seen in the ICU and complicates nearly 30-50% ICU admissions. AKI is defined as deterioration of kidney function occurring rapidly over hours, or days to weeks. The common etiologies of AKI in these patients are chiefly due to hypovolemia or kidney hypoperfusion and ATN results due to ischemia, shock, inflammatory state/sepsis, or nephrotoxic drugs. Common causes of AKI in tropical countries like India are snake bites, malaria, leptospirosis, or obstetric causes. AKI is a syndrome not just limited to the kidneys but also causes distant organ dysfunction. Early diagnosis of AKI should be done by careful review of history, hospital course, and physical examination, including volume assessment. This should be complemented by various biochemical and urinary tests including FENa. Primary prevention and early diagnosis of AKI are of importance. To prevent AKI, hypotension, hypovolemia, and sepsis should be quickly addressed. All correctable causes should be treated and any potential nephrotoxic agent or new insult should be avoided to further hamper renal recovery. RRT is an important supportive and therapeutic modality used commonly in clinical practice. However, uncertainty still remains about the ideal circumstances when to initiate RRT, the ideal modality and indications when RRT should be done **(Flowchart 1)**. This process of selection of various factors for RRT is influenced by numerous factors. The strategies for the use

Flowchart 1: Implied algorithm for management of AKI in critically ill patient in ICU.

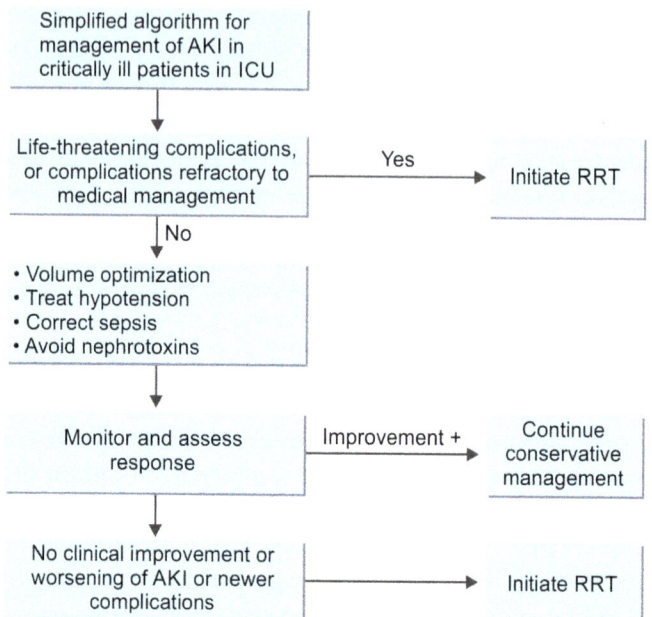

(AKI: acute kidney injury; ICU: intensive care unit; RRT: renal replacement therapy)

of RRT in AKI are dynamic and constantly evolving. Continuous therapies are preferred over intermittent ones in patients with hemodynamic instability, cerebral edema, or liver failure, though no robust evidence exists for the same. Any mode of the chosen RRT should be able to achieve desired solute and water clearance while maintaining hemodynamic stability have a positive effect on nutrition and have low complication rates.

■ SUGGESTED READING

1. Ahmed AR, Obilana A, Lappin D. Renal replacement therapy in the critical care setting. Crit Care Res Pract. 2019;2019:6948710.
2. Asfar P, Meziani F, Hamel J-F, Grelon F, Megarbane B, Anguel N, et al. High versus low blood-pressure target in patients with septic shock. N Engl J Med. 2014;370(17):1583-93.
3. Bagshaw SM, Wald R, Adhikari NKJ, Bellomo R, da Costa BR, Dreyfuss D, et al. Timing of initiation of renal-replacement therapy in acute kidney injury. N Engl J Med. 2020;383(3):240-51.
4. Bhargava S, Jain A, Gupta V. Fractional excretion of sodium—a simple test for the differential diagnosis of acute renal failure. Clin Nephrol. 2002;58(1):79-80.
5. Druml W. Systemic consequences of acute kidney injury. Curr Opin Crit Care. 2014;20(6):613-9.
6. Feehally J. Acute kidney injury. In: Feehally J (Eds). Comprehensive Clinical Nephrology, 6th edition. Amsterdam: Elsevier; 2019.
7. Grams ME, Rabb H. The distant organ effects of acute kidney injury. Kidney Int. 2012;81(10):942-8.
8. Hoste EA, Maitland K, Brudney CS, Mehta R, Vincent J-L, Yates D, et al. Four phases of intravenous fluid therapy: a conceptual model. Br J Anaesth. 2014;113(5):740-7.

9. Hsu CY, Ordoñez JD, Chertow GM, Fan D, McCulloch CE, Go AS. The risk of acute renal failure in patients with chronic kidney disease. Kidney Int. 2008;74(1):101-7.
10. Jha V, Parameswaran S. Community-acquired acute kidney injury in tropical countries. Nat Rev Nephrol. 2013;9(5):278-90.
11. Judd PW, Sanders AA. Diagnosis and Clinical Evaluation of Acute Kidney Injury. In: Feehally J (Eds). Comprehensive Clinical Nephrology, 6th edition. Amsterdam: Elsevier; 2019. pp. 810-9.
12. Kellum JA, Lameire N, Aspelin P, Barsoum RS, Burdmann EA, Goldstein SL, et al. Kidney disease: improving global outcomes (KDIGO) acute kidney injury work group. KDIGO clinical practice guideline for acute kidney injury. Kidney Int Suppl. 2012;2:1-138.
13. Koyner JL. Assessment and diagnosis of renal dysfunction in the ICU. Chest. 2012;141(6):1584-94.
14. Lameire N. Acute kidney injury. In: Turner NN, Lameire N, Goldsmith DJ, Winearls CG, Himmelfarb J, Remuzzi G (Eds). Oxford Textbook of Clinical Nephrology, 4th edition. Oxford: Oxford University Press; 2015.
15. Leah Haseley JAJ. Pathophysiology and etiology of acute kidney injury. In: Feehally J (Eds). Comprehensive Clinical Nephrology, 6th edition. Amsterdam: Elsevier; 2019. pp. 786-801.
16. Levy MM, Evans LE, Rhodes A. The Surviving Sepsis Campaign Bundle: 2018 update. Intensive Care Med. 2018;44(6):925-8.
17. Lobo VA. Renal replacement therapy in acute kidney injury: which mode and when? Indian J Crit Care Med. 2020;24(Suppl 3):S102-6.
18. Lopes JA, Jorge S. The RIFLE and AKIN classifications for acute kidney injury: a critical and comprehensive review. Clin Kidney J. 2013;6(1):8-14.
19. Malhotra R, Kashani KB, Macedo E, Kim J, Bouchard J, Wynn S, et al. A risk prediction score for acute kidney injury in the intensive care unit. Nephrol Dial Transplant. 2017;32(5):814-22.
20. Mehta RL, Burdmann EA, Cerdá J, Feehally J, Finkelstein F, García-García G, et al. Recognition and management of acute kidney injury in the International Society of Nephrology by 25 Global Snapshot: a multinational cross-sectional study. Lancet. 2016;387(10032):2017-25.
21. Mehta RL, Cerdá J, Burdmann EA, Tonelli M, García-García G, Jha V, et al. International Society of Nephrology's by 25 initiative for acute kidney injury (zero preventable deaths by 2025): a human rights case for nephrology. Lancet. 2015;385(9987):2616-43.
22. Mårtensson J, Martling C-R, Bell M. Novel biomarkers of acute kidney injury and failure: clinical applicability. Br J Anaesth. 2012;109(6):843-50.
23. National Heart, Lung, and Blood Institute Acute Respiratory Distress Syndrome (ARDS) Clinical Trials Network, Wiedemann HP, Wheeler AP, et al. Comparison of two fluid-management strategies in acute lung injury. N Engl J Med. 2006;354(24):25642575.
24. Neri M, Villa G, Garzotto F, Bagshaw S, Bellomo R, Cerda J, et al. Nomenclature for renal replacement therapy in acute kidney injury: basic principles. Crit Care. 2016;20(1):318.
25. Ostermann M, Joannidis M, Pani A, Floris M, De Rosa S, Kellum JA, et al. Patient selection and timing of continuous renal replacement therapy. Blood Purif. 2016;42(3):224-37.
26. Perez Valdivieso JR, Bes-Rastrollo M, Monedero P, De Irala J, Lavilla FJ. Evaluation of the prognostic value of the risk, injury, failure, loss and end-stage renal failure (RIFLE) criteria for acute kidney injury. Nephrology (Carlton). 2008;13(5):361-6.
27. The 2012 Kidney Disease: Improving Global Outcomes (KDIGO) Clinical Practice Guideline for Acute Kidney Injury (AKI).

CHAPTER 8

Coma in the ICU: A Clinical Approach

Sarosh M Katrak

■ INTRODUCTION

In this era of improved resuscitation and support systems, one of the most common problems facing a clinical neurologist is the assessment, diagnosis, and management of a patient in an altered state of consciousness. Assessment of coma is always a medical emergency. This is always a taxing problem, as time is of essence to achieve many goals. Often the history is not available but the clinician has to make a prompt diagnosis, order relevant investigations, and start appropriate therapy to avoid morbidity and more importantly mortality. A classical example is a subdural hematoma in an elderly patient. If it is not promptly diagnosed and evacuated, there may be residual neurological deficit, where none should be present.

■ PATHOPHYSIOLOGY OF CONSCIOUSNESS

Before we dwell on coma, one must understand the normal pathophysiology of consciousness. Consciousness depends on two factors, i.e., arousal and the content of consciousness. Arousal is linked to the ascending reticular formation, a series of neurons in the rostral brainstem, which projects to the diencephalon and cerebral cortex. The content of consciousness, simply put, is awareness of self and environment. It is the exclusive function of the integrated activity of the cortical neurons in both hemispheres. Since both hemispheres are involved, consciousness is not localized to any hemisphere or to one or more lobes of a hemisphere. This results in three states: (1) awake and aware which is the normal level of consciousness, (2) awake but not aware, and (3) not awake and not aware. The last category involves stupor and coma. Hence, in the initial approach to a patient in the intensive care unit (ICU), the clinician should categorize his/her patient into one of these three categories.

When the central nervous system (CNS) is affected by a disease process, the level of consciousness deteriorates. This is assessed by two parameters: Cognitive and motor functions **(Fig. 1)**. Hypersomnia, acute confusional state, delirium, and severe cognitive disability/akinetic mutism are a continuum of deterioration in which the patient is awake but not aware. If the disease progresses, the patient deteriorates into stupor or coma and is not awake and not aware. If the coma is very severe and prolonged, the patient may be brain dead; if severe but not prolonged, he/she may improve partially into a persistent vegetative state (PVS) or a minimally conscious state (MCS), putting them again in the category of awake but not aware.

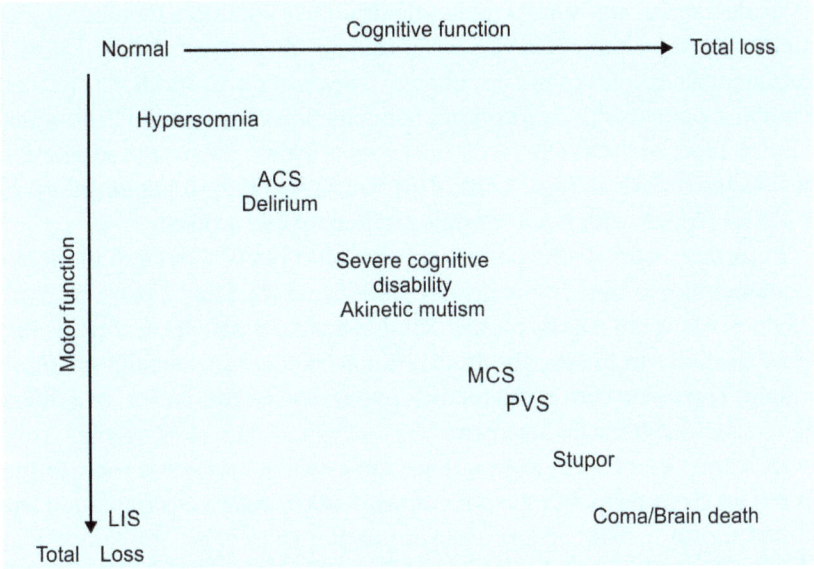

Fig. 1: Cognitive and motor function. (ACS: acute confusional state; LIS: locked-in state; MCS: minimally conscious state; PVS: persistent vegetative state)

As mentioned earlier, a normal individual is awake and aware. In **Figure 1**, there is one exception to the rule—the locked-in state (LIS). This condition was described by Plum and Posner in their classic monograph: The Diagnosis of Stupor and Coma in 1966. There is a lesion in the ventral pons sparing the paramedian and lateral tegmentum. This results in severe quadriplegia and anarthria with preserved consciousness, voluntary eye movements, and blinking. Clinically corticospinal, corticobulbar, and corticopontine tract signs are elicited. In the acute phase, such patients have a high mortality. If they survive, they are left behind with severe disability. It may be of interest to know that in the Count of Monte Cristo, Alexandre Dumas in 1884, described a character, Monsieur Noirtier as "immovable as a corpse...... sight and hearing were the only senses remaining...... which gave the impression of a *"corpse with living eyes"*. What a beautiful description of a locked-in state. This state must be distinguished from an akinetic mute state in which the patient is not aware and has no clinical signs, in sharp contrast to the locked-in state where there are plenty of clinical signs and the patient is appropriately aware. As mentioned earlier, the neurological states in which the patient is awake but not aware are hypersomnia, acute confusional state, delirium, akinetic mutism, PVS, and MCS. The latter two will be discussed later.

Hypersomnia, as the name suggests is a condition in which the patient sleeps excessively but can be aroused easily with verbal or painful stimulus. Once the stimulus stops, he falls back to sleep. This occurs early when the diencephalon is involved in a disease process.

Acute confusional "state" entails impairment of attention, memory, logical thinking, and lack of recall of part of the day or location. A key feature is prominent distractibility and no coherent conversation. In addition to all these features, a patient with *delirium* has hallucinations and systemic autonomic manifestation, such as tachycardia, tachypnea, hypertension, and sweating. In these states, there is a diffuse cortical involvement and the brain misinterprets all sensory inputs with inappropriate excitement and arousal.

In *akinetic mutism,* the patient appears alert but is silent and immobile. Spontaneous eye opening is present and visual tracking is preserved, but defective. Alertness may be partial. There is a relative paucity of corticospinal signs. The best way to describe this condition is seeming wakefulness without content. The lesions are in the medial frontal lobe, limbic cortex, or a diffuse bilateral hemispheric involvement.

In *stupor and coma*, the patient is not awake and not aware. Stupor resembles deep sleep, but the patient responds to vigorous stimulation with limited motor activity. When the stimulation ceases, he/she lapses back into the sleep-like state. Stupor should be differentiated from psychogenic unresponsiveness (PUR). The differentiating features in PUR are resistance to eyelid opening, absence of long tract signs, and optokinetic nystagmus can be elicited. In very difficult cases, ice-cold caloric test will produce a nystagmus in PUR whereas there will be tonic deviation of the eyes to the side of the irrigated ear in stupor. Of course, the electroencephalogram (EEG) will be abnormal in stupor and entirely normal in PUR.

Coma is the main focus of this chapter. Coma is a state of unresponsiveness from which the patient cannot be aroused with deep painful stimulus. The eyes are closed but rarely may be open but without any fixation or tracking. On deep painful stimulus, the response is reflex-flexion of the upper limbs or extension of all four limbs. With further deterioration, there is no motor response with flaccidity of the limbs. Severe and irreversible coma results in brain death. If the coma is severe but transient, the patient may survive in a PVS, or with less severe coma, in an MCS.

ETIOLOGIES OF COMA

The etiologies of coma are (1) large unilateral hemispheric lesion with mass effect; (2) diffuse bilateral hemispheric abnormalities; (3) discrete or diffuse upper brainstem lesion; or (4) cerebellar lesions. In a review of 14 studies between 1981 and 2013, regarding the etiology and outcome of nontraumatic coma, the two most common etiologies were strokes and hypoxic-anoxic encephalopathy. In the African countries, involved in this study, 10–51% of admissions were due to CNS infection, a common feature in developing countries like India. The key component of the pathogenesis of coma is cerebral or cerebellar edema and the resultant herniation of the brain. The main sites of herniation in the supratentorial compartment are transfalcine herniation of the medial part of the temporal lobe—uncal herniation, rostral to caudal herniation of the cerebral hemispheres, and ultimately in the infratentorial compartment, tonsillar herniation through the foramen magnum. It is important to pick up the early signs of central and uncal herniation. In the early stages of central herniation, the patient becomes drowsy with long cycle Cheyne-Stokes respiration, small but reactive pupils, preserved ciliospinal reflex, intact oculocephalic maneuver (OCM) with mildly impaired upward gaze and localization or flexion response to pain. In the early stages of uncal herniation, the respiration is regular but rapid, an ipsilateral partial third nerve palsy, an early loss of OCM and oculovestibular reflex (OVR) and unilateral or bilateral pyramidal tract signs. The clinician should be alert to these early signs and take appropriate action. If the condition deteriorates, the coma may become irreversible with late signs of central herniation. There is hyperventilation or short cycle Cheyne-Stokes respiration, fixed midposition/dilated pupils, loss of OCM and OVR, and flexion to extension reflex response to pain or total flaccidity. In the late stages of uncal herniation, there is a total third nerve palsy before the other features merge with those of central herniation.

Coma due to an *infratentorial lesion*, may be due to a small discrete brainstem or cerebellar lesion. There are a few distinguishing features which may be overlooked if one is not aware of them. These signs are ataxia just prior to the onset of coma, abnormalities of external ocular movements (EOMs), and very early loss of OCM and OVR. In this context, I would like to stress on the "pseudotumoral" presentation of a cerebellar infarct. This is usually a large cerebellar hemispheric infarct, involving the complete posterior inferior cerebellar artery (PICA) territory. Uncommonly, it can be due to a cerebellar hemorrhage. The initial symptoms may be nonspecific to the cerebellum, such as headache and persistent vomiting. Ocular signs are ocular gaze or 6th nerve paresis. As the brainstem gets compressed by the edematous cerebellum, bilateral gaze palsy and/or ocular bobbing occurs. The patient is initially drowsy and deteriorates into stupor or coma over 1-3 days. The CT scan may be normal in 25% of cases in the initial stages but the MRI is invariably abnormal. If the patient becomes comatose, 85% will die without surgery. Suboccipital craniectomy is the procedure of choice. Not only is it life-saving but the results are excellent if it is done before the patient becomes comatose. This is the reason why the treating clinician must be aware of this entity.

The clinician should also be aware of *brainstem depression due to sedative drugs* or intoxication. The danger here lies in the premature diagnosis of brain death. Sedative drugs selectively "paralyze" the median longitudinal fasciculus (MLF) which connects the 6th nerve nucleus to the appropriate part of the 3rd nerve nucleus for conjugate horizontal eye movements. Hence, on eliciting brainstem reflexes, the pupillary and corneal reflexes are preserved out of proportion to the OCM and OVR. In a normal individual, irrigation of both ears with ice-cold water results in upward deviation of the eyes. When the

MLF is "paralyzed" by sedative drugs, horizontal ocular deviation is no longer possible, and vertical ocular deviation does not need the MLF. Thus, ice-cold irrigation of one ear produces upward deviation of the eyes. This test confirms brainstem depression by sedative drugs.

■ NEUROLOGICAL EXAMINATION

Neurological examination in a comatose patient is limited and essentially consists of good observation and eliciting reflex responses. A structured neurological examination involves observing first the position and posture of the patient and then the respiratory pattern. The respiratory pattern is a good indicator of the level of the brain that is malfunctioning. Diffuse hemispheric dysfunction produces Cheyne-Stokes respiration and midbrain involvement, hyperventilation. The rostral pons may produce a peculiar pattern called apneusis, in which breathing halts briefly in full inspiration, whereas in the lower pons or upper medullary lesions the respiration becomes irregular and of uneven depth—ataxic breathing. This pattern often heralds a respiratory arrest. The value of identifying these different types of respiration has probably been overestimated, and assisted ventilation has perhaps made this exercise superfluous. Once this is done, one should rule out a fracture of the skull or cervical spine and then check for neck stiffness. Look closely for the Battle's sign, which is a discoloration along the course of the posterior auricular artery with ecchymosis near the tip of the mastoid process, indicating a fracture of the base of the skull. The next step is the fundus examination, which may show evidence of hypertension or diabetes. A subhyaloid hemorrhage on fundus examination is practically diagnostic of subarachnoid hemorrhage (SAH). Once this is done, one should judge the level of consciousness, signs of lateralization, and reflexes to establish brainstem activity. The level of consciousness is judged by either the Glasgow Coma Scale (GCS) or the more recent Full Outline of UnResponsiveness (FOUR) score. The FOUR score involves eye responses (0-4), motor responses (0-4), brainstem reflexes (0-4), and respiration (0-4). The main advantage of the FOUR score is in patients who are intubated or have a tracheostomy, as there is no verbal response score.

Lateralizing and motor signs are easily established by good observations at the bedside. Weakness, unilateral grasp reflex, and focal clonic or myoclonic seizure activity establish the abnormal side. If a patient is agitated and plucking or clutching at his clothes, the corticospinal tracts are intact. Grimacing to deep painful supraorbital stimulus indicates that the corticobulbar tracts up to the pons are intact. Roving eye movements mean an intact midbrain and pons. Lastly multifocal myoclonus and orofacial dyskinesia are seen in hypoxic-ischemic and metabolic encephalopathy, respectively.

Brainstem function is judged by the brainstem reflexes—pupillary reaction, the corneal reflex, spontaneous (roving) and reflex (OCM and OVR) eye movements, gag reflex, and respiration. While examining the pupils also note for any asymmetry in the position of the two upper eyelids to detect subtle ptosis. It is beyond the scope of this chapter to go into the details of brainstem reflex examination.

■ CLINICAL CLASSIFICATION OF COMA

Once the neurological assessment is complete, one can categorize the patient into three clinical groups:
1. Coma with focal signs
2. Coma without focal signs but with meningeal signs
3. Coma without focal and meningeal signs.

Coma with Focal Signs

The various etiologies are focal trauma, cerebral or cerebellar ischemic or hemorrhagic strokes, neoplasms or space occupying lesions (SOLs) like subdural hematoma, abscess or herpes simplex virus (HSV) encephalitis, and rarely, hypoglycemic hemiplegia. Focal trauma is easily diagnosed by the appearance of the patient and the history of trauma. Strokes usually have associated risk factors—hypertension, diabetes or dyslipidemias, and are acute in onset. Neoplasms or SOL have a subacute or insidious onset and may be associated with signs of rise of intracranial pressure. Abscesses or HSV encephalitis may have an acute or subacute onset but are usually associated with fever, headache, and other signs of infection. Rarely, a pitfall in this diagnostic algorithm may be hypoglycemic hemiplegia. The neuroimaging is very useful in this category of patients and shows a variety of abnormalities, which confirm the diagnosis. The exception to the rule is hypoglycemic hemiplegia, where the neuroimaging is normal and the diagnosis is made on the blood glucose levels.

Coma without Focal Signs but with Meningeal Signs

In this category, the main differentiating symptom is fever. With fever, one should consider meningitis/encephalitis be it viral, bacterial, fungal, or protozoal. Without fever, consider SAH. Further investigations such as cerebrospinal fluid (CSF) examination, CT scan, MRI, MRA, and four-vessel digital subtraction angiography (DSA) aid in arriving at the diagnosis.

Coma without Focal or Meningeal Signs

This is the main category in which general physicians are involved. It includes anoxic-ischemic, metabolic and toxic encephalopathy, nonconvulsive status epilepticus (NCSE), drug intoxication or poisoning, and hypo- or hyperthermic brain damage. Here neuroimaging may be normal or show nonspecific changes. The EEG is more useful particularly in NCSE. Anoxic-ischemic encephalopathy is diagnosed because of a history of cardiac arrest and cardiopulmonary resuscitation. The diagnosis of metabolic/toxic encephalopathy is made by the

TABLE 1 Drug-induced seizures and coma.

Antibiotics	Encephalopathy	Seizures	Nonconvulsive status epilepticus	Delirium/ psychosis	Coma
Cephalosporins (cefepime)	+	++	+	+	- +
Piperacillin and tazobactum	+	+	+	+	-
Carbapenems	-	++	-	-	-
Quinolones	+	++	+	++	-
Linezolid	+	-	-	-	-
Metronidazole	+	+	-	-	-

(*Source*: Adapted from Grill MF, Maganti RK. Neurotoxic effects associated with antibiotic use: management considerations. Br J Clin Pharmacology. 2011;72:381-93.)

EEG and laboratory investigations. In hypo- or hyperthermic brain damage, there is a prior history of exposure to extremes of temperature.

Nonconvulsive status epilepticus needs a high index of suspicion for diagnosis. In NCSE, motor symptoms may be absent or minimal. The patient may present with mild confusion or even coma. Negative symptoms like aphasia, mutism, or amnesia can be the initial presentation. At times, positive symptoms like tonic eye deviation or nystagmoid jerking of the eyes may lead to the diagnosis. The common underlying etiologies are strokes, SAH, infections, trauma or anoxic-ischemic, and metabolic or toxic encephalopathies (sepsis). Multiagent chemotherapy and beta-lactam antibiotics in conjunction with chronic kidney disease can also precipitate NCSE. In a study of EEG monitoring in coma, 8-20% of patients had NCSE. The clinician must have a high index of suspicion for NCSE in any patient with unexplained alteration in behavior or consciousness. In this situation, an EEG is warranted.

Table 1 outlines all the adverse effects of antibiotics in the ICU. The risk factors for these adverse effects are old age, chronic kidney disease, prior CNS disease, and chronic liver disease for metronidazole. Among the cephalosporins, cefepime is the only one which can produce coma. This happens after 1-10 days of administration and resolves in 2-7 days after stopping the drug. Awareness of this adverse effect of cefepime will prevent a disastrous outcome.

OUTCOME OF COMA

The outcome of coma depends on many factors—etiology, duration, the presence or absence of the pupillary and corneal reflexes, OCM, OVR, the motor response to pain, or a combination of all the above. Factors predictive of a good outcome are traumatic etiology, a shorter duration of coma, and early return of the pupillary and corneal reflexes. Localization of a painful stimulus and grimacing are good prognostic signs whereas flaccidity or extensor response to pain elude to a poor outcome. In a prospective study of 310 patients of nontraumatic coma, Bates et al. found that 25% of patients who were comatose for 6 hours or more had severe disability or PVS. This increased to 79% of those still in coma after a week. The chances of regaining independent existence was greater in patients who obeyed commands, or moved the limbs appropriately to painful stimuli by one day, or had normal EOM, OCM, or OVR. The American Academy of Neurology practice parameters: prediction of outcome in comatose survivors after cardiopulmonary resuscitation concluded that the absence of the pupillary and corneal reflexes and the motor response to pain accurately predicted poor outcome in these patients.

Persistent Vegetative State

If the coma is severe but not unduly prolonged, the patient is likely to go into PVS. In PVS, arousal, sleep/wake cycle, and respiration are preserved. The eyes are open but there is no fixation or tracking. Initially when the patient is emerging from the coma, roving eye movements are seen. Motor function is not purposeful and there is no higher level of communication, intellectual thinking, or recall. Also there is no response to external stimuli. The diagnosis of PVS is made after several weeks of observation and if it persists after 1 year, it is likely to be irreversible.

Minimally Conscious State

The boundaries between PVS and MCS are difficult to define. All the features of PVS are present in MCS with three exceptions. The eyes may open on prodding and there may be ill-sustained tracking. Motor functions may be intermittently purposeful.

■ EMERGENT THERAPY

The principles of emergent therapy in a comatose patient are:
- Ensure and maintain airway, breathing, and circulation
- Maintain adequate nutrition and supplement vitamins
- Lower intracranial pressure, medically or surgically
- Control seizures and infection
- Maintain fluid, electrolyte, and acid/base balance
- For poisoning, give the specific antidote
- Control agitation and pain
- Protect the eyes.

The last point is important as many patients have improved and regained independent or semi-independent existence only to complain of impaired vision due to exposure keratitis. In a comatose patient, the upper eyelid can be pulled down over the eyeball and kept fixed by a 3M or sticky tape or a cello tape. This simple measure will protect the eyes.

SUGGESTED READING

1. Bates D, Caronna JJ, Cartlidge NE, Knill-Jones RP, Levy DE, Shaw DA, et al. A prospective study of non-traumatic coma: methods and results in 310 patients. Ann Neurol. 1977;2:211-20.
2. Bates D. Coma in Clinical Neurology. New York: Churchill Livingstone; 1991. pp. 188-204.
3. Edlow JA, Newman-Toker DE, Savitz SI. Diagnosis and initial management of cerebellar infarction. Lancet Neurol. 2008;7:951-64.
4. Grill MF, Maganti RK. Neurotoxic effects associated with antibiotic use: management considerations. Br J Clin Pharmacol. 2011;72:381-93.
5. Hosting MWB, Franken MD, Meulenbelt J, van Klei WA, de Lange DW. The etiology and outcome of non-traumatic coma in critical care: a systemic review. BMC Anesthesiol. 2015;15:65.
6. Multi-Society Task Force on PVS. Medical aspects of the persistent vegetative state (1). N Engl J Med. 1994;330:1499-508.
7. Plum F, Poser JB. The diagnosis of stupor and coma. Brain Nerve. 2015;67(3):344-5.
8. Wijdicks EF, Hijdra A, Young GB, Bassetti CL, Wiebe S. Practice parameters: prediction of outcome in comatose survivors after cardiopulmonary resuscitation (an evidence-based review): report of the Quality Standards Subcommittee of the American Academy of Neurology). Neurology. 2006;67:203-10.
9. Wijdicks EFM, Bamlet WR, Maramattom BV, Manno EM, McClelland RL. Validation of a new coma scale: the FOUR score. Ann Neurol. 2005;58:585-93.

CHAPTER 9

Stroke for Physicians and Intensivists

Fali Poncha, Azad Marazban Irani, Vibhor Pardasani

■ INTRODUCTION

Stroke is defined as an abrupt onset of a focal neurological deficit corresponding to a vascular territory lasting >24 hours. It is an acute event resulting in sudden/rapidly developing weakness of a limb/limbs or the face, impairment of sensation, mental confusion, alteration in speech, loss of balance, or visual blurring.

■ CLINICAL APPROACH TO ACUTE STROKE

In the emergency room, any patient who presents with sudden or rapidly developing neurologic deficit that can clinically be localized to a vascular territory should be suspected to be having stroke.

Localization to a vascular territory implies that patients presenting with acute sensory-motor paraplegia or rapidly ascending weakness in the limbs or rapid painful unilateral visual loss or sudden bilateral hearing loss are all unlikely to be having stroke since the clinical syndromes would not correspond to defined vascular territories.

A rapid neurologic examination to confirm the presence, nature, and extent of neurologic deficit is mandatory in all patients even in those arriving in the window period. Airway, breathing, and circulation (ABC) remains of primary importance as in any other medical emergency. Patients with hypoglycemia present not just with dizziness, loss of awareness, and seizures but also at times with focal neurologic deficits. Detection and rapid reversal of hypoglycemia would spare neuroimaging in many patients. Post-seizure Todd's paresis is another important and common stroke mimic and makes current and past history of seizures indispensable. Inconsistencies in neurologic examination, absence of vascular risk factors, and previous history of spontaneously improving neurologic deficits with normal neuroimaging together may point towards a functional disorder rather than true neurologic deficit.

The National Institutes of Health Stroke Scale (NIHSS) is a validated and standardized way to measure the severity of a stroke on a 0–42 point scale (normal to worst). Once a clinical diagnosis of stroke is being considered, applying the NIHSS helps in further decision making in choosing the correct intervention for the patient who has arrived in the window period.

NEUROIMAGING

Once hypoglycemia has been excluded, the next important step in stroke management is neuroimaging. A plain CT scan of the brain is an easily available and interpretable rapid method of neuroimaging. It effectively diagnoses intracranial bleeds and obviates the need for a longer and less easily available modality of MRI. In clinically typical cases (sudden onset neurologic deficit in vascular territory), a noncontrast CT that shows no other explanation for the neurologic deficit is sufficient to diagnose acute ischemic stroke (AIS) so as to initiate immediate management including intravenous (IV) thrombolysis. However, in patients in whom the clinical presentation is atypical or the history unclear; MRI of the brain is necessary. The MRI sequences can be tailored so as to provide the essential information without consuming excessive time. These sequences include diffusion-weighted images (DWIs) and corresponding apparent diffusion coefficient (ADC) maps to detect acute infarct, gradient echo images to diagnose acute hemorrhages/hemorrhagic changes in an infarct, and fluid-attenuated inversion recovery (FLAIR) images to detect established infarcts and small acute subarachnoid hemorrhages (SAHs).

Some patients require further neuroimaging to determine eligibility for some interventions. Diffusion-weighted MRI and perfusion MRI/CT measurements are used to define ischemic brain tissue that is probably irreversibly damaged ("core") and the ischemic tissue that is potentially salvageable ("penumbra"). The mismatch between diffusion and perfusion would determine eligibility for IV thrombolysis and mechanical thrombectomy in selected patients who present beyond the thrombolytic window or in whom the time of onset of stroke is unclear. Patients with large neurologic deficit who are candidates for mechanical thrombectomy should undergo MR angiography (MRA) or CT angiography (CTA) in order to visualize the location of intracranial arterial occlusions.

It must be remembered that patients of AIS presenting within the window period may benefit with recanalization procedures such as IV thrombolysis and mechanical thrombectomy and the initial clinical and radiologic evaluation needs to be hastened so as to initiate such interventions at the earliest. IV thrombolysis can be offered to eligible patients for up to 4.5 hours from time of symptom onset while mechanical thrombectomy can be offered for up to 24 hours in correctly selected patients.

INTRAVENOUS THROMBOLYSIS WITHIN 4.5 HOURS AFTER STROKE ONSET

Patients presenting to the health facility within 4.5 hours of onset of symptoms are eligible for IV thrombolysis once intracranial hemorrhage (ICH) has been ruled out with a CT scan. IV alteplase (0.9 mg/kg body weight over 60 minutes (maximum total dose, 90 mg), with the first 10% of the dose given as a single bolus over 1 minute has been proven to reduce disability from AIS.

Eligibility criteria must be fulfilled before alteplase is offered. It is usually not recommended for those with nondisabling stroke regardless of NIHSS score.

While offering IV thrombolysis, it is important to make the patient as well as the care givers aware of the potential risks and benefits. For treatment within 3 hours of stroke onset, alteplase can lead to a good outcome for 33%, versus 23% for controls [odds ratio (OR) 1.75, 95% confidence interval (CI) 1.35–2.27]. The number needed to treat (NNT) for one additional patient to achieve a good outcome is 10. This implies that for every 10 patients undergoing IV thrombolysis, 1 patient shall have a good outcome. The good outcome is defined as per the score on Modified Rankin Score (mRS). For treatment from 3–4.5 hours, the proportion with a good outcome in the alteplase and control groups was 35 and 30% (OR 1.26, 95% CI 1.05–1.51, NNT 20). The benefit of alteplase was similar regardless of patient age or stroke severity. Clearly, the sooner the patient undergoes IV thrombolysis, the higher the chances of good neurological recovery.

While considering IV thrombolysis in a patient with AIS, it is important to run through the inclusion and exclusion criteria. Broadly, any patient with measurable neurologic deficit, presenting within 4.5 hours of stroke onset should be offered IV thrombolysis unless the infarct is already established in the CT scan or the MRI shows the infarct size to be more than two-thirds the vascular territory or the neurologic deficit has improved to the degree of not causing any disability.

What is the risk of hemorrhage following intravenous thrombolysis?
With alteplase, the risk of ICH is 5.8%. Out of every 18 patients who receive alteplase, 1 would develop ICH. Around 40% of patients developing ICH do not survive.

Can intravenous thrombolysis be offered after 4.5 hours of stroke onset if mechanical thrombectomy is not available?
If a patient presents >4.5 hours after stroke onset and thrombectomy is not available, IV thrombolysis can only be considered if certain radiologic features establish that there is a sizable "at-risk" penumbra which can be salvaged with thrombolysis. The usual considerations are:
- An abnormal signal on diffusion-weighted MRI (DWI) without any visible signal change on FLAIR imaging
- DWI lesion not larger than one-third of the territory of the middle cerebral artery (MCA)
- NIHSS score of 25 or lower
- A penumbra-to-core ratio of >1.2 and a core volume of <70 mL (as shown on perfusion CT or diffusion-weighted MRI with perfusion MRI)

ROLE OF THROMBECTOMY IN ISCHEMIC STROKES
Mechanical thrombectomy entails removing an occluding thrombus from an intracranial artery by passing a peripheral intra-arterial catheter. When

performed within 6 hours of onset of stroke in patients with occlusion of the internal carotid artery (ICA) or the first segment of the MCA (M_1), it significantly improves the chances of a better clinical outcome (OR, 2.49; 95% CI, 1.76-3.53). The NNT for functional benefit with mechanical thrombectomy has ranged from 2.6 to 4 in various clinical trials. Mechanical thrombectomy can be performed in patients with major artery occlusion who are receiving IV thrombolysis. It can be used as the sole measure in patients who are ineligible for IV alteplase. Current guidelines recommend that patients who are eligible for alteplase receive it even if mechanical thrombectomy is still under consideration.

ROLE OF ANTIPLATELETS AND STATINS

Most patients with AIS would require initiation of antiplatelets almost immediately. There is no convincing evidence that antiplatelets limits the size of an acute infarct and therefore improve neurological outcome of stroke in a direct way. However, since the risk of recurrent strokes is maximum in the initial few days of an ischemic stroke and tends to decrease with time, early institution of antiplatelets improves long-term outcome through secondary prevention. The role of high loading doses of antiplatelets (as in acute coronary syndromes) is uncertain due to lack of evidence but very unlikely to help considering that loading doses shall expose patients to higher risk of bleeding. Clopidogrel is slightly superior to aspirin in secondary stroke prevention but is costlier. Dual antiplatelets are superior to single antiplatelet for the initial 3 months. There is no added advantage of using two agents for long-term stroke prophylaxis. In large hemispheric infarcts, dual antiplatelets carry additional risk of hemorrhagic transformation and hence are best avoided in the first 1 week. Statins are usually initiated from day one for their role in secondary stroke prevention, both by way of improving the lipid profile as well as by way of plaque stabilization.

MANAGEMENT OF BLOOD PRESSURE

Blood pressure (BP) is usually elevated in patients with AIS. This may be due to chronic hypertension, an acute sympathetic response, or other stroke-mediated mechanisms to protect cerebral perfusion. The acute hypertensive effect is transient, as BP can normalize in a lot of patients within 10 days. In patients with AIS, the cerebral perfusion distal to the obstructed vessel is low. Since cerebral autoregulation gets impaired in acute stroke, blood flow in the dilated distal vessels gets dependent upon the systemic BP. Lowering the BP too rapidly can impair the perfusion and worsen the neurologic deficit.

If a patient presents with AIS within 4.5 hours of symptom onset, it is mandatory to reduce the systolic BP below 185 mm Hg and diastolic BP below 110 mm Hg before thrombolytic therapy can be initiated. This reduces the risk of thrombolysis-related ICH. BP should be stabilized and maintained at or below 180/105 mm Hg for at least 24 hours after thrombolytic treatment. The same principle also applies to patients with acute large artery thrombosis, who are being considered for mechanical thrombectomy.

If a patient with AIS is not considered for thrombolytic therapy, BP should be lowered only if it is extreme (systolic >220 mm Hg or diastolic >120 mm Hg), or in case of acute coronary syndrome, heart failure, aortic dissection, hypertensive encephalopathy, or preeclampsia/eclampsia. In such patients, BP should be lowered gradually and cautiously by approximately 15% during the first 24 hours after stroke onset. For AIS patients with stable neurologic deficit, who remain hypertensive (≥140/90 mm Hg) >3 days after the event, anti-HT should be initiated/reintroduced. The BP should be lowered gradually over 7–14 days in AIS patients with large artery stenoses. The choice of antihypertensive drug in this situation and for secondary prevention is guided by the patient profile and the comorbidities. There is no definite evidence suggesting superiority of one antihypertensive class over another.

When immediate antihypertensive therapy is needed, IV agents are recommended owing to the rapid onset of action, short half-lives, and thereby ease of titration. Labetalol is the agent of choice. It is given in a dose of 10–20 mg IV over 2 minutes; can be repeated in double dose (maximum: 80 mg/dose) at 10-minute intervals to achieve the target BP; total maximum dose: 300 mg. Alternatively after the initial bolus, a continuous infusion can be started at 0.5–2 mg/minute. IV nitroprusside and nitroglycerin are generally avoided since they can potentially elevate the intracranial pressure (ICP). Sublingual nifedipine which is commonly used in general practice for accelerated hypertension can cause a prolonged or precipitous decline in BP which can worsen the neurologic deficit. It should therefore be avoided.

If a patient with AIS is neurologically worsening or is unstable, antihypertensive therapy should be delayed till the stroke-related deficits have stabilized.

SURGERY IN LARGE HEMISPHERIC STROKE

Hemicraniectomy may be required for uncontrolled edema or malignant MCA infarction. This is a lifesaving measure, especially if performed within 24–48 hours of stroke, but it may leave up to 40% of survivors severely disabled (mRS 4). So the decision to decompress must be discussed in detail with the family after explanation of realistic expectations of outcome. Large cerebellar strokes with edema causing compression of the 4th ventricle require urgent posterior fossa decompression.

LATE COMPLICATIONS OF ACUTE STROKE

Pneumonia is the most common cause of non-neurological mortality in acute stroke patients after the second week. Most cases of pneumonia are caused by aspiration of food, saliva, or regurgitated gastric secretions. Proper and timely measures to prevent aspiration go a long way in preventing mortality and curtailing hospital stay in acute stroke patients.

Seizures occur in <5% of patients after an ischemic stroke and there is no role of prophylactic antiseizure medications irrespective of the size of the infarct. Antiseizure medications should be initiated only if a seizure occurs.

■ INTRACEREBRAL HEMORRHAGE

Intracerebral hemorrhage (ICH) comprises 10-20% of all strokes, with up to 50% of the patients dying within 30 days of experiencing an ICH. The clinical presentation of an ICH is largely similar to an ischemic stroke with a sudden onset neurological deficit. Reliably distinguishing between ICH and AIS can only be done through neuroimaging. Patients with ICH may have a decreased level of consciousness. Headache at stroke onset is more common in SAH and in ICH than in AIS or transient ischemic attack (TIA). Persons with ICH may have gradual worsening of symptoms after the abrupt onset, reflecting an increasing size of the hematoma.

Hypertension is the most common etiology of an intracerebral (IC) bleed, the usual locations being the basal ganglia (putamen and caudate), pons, thalamus, and cerebellum. Hemorrhages occurring in locations other than these should be suspected to be due to secondary causes rather than related to hypertension alone. Secondary causes/processes leading to ICH include amyloid angiopathy, tumors, hemorrhagic transformation of an ischemic stroke, cerebral venous thrombosis, vasculitis, and vascular malformations such as cavernous malformations, arteriovenous malformations, and ruptured saccular aneurysms.

Initial management of ICH focuses on standard principles of critical care such as stabilization of the patient's ABC. Frequent neurologic examinations ensure that any hematoma expansion or continuous bleeding is recognized early and managed appropriately. One must ensure that any antiplatelets/anticoagulation that the patient might be taking is immediately stopped.

An important differential of ICH is acute hemorrhagic infarction (usually embolic). Patients with hemorrhagic infarction usually have a maximal deficit at onset and do not progress. They usually do not have signs of raised ICP and have an obvious embolic source. CT scan usually shows a spotted mottled type of hyperdensity with no or mild mass effect. CT scan in ICH patients shows dense homogenous hyperdensity in subcortical regions not respecting arterial territories with prominent mass effect. If the patient has a depressed level of consciousness and a Glasgow Coma Scale score of 8 or less, endotracheal intubation should not be delayed.

Control of Hypertension

Unlike the situation in ischemic strokes, the rapid lowering of BP does not seem to have a significant effect on perihematomal cerebral perfusion in patients with ICH. Rapid correction of severe hypertension prevents hematoma expansion and is recommended in the acute phases of ICH with target BP of 160/90 mm Hg. Further reduction of systolic BP to 140 mm Hg is known to improve clinical outcome in patients presenting with systolic BP of 150–220 mm Hg. The antihypertensive agent of choice is the IV beta- and alpha-blocking agent labetalol, often used in combination with loop diuretics.

Management of Patients Who Are on Anticoagulants

Coagulation abnormalities in patients receiving anticoagulants should be treated emergently so as to prevent progressive enlargement of the hematoma. Patients with ICH in the setting of heparin anticoagulation should be treated with protamine sulfate, 1 mg per 100 units of heparin estimated in plasma. Patients who are on warfarin should receive 5–25 mg of IV vitamin K1 and, most important, fresh frozen plasma (10–20 mL/kg) or prothrombin complex concentrate (PCC).

Direct oral anticoagulants, which include direct thrombin inhibitors and factor Xa inhibitors, are used increasingly over warfarin because of their more stable pharmacokinetics. Currently, only dabigatran has a reversal agent (idarucizumab, a humanized monoclonal antibody fragment against dabigatran). For the remaining agents in this group, current anticoagulation reversal options include PCC, antifibrinolytic agents, and prohemostatic therapies such as desmopressin; dialysis is not useful because of low renal excretion of the factor Xa inhibitors. Reversal of factor Xa inhibitors is typically managed with PCC at this time.

Management of Patients with Intracranial Hemorrhage Who Are on Antiplatelets

Platelet transfusion is not known to benefit and is therefore not indicated in conservatively managed patients with ICH. It is considered in patients who have to undergo neurosurgical intervention.

Seizure Management

Seizures, a feature of the lobar/cortical rather than deep ganglionic varieties of ICH, typically occur at onset. Routine prophylactic use of antiseizure medications is not justified in patients with ICH. Tonic-clonic convulsions need immediate control as they can contribute to increased ICP and worsen the prognosis. No single antiseizure drug is superior to others in this situation. In patients with obtunded consciousness that is out of proportion to the size and location of ICH, nonconvulsive seizures must be excluded by an electroencephalogram (EEG).

Which patients benefit with surgery?
A direct surgical approach is usually considered in patients with moderate to large superficial (lobar) hematomas of the cerebral hemispheres or with

cerebellar hemorrhage. Patients with deep hemorrhages (caudate, thalamic, pontine, mesencephalic, and medullary in location) rarely benefit with surgery. Putaminal hemorrhage occupies an intermediate position and is most controversial. Few scientific data are available to assist the clinician in this therapeutic choice.

There is a definite lack of benefit of surgical treatment for most varieties of supratentorial ICH.

Most patients are currently treated nonsurgically, with the exception of those with lobar hemorrhage with progressive deterioration in the level of consciousness, and most instances of cerebellar hemorrhage. Occasional patients with putaminal ICH with clinical worsening are treated surgically with a slight improvement in survival rates but without any improvement in functional outcome. One needs to discuss and guide families in making their choice between early mortality with conservative treatment and improved survival with poor quality of life in patients with massive basal ganglionic ICHs, in whom severe hemiplegia, hemisensory loss, and aphasia or hemi-inattention syndromes are the expected lifelong disabling sequelae.

Surgery for lobar or cerebellar hematomas larger than 3 cm, in patients who deteriorate clinically, is supported by current guidelines. However, it is necessary to explain to the family that this may/may not change the functional outcomes. Here, the end-of-life care concepts and the patient's decision, if he had made any during his life, should be considered.

Uncertainty remains regarding deep hemorrhages where the parenchymal injury required to access the hematoma, appears to have been a limiting factor.

Another surgical intervention commonly used as a lifesaving measure is craniectomy to relieve the effects of raised ICP. Hemicraniectomy and suboccipital craniectomies are known.

Microsurgical clot evacuation and newer techniques like sonothrombolysis are also under constant study and are being used at some centers.

Close frequent neuromonitoring is needed. This includes sensorium monitoring, pupillary size monitoring with symmetry, and checking the plantar responses (especially of the side contralateral to the hemiparesis).

■ MANAGEMENT OF INTRAVENTRICULAR HEMORRHAGES

Primary intraventricular bleed or intraventricular extension in an IC bleed is rather common and portends a higher mortality risk. External ventricular drain (EVD) insertion, with or without use of a local thrombolytic agent for treatment of obstructive hydrocephalus is the standard of treatment in such situations. Management of BP, seizures, and other complications remains the same as in IC bleed. Studies demonstrate mortality reduction (by nearly half), with intraventricular thrombolysis (as compared to EVD alone), but whether the overall functional outcomes improve, or patients remain with a poor mRS scores (a functional disability score), remains uncertain. Subsequently few patients may need insertion of a permanent ventriculoperitoneal (VP) shunt.

■ SUBARACHNOID HEMORRHAGE

Subarachnoid hemorrhage remains one of the neurological emergencies with a high mortality and morbidity rate even in the best centers.

Spontaneous SAH is most commonly due to the rupture of saccular (berry) aneurysms (85%). 10% of SAHs may not reveal a bleeding source even with the best neurovascular imaging modalities. A minority of cases (5%) may be due to other vascular causes [e.g., arteriovenous malformation, arteriovenous fistula, reversible cerebral vasoconstriction syndrome (RCVS)].

Subarachnoid hemorrhage is clinically suspected when a patient presents with sudden onset of very severe headache, often referred to as thunderclap headache, defined as reaching maximum severity within a flash of a second. Associated with the headache there may be nausea, vomiting, photophobia, nuchal rigidity, or meningismus and loss of consciousness or coma. Unlike AIS and parenchymal hemorrhage, patients with SAH do not have focal deficits like hemiparesis at the onset of the event.

Common scales used to define severity of SAH include World Federation of Neurological Surgeons (WFNS) scale, Hunt and Hess scale, and the modified Fisher scale. Clinical grading is important as it influences recommendations for the acute management of SAH and is the most powerful prognostic factor for outcome.

Once suspected, the investigation of choice for confirmation of SAH is a plain CT scan of the brain. A CT scan is able to detect SAH rapidly after onset and blood can be seen in the subarachnoid spaces for several days. Acute blood in the cisterns and the sulci appears hyperdense and the hemorrhage pattern may indicate the location of the ruptured aneurysm while also showing other acute complications of SAH such as hydrocephalus and ICH. MRI is considered to be equally sensitive in detecting SAH in the first 2 days. However, in the hyperacute first 6 hours after SAH, CT may miss a small proportion of SAHs and MRI is slightly superior. Once SAH is diagnosed, a rapid search for the bleeding aneurysm is needed. This includes CTA or MRA or directly a digital subtraction angiography (DSA).

In cases of negative or equivocal head CT findings where a high suspicion for SAH still exists, a lumbar puncture aids diagnosis. It is one of the most sensitive tests to confirm SAH by detecting xanthochromia in the cerebrospinal fluid (CSF). Xanthochromia is yellow discoloration of CSF >12 hours after SAH due to formation in vivo of bilirubin. The CSF sample should be centrifuged immediately, stored in the dark and analyzed as soon as possible. To differentiate a traumatic tap from true SAH, CSF should be collected in four consecutive tubes. The red blood cell (RBC) count remains constant in tubes one and four in SAH patients while it falls in CSF samples with traumatic tap.

Following detection of SAH and the ruptured aneurysm, all patients should be monitored in an intensive care unit (ICU) until endovascular or surgical repair of the aneurysm. Patients with impaired consciousness usually receive an EVD for CSF drainage. Patients with acute subdural hemorrhage and/or ICH (commonly due to MCA aneurysms) may require surgical clot removal and simultaneous clipping of the ruptured aneurysm.

A ruptured aneurysm is the cause in 85% of spontaneous SAH cases and preventing a rebleed is of prime importance. Rebleeding is a life-threatening complication with a mortality rate of 20-60% and has its highest occurrence rate (8-23%) within the first 72 hours after SAH. Majority of rebleeding (50-90%) occurs within the first 6 hours, not including patients who die before hospital arrival.

Endovascular coiling is superior to microsurgical clipping in patients with high-grade SAH, those with poor medical condition aneurysms in posterior circulation, narrow neck aneurysms or aneurysms with one/more vessels arising from their neck, and in the presence of vasospasm. Patients with wide neck aneurysms in the anterior circulation and those with inadequate endovascular access benefit with clipping more than coiling.

Delayed Cerebral Ischemia

Subarachnoid hemorrhage is unique in that there is a secondary phase, commonly 3-14 days after ictus, during which delayed cerebral ischemia (DCI) can result in cerebral infarction. While angiographic vasospasm is correlated with delayed cerebral infarction after SAH, other factors include amount of hemorrhage, seizures, and hyponatremia. Seventy percent of patients with SAH develop angiographic vasospasm; 30% of these patients develop clinical symptoms for DCI and/or cerebral infarction.

Delayed cerebral ischemia should be suspected if patients with SAH develop a focal or global neurologic deficit, or have a decrease of 2 or more points on the Glasgow Coma Scale lasting for at least 1 hour and which cannot be explained by another cause. CT or MRI to confirm new infarcts if symptoms appear and CTA or MRA to suggest vasospasm. Transcranial Doppler (TCD) is the most useful noninvasive approach to monitor vasospasm. The sensitivity of TCD is good for the middle cerebral and internal carotid arteries, but is much lower for the anterior cerebral arteries and the posterior circulation arteries.

Digital subtraction angiography is the gold standard for detection of large artery vasospasm. In patients who are comatose or obtunded, a reliable neurologic examination is usually difficult and therefore regular TCD and, in addition, CTA/CT perfusion (CTP) or DSA for vasospasm screening may be even more useful.

Medical Management

All patients must receive nimodipine and maintain euvolemia.

Administration of oral nimodipine (60 mg every 4 hours, for a period of 21 days after SAH) and maintenance of normal intravascular volume status have the strongest evidence of beneficial prophylactic interventions for the prevention of DCI. A common side effect is hypotension, which may lead to hypoperfusion, and decreased cerebral perfusion pressure. In such scenarios, nimodipine dose reduction or adding an alpha-1 receptor agonist vasopressor may become mandatory.

Only symptomatic vasospasms (30% of all vasospasms) should be treated. Such patients should undergo a trial of induced hypertension. This is done by initiating IV fluids and maintaining euvolemia or mild hypervolemia. Hypertension is preferably induced using α-1 receptor agonist infusions (norepinephrine or phenylephrine). With these, systemic vasoconstriction is selectively achieved and cerebral vasoconstriction is avoided.

Triple H (HHH—hypervolemic, hypertensive, and hemodilutional) therapy is no longer supported because of the existing evidence of its adverse associations with outcomes after the use of hemodilution. The current standard treatment is the hypertensive and mild hypervolemic therapy (HHT). If neurologic deficits persist despite induced hypertension, DSA and endovascular treatment using intra-arterial vasodilators (nimodipine, nicardipine, milrinone, and verapamil) and/or angioplasty may be considered for vasospasm-related DCI.

The magnitude of BP control to reduce the risk of rebleeding has not been established, but a decrease in systolic BP to <160 mm Hg is reasonable.

Another strategy to reduce rebleeding is to administer antifibrinolytic drugs. The rationale is data suggesting that aneurysm rupture is associated with activation of fibrinolysis in clot surrounding the aneurysm. Patients treated with or without tranexamic acid or E-aminocaproic acid report a significant reduction in rebleeding but an increase of cerebral infarctions such that there was no overall effect on outcome. The right indication and timing for antifibrinolytic agents still needs to be ascertained through trials.

Cardiopulmonary complications are mediated through the hypothalamus. Sympathetic release can result in cardiac and pulmonary complications, including neurogenic ECG changes, arrhythmias, diminished cardiac contractility [stress (takotsubo) cardiomyopathy], troponin leaks, and myocardial contraction band necrosis. The early recognition and treatment of these complications is crucial in achieving the best possible outcome.

Hydrocephalus occurs in 20% of patients with SAH and is more common in those with poor grade SAH. Clinically one should suspect hydrocephalus if there is alteration in the level of consciousness, impaired upgaze, hypertension, and delirium. The diagnosis is made by repeat head CT. Insertion of an EVD or of a VP shunt (in chronic cases) may be required. Complications associated with inserting an EVD includes the risks of infection, bleeding (IC or intraventricular), and changes in the transmural pressure precipitating rebleeding of an unsecured aneurysm.

Seizures are common in poor grade SAH. Seizures occurring in the initial phase, prior to aneurysm securement, are usually a sign of early rebleeding. In severe SAH cases, prophylactic short-term use of anticonvulsants (for 3–7 days), especially with the newer antiepileptic drugs (AEDs), is very often used. A high index of suspicion for nonconvulsive seizures/status epilepticus must always be maintained for poor grade SAH patients who are already semiconscious.

Measures to prevent deep vein thrombosis should be employed in all patients with SAH right from day one. Unfractionated heparin for prophylaxis can be started 24 hours after undergoing aneurysm obliteration, after making sure there is no other bleeding diathesis. Sequential compression devices (SCDs) can be used at all stages.

Hyponatremia can occur in up to 30% of SAH patients. Its cause is presumed to be hypothalamic dysfunction, most commonly from cerebral salt-wasting due to an increase in circulating brain natriuretic peptide levels. The syndrome of inappropriate secretion of antidiuretic hormone (SIADH) should always be considered, but is generally uncommon in patients with SAH.

In both cerebral salt-wasting and SIADH, the laboratory findings are similar viz. low serum sodium, low serum osmolality, high urine sodium, and high urine osmolality. The only differentiating finding is the patient's intravascular volume status—cerebral salt-wasting is a hypovolemic state, while patients with SIADH are euvolemic or even hypervolemic. Cerebral salt-wasting is treated with fluid administration and sometimes a continuous infusion of hypertonic saline (1.5–3%) and fludrocortisones. However, patients with SIADH are treated with fluid restriction and sometimes diuresis with loop diuretics.

Patients with a negative initial DSA should have a repeat study 7–14 days after the initial one. In addition, in those with negative initial DSA/MRI of the brain and depending on the location of the SAH, MRI of the cervical spine should be performed to search for a possible arteriovenous malformation of the brain, brainstem, or spinal cord.

Nonaneurysmal perimesencephalic subarachnoid hemorrhage (PMSAH) is a special benign form of SAH with hemorrhage restricted to the perimesencephalic cisterns. Approximately 15% of patients with SAH will have negative imaging studies for a source of bleeding, of which approximately 38% have nonaneurysmal perimesencephalic SAH.

■ SUGGESTED READING

1. Andreasen TH, Bartek J Jr, Andresen M, Springborg JB, Romner B. Modifiable risk factors for aneurysmal subarachnoid hemorrhage. Stroke. 2013;44(12):3607-12.
2. Connolly ES Jr, Rabinstein AA, Carhuapoma JR, Derdeyn CP, Dion J, Higashida RT, et al. Guidelines for the management of aneurysmal subarachnoid hemorrhage: a guideline for healthcare professionals from the American Heart Association/American Stroke Association. Stroke. 2012;43(6):1711-37.
3. Diringer MN, Bleck TP, Hemphill JC, Menon D, Shutter L, Vespa P, et al. Critical care management of patients following aneurysmal subarachnoid hemorrhage: recommendations from the Neurocritical Care Society's Multidisciplinary Consensus Conference. Neurocrit Care. 2011;15(2):211-40.

4. Edlow JA, Malek AM, Ogilvy CS. Aneurysmal subarachnoid hemorrhage: update for emergency physicians. J Emerg Med. 2008;34(3):237-51.
5. Feigin VL, Lawes CM, Bennett DA, Barker-Collo SL, Parag V. Worldwide stroke incidence and early case fatality reported in 56 population-based studies: a systematic review. Lancet Neurol. 2009;8(4):355-69.
6. Goyal M, Menon BK, van Zwam WH, Dippel DWJ, Mitchell PJ, Demchuk AM, et al. HERMES collaborators. Endovascular thrombectomy after large-vessel ischaemic stroke: a meta-analysis of individual patient data from five randomised trials. Lancet. 2016;387(10029):1723-31.
7. Hemphill JC 3rd, Greenberg SM, Anderson CS, Becker K, Bendok BR, Cushman M, et al. Guidelines for the management of spontaneous intracerebral hemorrhage: a guideline for healthcare professionals from the American Heart Association/American Stroke Association. Stroke. 2015;46(7):2032-60.
8. Kapadia A, Schweizer TA, Spears J, Cusimano M, Macdonald RL, et al. Nonaneurysmal perimesencephalic subarachnoid hemorrhage: diagnosis, pathophysiology, clinical characteristics, and long-term outcome. World Neurosurg. 2014;82(6):1131-43.
9. Kasprowicz M, Lalou DA, Czosnyka M, Garnett M, Czosnyka Z. Intracranial pressure, its components and cerebrospinal fluid pressure-volume compensation. Acta Neurol Scand. 2016;134(3):168-180.
10. Molyneux A, Kerr R, Stratton I, Sandercock P, Clarke M, Shrimpton J, et al. International Subarachnoid Aneurysm Trial (ISAT) of neurosurgical clipping versus endovascular coiling in 2143 patients with ruptured intracranial aneurysms: a randomized trial. J Stroke Cerebrovasc Dis. 2002;11(6):304-14.
11. Muehlschlegel S. Subarachnoid Hemorrhage. Continuum (Minneap Minn). 2018;24(6):1623-57.
12. Suarez JI, Qureshi AI, Yahia AB, Parekh PD, Tamargo RJ, Williams MA, et al. Symptomatic vasospasm diagnosis after subarachnoid hemorrhage: evaluation of transcranial Doppler ultrasound and cerebral angiography as related to compromised vascular distribution. Crit Care Med. 2002;30(6):1348-55.
13. Suarez JI. Diagnosis and management of subarachnoid hemorrhage. Continuum (Minneap Minn). 2015;21(5 Neurocritical Care):1263-87.
14. Wijdicks EF, Sheth KN, Carter BS, Greer DM, Kasner SE, Kimberly WT, et al. Recommendations for the management of cerebral and cerebellar infarction with swelling: a statement for healthcare professionals from the American Heart Association/American Stroke Association. Stroke. 2014;45(4):1222-38.
15. Yaghi S, Willey JZ, Cucchiara B, Goldstein JN, Gonzales NR, Khatri P, et al. Treatment and Outcome of Hemorrhagic Transformation after Intravenous Alteplase in Acute Ischemic Stroke: A Scientific Statement for Healthcare Professionals from the American Heart Association/American Stroke Association. Stroke. 2017;48(12):e343-e361.

CHAPTER 10

Acute Liver Failure

Amey Sonavane, Aabha Nagral

■ DEFINITION, EPIDEMIOLOGY, AND ETIOLOGY

Acute liver failure (ALF) is characterized by a sudden insult to a healthy liver with catastrophic consequences and high short term mortality. The cardinal features of ALF include coagulopathy and encephalopathy. It is an umbrella term that includes fulminant, subfulminant, and late-onset hepatic failure. ALF is defined as presence of encephalopathy (any grade) and coagulopathy [International Normalized Ratio (INR) > 1.5 or prothrombin time (PT) > 15 seconds] in the absence of preexisting liver disease/cirrhosis. The time interval between onset of jaundice and encephalopathy varies across various definitions described across the globe **(Table 1)**. The Indian guidelines suggest development of encephalopathy within a period of 4 weeks from the onset of jaundice, although, few patients presenting like ALF secondary to drug-induced liver injury, can develop encephalopathy up to 8 weeks after the onset of jaundice.

The exact burden of ALF in India is unknown. The most common causes of ALF in India include viral hepatitis and drug-induced hepatitis due to antitubercular therapy. In about 15–47% of adults with ALF in India, the etiology is indeterminate. It is likely that these patients probably suffer from infections due to other rare viruses that are not routinely tested, for example, dengue virus, herpes simplex virus, Epstein–Barr virus, varicella zoster virus.

TABLE 1 Definition of ALF as per various authors and guidelines across the world.

	Coagulopathy	Encephalopathy	Interval between jaundice and encephalopathy
American Association for the Study of Liver Diseases	INR >1.5 or PT >15 seconds	Any grade	26 weeks
Trey and Davidson	INR >1.5	Any grade	8 weeks
O'Grady	INR >1.5	Any grade	12 weeks
Indian National Association for Study of the Liver	INR >1.5	Any grade	4 weeks

(ALF: acute liver failure; INR: International Normalized Ratio; PT: prothrombin time)

> **BOX 1** Causes of acute liver failure.
>
> *Viral hepatitis*:
> - Hepatitis A, B, and E (hepatotropic viruses)
> - Herpes simplex virus
> - Epstein–Barr virus
> - *Cytomegalovirus*
> - Parvovirus B19
> - Dengue virus
> - Varicella zoster virus
>
> *Drug-induced liver injury*:
> - Paracetamol
> - Antituberculosis drugs (isoniazid, rifampicin, and pyrazinamide)
> - Antibacterials (dapsone, sulfonamides, and cotrimoxazole)
> - Nonsteroidal anti-inflammatory drugs
> - Antiepileptic drugs (aromatic)
> - Antiretroviral dugs
> - Halothane
> - Methylenedioxy-N-methylamphetamine (MDMA)
> - Herbal and dietary supplements
> - Complementary and alternative medications
>
> *Pregnancy*:
> - Hepatitis E virus
> - Acute fatty liver of pregnancy
> - Preeclampsia
> - HELLP syndrome
>
> *Toxins*:
> - Yellow phosphorus (aluminumphosphide and rat poison)
> - Amanita phyllodes (mushroom poisoning)
> - CCl_4
>
> *Vascular*:
> - Budd–Chiari syndrome
> - *Autoimmune hepatitis*
> - *Wilson's disease*
> - Ischemic hepatitis
> - Reye syndrome
> - Hemophagocytic lymphohistiocytosis
> - *Extensive malignant infiltration of liver*

Furthermore, use of indigenous medicines as an associated cofactor cannot be ruled out. The causes of ALF are depicted in **Box 1**.

■ PATHOGENESIS

The cornerstone pathological feature in ALF is massive hepatocyte death due to apoptosis, necrosis, and immune damage. This is associated with an immune and inflammatory response in both hepatic microenvironment and systemic circulation. Activated immune cells, dying hepatocytes, and stromal cells secrete chemokines that lead to recruitment and retention of effector T and natural killer cells. This amplifies the inflammatory response and leads to a systemic inflammatory response syndrome (SIRS) which is the most common cause of death.

Hepatic encephalopathy is an integral component at presentation, the pathogenesis of which is multifactorial. Necroinflammation and rising ammonia levels cause astrocyte swelling and resultant cerebral edema and intracerebral hypertension. Ammonia also alters neurotransmission and affects mitochondrial function. Cerebral complications determine the outcome of disease and prognosis of the patient.

Acute kidney injury can be associated with ALF, especially in cases of paracetamol poisoning. Risk factors include older age, SIRS, development of sepsis, hypotension with resultant vasopressor support and severity of ALF. Mechanisms of acute kidney injury include toxic or ischemic acute tubular necrosis and systemic inflammation. Hepatorenal syndrome may also occur in a few cases of ALF. Acute kidney injury is also associated with poorer prognosis.

Emerging evidence has demonstrated that there is a close entwined connection between the liver, the gut, and the immune system. A "leaky" gut is instrumental in the pathogenesis of sepsis associated multiorgan failure. Uncontrolled release of inflammatory cytokines secondary to bacterial endotoxins and damage-associated molecular patterns (DAMPs) are responsible for multiorgan failure. Once multiorgan dysfunction sets in, the prognosis worsens.

■ CLINICAL FEATURES

Acute liver failure may manifest initially with constitutional symptoms that include malaise, fever, nausea, vomiting, fatigue, anorexia, upper abdominal pain, and arthralgias. The symptoms evolve to hepatic encephalopathy, hypotension, and those related to multiorgan failure. More than 80% patients develop encephalopathy within 2 weeks of the onset of icterus, and all patients present within 4 weeks of onset of jaundice. Hepatic encephalopathy can have varied clinical manifestations ranging from altered sensorium, drowsiness, slowed mentation, cognitive impairment and confusion to deep coma. It is classically graded on a scale from 1 to 4, with 4 pronouncing deep coma and thus poorer prognosis.

After acute liver injury, circulating levels of fibrinogen, prothrombin, and factors V, VII, IX, and X fall. Synthesis of anticoagulant proteins (e.g., proteins C and S), as well as antithrombin also reduces, and often remains in physiologic balance with the levels of coagulation factors. Thus, though the patients have elevated prothrombin and partial thromboplastin times, clinically significant spontaneous bleeding is rare. Less than 1% of patients may have spontaneous intracranial bleed.

Bacterial and fungal infections are common secondary to altered immune defense mechanisms. Bacterial pneumonias, urinary tract infections, and intravenous catheter-induced sepsis are common. The predominant bacteria include *Staphylococcus aureus*, streptococci, and coliform bacteria, whereas *Candida* species accounts for most of the fungal infections. Fungal sepsis indicates extremely poor prognosis.

Hypoglycemia is an important feature and is a result of impaired gluconeogenesis in the affected liver and reduced uptake of insulin by the hepatocytes. Impaired systemic microcirculation and failure of the liver to clear lactate are important reasons for hyperlactatemia. Common electrolyte abnormalities include hyponatremia, hypokalemia, and hypophosphatemia. This can result in cardiac arrhythmias.

Circulatory dysfunction ensues, initially due to hypovolemia and later fuelled by cytokine and inflammatory mediators. This results in low systemic vascular resistance, systemic hypotension, and increased cardiac output. These hemodynamic derangements lead to decreased peripheral tissue oxygenation and eventually multiorgan failure.

■ EVALUATION AND MONITORING OF PATIENTS WITH ACUTE LIVER FAILURE

Box 2 includes the baseline laboratory tests and **Table 2** summarizes tests used to determine the etiology of ALF, depending upon the clinical presentation.

After a diagnosis of ALF is established, the components of monitoring a patient with ALF can be broadly classified into biochemical parameters, hemodynamic monitoring, and neurological monitoring **(Table 3)**.

The role of liver biopsy in the diagnosis and management of ALF is limited and biopsy is not performed routinely. If performed, the findings on biopsy may support specific diagnosis such as autoimmune hepatitis (interface hepatitis and characteristic inflammation are typical; although autoimmune ALF shows characteristic necrosis and not typical features), pregnancy-related syndromes (fatty infiltration characteristic of acute fatty liver of pregnancy or fibrin microthrombi and necrosis secondary to preeclampsia or eclampsia),

---

BOX 2 Baseline laboratory tests to be performed in a patient with acute liver failure (ALF).

- Complete blood count
- Liver function tests
- Renal function tests
- Prothrombin time (International Normalized Ratio)
- Serum lipase
- Serum phosphorus
- Arterial blood sample for arterial blood gas (ABG); lactate level and ammonia level
- Urine routine and culture
- Blood culture set (BACTEC Plus if patient has received prior antibiotics)
- Abdominal ultrasound with Doppler examination
- Chest X-ray
- Electrocardiogram
- Two-dimensional echocardiogram

TABLE 2 Summary of tests used to evaluate the probable etiology of ALF.

Viral etiology	Anti-HAV IgM, anti-HEV IgM, HBsAg, anti-HCV, and anti-HBc IgM
Autoimmune markers	Antinuclear antibody, serum immunoglobulin G, and anti-smooth muscle antibody (if needed)
Other infective workup	Rapid malaria test, rapid dengue test, and anti-*Leptospira* IgM
In selected cases	β-hCG and uric acid (females of child-bearing age; if indicated), serum ceruloplasmin (if Wilson's disease suspected, not recommended), Serum acetaminophen level and urine toxic screen, CT/MRI venography of abdomen (in suspected cases of Budd–Chiari syndrome), anti-HSV IgM, CMV DNA viral load quantitative, anti-parvovirus IgM, anti-EBV IgM, and anti-VZV IgM (depending on clinical presentation, especially when SGOT >> SGPT)

(ALF: acute liver failure; β-hCG: β-human chorionic gonadotropin; CMV: cytomegalovirus; DNA: deoxyribonucleic acid; EBV: Epstein–Barr virus; HAV: hepatitis A virus; HBc: hepatitis B core antigen; HBsAg: hepatitis B surface antigen; HCV: hepatitis C virus; HEV: hepatitis E virus; HSV: herpes simplex virus; IgM: immunoglobulin M; SGOT: serum glutamic oxaloacetic transaminase; SGPT: serum glutamic pyruvic transaminase; VZV: varicella zoster virus)

TABLE 3 Components of monitoring a patient with ALF.

Parameters	*Frequency of monitoring*
Biochemistry:	
• PT/INR	• 12th hourly
• Blood sugar levels	• Hourly—4th hourly
• Arterial ammonia	• 12th hourly
• Serum lactate levels	• 12th hourly
• Serum sodium levels	• 12th hourly
• Liver and kidney function tests	• 12th hourly—daily
• Surveillance blood, urine, and ET cultures	• Every 48 hours
• Thromboelastogram (TEG)	• If bleeding—decision on appropriate blood products
Hemodynamic monitoring:	
• Blood pressure	• Continuous
• Core body temperature	• Continuous
• Urine output	• Hourly
Neurological monitoring: Intracerebral pressure	Invasive methods not recommended; noninvasive monitoring may be considered (optic nerve sheath diameter and transcranial Doppler)

(ALF: acute liver failure; ET: Endotracheal tube; INR: International Normalized Ratio; PT: prothrombin time) valproic acid toxicity (microvesicular steatosis) and Budd–Chiari syndrome (venous congestion and sinusoidal dilatation).

Over the last few decades, multiple prognostic scores have been developed and validated. Leading examples include King's College criteria (KCC), Clichy criteria, model for end-stage liver disease (MELD) score, MELD-Sodium (MELD-Na) score, clinical prognostic indicator (CPI) score, and acute liver failure early dynamic (ALFED) score. Common variables to these scores are coagulopathy, grades of encephalopathy, bilirubin, presence or absence of raised intracranial pressure (ICP), underlying etiology, age, and jaundice to encephalopathy interval.

The KCC **(Box 3)** was developed by O'Grady et al. for paracetamol and nonparacetamol-induced liver failure. Its sensitivity ranges between 68–69% and specificity from 82% to 92%. Liver transplantation (LT) should be considered in patients satisfying the KCC.

The Clichy criteria also effectively determine the outcomes. These criteria are based on factor V levels, with discriminatory values <20% in patients under 30 years of age, and <30% in older patients. These criteria are applicable once grade 2 encephalopathy has developed.

The ALFED score **(Table 4)** is the first model to assess and stratify patients with ALF dynamically over a period of 3 days. This was described in Indian patients with mainly viral etiology unlike the KCC. ALFED score is found to be superior to KCC and MELD scores. ALFED score ≥4 has a high positive predictive value (85%) and negative predictive value (87%) in the validation cohort. An arterial ammonia level of >123 µmol/L was found to predict mortality with 78.6% sensitivity and 76.3% specificity and had 77.5% diagnostic accuracy. Higher ammonia levels are associated with deeper encephalopathy, cerebral edema, need for ventilation, and seizures.

BOX 3 The King's College criteria (used to determine consideration for liver transplantation).

King's College Hospital Indicators of a poor prognosis in acute liver failure
Acetaminophen cases:
- Arterial pH < 7.25 more than 24 hours after drug ingestion

All of the following:
- Prothrombin time > 100 seconds or INR > 6.5
- Serum creatinine level > 3.4 mg/dL (300 µmol/L) or anuria
- Grade 3 to 4 encephalopathy

Nonacetaminophen cases
- Prothrombin time > 100 seconds or INR > 6.5

Any three of the following:
- Unfavorable etiology (seronegative hepatitis or drug reaction)
- Age < 10 or > 40 years
- Acute or subacute category (duration of jaundice > 7 days)
- Serum bilirubin level > 17.5 mg/dL (300 µmol/L)
- Prothrombin time > 50 seconds or INR > 3.5

(INR: International Normalized Ratio)

TABLE 4 The dynamic ALFED score to assess and stratify patients with ALF.

ALFED model

Variables over 3 days	Score assigned
• Hepatic encephalopathy (persistent or progressed to grade >2)	2
• INR (persistent or increased to ≥5)	1
• Arterial ammonia (persistent or increased to ≥123 mmol/L)	2
• Serum bilirubin (persistent or increased to ≥15 mg/dL)	1

Those with a score of 1–3 had a survival probability of about 80% or more, and those with ≥4 had a mortality risk of >80%.

(ALF: acute liver failure; ALFED: acute liver failure early dynamic; INR: International Normalized Ratio)

BOX 4 Clinical indications to determine urgent transfer to the intensive care unit.

- Hepatic encephalopathy grade 2 and higher or difficulty to manage the patient in the ward
- *Hypotension:* Mean arterial pressure (MAP) <60 mm Hg after adequate fluid resuscitation
- Oliguria despite fluid resuscitation
- Oxygen requirement > 6 L/min to maintain SpO_2 > 95
- Recurrent hypoglycemia

(SpO_2: peripheral oxygen saturation)

■ MANAGEMENT

Over the last few decades, the survival of patients with ALF has been improving. This seems to be a reflection of better intensive care and certain interventions in these patients. The pillar stones of management include (1) intensive care unit based aggressive supportive therapy including organ support systems; (2) identification and treatment of etiology; (3) elimination of toxic products like ammonia; and (4) prevention and treatment of fatal complications such as cerebral edema, sepsis, renal failure, and gastrointestinal bleeding. All patients with ALF should be hospitalized and monitored closely. Majority will need intensive care management. If the hospital does not have adequate facilities, transfer to a tertiary care/transplant centre should be initiated. The indications to transfer to the intensive care unit are summarized in **Box 4**.

Various specific aspects of management are discussed below.

Ventilation

Mechanical ventilation should be initiated once the patient has grade 3 or higher encephalopathy. The aim of ventilation should be to protect airways and ensure physiological oxygen concentration and normocapnia. Sedation with propofol, low tidal volumes (6-8 mL/kg predicted body weight), and minimum positive end-expiratory pressure (PEEP) is the preferred lung protective strategy in mechanically ventilated patients with ALF. Minute ventilation should be titrated to get a target partial pressure of carbon dioxide (PCO_2) of 30–40 mm Hg with avoidance of hypocarbia and hypercarbia. Agents to be used for analgesia and sedation include propofol and fentanyl. The aim must be to minimize tactile stimuli, avoid unnecessary neck rotation, dim ambient lights, and keep the head-end elevated (around 20–30°).

Hemodynamics

If the patient is hemodynamically unstable, fluid replacement should be initiated promptly (Plasmalyte, especially if serum lactate levels are high; avoid Ringer's lactate), followed by inotropes (norepinephrine and vasopressin). Care must be taken to avoid hypervolemia by using dynamic assessment of fluid status (inferior vena cava collapsibility, assessment of B lines in lung fields).

Renal Dysfunction

For renal dysfunction, it is ideal to institute early continuous renal replacement therapy (CRRT), especially in patients with progressive encephalopathy and hyperammonemia, severe metabolic acidosis, uremia, electrolyte imbalance (hyponatremia, hyperkalemia, and hypermagnesemia), and acetaminophen-related ALF. CRRT [high volume continuous veno-venous hemofiltration (CVVH)/continuous veno-venous hemodiafiltration (CVVHDF)], is better than the intermittent form in presence of severe hemodynamic instability. In patients with high arterial ammonia levels, progressive encephalopathy and increasing lactate levels, CVVH may be initiated even without evident renal dysfunction. It is advisable to use a bicarbonate based buffer solution instead of lactate/citrate-based solutions for CRRT. Anticoagulation with heparin is best avoided in presence of coagulopathy. The use of citrate-based solutions is recommended with strict monitoring of ionized calcium and acid base status. CRRT in ALF requires particular attention in terms of antibiotic dose adjustment, electrolyte correction, nutritional demand, and other drug dose adjustments.

Raised Intracranial Pressure

It is recommended to keep the head-end elevated (30–40°) and avoid ties around the neck or unnecessary neck movement and chest physiotherapy. For raised ICP, 3% NaCl is preferred, especially in hypotensive patients. A target serum sodium level of 145–155 mEq/L is aimed. Intravenous mannitol is another agent that can be used in raised ICP. The dose is 0.25–0.5 mg/kg boluses over 20–30 minutes, which can be repeated two to three times till serum osmolality reaches 320 mOsm. A fixed dose schedule is not preferred and is best avoided in patents with renal dysfunction. The usual practice is to use hypertonic saline as a continuous infusion and use mannitol as intermittent boluses for ICP surges. Noninvasive assessment by optic nerve sheath diameter and clinical parameters could be done in all intubated patients regularly.

Coagulopathy

Transfusion of blood products is indicated only if there is clinical evidence of bleeding or in case any invasive procedure is planned. Thromboelastogram-based blood product therapy is recommended. There is no role for prophylactic correction of deranged coagulation parameters as it affects prognosis, increases the risk of thrombosis, volume overload, and transfusion-related acute lung injury (TRALI). Also, INR is a good prognostic marker and administering fresh frozen plasma (FFP) can confound results.

Infection

Worsening hypotension or encephalopathy, renal failure, or development of metabolic acidosis could suggest sepsis in patients with ALF. Broad-spectrum antibiotics (beta-lactam and beta-lactamase inhibitors, e.g., piperacillin + tazobactam, cefoperazone + sulbactam) and antifungals should be started early in the course of the illness. However, the choice of empirical antibiotics should be guided by local microbiological profiles. The dosages of antibiotics need adjustment when the patient is initiated on CRRT, plasmapheresis, molecular adsorbent recirculating system (MARS), or any other form of extracorporeal treatment.

Electrolyte Balance

Hyponatremia is detrimental and the serum sodium must be maintained between 145 and 155 mEq/L. Hypokalemia or hyperkalemia should be aggressively treated to maintain the serum potassium level around 4-4.5 mEq/L. When CRRT is initiated, it is prudent to check serum magnesium and serum phosphate levels; if citrate-based anticoagulation is used, it is essential to monitor ionized calcium.

Hypoglycemia

The aim is to maintain euglycemia (140-180 mg/dL) using 25% or 50% dextrose infusion. Adrenal insufficiency should be looked for by random cortisol measurement, and if present, needs treatment.

Nutrition

Early enteral feeding (within 24 hours) is recommended. Ideal calorie intake target should be 25-30 kcal/kg/day along with a protein intake of 1.2-1.5 g/kg body weight/day of proteins. There is no role of restriction of dietary proteins. Use of branched-chain amino acid (BCAA)-enriched formulas may have some benefit in patients with hepatic encephalopathy.

General Care

Intravenous N-acetyl cysteine (NAC) should be used in all cases of ALF, although benefit has been shown only during early stages of encephalopathy.

The loading dose of NAC is 150 mg/kg over 1 hour, followed by 50 mg/kg over 4 hours, and then 100 mg/kg over 16 hours as a continuous infusion. Proton pump inhibitors should be used in prophylactic dosages to protect the gastric mucosa. If the patient has seizures, anticonvulsants should be started (levetiracetam/lacosamide). Lactulose should be used to ensure adequate bowel movements. Overzealous usage of lactulose can result in ileus. Polyethylene glycol is a good substitute/addition if the patient requires high doses of lactulose. Hemoglobin target for transfusion is 7 g/dL. Pancreatitis should be evaluated for and treated with supportive measures, especially in cases of acetaminophen/toxin injury. Hepatotoxic and nephrotoxic drugs are best avoided. All invasive lines should be ideally cannulated using ultrasound guidance. Fever or hypothermia should be promptly treated.

General Nursing Care

Care should be taken during Foley's catheterization. Administration of enema may be avoided as there is an increased tendency to bleed. Deep vein thrombosis (DVT) prophylaxis, using serial compression devices, should be initiated. Pressure sores/skin peels should be actively looked for and prevented. Aseptic precautions should be ensured while handling invasive lines, cannulas, and tubings.

Other Extracorporeal Treatments in Acute Liver Failure

High Volume Plasma Exchange

High volume plasma exchange (HPVE) may have potential benefit in patients where liver transplant is not possible or contraindicated. In HVPE, around 10-12 L of FFP is exchanged at the rate of 1-2 L/hour per session, for 3 consecutive days. HVPE causes significant reduction in bilirubin, INR, and increase in serum albumin levels. It has been used as a bridge to transplant. In fact, there have been a few anecdotal reports of patients even escaping liver transplant.

Molecular Adsorbent Recirculating System and Extracorporeal Albumin Dialysis

Decision to start therapy is taken on a case-by-case basis. These techniques may give some physiological stabilization in patients awaiting LT. The timing of initiation is not well defined; however, early initiation at lower sequential organ failure assessment (SOFA) score (<7) may be beneficial in sicker patients. CRRT/HVPE seems more economical and equally beneficial in the Indian setting.

Liver Transplantation in Acute Liver Failure

Liver transplantation in ALF is a lifesaving intervention if performed on time. LT for ALF has evolved as an established treatment in selected cases of ALF and has led to a reduction in mortality from 80% to 30%. LT can be considered as a possible option in those patients who fulfill the King's College/ALFED criteria.

> **BOX 5** Contraindications for liver transplantation.
>
> *Absolute contraindications*
> - Severe cardiopulmonary disease
> - Extrahepatic malignancy (oncologic criteria for cure not met)
> - Active alcohol/substance abuse
> - Active infection/uncontrolled sepsis
> - Lack of psychosocial support/inability to comply with medical treatment
> - Irreversible brain damage
>
> *Relative contraindications*
> - Advanced age
> - Acquired immune deficiency syndrome
> - Systemic disease (e.g., dengue virus-related ALF)
> - Diffuse mesenteric and portal vein thrombosis

The criteria should be reviewed regularly. Dynamic models like ALFED score should be employed and LT should not be performed if the patient is recovering clinically. Counseling of relatives regarding possible need of transplant should be done as early as feasible after admission to hospital.

Patients of ALF with more than three organ failure, circulatory failure with the requirement of two vasopressors, both with limited responses to further dose escalation, absence of brainstem reflexes, severe respiratory failure requiring maximum ventilator support [fraction of inspired oxygen (FiO_2) > 0.8 and high PEEP), or on extracorporeal membrane oxygenation (ECMO) should be considered as contraindications for LT. Relative contraindications to LT include ongoing severe sepsis and tissue invasive fungal infection **(Box 5)**.

■ CONCLUSION

With progress in our understanding of the pathogenesis and improving intensive care, ALF is now better managed and treated, with or without the need for LT.

■ SUGGESTED READING

1. Acharya SK, Dasarathy S, Kumer TL, Sushma S, Prasanna KS, Tandon A, et al. Fulminant hepatitis in a tropical population: clinical course, cause, and early predictors of outcome. Hepatology. 1996;23:1448-55.
2. Anand AC, Garg HK. Approach to clinical syndrome of jaundice and encephalopathy in tropics. J Clin Exp Hepatol. 2015;5:S116-S130.
3. Anand AC, Nandi B, Acharya SK, Arora A, Babu S, Batra Y, et al. Indian National Association for the Study of Liver Consensus Statement on Acute Liver Failure (Part-2): Management of Acute Liver Failure. J Clin Exp Hepatol. 2020;10(5):477-517.
4. Bernal W, Auzinger G, Sizer E, Wendon J. Intensive Care Management of Acute Liver Failure. Semin Liver Dis. 2008;28(2):188-200.
5. Bernal W, Hyyrylainen A, Gera A, Audimoolam VK, McPhail MJW, Auzinger G, et al. Lessons from look-back in acute liver failure? A single centre experience of 3300 patients. J Hepatol. 2013;59:74-80.
6. Cardoso FS, Gottfried M, Tujios S, Olson JC, Karvellas CJ. Continuous renal replacement therapy is associated with reduced serum ammonia levels and mortality in acute liver failure. Hepatology. 2018;67:711-20.

7. Choudhary NS, Saigal S, Saraf N, Rastogi A, Goja S, Bhangui P, et al. Good outcome of living donor liver transplantation in drug-induced acute liver failure: a single-center experience. Clin Transplant. 2017;31(3).
8. Cordoba J, Dhawan A, Larsen FS, Manns M, Samuel D, Simpson KJ, et al. EASL Clinical Practical Guidelines on the management of acute (fulminant) liver failure. J Hepatol. 2017;66:1047-81.
9. Donnelly MC, Hayes PC, Simpson KJ. The changing face of liver transplantation for acute liver failure: Assessment of current status and implications for future practice. Liver Transplant. 2016;22(4):527-35.
10. Kaido T, Ogawa K, Ogura Y, Hata K, Yoshizawa A, Yagi S, et al. Liver Transplantation in Adults with Acute Liver Failure: A Single Center Experience over A Period of 15 Years. Hepatogastroenterology. 2015;62:937-41.
11. Khuroo MS, Kamili S. Aetiology and prognostic factors in acute liver failure in India. J Viral Hepat. 2003;10:224-31.
12. Koch DG, Speiser JL, Durkalski V, Fontana RJ, Davern T, McGuire B, et al. The natural history of severe acute liver injury. Am J Gastroenterol. 2017;112:1389-96.
13. Kumar R, Bhatia V. Structured approach to treat patients with acute liver failure: A hepatic emergency. Indian J Crit Care Med. 2012;16(1):1-7.
14. Kumar R, Sharma H, Goyal R, Kumar A, Khanal S, Prakash S, et al. Prospective derivation and validation of early dynamic model for predicting outcome in acute liver failure. Gut. 2012;61(7):1068-75.
15. Lee HS, Choi GH, Joo DJ, Kim MS, Kim SI, Han KH, et al. Prognostic value of model for end-stage liver disease scores in patients with fulminant hepatic failure. Transplant Proc. 2013;45:2992-4.
16. Lee WM, Stravitz RT, Larson AM. Introduction to the revised American Association for the Study of Liver Diseases Position Paper on acute liver failure 2011. Hepatology. 2012;55:965-7.
17. O'Grady JG, Alexander GJ, Hayllar KM, Williams R. Early indicators of prognosis in Liver. Gastroenterology. 1989;97:439-45.
18. Pamecha V, Vagadiya A, Sinha PK, Sandhyav R, Parthasarthy K, Sasturkar S, et al. Live donor liver transplantation for acute liver failure—donor safety and recipient outcome. Liver Transplant. 2019;25(9):1408-21.
19. Samuel D, Saliba F, Ichai P. Changing outcomes in acute liver failure: Can we transplant only the ones who really need it? Liver Transplant. 2015;21:S36-8.
20. Shalimar, Sonila U, Kedia S, Mahapatra SJ, Nayak B, Yadav DP, et al. Comparison of dynamic changes among various prognostic scores in viral hepatitis-related acute liver failure. Ann Hepatol. 2018;17:403-12.
21. Stravitz RT, Kramer AH, Davern T, Shaikh AO, Caldwell SH, Mehta RL, et al. Intensive care of patients with acute liver failure: recommendations of the U.S. Acute Liver Failure Study Group. Crit Care Med. 2007;35:2498-508.
22. Stravitz RT, Kramer DJ. Management of acute liver failure. Nat Rev Gastroenterol Hepatol. 2009:6:542-53.
23. Tujios SH, Hynan LS, Vazquez MA, Larson AM, Seremba E, Sanders CM, et al. Risk Factors and Outcomes of Acute Kidney Injury in Patients With Acute Liver Failure. Clin Gastroenterol Hepatol. 2015;13(2):352-9.
24. Vaquero J, Chung C, Cahill ME, Blei AT. Pathogenesis of hepatic encephalopathy in acute liver failure. Semin Liver Dis. 2003;23:259-69.
25. Zalewska K. POLICY POL195/6 Liver Transplantation: Selection Criteria and Recipient Registration. [online] Available from: http://odt.nhs.uk/pdf/liver_selection_policy.pdf. [Last accessed September, 2021].

SECTION 4

Infection

- **Sepsis and its Sequelae**
  Jamshed Sunavala

- **Antimicrobial Therapy in the Intensive Care Unit**
  Ayesha Sunavala

- **Optimal Usage of the Microbiology Laboratory in the ICU**
  Karuna Tiwari, Camilla Rodrigues

- **Invasive Fungal Infections in the ICU: Diagnosis and Management**
  Rajeev Soman, Rakshita Eashwernath

- **Ventilator-associated Pneumonia**
  Joanne Mascarenhas

- **Case Studies in ICU Infections**
  Rajeev Soman, Rakshita Eashwernath

CHAPTER 11

Sepsis and its Sequelae

Jamshed Sunavala

■ INTRODUCTION

The term "sepsis" is derived from the Greek word "sepo" meaning "decay" or "putrefaction" and the word "shock" is derived from the French word "choquer" meaning to "hit or collide". Throughout the history, sepsis was associated with some external agent or some form of infection. By the 16th century the confirmation of the Germ Theory and Koch's Postulates well established this concept and sepsis became synonymous with systemic infection. It was only in the 1970s that one realized that despite antibiotics and eradication of the pathogens along with successful resuscitation, many patients failed to survive. The NEJM publication in 1972 first alluded to the possible role of an inflammatory response to infection. Further studies reinforced the fact that the host's hyperinflammatory response to infection released cytokines which lead to organ dysfunction. However, it was not till 1991 at the ACCP/SCCM Consensus Conference that *Sepsis and its Sequelae* were first defined and published by Roger Bone and his colleagues in "Chest" in 1992.

■ DEFINITION

The 1992, definition of sepsis was described as two or more of the systemic inflammatory response syndrome (SIRS) following an infective pathology, manifest clinically or confirmed on culture. Severe sepsis was defined as infection-induced organ dysfunction or tissue hypoperfusion, and septic shock as hypotension persisting despite adequate volume challenge **(Table 1)**. This definition is now labeled as Sepsis-1. In 2006, an unsuccessful attempt was made to revise this definition by adding a few more clinical and laboratory variables and biomarkers and it was labeled as Sepsis-2 definition. However the Sepsis-1 definition of 1992 continued to be used for all clinical and academic purposes, as the additional parameters added in 2006, did not significantly contribute in increasing the sensitivity or specificity toward diagnosing sepsis; rather, the myriad additional investigations caused unwanted delay in the prompt treatment of a critically ill patient.

In 2016, the third Consensus Conference proposed a new definition labeled Sepsis-3, where the term severe sepsis was dropped and sepsis was redefined as a "life-threatening organ dysfunction caused by a dysregulated host response to infection" **(Table 2)**. Organ dysfunction was identified as an acute change in Sequential Organ Failure Assessment (SOFA) score by 2 or

TABLE 1	Sepsis-1 (1992) definition.
Sepsis	Systemic infection manifested by two or more of the SIRS criteria, secondary to a suspected or known source of infection
SIRS	Systemic inflammatory response syndrome (SIRS): • WBC > 12,000 mm³ or <4,000/mm³ or > 10% immature bands • Respiratory rate > 20 or $PaCO_2$ < 32 mm Hg • Body temperature > 38°C or < 36°C • Hear rate > 90/minute
Severe sepsis	Sepsis with any organ dysfunction (including hypotension, lactic acidosis, oliguria or altered mental status)
Septic shock	Sepsis + systolic BP < 90 mm Hg despite adequate volume challenge and requiring vasopressor support

TABLE 2	Sepsis-3 (2016) definition.
Sepsis	Life-threatening organ dysfunction caused by a dysregulated host response to an infection
Criteria of organ dysfunction	Acute change in the SOFA score by 2 or more points from the baseline
Septic shock	It is subset of sepsis with persistent hypotension requiring vasopressors to maintain MAP ≥ 65 mm Hg and serum lactate ≥ 2 mmol/L despite adequate volume resuscitation

(SOFA: Sequential Organ Failure Assessment)

more from the baseline and septic shock was considered a subset of sepsis where the underlying circulatory compromise and the cellular/metabolic abnormalities were serious enough to substantially increase mortality. However many centers continue to use the Sepsis-1 definition of 1992 and not altogether without merit.

Features of sepsis are often confounded by pre-existing comorbidities and hence organ dysfunction may not be apparent in the early phase of sepsis which may delay prompt treatment, whereas Sepsis-1 with its less stringent criteria, remains a more sensitive definition. Thus to increase early diagnosis, a Sepsis-3 expert panel included a bedside early warning score called quick SOFA (q-SOFA) **(Box 1)**. To complement q-SOFA, the National Early Warning Score (NEWS) was devised adding a few more bedside parameters. Personally, we still prefer the Sepsis-1 definition rather than getting shackled with scoring systems thereby missing an impending catastrophe, especially in the fast track environment of an emergency medical service (EMS). We still feel that a patient with tachypnea, high fever and with clinical evidence of infection, deserves to be in the ICU and it would be unwise to wait for organ dysfunction to manifest. It is interesting to note that the International Classification of Diseases Codes and the latest standard *Textbook of Critical Care Medicine (Parillo and Dellinger, 2019 edition)*, however continue to use the 1992 Sepsis-1 definition.

> **BOX 1** Quick sequential organ failure assessment (qSOFA).
>
> The qSOFA is used to identify high-risk patients for in-hospital mortality with suspected infection at the bedside
> *Criteria:*
> - Respiratory rate ≥ 22/min
> - Acute change in mental state (GCS < 15)
> - Systolic BP ≤100 mm Hg
>
> *A positive qSOFA ≥ 2 suggests high risk of poor outcome in patients with suspected infection*

■ PATHOGENESIS

This chapter does not intend to go into a detailed discourse on the pathogenesis of sepsis; excellent and extensive material is available in standard textbooks. However, to briefly understand the complex interaction between the infecting organism and the host response, we have endeavored to simplify it by briefly explaining the progression of the invading organism crossing the mucosal barrier and attacking host defenses, thus creating a pro- and anti-inflammatory response, and finally leading to life-threatening organ failure.

Depending on the virulence/load of the organism and patient immunity, the host defenses are compromised, allowing the crossing of the pathogen through the mucosal barrier.

The host defense now recognizes the molecular component of the invading organism, more specifically called *pathogen activated molecular pattern (PAMP)* and these are immediately recognized by specialized host receptors called *pattern recognition receptors (PRRs)*. PRRs have four main families of receptors of which the best known are the *toll-like receptors (TLRs)*, activated by "ligands" presented by the organisms, and each TLR remains specific to either bacteria, virus or fungi. Stimulation of PRRs after recognizing the PAMP leads to activation of proinflammatory "cytokines".

These cytokines cause a systemic inflammatory response with vasodilatation and cardiac dysfunction leading to hemodynamic collapse and tissue damage. The damaged tissue in turn releases endogenous molecules called *damage associated molecular patterns (DAMPs)*, from the injured cells. Polytrauma, major surgery, extensive burns also release similar molecules. DAMPs are also recognized by the host receptors (PRRs), resulting in further increase of cytokines and producing a vicious cycle of perpetuation of inflammation. The end result of the hyperinflammation from both PAMP and DAMP molecules culminates in a cytokine storm with life-threatening organ failure (MODS).

■ COAGULATION AND SEPSIS

Coagulation abnormalities occur consistently in patients with sepsis and can range from subtle hemostatic changes which may be barely perceptible clinically, to somewhat more severe coagulation activation which manifests by a mild fall in platelet count. However, in severe sepsis one-third of the patients can succumb to fulminant disseminated intravascular coagulation (DIC), manifested by the microvascular thrombosis and simultaneous hemorrhage from different sites. In this case, hemorrhage is due to consumption of coagulation factors and platelets. Majority of septic patients will develop thrombocytopenia and the severity of the sepsis often correlates with the fall in platelet count. However, the thrombocytopenia may well be due to associated comorbidities and not necessarily due to severe sepsis such as medications (antibiotics) or heparin-induced thrombocytopenia (HIT) all of which often poses a problem in differentiating sepsis-induced thrombocytopenia from other causes. Abnormality of other coagulation assays such as a prolonged prothrombin time (PT) or activated partial thromboplastin time (aPTT) may not be apparent in every case of sepsis except when complicated with severe DIC.

The primary trigger in initiation of thrombus generation is a "tissue factor" which occurs due to a release of proinflammatory cytokines. Platelet activation can also be triggered by proinflammatory mediators which can also generate fibrin formation (fibrin-platelet clot). Basically the three important anticoagulant pathways which are responsible for preventing undue intravascular thrombosis, viz. the antithrombin system, the activated protein C system and the tissue factor pathway inhibitor, are deranged in sepsis.

Isolated thrombocytopenia has a dubious value in diagnosis of DIC as shown earlier. Prothrombin time can be falsely elevated due to an associated liver disease and measurement of fibrin degradation products (FDP) or fibrinogen levels may be useful but has its limitations. However, a scoring system devised by the International Society of Thrombosis and Hemostasis (ISTH), based on available laboratory data such as platelet count, PT (INR), D-dimer and fibrinogen levels, showed a reasonably high diagnostic accuracy.

■ DIAGNOSIS

The three definitions of sepsis **(Tables 1 and 2; Box 1)** vividly describe the clinical and biochemical manifestations of sepsis. However signs of SIRS are typical of early sepsis characterized by hypothermia or hyperthermia, tachypnea, tachycardia and elevation or reduction of white blood cell count. By Sepsis-1 definition, there should be at least two of the signs to suspect sepsis, provided there is a clinical or confirmed evidence of underlying infection. However using this criterion is to risk detecting a significant population with false positives because signs of inflammation are often commonly seen in patients with bloodstream infection with no evidence of sepsis. Nonetheless, it is a useful benchmark for physicians to detect early sepsis in the community or in the EMS.

Hypotension not responding to fluid challenge or signs of tissue hypoperfusion such as lactic acid acidosis and/or encephalopathy are the

TABLE 3	Hemodynamic profile in shock.			
Type of shock	CVP	PCWP	SVR	CO
Distributive (septic or anaphylactic)	↓N	↓N	↓↓	↑↑ (low in terminal stage)
Cardiogenic	↑↑	↑↑	↑	↓↓
Hypovolemic (hemorrhagic)	↓↓	↓↓	↑	↓↓
Pericardial tamponade	↑↑	↑↑	↑	↓ or ↓↓
Obstructive massive air embolism	↑↑	N↓	↑	↓↓

(CVP: central venous pressure; CO: cardiac output; PCWP: pulmonary capillary wedge pressure; SVR: systemic vascular resistance)

hallmark of severe sepsis and require prompt antibiotics and cardiorespiratory support. Multiorgan dysfunction may involve the respiratory, cardiovascular, renal and central nervous systems; liver failure, hematological and metabolic failure can also occur. Sepsis-3 uses the SOFA score as criteria to assess organ failure **(Table 2)**. Hyperglycemia or hypoglycemia and metabolic acidosis are common manifestations of metabolic abnormalities. Mild DIC in subclinical form may be present in all septic patients though in more severe cases, bleeding from various sites can also occur.

At times differentiating between sepsis-induced organ dysfunction and that resulting from associated comorbidities, may be difficult. For instance, a patient with prolonged PT (INR) and reduced platelet count, bleeding from a single site or a surgical wound need not necessarily be having DIC. Prolonged PT may be due to a previous liver problem and a low platelet count may be associated with a drug-induced worsening of thrombocytopenia. An experienced judgment call needs to be taken here as any delay in stopping the bleeder from a surgical site can prove fatal.

Similarly, diagnosis of shock remains in doubt if a background history or presenting clinical picture suggests a possibility of cardiogenic or hemorrhagic shock. To resolve the dilemma, a study of the patient's hemodynamic profile **(Table 3)** may help to differentiate between the types of shock, as is covered in detail in the Chapter on Hemodynamic Monitoring.

■ BIOMARKERS

Among the numerous biomarkers studied, *C-reactive protein (CRP) and procalcitonin (PCT)* are the most commonly used in clinical practice, wrongly or rightly, for the diagnosis of sepsis. CRP is nonspecific, in that it is increased in all inflammatory states and is not specific to infection. Thus, it may be already elevated in most ICU patients and further it is also found to be raised in the elderly. It also has the disadvantage of appearing late (about 12-24 hours) after the onset of sepsis, and peaking by 2-3 days. Further, CRP should not be used as a marker of infection in patients with hepatic failure, and in fact, a low or declining concentration of CRP in the presence of persistent septic shock, should raise suspicion of underlying hepatic failure. In general, CRP is an inferior marker of sepsis.

In contrast to CRP, PCT is more specific for bacterial infections as it surfaces early (by 3–4 hours), peaks within 6 hours and is not affected by age. Hence, it is superior to CRP for use in sepsis though it is definitely not a perfect marker for more reasons than one, which we will appreciate as we go further.

Procalcitonin is an acute phase protein and its production is governed by calcitonin-1 which is primarily expressed in the C-cells of the thyroid gland. Normally, the concentration of PCT in the circulatory blood is only 0.05–0.1 ng/mL. In serious bacterial infections and sepsis the levels rise due to release of PAMPs; however, it also rises in other noninfectious causes of inflammation such as trauma, burns, surgery, and pancreatitis as a result of DAMPs. In septic shock the levels are high (≥10 ng/mL) and can be even higher if associated with polytrauma or postsurgery. PCT can also rise marginally in fungal infections and in fact a sudden flattening of a declining trend in PCT following adequate treatment of septic shock, should raise suspicion of a concomitant fungal infection. PCT level is however, not elevated in viral infections as it is attenuated by the production of interferon Y. A bar diagram **(Fig. 1)** gives a rough estimate of PCT levels from various studies, across various conditions.

Though PCT is liberally used as a biomarker by all physicians in most hospitals, it is also misinterpreted widely. The following recommendations may prove useful as guidelines:

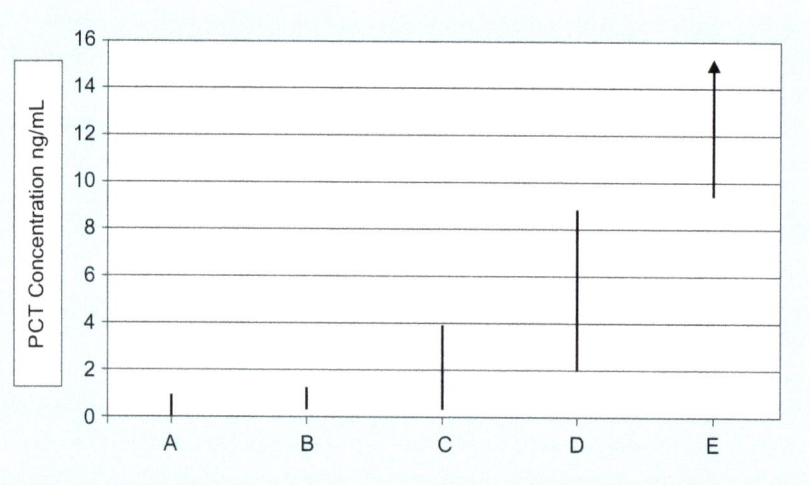

Fig. 1: Interpretation of procalcitonin (PCT) concentration in guiding therapy. (A = healthy adult; B = systemic infection unlikely; C = systemic infection possible and/or DAMP; D = high likelihood of systemic infection and sepsis; E = severe bacterial sepsis/septic shock)

- *"PCT as a biomarker, is more useful to rule out than to rule in"*—hence a normal PCT level would by and large exclude infection, but a raised PCT does not necessarily confirm infection because of its poor specificity; hence it is a poor indicator regarding decision to commence antibiotics
- *"Greater the concentration of PCT, greater the severity"*—hence it is useful for patient triage in identifying a high-risk group.
- *"Trend over time"*—it is useful to evaluate response to therapy reflected by a falling trend in the PCT levels
- *"PCT kinetics is the keyword"* for diagnosis of bacterial infection. Delta change in values (before and after the onset of fever) of over 0.76 ng/dL has a sensitivity of 80% and specificity of 86% (Trasy D et al., 2016)
- *PCT can remain normal in the early course of bacterial infections* and also in localized infections (empyema, osteomyelitis or localized collection, SBE)
- The following *noninfective causes of raised PCT* could be misleading:
  - Major surgery, trauma, burns
  - Drugs that stimulate cytokine release
  - Medullary thyroid and small cell lung carcinomas
  - Chronic kidney disease (CKD)
- *With recurrent infections* encountered during prolonged ICU stays, the value of PCT is unreliable and makes detection of new infection very difficult.
- *Finally, biomarkers cannot be used as standalone in decision making, they only complement clinical suspicion and other laboratory parameters.*

MANAGEMENT

Every physician caring for the critically ill should be familiar with the surviving sepsis campaign (SSC) guidelines; hence, throughout the discussion on management we have tried to adhere to the main facets of the guidelines.

Early Resuscitation

Early resuscitation includes stabilization of a hemodynamically compromised patient and respiratory support and this involves fluid challenge, inotropic and ventilator support, as described further in this chapter. Timing is of essence here and early intervention is of prime importance and improves survival of patients with sepsis. Early-goal directed therapy (EGDT) for severe sepsis by Rivers and colleagues, involved early resuscitation, targeting predefined parameters such as CVP, SvO_2 and MAP, achieving predefined end-points within a predefined period of 6 hours. This was a landmark study published in NEJM in 2001, but later studies showed conflicting results as some of the therapeutic and monitoring interventions in EGDT used for optimization of oxygen delivery were rarely required to achieve therapeutic goals in sepsis resuscitation. Further studies showed that the EGDT protocol of Rivers revealed no survival benefit as compared to usual care. However, the fact remains that earlier the therapeutic intervention for resuscitation, the greater the benefit, and that stands as Rivers's important contribution.

Fluid Resuscitation

Septic shock is defined as hypotension not responding to fluid challenge; hence the initial approach should be toward volume resuscitation. A rapid infusion of 30 mL/kg of crystalloid fluid (Normal Saline or Ringer Lactate) should be given within the first 3 hours and once the hemodynamic stability is achieved, further aggressive fluid resuscitation is not necessary and in fact, could be harmful; of course, maintenance fluids need to be continued. There is no particular type of fluid, crystalloid or colloid, that has shown any superiority in outcomes; however, starch-containing colloids should be avoided in the resuscitation phase as they have been reported to be associated with kidney injury. As of date, the recommendation is to prefer balanced crystalloids (Ringer Lactate or Ringer Acetate) for fluid resuscitation; normal saline (0.9 % NaCl), if given rapidly in larger volumes is associated with metabolic acidosis due to the chloride load and there is also a concern for potential chloride-induced nephropathy. Albumin (4%) may be used for resuscitation if there is a poor response to crystalloids.

The clinical end-point of fluid resuscitation should be stabilization of BP and HR, improving cognition and urine output and presence of capillary refill. More demanding targets include monitoring of Serum Lactate, CVP, $ScvO_2$, IVC collapsibility index by Echo and CO; though, studies from USA / UK (PROMISE) and Australia/New Zealand (PROCESS) have shown that using these parameters alone cannot replace good clinical assessment. In the elderly population and in those with a background history of cardiac dysfunction, it is important to monitor CVP in addition to clinical parameters, especially if there is a high risk of volume overload. Appearance of pulmonary edema from acute cardiac decompensation or from alveolar capillary leak, may require hemodynamic monitoring to predict fluid responsiveness. The different methods of predicting fluid responsiveness are stroke volume variation (SVV), bilateral passive leg raising and IVC collapsibility index by echocardiography, but each has its merits and demerits.

Lastly it is important to understand that volume challenge beyond the early stage of sepsis (beyond 24 hours), may be associated with harm, hence one needs to avoid aggressive fluid resuscitation by limiting the volume of fluid infusion given under close monitoring. Volume challenge alone may not suffice to maintain the blood pressure and early vasopressor support should be seriously considered. Patients should be closely monitored throughout, to avoid fluid overload. The maxim here is to give larger fluid volumes in the early phase of sepsis and to avoid positive fluid balance in later stages of sepsis when alveolar capillary leaks become more prominent.

Vasopressor Support

Vasopressors are considered at a point when fluid challenge has failed to correct hypotension during resuscitation, or hypotension has failed to remain corrected post-resuscitation. Hypotension, if persistent, may contribute to impaired oxygenation and poor peripheral tissue perfusion and hence it is imperative to target a mean arterial pressure (MAP) of 65–70 mm Hg. Studies have revealed that targeting a lower MAP was associated with an increased incidence of acute kidney injury (AKI); however, targeting a higher MAP in the range of 75–85 mm Hg has not show any survival benefit. The possible reasons may be that excessive vasoconstriction for prolonged periods would cause increased afterload and impair LV function or result in vasopressor associated side-effects such as arrhythmias and impaired splanchnic perfusion. On the other hand, elderly and hypertensive patients may benefit from a higher MAP but this is variable in different individuals.

Universally, *noradrenaline* is the preferred vasopressor because of its predominant alpha-adrenergic stimulation which increases the vascular tone and BP, and its modest beta-adrenergic effect which helps in maintaining the cardiac output; also, it has little effect on heart rate. The usual dose is 0.1–0.2 µg/kg/min to start with, and titrated upward or decreased to maintain mean BP of 65 mm Hg. To avoid adverse effects such as tissue necrosis and intense vasoconstriction causing organ dysfunction, the drug should be given through a central vein and the maximum dose should be maintained between 2 and 3 µg/kg/min.

Epinephrine has strong alpha and beta-adrenergic effects and in low doses it is effective for hypotension, but in higher doses it produces strong metabolic effects, tachycardia and arrhythmias. In fact, a large multicenterd double-blind RCT by Myburgh JA and colleagues comparing epinephrine with noradrenaline, had to be terminated as patients receiving epinephrine experienced transient tachycardias, increased insulin requirements and lactic acid acidosis.

Dopamine is no longer recommended as a vasopressor in patient with septic shock as it has a strong negative impact on the heart rate producing tachycardia and arrhythmias and moreover, meta-analysis of several large RCTs has associated it with higher mortality when compared to noradrenaline.

Vasopressin is another vasoconstrictor that acts by directly constricting vascular smooth muscles. Vasopressin reduces the need for the increasing use of noradrenaline. In patients not responding to noradrenaline, vasopressin may be added to achieve the target MAP avoiding high doses of noradrenaline. Vasopressin dose should not exceed 0.03–0.04 µg/min, as higher doses impair splanchnic perfusion and cause ischemia of the intestines. Further, it should not be used in suspected low cardiac output states as it tends to decrease the blood flow to the heart and kidneys. In conclusion, most trials have shown that vasopressin in appropriate doses can be used in patients with limited response to noradrenaline and is safe with little or no side effects, if used in the recommended dose and not for prolonged periods. However, there is no data to support vasopressin as first-line therapy. The doses and effects of vasopressors are given in **Box 2**.

> **BOX 2** Doses and effects of vasopressors.
>
> *Norepinephrine*
> *Effect:* Mainly vasopressor effect
> *Dose:* 0.1 µg/kg/min as starter and increase as needed up to 3 µg/kg/min
> *Remarks:* It is the first drug of choice.
>
> *Dopamine*
> *Effect:* Dopaminergic effect
> Probable splanchnic and renal perfusion in dose upto 5 µg/kg/min
> Vasoconstriction is predominant effect in dose up to 10 µg/kg/min
> *Dose:* 5 µg/kg/min up to 15 µg/kg/min
> *Remarks:* Tachycardia and arrhythmias
>
> *Vasopressin*
> *Effect:* Vasopressor effect
> *Dose:* 0.01–0.03 units/min
> *Remarks:* Pure vasoconstrictor and can promote splanchnic and digital ischemia if given in higher doses or for prolonged period
> It is always given in addition to norepinephrine and not alone
>
> *Epinephrine*
> *Effect:* Strong alpha and beta adrenergic effects
> *Dose:* The initial dose recommended is 0.01–0.02 µg/kg/min and the usual effective dose to correct hypotension or augment cardiac output is 0.1–0.2 µg/kg/min
> *Remarks:* Main side effects—tachycardia, increased insulin requirement and lactic acid acidosis when given in higher doses

Antibiotics

Early empirical therapy and source control is imperative in sepsis, in order to improve survival. The choice of antibiotic is empirical because the offending organism is yet not identified and the antibiotic needs to be given without delay.

The thorny issue here is not just the selection of an antibiotic agent but the overall concerns about timing, choice of antibiotic, correct dosing and duration of treatment and this is best described as appropriateness in antimicrobial administration.

Timing: Barring a few criticisms, there is overwhelming evidence in clinical studies indicating the urgent administration of an appropriate antimicrobial agent and the first dose should be within 1 hour of sepsis detection, or on arrival in EMS/ICU or any responsible healthcare facility. This should of course be preceded by collection of blood and other relevant specimens for aerobic, anaerobic and fungal cultures. Preferably the detection of sepsis should be based on the SIRS criteria of Sepsis-1 definition, as it would be unwise to wait for microcirculatory tissue perfusion abnormalities and organ dysfunction to manifest (Sepsis-3 definition). A strong association has been noted between delay in antibiotic timing and an increased risk adjusted in-hospital mortality. Most studies have shown that beyond 2 hours, each elapsed hour was associated with increasing hospital mortality. Surviving

TABLE 4	Choice of antimicrobials for empiric therapy in sepsis using the mnemonic "SEPSIS".
Site	• Location of infection is specific to contain pathogens which are susceptible to selective antibiotics which should be used in symptomatic patients • These sites are also home to colonizers; hence disregard cultures in asymptomatic patients, e.g., UTI with Foley's catheter, wounds with nonpurulent discharge, respiratory secretions in intubated patients with no imaging evidence of LRTI
Environment	• Community, health care facility or ICU acquired infections including VAP; to be familiar with hospital flora and antibiogram—community and regional flora
Previously used antibiotics	Best to avoid antibiotics used in last 3 months
Severity	• In patients with septic shock and severe sepsis a multidrug approach – covering GNB + *Pseudomonas* (if strongly suspected also to cover MRSA and antifungal) • Using blanket, broad-spectrum combination therapy for all patients admitted to ICU with severe sepsis may be counter-productive. Empiric treatment must be based on the host factor/community-hospital acquired and site of infection regardless of severity
Immunologically compromised	• Age, comorbidities, depressed immunity • Broad-spectrum coverage with GNB + *Pseudomonas* cover, (if indicated antifungal and MRSA cover)
Side effects	• Avoid nephrotoxic drugs (aminoglycosides, colistin in patients with kidney dysfunction or high serum creatinine)

sepsis campaign recommends early IV antimicrobial therapy, preferably within 1 hour of recognition of sepsis and septic shock.

Choice of Antibiotics

We have coined an appropriate mnemonic termed "SEPSIS" **(Table 4)** to help one's memory to remember the 6 principles guiding the selection of an appropriate antimicrobial for an empiric therapy.

Dosing Strategies

Dosing Strategies of drugs should be based on accepted pharmacokinetic/pharmacodynamics (PK/PD) properties of the drug. The concentration of the drug in the serum is also affected by the serum half-life, protein-binding and renal and hepatic function. More importantly drug usage may have to be increased in solid organ infections where the optimum tissue concentration is required for penetration of the antibiotic to reach therapeutic levels. PK/PD properties of antimicrobial display either concentration killing or time-dependent killing. Antimicrobials that exhibit concentration dependency such as aminoglycosides, need to be given in a higher once-a-day dose to achieve maximum serum concentration over the minimum inhibitory concentration of the drug (Cmax/MIC). On the other hand, antimicrobials that display time-dependent killing, work best by keeping the blood levels close to MIC levels as long as possible; hence one advocates a prolonged infusion and we see this in practice in giving meropenem infusion over 3-4 hours, thrice a day.

Critically ill patients with diverse host factors have dynamic physiological fluctuations due to organ dysfunction, variable volumes of distribution and renal clearance, leading to unpredictable PK alterations. Dosing strategies in these patients may need to be augmented to ceiling doses or greater, to overcome organism burden, achieve target site concentration and require to be carefully titrated to account for patient variations and organ dysfunction.

Duration

Duration of antibiotics in critically ill patients is based on the same principles as in other patients. It is a decision based on the site of infection, ability or inability to achieve complete source control, host factors and clinical response to appropriate antimicrobials. Hence, unwarranted prolonged courses of antimicrobials should be avoided, except in cases where source control is inadequate and target site concentrations are difficult to achieve, or in immunosuppressed hosts.

De-escalation of antibiotics to targeted narrow spectrum agents based on appropriate cultures is strongly recommended. However, final discontinuation of antimicrobials at the earliest opportune time, is the only real de-escalation strategy. (For details refer to Chapter 12, Antimicrobial Therapy in the ICU)

Mechanical Ventilation

All patients in septic shock with respiratory distress should be intubated and supported on mechanical ventilation as part of early resuscitation, because hypoxia and increased respiratory workload can be detrimental with poor outcome. However, patients with sepsis but hemodynamically stable with no serious respiratory affliction, can be maintained on nasal oxygen or NIV, but with worsening of sepsis-associated lung injury, timely intubation and mechanical ventilation is important. Delaying intubation and ventilation by using NIV in patients with persistent hypoxia, is not buying time as many advocate, but is an unwise move, which will adversely influence outcome. For lung protection ventilation and recruitment strategies including maneuvers like *proning* for severe acute respiratory distress syndrome (ARDS), and for all guidelines to prevent VAP, refer to appropriate chapters.

Corticosteroids in Septic Shock

There is a general acceptance that steroids mitigates shock and that the risk of secondary infection is minimal if given in small doses for a short period. Most guidelines, however, are against using IV hydrocortisone to treat septic shock if adequate fluid replacement and vasopressors are able to stabilize the hemodynamics, but if this cannot be achieved, the guidelines advocate using hydrocortisone in a dose of 200 mg/day.

Source Control

The site of infection should be identified at the earliest and required source control should be implemented as soon as possible. Prompt withdrawal of central lines and other indwelling catheters is mandatory, if suspected to be a source of infection. Major surgical interventions may not be possible till the patient is reasonably stable, but abscesses and collections should be drained or aspirated using minimal intervention.

Glucose Control

Critically-ill patients tend to be hyperglycemic and blood sugars may rise to very high levels particularly in hypermetabolic states because of insulin resistance. Initial trials recommended an upper level to not exceed 110 mg%, but further studies revealed poor outcome and hence, present guidelines recommend targeting the upper level below 180 mg%. If the patient's blood sugar levels are uncontrolled, the best practice is to start insulin by IV infusion, monitoring blood sugar values 2 hourly and adjusting the dose by a protocolized scale keeping the blood sugar values between 150 and 180 mg%.

DVT Prophylaxis

All patients with sepsis are at risk of developing deep vein thrombosis. Therefore, they should receive prophylaxis in some form, be it mechanical (sequential compression devices or stockings) or pharmacological (low molecular weight heparin such as enoxaparin, or unfractionated heparin). The choice of drug and dosage depends on the renal and liver functions as well as the coagulation parameters.

■ SUGGESTED READING

1. Angus DC, van der Poll T. Severe sepsis and septic shock. N Engl J Med. 2013;369(9):840-51.
2. Bone RC, Balk RA, Cerra FB, Dellinger RP, Fein AM, Knaus WA, et al. Definitions for sepsis and organ failure and guidelines for the use of innovative therapies in sepsis. The ACCP/SCCM Consensus Conference Committee. American College of Chest Physicians/Society of Critical Care Medicine. Chest. 1992;101(6):1644-55.
3. Bone RC. Sir Isaac Newton, Sepsis, SIRS and CARS. Crit Care Med. 1996;24(7):1125-8.
4. Dellinger P, Roy A, Paririllo J. Severe sepsis and septic shock. In: Parrillo J, Dellinger P (Eds). Critical Care Medicine: Principles of Diagnosis and Management in Adults, 5th edition. New York: Elsevier; 2019.

5. Dellinger RP, Schorr CA, Levy MM. A users' guide to the 2016 Surviving Sepsis Guidelines. Intensive Care Med. 2017;43(3):299-303.
6. Devlin D, Deutschman C, Neligan PJ. What is the role of vasopressors and inotropes in septic shock? In: Deutschmanand Neligan's Evidence Based Practice of Critical Care, 3rd edition. New York: Elsevier; 2020.
7. Ferreira FL, Bota DP, Bross A, Mélot C, Vincent JL. Serial evaluation of the SOFA score to predict outcome in critically ill patients. JAMA. 2001;286(14):1754-8.
8. Levi M, van der Poll T. Coagulation and sepsis. Thromb Res. 2017;149:38-44.
9. Levy MM, Evans LE, Rhodes A. The surviving sepsis campaign bundle: 2018 update. Intensive Care Med. 2018;44(6):925-8.
10. Machado FR, Azevedo LCP. Sepsis: a threat that needs a global solution. Crti Care Med. 2018;46(3):454-9.
11. Marik PE, Preiser JC. Toward understanding tight glycemic control in the ICU: a systematic review and meta-analysis. Chest. 2010;137(3):544-51.
12. Paltan ID, Vincet JL. Does the timing of antibiotics administration matter in sepsis. In: Deutschman and Neligan's Evidence Based Practice of Critical Care, 3rd edition. New York: Elsevier; 2020.
13. Rhodes A, Evans LE, Altazzani W, Levy MM, Antonelli M, Ferrer R, et al. Surviving Sepsis Campaign: International Guidelines for Management of Sepsis and Septic Shock: 2016. Intensive Care Med. 2017;43(3):304-77.
14. Singer M, Deutschman CS, Seymour CW, Shankar-Hari M, Annane D, Bauer M, et al. The third international consensus definitions for sepsis and septic shock (sepsis-3). JAMA. 2016;315(8): 801-10.
15. Vincent JL, Brealey D, Libert N. Rapid diagnosis of infection in the critically ill, a multicenter study of molecular detection in bloodstream infections, pneumonia, and sterile site infections. Crit Care Med. 2015;43(11):2283-91.

CHAPTER 12

Antimicrobial Therapy in the Intensive Care Unit

Ayesha Sunavala

■ INTRODUCTION

The practice of modern medicine has been singularly transformed by the discovery of antimicrobials in the last century. Apart from reducing mortality due to infectious diseases, the unparalleled discovery of these "magic bullets" has enabled us to perform complex and invasive surgeries, organ and stem cell transplants, administer immunosuppressive therapies for neoplastic and autoimmune conditions and subject critically ill patients to life-saving procedures such as mechanical ventilation and intravascular device placement. In short, it would be impossible to conceive the functioning of a modern intensive care unit (ICU) in present times without the backbone of the antimicrobial armamentarium.

There are two scenarios that fundamentally underscore antimicrobial therapy in the ICU-empirical antimicrobial therapy for sepsis and targeted/directed antimicrobial therapy against a pathogen isolated on culture.

■ EMPIRICAL ANTIMICROBIAL THERAPY

Empirical therapy in the ICU is generally deployed for the hemodynamically unstable, septic patient in whom appropriate agents are administered as early as possible. Empirical therapy in this situation is typically broad spectrum, taking into account individual host factors, epidemiology, the likely site of infection and recent receipt of antimicrobials. It must be emphasized though that collection of blood cultures and other easily obtained, appropriate samples for culture, are the prerequisite before empirical therapy as well, regardless of the urgency of the situation. Cultures of body fluids that require invasive procedures, e.g., cerebrospinal fluid (CSF), drainage of abscesses, etc., may be procured in a timely manner, after the first dose of empirical therapy in critically unwell patients.

Needless to say, empiric therapy must be discouraged in clinically stable ICU patients, in whom thorough evaluation of fever, or suspected infection is warranted prior to starting antibiotics.

General Principles of Empirical Antimicrobial Selection in the ICU

The intensivist unlike other clinicians often cannot afford the luxury of observation and restraint while awaiting investigations, or a clinical syndrome to completely evolve. Additionally, empiric choices are often restricted as the patient has already received end of the line, broad spectrum antibiotics prior to admission to the ICU. Nevertheless, the optimal empirical selection of antimicrobials and optimization of their pharmacokinetic-pharmacodynamics (PKPD) characteristics are paramount in improving outcomes in sepsis.

The following simplistic approach to empirical therapy is proposed as a means of reducing errors in our day-to-day antimicrobial decision making.

Host Assessment

Even in the era of advanced radiodiagnostics and molecular testing, a thorough assessment of the patient's history and risk factors provides invaluable clues and can dramatically alter the diagnostic thought process. Extremes of age, uncontrolled diabetes mellitus, chronic organ dysfunction, dementia, alcoholism, prior receipt of steroids and other immunosuppressive medications, are among the many significant host factors that can affect the immune system and predispose the individual to different microorganisms, as well as diverse manifestations of the same infection. Bearing the above in mind, an empirical antimicrobial regimen should only be as broad as necessary. Widening the spectrum to treat unlikely organisms, even in a critically ill patient, are likely to do more harm in terms of selecting resistance and potential drug toxicity.

For example, empirical treatment of community acquired acute bacterial meningitis in an elderly or immunosuppressed patient, must include a listerial cover. However, broad-spectrum gram-negative drugs would be inappropriate for a community-acquired meningitis regardless of clinical severity, unless the patient has risk factors for a resistant gram-negative infection.

Advances in hemato-oncology and transplant medicine have inevitably led to an increased population of chronically immunosuppressed individuals. Caring for the immunosuppressed host in the ICU is often fraught with multiple challenges and surprises. Empirical selection of antimicrobials in this population, must account for opportunistic bacteria, viruses, fungi and parasites. The presentation and course of infection in an immunocompromised host may be atypical and diverse. A seemingly stable patient may dramatically deteriorate within hours. On the other hand, clinical signs and symptoms other than fever may be absent in a profoundly neutropenic patient, *who is* too immunosuppressed to mount an inflammatory response to infection.

For example, the clinical finding of a pyogenic abscess in a patient with gram-negative sepsis, or retinal deposits in a candidemic patient, may be appreciated only after the neutrophil count starts recovering.

By and large, opportunistic bacterial and viral illnesses have an acute onset as compared to fungal and parasitic infections which may have a subacute to chronic course in these patients. However, as it is impossible and irrational to cover all opportunistic pathogens, the physician must have a basic knowledge of the spectrum of opportunistic infections seen with various immunosuppressed states.

For example, neutropenic patients are at high risk of acute hospital-acquired bacterial infections and subsequent invasive mold infections. In contrast, defects in cell-mediated immunity pose a risk of chronic infections such as pneumocystis pneumonia, mycobacterial infections, toxoplasmosis and cryptococcosis.

Finally, the rule of parsimony (principle of using the least resources or explanations to solve a problem), often does not apply to immunosuppressed individuals who may present with multiple opportunistic infections simultaneously. Hence, therapeutic trials in these patients are often unsuccessful and every attempt should be made at obtaining appropriate specimens despite diagnostic obstacles like cytopenias in this population.

Epidemiology

For syndromes such as acute undifferentiated fevers, pyrexia of unknown origin, or subacute to chronic meningoencephalitis, the patient's residence (past and present), occupation, exposure and travel history may assume tremendous significance. Exposures, however remote, may be of importance in infections with prolonged incubation periods, or the potential to reactivate after protracted periods of time, e.g., in tuberculosis, brucellosis, melioidosis, HIV, rabies.

Risk Factors for Drug-resistant Pathogens

Evaluating the patient for risk factors for drug-resistant (DR) pathogens is crucial in empiric decision making. History of recent healthcare contact, antimicrobials in the past three months, surgery or invasive procedures, hemodialysis, presence of indwelling devices, prosthetic joints, are some of the more widely accepted risk factors that predispose an individual to DR pathogens. Of these, receipt of antimicrobials in the past 3 months is considered the strongest risk factor for multidrug-resistant (MDR) pathogens. Prescriptions and discharge papers seldom have complete information on antimicrobials used and the response to initial treatment. However, if this information is carefully extracted from the patient, caregiver or treating physician, it can yield vital clues as to the original pathogen and possible development of resistance.

On the other hand, after careful evaluation, if the above risk factors for resistant pathogens are absent, then antimicrobial selection for community-acquired infections must be based on the syndrome and not the clinical severity.

For example, septic shock due to community-acquired pneumonia or urinary tract infection does not warrant empirical use of carbapenems in the absence of risk factors for MDR infection.

Reviewing the Syndrome

Straightforward syndromes that have a clear localization to skin and soft tissue, meninges, respiratory tract or urinary tract, have well developed guidelines for their management.

On the other hand, acute undifferentiated fevers, fevers with rash, encephalitis, and hemorrhagic fevers, often have overlapping features and pose serious diagnostic challenges. Clinical suspicion in such cases should be driven by predisposing factors in the patient, regional disease burden, geography, seasonality of transmission, and spectrum and severity of the disease. Often repeated history and clinical examination, and the re-evaluation of an earlier made diagnosis or an evolving syndrome, is imperative to differentiate between various infections as well as noninfectious causes, rather than irrational escalation of antibiotics.

For example, a young nature enthusiast was transferred from a nursing home with a diagnosis of cerebral malaria on the basis of a rapid malarial antigen test positive for *P. vivax*. Despite completing a course of IV artesunate prior to admission, he presented with fever, shock, seizures and encephalitis. Multiple peripheral smears for malarial parasites were negative. History of fever that began 1 week after returning from a forest trek and identification of the pathognomonic inoculation eschar in the patient's groin, clinched the diagnosis of scrub typhus. He was treated successfully with doxycycline for 7 days.

Identifying and Controlling the Source of Infection

One of the most important causes of failure of appropriate antimicrobial therapy is an unidentified and/or an untreated focus of infection. Some foci may be especially difficult to address in hemodynamically unstable patients who are unable to undergo surgical intervention, or removal and reinsertion of critical lines in patients with coagulopathy and platelet dysfunction. However, the burden of infection and the development of biofilms on lines and devices greatly impacts antimicrobial penetration and concentration at the desired site, with eventual development of drug resistance. Hence, every attempt should be made, even in unstable patients, to achieve source control through minimally invasive bedside procedures such as ultrasound-guided pigtail drainage of a postsurgical collection for both diagnostic and therapeutic success.

■ ANTIBIOTIC SELECTION AND DOSING IN CRITICAL ILLNESSES

The systemic exposure to a drug based on its absorption, distribution, metabolism, and excretion, is termed as pharmacokinetics (PK). *Pharmacodynamics* (PD) describes the mechanism of action of the drug with respect to the biochemical and physiologic response that the drug exerts in the body.

For maximal efficacy and safety, it is imperative that the right drug against the right pathogen is chosen at the optimal dose for an optimal duration. The

Flowchart 1: PKPD alterations in sepsis.

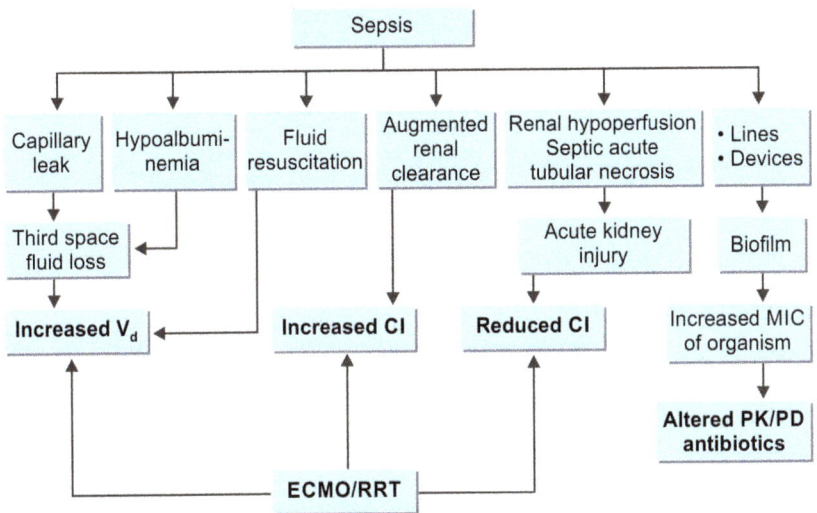

(V_D: volume of distribution; Cl: clearance; MIC: minimum inhibitory concentration; ECMO: extracorporeal membrane oxygenation; RRT: renal replacement therapy; PKPD: pharmacokinetics-pharmacodynamics)
Source: Sunavala A, Agrawal U, Gala P. TDM: Is it Ready for Prime Time? In: Todi S, Dixit SB, Zirpe K, Mehta Y (Eds). Critical Care Update 2019. New Delhi: Jaypee Brothers Medical Publishers (P) Ltd.; 2019.

mathematical framework for this rational selection and dosing is provided by the knowledge and application of PKPD principles **(Flowchart 1 and Fig. 1)**.

Unlike other pharmacological agents, anti-infective PKPD is particularly unique owing to its effects on the infective pathogen, the host, as well as collateral impact on the microbiome. The need for nontoxic but higher doses of antimicrobials in order to destroy nonmammalian target sites, and the relentless battle against emergence of resistance over time, are the most significant PKPD challenges associated with anti-infective drugs.

Diverse host factors that alter PKPD in septic patients include extremes of age, obesity, organ dysfunction, immunosuppression, long standing catheters, devices and sophisticated hemodynamic and ventilatory support systems and extracorporeal therapies like continuous renal replacement therapy (CRRT). Additionally, organ dysfunction in these patients leads to dynamic physiological fluctuations, variable volumes of distribution, hypoalbuminemia and augmented renal clearance which can lead to unpredictable PK alterations. Hence, the practice of protocolized antimicrobial dosing in the ICU has fallen out of favor with an emphasis now on individualized therapy, with a pivotal focus on applying PKPD knowledge at the bedside.

A combination of diverse factors that contribute to altered PKPD in critically ill patients is shown in **Flowchart 1**.

The minimum inhibitory concentration for 50% or 90% of all isolates of a bacterial species (MIC_{50} or MIC_{90}) and the inhibitory or effective concentration

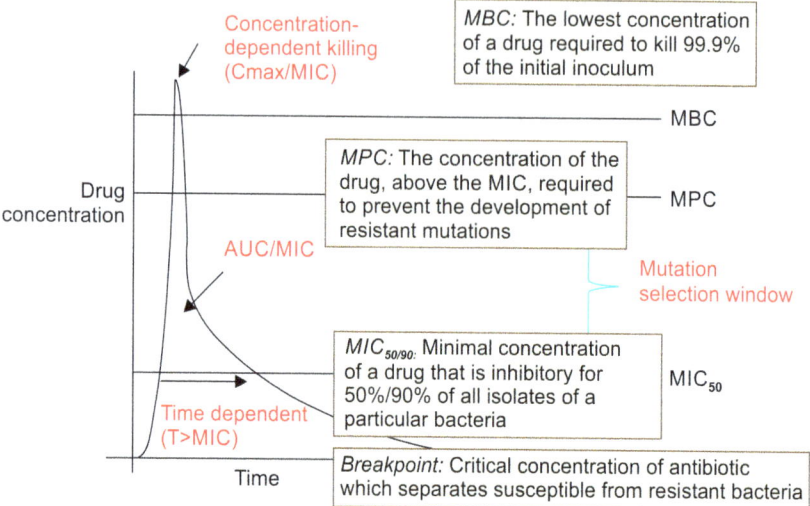

Fig. 1: Principles of PKPD of antimicrobials. (MIC: minimum inhibitory concentration; MBC: minimum bactericidal concentration; MPC: mutant prevention concentration; C_{max}: maximum concentration; AUC: area under curve; T: time; PKPD: pharmacokinetics-pharmacodynamics)
Source: Sunavala A. Rational Use of Antibiotics in Intensive Care Unit. In: Patel M (Ed). ICP Monograph, Critical Care Medicine 2017. New Delhi: Jaypee Brothers Medical Publishers (P) Ltd.; 2019.

for 50% of all isolates of a virus (IC_{50} or EC_{50}), are considered the conventional standards used to describe drug activity against pathogens. In simple terms, they are defined as the lowest concentration of a drug required to inhibit visible growth in vitro.

The minimal bactericidal concentration (MBC) provides information on the lowest concentration at or above the MIC required to kill 99.9% of the inoculum of the given microorganism. Antimicrobials are considered bactericidal if the MBC is no more than four times the MIC.

The mutant prevention concentration (MPC) is the required concentration of the drug above the MIC, to prevent the development of resistant mutations. The area on the graph between the MIC and MPC, is known as the mutant selection window (MSW). This window denotes the antimicrobial concentration range in which evolution of resistance can occur during therapy, by selecting the mutant or resistant organisms in the population.

These in vitro parameters are extremely important as standard epidemiological tools that govern PK principles. However, they are fraught with limitations in the dynamic in vivo environment of the body and do not take into account factors like the postantibiotic effect (persistent suppression of bacterial growth even after the concentration of the drug at the site has decreased below the MIC), or the interaction of the immune system with the drug, and more importantly, the effect of antimicrobial combinations used in critically ill patients.

Antimicrobial combinations are often used empirically in the ICU to enhance efficacy in life-threatening infections, e.g., polymyxins plus carbapenem or tigecycline for suspected CRE sepsis, or to broaden the spectrum of coverage in polymicrobial infections, e.g., combination of penicillin plus metronidazole for necrotizing fasciitis.

However, a thorough understanding of antimicrobial combinations is essential to prevent antagonism, drug interactions and toxicity.

Combination therapy may result in:
- Antimicrobial synergism means that the sum of the activity of the agents used in combination is greater than the individual activity of the agents if used alone. This concept has been well established and standardized for antitubercular and antiretroviral treatment, as well as in specific infections such as cryptococcal meningitis where a combination of amphotericin b and 5 flucytosine/fluconazole have been found to be superior to use of a single agent. Another example is the treatment of methicillin-resistant *Staphylococcus aureus* (MRSA) prosthetic valve endocarditis, where a synergistic combination of vancomycin and gentamicin is recommended for bactericidal killing in the vegetation and the addition of rifampicin is recommended for its antibiofilm property in the presence of prosthetic material.
- Antimicrobial antagonism as the name suggests, means that the sum of the activity of two or more antimicrobial agents given together is lower than the activity of the most active agent given alone. For example, the antiretroviral zidovudine has been found in animal studies to antagonize the anti-CMV effects of ganciclovir.

Dosing Principles based on PKPD

The Loading Dose

The loading dose (LD) is a product of the volume of distribution and desired plasma concentration. Renal function plays no role in the calculation of a loading dose.

$$LD = V \times Cp$$

For hydrophilic drugs such as beta lactams and glycopeptides, the volume of distribution is usually small. However, this may be increased in early sepsis due to extravascular space expansion. Thus, a high loading dose is optimal for these drugs.

The second critical factor, plasma concentration, is based on the MIC of a particular antimicrobial for a susceptible pathogen. However, with empirical therapy this information is not available beforehand. Therefore, a high initial dose is recommended for both concentration-dependent antibiotics for maximum bactericidal effect, as well as time-dependent antibiotics to ensure adequate tissue penetration.

The Maintenance Dose

Maintenance dosing strategies vary based on the mode of action of the drug as well as individual patient factors that influence its PKPD interactions **(Table 1)**.

The benefit of prolonged β-lactam infusions to improve outcomes in critically ill patients has been validated in various studies. However, it must

TABLE 1 Dosing strategies based on PKPD characteristics of antimicrobials.

Mode of action	PKPD target	Dosing inference	Remarks
Concentration dependent drugs For example, aminoglycoside, metronidazole, daptomycin, Amphotericin B, echinocandins	Maximum concentration (C_{max}) C_{max}/MIC	• High dose • Extended interval/ once daily dosing • Increase dosing intervals in renal dysfunction	• Toxicity correlates to trough and not peak concentration • Less frequent dosing supported by post-antibiotic effect
Time dependent For example, Beta-lactams, macrolides, clindamycin, tetracyclines, aztreonam, linezolid	Time above MIC Maximum bactericidal effect is usually achieved at 3–4 times the MIC with BL concentration above the MIC (f T>MIC) for 40–70% of the dosing interval*	• High LD followed by frequent maintenance doses • Benefit of extended infusions is considered in patients with high APACHE scores, high V_d, augmented renal clearance and high organism burden	LD may be essential prior to extended infusions to ensure rapid antimicrobial action especially in pharmacologically protected sites such as CNS, bone and joint
Area under curve (AUC) For example, polymixins, FQNs, azithromycin, tetracyclines, glycopeptides, tigecycline, linezolid	AUC/MIC AUC takes both the antimicrobial concentration and time into account	• High doses plus frequent dosing intervals • Target AUC/MIC ratios to be achieved for greatest efficacy. For example, AUC/MIC ratio > 400 for vancomycin	

*It has been suggested however that to obtain a similar therapeutic response in a critically ill patient, higher exposures (100% *f* T>MIC) may be needed in view of immunological impairment and/or high inoculum effect as shown in **Figure 2**.
Source: Modified from Amsden GW, Ballow CH, Bertino JS. Pharmacokinetics and Pharmacodynamics of Anti-infective Agents. In: Mandell GL (Ed). Principles and Practice of Infectious Diseases, 7th edition. Philadelphia, PA: Churchill Livingstone/ Elsevier; 2010. pp. 297-307.
(LD: loading does; BL: beta lactams; V_d: volume of distribution; fT>MIC: fractional tine over MIC; FQN: fluoroquinolones; PKPD: pharmacokinetics-pharmacodynamics)

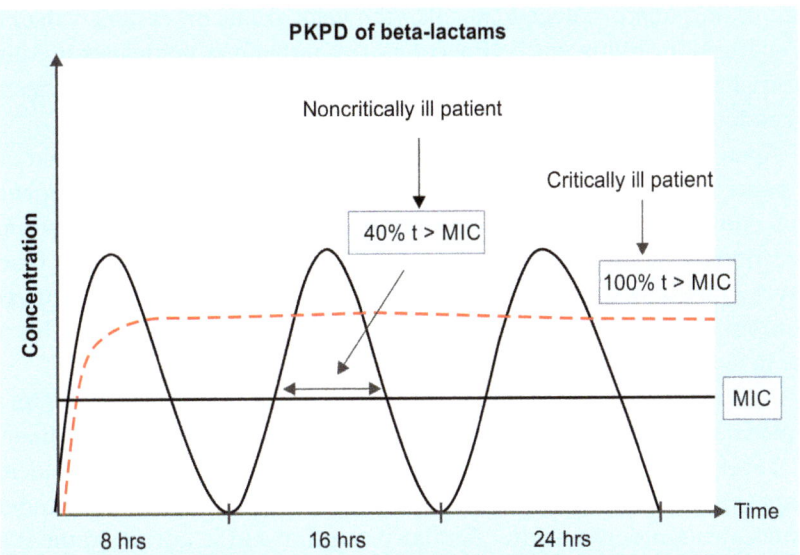

Fig. 2: Desired pharmacokinetics-pharmacodynamics (PKPD) parameters for beta-lactams in critically ill patients.
Source: Sunavala A, Agrawal U, Gala P. TDM: Is it Ready for Prime Time? In: Critical Care Update 2019.Todi S, Dixit SB, Zirpe K, Mehta Y (Eds). New Delhi: Jaypee Brothers Medical Publishers (P) Ltd.; 2019.

be kept in mind that prolonged infusions alone result in lower peak drug concentrations. Although the PKPD target for these agents is time above MIC, for organisms with intermediate-high MICs, prolonging the infusion may reduce efficacy by preventing the achievement of antibiotic concentrations above the MIC. In these circumstances, starting with a standard bolus loading dose followed by prolonged infusions, or intermittent doses to achieve peak concentration above the MIC, may be preferred.

For example, the CLSI resistance breakpoint for Meropenem is ≥4 µg/mL for *Klebsiella penumoniae*. It has been found that if the Meropenem breakpoint for a carbapenem-resistant *Klebsiella* isolate is ≥16 µg/mL, prolonging the infusion of the carbapenem may be counterproductive as it may prevent the drug from achieving concentration above the MIC, and hence diminish bacterial killing.

Antimicrobials are commonly classified as "static-inhibiting growth and replication", or "cidal-causing bacterial cell death". However, these are relative terms rather than water tight compartments. The cidal or static property of each antimicrobial may vary depending on the dose, the concentration achieved at the site of infection, the organism in question, the inoculum density or burden of infection and finally the environmental conditions such as pH and protein concentration.

Contrary to conventional belief, there is no concrete scientific data to suggest clinical evidence of the benefit of cidal agents over static agents for most conditions even in the critically ill. However, this dogma may still hold true in immune privileged sites like the vegetations on cardiac valves in infective endocarditis, or CNS infections, as international guidelines continue to emphasize the importance of parental, bactericidal and fungicidal agents for endocarditis and meningitis.

Apart from the in vitro properties of the drug, the ability of the antimicrobial to penetrate a particular site or body compartment and achieve therapeutic concentrations must be considered during drug selection. Bloodstream infections warrant the selection of antibiotics that achieve higher blood levels. Antibiotics such as macrolides and tetracyclines have large volumes of distribution and achieve excellent tissue levels, but may be less favorable for use in bacteremia.

Apart from the concentration at a desired site of action, it is important to understand the antimicrobial properties of a drug in a specific environment.

For example, the use of an aminoglycoside to treat an abscess is considered inappropriate as the low pH and low oxygen tension in this environment inactivates aminoglycosides. Similarly, daptomycin is not recommended for the treatment of community-acquired pneumonia, as it is inactivated by pulmonary surfactant.

It is believed that conventional doses of many antimicrobials are unlikely to eradicate severe infection and overcome the emergence of resistance due to extensive PKPD variability in the critically ill population, and in protected compartments such as the CNS, bone and joint, or other deep-seated infections. In these situations, the use of bactericidal agents in supranormal doses to optimize drug levels is advised.

For example, the recommended doses of the glycopeptides (Vancomycin and Teicoplanin) for MRSA bone and joint infections:

Vancomycin 20–30 mg/kg (loading dose) followed by 15–20 mg/kg 8–12 hourly to target trough concentration of 15–20 µg/mL

Teicoplanin 12 mg/kg 12-hourly × 3 doses (loading dose), followed by 12 mg/kg/day (recommended for MRSA septic arthritis/ endocarditis).

Principles of Targeted Antimicrobial Therapy
- *Colonization versus infection* (**Table 2 and Flowchart 2**)

    Due to the widespread use of empirical antimicrobials in our community and institutions, clinicians often struggle with negative cultures despite multiple diagnostic attempts at a microbiological result. On the other hand, a positive culture report can be grossly misleading if the isolated organism is a contaminant or colonizer, rather than the true pathogen. Separating the wheat from the chaff requires a discerning, multidisciplinary approach.

    A patient who has either received multiple antibiotics for prolonged periods, has no compatible syndrome, or has an alternative explanation for the clinical signs and symptoms, is likely to be colonized rather than truly infected. The most common examples of this in the ICU are:

TABLE 2	Colonization versus Infection.	
	Colonization	**Infection**
Definition	• Host-microbe association with growth and multiplication of the microbe but without tissue invasion or damage • Does not result in sufficient tissue damage to cause clinical disease	• Host-microbe association that results in clinical symptoms and signs of disease *or* • Radiological, microbiological or histopathological evidence of invasion, inflammation and tissue reaction
Pathogenesis	• Usually harmless commensals • Maybe protective against invading pathogens • May invade under some circumstances (breach of skin, mucosa, immunosuppression)	• Invasive • Host tissue destruction
Diagnosis	• Organism usually identified from nonsterile site (swab, tracheal aspirate, drain, urinary catheter) • May be true pathogens if repeatedly isolated, protected specimens or colony counts above certain specified limits	• Organism isolated from sterile site (blood, CSF, USG/CT guided aspirate, surgical specimen)
Role of treatment	Usually none Source control in presence of device/catheter	Antimicrobials usually required for cure

Source: Sunavala A. Rational Use of Antibiotics in Intensive Care Unit. In: Patel M (Eds) ICP Monograph, Critical Care Medicine 2017. New Delhi: Jaypee Brothers Medical Publishers (P) Ltd.; 2017.

- *Candida spp.* are frequently isolated from urine, sputum, tracheal secretions and BAL, especially in antibiotic treated patients and are almost always colonizers. This fungal colonization is best considered as a risk factor for candidemia rather than as a disease state. On the other hand, isolation of the same organism from the urine of a neutropenic host or a patient due to undergo urological instrumentation warrants prompt treatment.
- Blood cultures detect bacteremia in only about half of the patients with clinically suspected sepsis, the positivity rate is much lower when drawn in the presence of ongoing antibiotic therapy. Nevertheless, a positive blood culture is generally considered an alarm bell that warrants immediate appropriate antimicrobials and source control. However, the isolation of coagulase negative *Staphylococcus aureus* (CONS) from a single blood culture sample, usually represents contamination of the culture by skin colonizers, due to inadequate infection control practices during sample collection. However, in patients with intravascular access devices, prosthetic valves, pacemakers, orthopedic implants

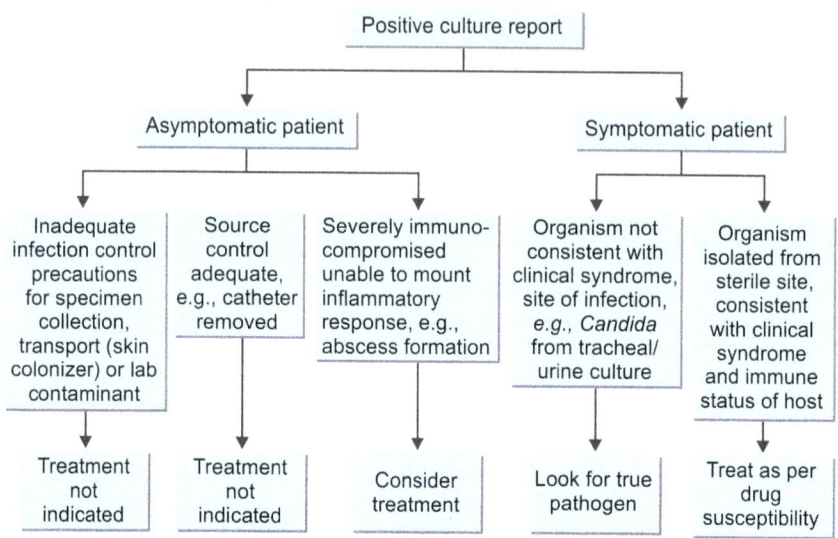

Flowchart 2: Algorithmic approach to colonization vs. infection.

Source: Modified from Sunavala A. Rational Use of Antibiotics in Intensive Care Unit. In: Patel M (Ed). ICP Monograph, Critical Care Medicine 2017. New Delhi: Jaypee Brothers Medical Publishers (P) Ltd.; 2017.

etc., isolation of CONS can have sinister implications and simultaneous, paired cultures should be repeated from both intravascular central catheters and percutaneously to differentiate colonization from true infection in these patients.
- Accurate interpretation of culture and drug susceptibility tests

There are several phenotypic antimicrobial susceptibility testing platforms available such as disk-diffusion method, macro and microdilution methods, determination of minimum inhibitory concentrations (MIC) by E-test, automated methods such as MicroScan, VITEK and mass spectrometry methods using MALDTI-TOF MS. Several molecular genotypic PCR-based platforms are also commercially available for identification and susceptibility testing. Each method has its advantages and limitations, but they all have a common purpose, viz. to provide a reliable prediction of whether an infection caused by a particular organism will respond therapeutically to a particular antimicrobial agent.

While interpreting a culture report, the clinician must bear in mind certain universal principles:
– Antimicrobial susceptibility testing is an in vitro phenomenon, performed under controlled conditions of temperature, pH, use of selective media, etc., and cannot indisputably predict in vivo efficacy. The clinical must take into account the site of infection, host factors, potential for drug interactions and toxicity when selecting a drug.
– For serious, deep seated infections such as infective endocarditis, meningitis, endophthalmitis, osteomyelitis, implant-related infections,

severe sepsis and infections in the immunocompromised host, susceptibility testing by determination of MICs is a must. Drug susceptibility by MICs is mandatory for certain organisms and antimicrobials for which there are no established disc diffusion criteria.

For example, Vancomycin, teicoplanin, daptomycin for all Staphylococcal species. Susceptibility of polymyxins for all GNB should be based on MICs by broth microdilution technique only.

A culture report that does not report MICs for these organisms cannot be interpreted and often a repeat diagnostic procedure and culture by accepted laboratory standards may be warranted for appropriate interpretation in serious infections.

The zone diameters or MICs of one antibiotic on the culture report cannot be compared with the zone diameter or MIC of another antibiotic. It is a common, erroneous practice to choose the antibiotic with the lowest MIC value on the culture report. The MIC value given on a report is specific for a given antimicrobial in relation to the microorganism isolated. However, it cannot be interpreted based on this absolute value alone and must be interpreted in relation to its breakpoint.

The breakpoint for a particular drug is the highest plasma concentration that can be achieved safely and defines whether an organism is susceptible or resistant to the drug. Clinical breakpoint values are predetermined by international bodies such as the Clinical Laboratory Standards Institute (CLSI) and European Union Committee on Antimicrobial Susceptibility Testing (EUCAST) based on extensive criteria including PKPD, toxicity and resistance mechanisms.

Susceptible (S) on a culture report indicates that the MIC of the drug is less than the breakpoint of the given organism and is hence likely to be effective in vivo.

Intermediate (I) indicates that the MIC is very close to or equal to the breakpoint and hence the drug may work at higher doses or if it concentrates particularly well at a given site.

Resistant (R) indicates that the MIC of the drug is greater than the breakpoint for the given organism and hence it is unlikely that the drug will achieve effective levels at a therapeutic dose.

- Using surveillance data and antibiograms to guide empirical antimicrobial choice

    Regular collection of antibiotic resistance surveillance data at all levels—institutional, regional and national, are invaluable for creating antibiograms that effectively influence empiric antibiotic prescribing trends.

    Although an integral part of a larger functioning hospital, the ICU environment is unique. Prolonged illness, greater morbidity, use of indwelling devices, mechanical ventilation, and the burden of

TABLE 3 Exemplar of unit-based antibiogram for blood isolates in the ICU.

ICU Site: Blood

	Community acquired (within 48 hours of admission)			Hospital associated (>48 hours of admission)	
Risk category	• Type 1 (Low risk) • No healthcare contact/antibiotics in last 90 days • No comorbid conditions	• Type 2 (Moderate risk) • Contact with healthcare/antibiotics in last 90 days (No invasive devices/procedures) OR <2 comorbid conditions	• Type 3 (High risk) • Hospitalization in last 90 days with invasive procedure/device OR • >2 antibiotics within 90 days OR • >2 comorbidities	• Type 2 (Moderate risk) • Contact with healthcare/antibiotics in last 90 days (No invasive devices/procedures) OR <2 comorbid conditions	• Type 3 (High risk) • Hospitalization in last 90 days with invasive procedure/device OR >2 antibiotics within 90 days OR >2 comorbidities
Most common organisms isolated	• *Streptococcus pneumoniae* • *Escherichia coli* • *Klebsiella pneumoniae*	• *Escherichia coli* • *Salmonella* spp. • *Staphylococcus aureus* • *Enterococcus* spp.	• *Escherichia coli* and *Klebsiella* spp. • *Acinetobacter* spp. • *Staphylococcus aureus*	• *Escherichia coli* • *Acinetobacter* spp. • *Salmonella* spp. • *Enterococcus* spp.	• *Klebsiella* spp. • *E. coli* • *Pseudomonas* spp. • *Candida* spp. • *Enterococcus* spp. • *Enterobacter* spp.
Resistance rates	ESBL rate: 33% CRE rate: Nil VRE rate: Nil MRSA: Nil	ESBL rate: 49% CRE rate: Nil VRE rate: Nil MRSA: 50%	ESBL rate: 45% CRE rate: 40% VRE rate: Nil MRSA: 50%	ESBL rate: 39% CRE rate: Nil VRE rate: Nil MRSA: 35%	ESBL rate: 46% CRE rate: 44% VRE rate: 5% MRSA: 33%

(ESBL: extended-spectrum beta-lactamases; MRSA: methicillin-resistant *Staphylococcus aureus*)

broad-spectrum antimicrobials, create an ideal sanctuary for microorganisms with resistance patterns which are uncommon in other areas of the hospital. As a result, *unit-based antibiograms* specific to the ICU, have been shown to have substantially different antibiotic susceptibility patterns as compared to hospital-wide antibiograms.

For example, the **Table 3** is an exemplar of surveillance data from blood isolates in an ICU. The hospital infection control and antibiotic stewardship teams must be encouraged to regularly extract this data and update unit-based antibiograms. This **Table 3** highlights the most common pathogens for different risk groups and their varied resistance patterns, based on which the intensivist can make informed empirical choices. Note how the resistance rates may vary for carbapenem-resistant Enterobacteriaceae (CRE) or methicillin-resistant *Staphylococcus aureus* (MRSA), when patients are risk stratified as per their comorbid conditions, even within the ICU setting.

Flowchart 3: Algorithmic approach to DE of antimicrobials.

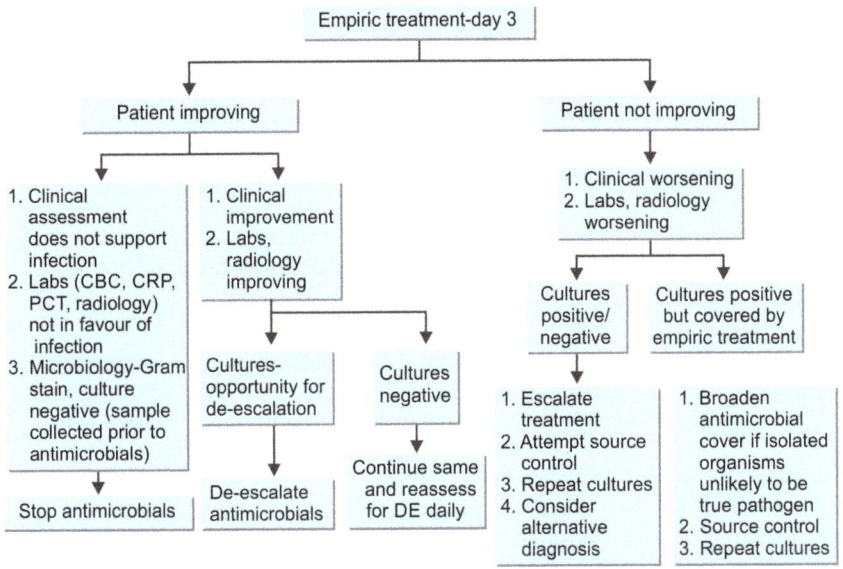

(CBC: complete blood count; CRP: C-reactive protein; PCT: procalcitonin test)
Source: Sunavala A. Rational Use of Antibiotics in Intensive Care Unit. In: Patel M (Ed). ICP Monograph, Critical Care Medicine 2017. New Delhi: Jaypee Brothers Medical Publishers (P) Ltd.; 2017.

- *De-escalation (DE) principles and myths:* Streamlining antimicrobial Use It is a strongly recommended stewardship objective in most practice guidelines. It may be described as the discontinuation of one or more components of an empirically prescribed antimicrobial combination, or the change from a broad-spectrum to a narrower spectrum antimicrobial **(Flowchart 3, Table 4)**.

  Key features integral to DE:
  – Intent to narrow the spectrum of antimicrobial coverage depending on clinical response, microbiological identity and susceptibility of the offending pathogen.
  – Commitment to stop antimicrobial treatment if no infection is established.

Anticipated benefits of DE:
- Decrease in antibiotic-related adverse events and superinfections, e.g., *C. difficile infection* or superinfection due to selection of resistant bacteria.
- Reduction in overall antimicrobial costs
- Overall antimicrobial consumption is directly proportional to antimicrobial resistance (AMR). DE with the aim of reducing antibiotic exposure and thus selection pressure in the ICU, should be an ongoing practice.

Drawbacks and challenges in the implementation of DE strategies:
- DE is considered as an effective strategy to mitigate the effects of empirical broad-spectrum agents with the assumption that short courses of these

TABLE 4: Adjusting antimicrobial therapy with the aid of microbiology results.

Stage 1: Organisms seen on Gram stain of appropriate specimen (cultures from sterile sites/blood culture)	*Clinical implications:* • Indicate high inoculum infection. Can give information on additional need for gram-positive or yeast cover • Morphology of organism on Gram stain gives initial clues, e.g., gram-positive cocci (GPC) in pairs/chains versus clusters to differentiate streptococci/enterococci from staphylococci • Possibility of de-escalation if clinical improvement, e.g., gram-negative cover may be discontinued if GPC is seen in clusters on a Gram stain with a compatible clinical syndrome
Stage 2: Organism identified; susceptibility awaited	• Treating organisms not routinely covered by empiric treatment, e.g., *S. maltophilia* with TMP SMX • Earlier appropriate antimicrobial initiated for classical MDR pathogens, e.g., *A. baumannii* • Altering treatment for organisms intrinsically resistant to certain antibiotics, e.g., *Proteus, Morganella, Serratia* spp. resistant to polymyxins
Stage 3: Organism identified, susceptibility complete	• Fine tuning antimicrobial as per susceptibility pattern, e.g., Cloxacillin, cefazolin known to be superior to vancomycin/teicoplanin for the treatment of MSSA infections. • Switching between susceptible agents based on drug penetration into site of infection, drug toxicity and cost

Source: Sunavala A. Rational Use of Antibiotics in Intensive Care Unit. In: Patel M (Ed). ICP Monograph, Critical Care Medicine 2017. New Delhi: Jaypee Brothers Medical Publishers (P) Ltd.; 2017.

agents have little impact on the development of AMR. However, recent research has clearly shown that AMR can appear within the first few days of treatment. Hence, the eventual strategy of DE cannot be used as a crutch for the indiscriminate prescription of broad-spectrum antimicrobial regimens to all patients who present with fever in the ICU. It must be reserved for those who present with severe sepsis alone.

- DE invariably involves the use of more than one antimicrobial agent, either as an initial combination therapy or serially during a step-down approach. It has been considered that two antimicrobials may actually cause more harm than one.
- Additionally, the principles of DE from broad to narrow may not be applicable in all situations. For example, when empirical treatment with meropenem is de-escalated to ciprofloxacin for a susceptible *pseudomonas* infection, this may be considered as narrowing of the spectrum, but the patient is exposed to two courses of short duration antimicrobial therapy, each with a different, and potentially cumulative damaging effect on the microbiome.
- DE has been found to be associated with an increase in the total duration of antimicrobial therapy. Various explanations have been postulated for this finding, including potential "errors in counting total days of therapy," where

initial broad spectrum empiric therapy days may not have been taken into account, and the false perception that narrow-spectrum antimicrobials are harmless and can be continued for longer periods of time.
- It must be remembered that narrower agents also have an impact on the individual microbiome, emergence of AMR, the ability to cause adverse effects and provide a false sense of security to the treating physician. Hence, the most optimal strategy for DE begins with effective source control where applicable, followed by the timely discontinuation of antimicrobials after they have served their purpose. The possibility of discontinuation must be thoroughly considered on a daily basis.

ANTIMICROBIAL RESISTANCE MECHANISMS AND THEIR CLINICAL APPLICATION

Advances in the medical field over the past few decades are unparalleled-genome sequencing, nanomedicine, robotics, brain mapping, stem cell transplantation, immunotherapy, are among the many rapidly evolving innovations entering our realm of practice. It seems ironic that a patient with access to cutting edge medical therapeutics in a modern tertiary care ICU should eventually succumb to an infection for which we have run out of effective antimicrobials. Yet, intensivists across the world will agree that sepsis due to extensively drug-resistant (XDR) pathogens and pandrug-resistant pathogens remains one of the most overwhelming challenges of contemporary critical care practice.

Antimicrobial resistance appears to be a natural phenomenon with resistant organisms discovered in remote uninhabited locations of the Earth. However, the overwhelming burden and rate of increase in resistant organisms over the last couple of decades appear to be the fall outs of an exponential increase in antimicrobial consumption across the world.

India's antibiotic use has more than doubled in the last decade, giving it the dubious distinction of the world's largest consumer of antibiotics. Our rates of antimicrobial resistance are equally alarming with carbapenem resistance seen in up to 50% of hospital-acquired *Klebsiella* spp. and more than 70% of hospital-acquired *Acinetobacter* spp. The increasing prevalence of azole-resistant *Candida auris* in ICUs across the country with some centers reporting it as the predominant isolate, serves as a grim reflection of the many potential fall outs of the unregulated, widespread use of broad-spectrum antibiotics.

Types of Antimicrobial Resistance

Antimicrobial resistance is primarily classified into two broad types:
1. *Intrinsic resistance* is chromosomally mediated (universally found within the genome of the species), wherein the antimicrobial is inherently resistance to a particular microorganism.

For example, polymyxins and the new β-lactam/β-lactamase inhibitors (BLBLI) ceftazidime avibactam have broad activity against drug-resistant gram-negative isolates. However, they have no anaerobic activity and this must be kept in mind when selecting empirical cover for a patient with intraabdominal sepsis or other sites with likely anaerobic infection.

Additionally, the knowledge of distinctive intrinsic resistance in certain pathogens can offer clues to a discerning clinician as to what the true pathogen may be.

For example, in this uncontrolled diabetic from the Konkan region, who presented with fulminant pneumonia and shock, with a blood culture report showing *Acinetobacter* spp., a closer look at the resistance pattern indicated the strong likelihood of species misidentification by the laboratory. He was confirmed to have melioidosis caused by *Burkholderia pseudomallei* which has a unique pattern of intrinsic resistance to polymyxins and aminoglycosides as seen in this report **(Table 5)**. This pattern of susceptibility would be unusual for *Acinetobacter* spp.

The **Table 6** is a compilation of the important intrinsic resistance patterns in commonly encountered ICU pathogens that the clinician should be aware of when making empirical choices in the critically ill patient.

2. *Acquired resistance,* on the other hand, is a highly efficient process whereby a resistance trait is transferred horizontally from one bacterium to the other.

    This is achieved through the transfer of genetic material carried on plasmids. Plasmids are small, circular, double-stranded DNA molecules that can be efficiently transferred from one bacterium to another even between bacteria of different species.

    Bacteria may employ various strategies encoded on these plasmids to develop acquired resistance. These are broadly classified into: (1) Reduced cell wall permeability to antibiotics; (2) Enzyme modification to inactivate antibiotics; (3) Drug target site alterations; and (4) Efflux pumps that remove antibiotics from the cell.

    The acronym ESKAPE has been coined to denote pathogens that are particularly notorious in terms of antibiotic resistance. These are *Enterococcus faecium, Staphylococcus aureus, Klebsiella pneumoniae, Acinetobacter baumannii, Pseudomonas aeruginosa*, and *Enterobacteriaceae*. The antibiotic resistance mechanisms of these important ICU pathogens and their clinical correlation will be emphasized in the following paragraphs.

ESKAPE Pathogens

Multidrug-resistant Enterococcus spp.: The phenomena of both intrinsic and acquired antibiotic resistance mechanisms may be best described in Enterococci.

These organisms are intrinsically resistant to cephalosporins, oxacillins, aztreonam, Ertapenem, TPM SMX, clindamycin and macrolides. Hence these

TABLE 5: Sensitivity of the blood culture (Aerobic: BACTEC).

Test	Result
Antibiotic Susceptibility Test	*Acinetobacter species*
Amikacin (Ak)	Resistant
Cefepime (Cpm)	Susceptible
Ceftazidime (Caz)	Susceptible
Co-Trimoxazole (Cot)	Susceptible
Gentamicin (Gen)	Resistant
Imipenem (Ipm)	Susceptible
Levofloxacin (Le)	Susceptible
Magnex (Cefoperazone/Sulbactam) 75-30	Susceptible
Meropenem (Mr)	Susceptible
Ofloxacin (Of)	Susceptible
Piperacillin/Tazobactam (P4)	Susceptible
Polymyxin B (PB)	Resistant
Tetracycline (T)	Susceptible

Comments:
Ciprofloxacin: Susceptible
Tigecycline: Susceptible
Ceftriaxone/EDTA/Sulbactum: Susceptible
Azithromycine: Susceptible
Colistin: Resistant (MIC = > 5 µg/mL)*
*MIC done using Hicomb strip Test (HIMEDIA) interpreted as per CLSI guidelines 2016
Kindly Correlate Clinically

TABLE 6: Intrinsic resistance patterns of common organisms.

Organism	Intrinsically resistant antimicrobial
Enterococcus spp.	Cephalosporins, fluoroquinolones, macrolides, TMP-SMX, clindamycin, ertapenem
Pseudomonas spp.	Tetracyclines, many beta-lactams, ertapenem, TMP-SMX
Acinetobacter spp..	Ertapenem, ampicillin, amoxicillin, Fosfomycin, ceftazidime avibactam
Anaerobes	Aminoglycosides, polymyxins, ceftazidime avibactam
Proteus, Providencia, Serratia, Morganella, Burkholderia, Salmonella spp.	Polymyxins
Trichosporon, Cryptococcus, Histoplasma capsulatum, Mucorales	Echinocandins

drugs should not be chosen as empirical monotherapy in likely enterococcal infections.

The predominant species *Enterococcus faecalis* and *Enterococcus faecium* display multiple acquired resistance mechanisms, which can result in multidrug resistance.

- Enterococci are relatively resistant to all penicillins. Altered penicillin binding proteins (PBPs) are the prime drivers of resistance in these organisms with beta-lactamase production seen less often, but resulting in high level resistance to beta-lactams. This is much more common in *E. faecium* strains.
- Enzymatic degradation is implicated in aminoglycoside resistance. Enterococci are intrinsically resistant to low to moderate levels of aminoglycosides. However, synergism is generally seen when aminoglycosides are combined with a cell wall active agent and this bactericidal combination has been the standard of care for enterococcal endocarditis. However, certain enzyme modifications and ribosomal mutations have led to high level aminoglycoside resistance resulting in loss of expected synergism between gentamicin or streptomycin and a cell wall-active agent such as penicillin or vancomycin.
- Changes in peptidoglycan synthesis results in high level vancomycin-resistant enterococci (VRE) more commonly seen in *E. faecium* strains. Different vancomycin resistance gene clusters (e.g., *VanA, B, D,* and *M*) result in varying resistance levels and phenotypes.

Class A resistant strains (VanA) of *E. faecium* and *E. faecalis* confer high-level resistance to vancomycin and teicoplanin.

Class B resistance strains (VanB) show variable resistance to vancomycin but are susceptible to teicoplanin.

All isolates of *E. gallinarum, E. casseliflavus,* and *E. flavescens* possess unique inherent low-level resistance to vancomycin and are susceptible to teicoplanin (class C phenotype). The resistance is mediated by chromosomal genes known as *VanC*.

Methicillin-resistant Staphylococcus aureus: The property of methicillin-resistance in *S. aureus* is chromosomally mediated, the bacterium must possess the *mecA* gene, which encodes for a structural change in penicillin-binding protein 2a (PBP2a). The structural change conferred by PBP2a prevents beta-lactam antibiotics from binding to the cell wall. This cannot be selected by antibiotic pressure on a methicillin susceptible *Staphylococcus aureus* strain during treatment.

Methicillin susceptible *Staphylococcus aureus* isolates with variable resistance to vancomycin have been reported (VISA, VRSA). These are possibly selected by prolonged exposure to suboptimal concentrations of vancomycin. Phenotypically, VISA clones express unusually thick peptidoglycan cell walls that are not completely cross-linked and display an increased number of false binding sites to vancomycin. The vancomycin molecules are trapped at these excess binding sites, preventing the antibiotic from reaching its target.

Gram-negative Resistance in Enterobacteriaceae: The Enterobacteriaceae are a group of gram-negative rods that commonly inhabit the human intestinal and genitourinary tract. They are also widely found in the environment (soil, water and sewage) and are an important cause of drug-resistant community and hospital-acquired infections worldwide. Some of the commonly isolated members of this family are *Klebsiella* spp., *E. coli*, *Enterobacter* spp., *Proteus* spp., *Serratia* spp., *Citrobacter* spp., *Salmonella* spp., and *Shigella* spp.

Resistance among enterobacteriaceae is predominantly acquired through the production of beta-lactamases.

β-lactamases: These enzymes split the amide bond of the β-lactam ring thereby deactivating the beta-lactam antibiotics. These can be encoded by chromosomal genes or more commonly by transferable genes located on plasmids, transposons and integrons leading to widespread dissemination of multidrug resistance among different bacterial species.

Extended-spectrum beta-lactamases (ESBL) are a heterogeneous group of enzymes that confer resistance to most beta-lactam antibiotics, including penicillins, cephalosporins, and the monobactam aztreonam. They retain susceptibility to cephamycins (cefoxitin, cefotetan and cefmetazole) and the carbapenems (imipenem, meropenem, doripenem, and ertapenem). They are also generally susceptible to beta-lactamase inhibitors, such as sulbactam, and tazobactam.

Carbapenemases are carbapenem-hydrolyzing enzymes that confer resistance to most beta-lactam antibiotics including carbapenems. This mechanism is distinct from other mechanisms of resistance exhibited by carbapenems such as impaired permeability due to porin channel mutations and efflux. However, on a culture report the phenotypical susceptibility patterns for isolates with carbapenem resistance may be identical, regardless of the underlying mechanism of resistance.

Ambler classified the β-lactamases into four major classes based on their molecular structure—Class A, C, and D β-lactamases hydrolyze the β-lactam ring by means of a serine residue at their active site, whereas class B enzymes (metallo-β-lactamases), use zinc to destroy the amide bond **(Table 7)**.

Knowledge of the Ambler classification finds clinical applicability in early optimization or de-escalation of antibiotics based on the rapid detection of resistance genes on molecular detection platforms.

For example, a hemodynamically unstable patient with VAP is found to have a CRE on tracheal culture. He was empirically started on Teicoplanin, Meropenem and Polymyxin B. An XpertCarba-R (rapid cartridge-based PCR), is performed on the sample which detects the *OXA-48 carbapenemase* gene with a turnaround time of 1 hour. The intensivist stops the ongoing medications and rapidly optimizes treatment to Ceftazidime avibactam which will be effective against this carbapenemase (OXA-48), and achieves superior lung concentrations as compared to polymyxin B, thus reducing the potential for nephrotoxicity with polymyxin use, and sparing additional carbapenem use.

On the other hand, if the same patient's XpertCarba-R detects the *NDM carbapenemase* gene, a polymyxin-based combination therapy, preferably with a carbapenem may be used. However, if the carbapenem MIC ≥16 mg/L for

TABLE 7 Ambler classification of β-lactamases.

Class Active site	β-lactamase enzyme	Target antibiotics	Examples
A Serine	*Penicillinases*: • Broad spectrum • Extended spectrum (ESBL) • Carbapenemases	• Penicillins • Narrow-spectrum cephalosporins • Substrates of broad spectrum plus • 3rd, 4th generation cephalosporins • Aztreonam • Substrates of extended-spectrum plus • Cephamycins • Carbapenems	*GNB:* TEM 1, SHV 1 • *Enterobacteriaceae*: TEM-derived, SHV-derived, CTX-M–derived • *Pseudomonas aeruginosa:* PER-1, VEB-1, VEB-2, GES-1, GES-2 • *K. pneumoniae*: KPC-1, KPC-2, KPC-3
B Metallo-β-lactamases (Zn^{2+})	Carbapenemases	Substrates of extended-spectrum plus • Cephamycins • Carbapenems	• *Enterobacteriaceae*: NDM-1 • *P. aeruginosa, Acinetobacter spp.*: IMP, VIM, GIM, SPM, SIM
C Serine	Cephalosporinases	Substrates of extended-spectrum plus • Cephamycins	• Enterobacteriaceae, *Acinetobacter* spp. AmpC-type enzymes
D Serine	*Oxacillinases*: • Broad-spectrum • Extended-spectrum • Carbapenemases	• Penicillins • Narrow-spectrum cephalosporins • Substrates of broad spectrum plus • 3rd, 4th generation cephalosporins • Aztreonam • Substrates of extended-spectrum plus • Cephamycins • Carbapenems	• *P. aeruginosa:* OXA-family • *P. aeruginosa:* OXA-derived • *Acinetobacter spp.*: OXA-derived

the given isolate, this combination has not been found to be advantageous in reducing mortality. In this situation, other drugs like tigecycline or fosfomycin have been used in combination with polymyxins depending on the site of infection.

It must be kept in mind that class B metallo-beta-lactamases (MBL) confer resistance to all beta-lactam-type antibiotics except aztreonam and the novel agent cefiderocol. However, most MBL-producing isolates also produce other extended-spectrum beta-lactamases that will confer resistance to aztreonam if used alone. Hence, combining aztreonam with a BLBLI drug serves as a suitable alternative to polymyxin-based combinations.

Genotypic platforms often pick up the presence of two carbapenemases in the same isolate, usually NBM plus OXA-48. Extrapolating from the above, combination of Aztreonam with ceftazidime avibactam in this situation can have a synergistic effect, as the ceftazidime avibactam inactivates the OXA-48 carbapenemase, leaving aztreonam to act against the NDM MBL.

Drug-resistant Acinetobacter spp.: These bacteria efficiently display multiple antibiotic resistance genes to various groups of antibiotics simultaneously, leading to the development of multidrug-resistant or extensively drug-resistant strains.

Acinetobacter spp. have chromosomally encoded, intrinsic AmpC beta-lactamases which are usually expressed at a low level that does not cause clinically appreciable resistance. However, the addition of another promoter insertion gene next to the *ampC gene* increases beta-lactamase production, causing resistance to cephalosporins.

Carbapenemase production in *Acinetobacter* spp., both by serine and metallo-beta-lactamases is widespread in hospital-acquired infections resulting in XDR pathogens with virtually no treatment options. Mutations in porin channels and over expression of efflux pumps also contribute to clinical resistance.

Polymyxins are the mainstay of treatment for drug resistant *Acinetobacter* spp. Other drugs that often retain susceptibility to resistant isolates include minocycline and the beta-lactamase inhibitor sulbactam. Even strains that are resistant to carbapenems sometimes retain in vitro susceptibility to sulbactam.

Drug-resistant Pseudomonas aeruginosa: Pseudomonas aeruginosa displays intrinsic resistance to various antibiotics (Ertapenem, tigecycline and chloramphenicol), and efficiently acquires resistance to other agents during treatment. Even the use of drugs such as Ertapenem (which does not have antipseudomonal activity), has been repeatedly identified as a risk factor for emergence of carbapenem resistance.

Resistance is often acquired exogenously, and be mediated by multiple mechanisms, including degrading enzymes, reduced permeability, and active efflux.

With respect to degrading enzymes, the classical plasmid-mediated extended spectrum beta-lactamases (TEM, SHV, and CTX-M) have been reported in *P. aeruginosa*, but are uncommon. Distinctive ESBL genes such as VEB and PER are found in *Pseudomonas* isolates from different geographic regions. These enzymes confer high-level resistance to antipseudomonal cephalosporins, and some, such as PER-1, also degrade monobactams.

Carbapenem resistance, particularly imipenem, is most often due to a mutation resulting in the loss of a carbapenem-specific porin, OprD. The production of carbapenemases, especially the metallo-beta-lactamases, has also been reported though less often. Overexpression of efflux pumps on the bacterial surface is also considered to be major contributors to multidrug resistance.

As we continue to face everyday challenges at the bedside with drug resistant pathogens, we must keep in mind a fundamental principal, crucial to our appreciation of resistance. Microorganisms have existed on the planet, battling the forces of nature, far longer than any other life form. Hence, the dynamic phenomenon of resistance does not develop anew when we start an antibiotic in our ICUs. It is a pre-existing, preconceived marvel that has existed since prehistoric times, abundant in nature, and ever-evolving to outwit every existing drug and most likely every compound still to be invented. Our use or misuse of antimicrobials only results in compounding the selection of resistant strains already existing in nature. The anticipation of novel agents is therefore not a viable solution to the XDR crisis. The burden is on us to preserve existing antimicrobials as a nonrenewable resource, a powerful double edged weapon that undoubtedly saves lives but at the same time has inconceivable ecological ramifications that compromise the very future of modern medicine.

■ SUGGESTED READING

1. De Waele JJ, Schouten J, Beovic B, Tabah A. Antimicrobial de-escalation as part of antimicrobial stewardship in intensive care: no simple answers to simple questions – a viewpoint of experts. Intensive Care Med. 2020;46:236-44.
2. Opal SM, Pop-Vicas A. Molecular Mechanisms of Antibiotic Resistance in Bacteria. In: Bennett JE, Dolin R, Blaser MJ (Eds). Mandell Douglas and Bennett's Principles and Practice of Infectious Diseases, 9th edition. New York: Elsevier; 2020.
3. Osmon DR, Tande AJ. Nonvertebral Osteomyelitis in adults: treatment. UpToDate. 2021.
4. Pai MP, Cottrell ML, Bertino JS Jr. Pharmacokinetics and Pharmacodynamics of Anti-infective Agents. In: Bennett JE, Dolin R, Blaser MJ (Eds). Mandell Douglas and Bennett's Principles and Practice of Infectious Diseases, 9th edition. New York: Elsevier; 2020.
5. Soman R. Colonization versus Infection. API Medicine Update. 2008;18:330-3.
6. Spellberg B. Principles of Anti-infective Therapy. In: Bennett JE, Dolin R, Blaser MJ (Eds). Mandell Douglas and Bennett's Principles and Practice of Infectious Diseases, 9th edition. New York: Elsevier; 2020.
7. Walia K, Madhumathi J, Veeraraghavan B, Chakrabarti A, Kapil A, Ray P, et al. Establishing Antimicrobial Resistance Surveillance and Research Network in India: Journey so far. Indian J Med Res. 2019;149:164-79.

CHAPTER 13

Optimal Usage of the Microbiology Laboratory in the ICU

Karuna Tiwari, Camilla Rodrigues

■ INTRODUCTION

The modern microbiology laboratory offers a wide array of innovative methods of microbial detection, identification, and susceptibility to antimicrobials. Novel cutting-edge technology includes rapid microbiological methods with significantly reduced turnaround times when compared with conventional microbiological methods, point of care diagnostics and automated, miniaturized platforms that increase sensitivity, precision, and reproducibility.

The practicing clinician is spoilt for choice and yet often lost in a sea of cutting-edge microbiological methods, biomarkers, genetic testing, and polymerase chain reaction (PCR) panels that detect novel microorganisms with complex resistance patterns. A basic knowledge of the clinical applicability of these platforms is essential to rationalize the use of the various tests and accurately interpret their results. Needless to say, a multidisciplinary approach with regular communication between the clinical team and the microbiologist is a prerequisite for optimal management.

The rational application of the various common microbiological tests offered is explained through a clinically suspected syndromic approach in the course of this chapter.

■ SYNDROMIC APPROACH TO THE USE OF MICROBIOLOGICAL METHODS IN THE INTENSIVE CARE UNIT

Acute Undifferentiated Fever

Tropical Fever

Malaria is detected by conventional methods like thin and thick peripheral smears as well as rapid diagnostic tests (RDTs) like lateral flow tests, which detect malarial antigens with the ability to detect >100 parasites/mL in blood. These are rapid, simple, and easy to perform as well as interpret. As these are qualitative tests and cannot quantitate parasite index, they are not useful for prognostic purposes. RDTs have decreased sensitivity and can yield false-negative results in nonimmune patients who have low levels of parasitemia.

There are three types of antigens that are used in detection, namely parasite lactate dehydrogenase (pLDH), histidine-rich protein II (HRP II), and parasite aldolase. pLDH is produced by both sexual and asexual stages of the malarial parasite and is reported to have high sensitivity and specificity in high endemic regions. HRP II is produced by the asexual stage and young gametocytes of

Plasmodium falciparum. It is more sensitive than pLDH but has a disadvantage that the antigen persists at detectable levels even after 28 days of treatment. *Plasmodium* aldolase, an enzyme of the glycolytic pathway produced by all four species, has been recently developed.

In India, there are more than five types of RDTs available with various combinations of pLDH with or without HRP II. From the treatment perspective, the test chosen should be able to differentiate *Plasmodium* species, especially *P. falciparum* and *P. vivax,* as both are almost equally prevalent.

Dengue enzyme immunoassay (EIA) is valuable as it detects the NS1 antigen, prior to seroconversion. NS1 is a marker of early acute active infection and can be detected in serum from the day after onset of fever, up to the first week of illness. Immunoglobulin M (IgM) enzyme-linked immunosorbent assay (ELISA) has a role for detection of dengue after the NS1 antigen is negative.

The DENV-1-4 rRT-PCR multiplex assay is a nucleic acid test for detection and typing of dengue virus in suspected and symptomatic cases. The PCR test is useful for the rapid and accurate diagnosis in the first 7 days after onset of fever. It can also differentiate between serotypes of the dengue virus thus providing epidemiologic information for surveillance of circulating dengue viruses.

Multiplex real-time PCR assays are also available that can simultaneously detect ribonucleic acid (RNA) of chikungunya and dengue viruses and leptospiral deoxyribonucleic acid (DNA). Although not widely available, novel real-time PCR assays have been developed for the detection of *Rickettsia* spp. which otherwise remains a clinical diagnosis in patients who present with fever, rash, and/or classical eschar.

Serology is performed for various pathogens, which are fastidious, hazardous to grow, or take long to grow. This detects either the specific or nonspecific immune responses of the host or the presence of the antigen in the host. Serology detects antigen and antibodies to organisms indicating either current or past infection. These test results may be affected by the patient's immune status. False-positive tests may occur due to cross-reaction with other antibodies.

Specific IgG and IgM antibodies can be detected using immunological techniques against an increasing range of organisms, e.g., dengue, *Leptospira*, chikungunya, rickettsiae, hepatitis (A-G), human immunodeficiency virus (HIV), rubella, measles, Epstein–Barr, Cytomegalovirus (CMV), herpes simplex, etc. IgM antibodies are indicative of recent infection. The secondary response on reexposure to the same antigen is predominantly IgG driven. There are various types of serological reactions, such as precipitation, agglutination, complement fixation, immunofluorescence, ELISA, and Western blot.

Sepsis

Identification of the organism: Smear microscopy is the rapid and easy method to determine causative agents and the smears are made directly

from specimens, stained and seen under the microscope for specific staining characteristics and bacterial morphology. Commonly used stains are:
- *Gram stain*: This is the most rapid and useful bacterial staining method and can be performed on any specimen, e.g., lanceolate-shaped gram-positive diplococci are suggestive of *Streptococcus pneumoniae* on Gram stain.
- *Acid-fast stain*: Also known as Ziehl–Neelsen (ZN) stain. It is used to identify *Mycobacterium tuberculosis*. Modifications of the stain help to identify other acid-fast organisms, e.g., branching acid-fast bacilli on modified (1%) ZN stain are suggestive of *Nocardia* spp.
- Other stains include more sensitive auramine/rhodamine fluorochrome staining over traditional ZN stain for mycobacteria, Wright–Giemsa stain for malarial parasites and microfilaria in blood smears.

Blood cultures are indicated in all cases of undifferentiated fever prior to starting empiric treatment. They are especially indicated in infections where bacteremia is the hallmark, e.g., in infective endocarditis, where ideally three blood samples should be drawn at least half an hour apart and inoculated in a set of aerobic and anaerobic medium containing bottles.

Patients with central lines, hemodialysis (HD) catheters, or ports for chemotherapy must have paired blood culture samples of the same volume, collected simultaneously from the intravascular catheter and a percutaneous collection to assess for differential time to positivity (DTP). The bottles must be appropriately labeled as "catheter/HD/chemo port" and "percutaneous" before sending them to the laboratory.

Catheter-related bloodstream infection (CRBSI) is diagnosed on the basis of DTP when the growth blood drawn from a catheter hub detects the growth of microbes at least 2 hours before microbial growth is detected in blood samples obtained from a peripheral vein. The accurate diagnosis of a CRBSI is vital in the intensive care unit (ICU) for effective source control, as well as to prevent the unnecessary removal of vital lines in unstable patients with difficult intravenous (IV) access.

Although recovery of bacteria from blood during episodes of sepsis is not difficult, certain concepts need to be understood. Adequate skin preparation prior to venipuncture is of utmost importance to prevent contamination of the specimen with normal skin flora. The most important factor that affects the rate of blood culture is the volume collected. So, a minimum of 30–40 mL of blood should be cultured. Septic patients have less than one organism per mL of blood and there is a 40% increase in positivity when blood culture is filled the requisite volume. Also, if the patient is on antibiotic treatment, blood culture media containing resins should be used to enhance recovery. There is data to substantiate that two or three blood cultures are adequate for detecting common pathogens, as recovery in the first culture is 80%, 88% in two cultures, and 99% in all three cultures. Organisms such as *Brucella*, *Legionella*, some fungi, and mycobacteria should be incubated for longer than the traditional 5 days and suspicion of these organisms must be conveyed to the microbiologist.

Most modern laboratories now use automated blood culture systems. The continuous monitoring blood culture systems are modular with a single computer controlling the incubator units. Culture vials are incubated in individual cells and monitored at intervals of 10–15 minutes for evidence of microbial growth. Three such systems, the BACTEC™ blood culture system (BD Diagnostic Systems), the BacT/ALERT® (bioMérieux), and the TREK-ESP culture systems (TREK Diagnostic Systems) are available in India. Multiple studies have shown that the bottles need to be incubated for only 5 days.

Rapid Identification Methods

Automated instruments such as BD Phoenix and Vitek 2 identify the isolated organisms to species level by using biochemical tests. This usually takes 8–10 hours. The recently introduced matrix-assisted laser desorption and ionization–time-of-flight (MALDI-TOF) is a mass spectrometer that identifies organisms (bacteria and fungi) within minutes.

Matrix-assisted Laser Desorption and Ionization–Time-of-Flight Mass Spectrometry

Matrix-assisted laser desorption and ionization–time-of-flight mass spectrometry (MALDI-TOF MS) is a rapid and accurate method for identifying microorganisms by protein analysis. The bacterial colony is processed and then pulsed with a laser. The laser ionizes and vaporizes the microbial proteins, which travel through a charged vacuum chamber to a detector. The resulting protein pattern (or fingerprint) is compared with a library of known patterns for various microorganisms to identify the test organism. The primary clinical advantage of MALDI-TOF is that it takes only minutes to identify an organism, whereas several hours are needed for conventional phenotyping. MALDI-TOF is highly accurate for identification of most bacteria and yeasts grown on solid agar or in blood culture broth.

■ LABORATORY TESTING FOR ANTIMICROBIAL SUSCEPTIBILITY OF ORGANISMS

Once the organism is identified by conventional or automated techniques, the principal function of the laboratory is to carry out in vitro antimicrobial sensitivity testing (AST), which helps in guiding the clinician in choosing the right drug. There are different methods to perform antimicrobial susceptibility such as agar dilution, broth dilution (macrobroth dilution and microbroth dilution), disk diffusion, antibiotic gradient methods (e.g.. E-test) and nowadays, automated instrument methods (e.g., Vitek).

Disk Diffusion Susceptibility Tests

Different paper disks with specified concentration of antimicrobial agents are applied to agar medium inoculated with the test organism. Antibiotics from the disk start diffusing into the surrounding medium on contact. Bacterial growth occurs on the agar surface after a specified incubation period (16–18 hours), but growth is inhibited in an area around the disk if the organism is drug sensitive. The concentration of the antibiotic at this interface of growing and inhibited bacteria is known as the critical concentration and approximates the minimum inhibitory concentration (MIC) of the dilution tests. Zone diameters are measured with calipers and interpreted on the basis of standard international guidelines as susceptible, intermediate, or resistant to the antimicrobial agent tested. This test is inadequate for the detection of vancomycin intermediate *Staphylococcus aureus*, cefoxitin heteroresistant staphylococci, and low level (Van-B type) vancomycin-resistant enterococci. Also as it is a qualitative and not a quantitative test, MIC cannot be determined.

Dilution Methods

Dilution methods are well-standardized, reliable techniques, and can be used as reference for evaluating accuracy of other testing systems. These are of two types: agar dilution and broth dilution testing.

Agar Dilution Susceptibility Testing

Standardized suspension of bacteria is inoculated onto a series of agar plates, each containing a different concentration of antibiotic. Organisms sensitive to the concentration of the antibiotic contained in the given agar plate do not produce a circle of growth at the inoculum site, whereas if resistant, appear as circular colonies. For example, series of agar plates containing 1, 4, 8, 16, and 32 µg/mL of antibiotic are used to determine the susceptibility of the organism being tested. If the organism grows on the first three plates but not on the plate with 16 µg/mL of the antibiotic, the MIC value is 16 µg/mL.

Broth Dilution Susceptibility Testing

Macrodilution and microdilution tests employ serial dilutions of the antimicrobial agents made in broth after which a standard suspension of bacteria is added. A tube free of antibiotic serves as a growth control. The tubes are then incubated at 35°C for 16–20 hours. Cloudiness indicates bacterial growth that has not been inhibited by the concentration of the antibiotic contained in the particular tube. The MIC is determined as the lowest concentration of the antibiotic in µg/mL that prevents in vitro growth of bacteria in broth.

Gradient Diffusion Method

E-test (AB Biodisk, Solna, Sweden) method is a quantitative antimicrobial susceptibility method. A preformed antimicrobial gradient diffuses from a plastic-coated strip into an agar medium inoculated with the test organism. The MIC is directly read from a scale on the plastic strip at a point where the ellipse of the organism growth intercepts the strip. It is a simple but expensive method to get MICs of antibiotics.

Automated Instrument Methods

Many laboratories have automated MIC systems utilizing panels containing varying concentrations of several antimicrobial agents. Following inoculation, the panels are incubated in the instrument and MIC endpoints are read automatically. Inbuilt software enables MIC to be interpreted and reports are printed automatically. The most common automated platforms used in our country include (1) the Vitek 2 system (bioMérieux) which is an integrated modular system that detects bacterial growth and metabolic changes after short incubation periods with an accuracy of 93% and (2) Phoenix (BD Diagnostics System).

INTERPRETATION OF RESULTS

Laboratories worldwide adhere to standardized protocols in order to achieve reproducible results. Clinical and Laboratory Standards Institute (CLSI) (formerly National Committee for Clinical Laboratory Standards—NCCLS) is one such organization in USA that publishes standards for susceptibility testing on a continuing basis. The European Committee on Antimicrobial Susceptibility Testing (EUCAST) is a similar organization in Europe. Revised procedures and current recommendations should be promptly followed by all clinical laboratories. These standards provide clinical breakpoints to interpret susceptibility tests. Breakpoints are discriminatory antimicrobial concentrations used in the interpretation of results of susceptibility testing to define isolates as susceptible, intermediate, or resistant. Clinical, pharmacological, microbiological, pharmacokinetic (PK), and pharmacodynamic (PD) considerations are important in setting breakpoints.

Susceptible

There is a high probability that the patient will respond to treatment with the appropriate dosage of that antimicrobial agent.

Resistant

Treatment with the antimicrobial agent is likely to fail.

Intermediate

With the agents that can be safely administered at higher doses, this category implies that higher doses may be required to ensure efficacy, or that the agent may prove efficacious if it is normally concentrated in an infected body fluid, e.g., urine. For body compartments where drug penetration is restricted even in the presence of inflammation, e.g., cerebrospinal fluid (CSF), it suggests that extreme caution should be taken in the use of the agent. Thus, this category represents a "buffer" zone that prevents strains with borderline susceptibility from being incorrectly categorized as resistant.

Susceptible Dose Dependent

Susceptible dose dependent (SDD) implies that susceptibility of the organism depends on dosing regimen that is used in the patient. To achieve levels for clinical effectiveness, use a dosing regimen (i.e., higher doses, more frequent doses, or both) that results in higher drug exposure than that was achieved with the dose that was used to establish the susceptibility breakpoint.

■ TESTS USED TO DIAGNOSE DRUG RESISTANCE

Even with positive blood cultures results in septic patients, identification of the organism and its antibiotic sensitivity pattern may take up to 48 hours. The various molecular methods available, such as fluorescence in situ hybridization, point-of-care PCR, and microarrays, can be applied directly to the positive blood cultures to identify the pathogen and achieve a profile of antimicrobial sensitivity within 3–6 hours.

A novel PCR-based rapid diagnostic method by Cepheid diagnostics detects drug resistance by GeneXpert and results are available in 2–3 hours. Cartridges are available for detection of methicillin-resistant *Staphylococcus aureus* (MRSA) (*mecA* gene), vancomycin-resistant enterococci (VRE) (*vanA* gene) as well as carbapenemase production (bla_{KPC}, bla_{NDM}, bla_{VIM}, bla_{OXA-48}, and bla_{IMP} gene sequences). Additionally, many in-house multiplex PCR systems are available for rapid detection of beta-lactamase, as well as carbapenemase activity directly from the clinical sample. This rapid platform is especially useful in deciding antibiotic choices in critically ill patients.

Multiplex PCR systems identify organisms directly from the positive blood culture bottle. The FilmArray® Blood Culture Identification (BCID) Panel tests for a comprehensive list of 24 pathogens which includes all the common bacterial pathogens, five common *Candida* species and three antibiotic resistance genes including *mecA*, *Van A/B*, and *KPC* associated with bloodstream infections. This is a Food and Drug Administration (FDA) approved multiplex PCR system, which gives result in 1 hour.

Molecular methods have revolutionized microbiology. These are rapid and can be used to detect almost any pathogen. In the past, these tests required specialized laboratories with highly trained staff. The current tests such as GeneXpert [tuberculosis (TB), *Clostridium difficile*, MRSA, influenza, etc.) are extremely simple and require no skill or expensive infrastructure. They can be used as point-of-care tests and are ideal for the detection of microorganisms with slow growth (mycobacteria), difficult growth (viruses and Chlamydia), or fastidious growth (mycoplasma). Another advantage is the ability to detect low pathogen loads as in meningitis and also in monitoring response to treatment (viral load assays for hepatitis B, hepatitis C, and HIV).

BIOMARKERS FOR SEPSIS

An ideal biomarker for sepsis should facilitate early rapid diagnosis, predict the course and prognosis of the disease, and guide therapeutic decisions (e.g., antibiotic stewardship). Various biomarkers have been aggressively researched; however, only a few are presently available to us in day-to-day practice **(Table 1)**.

TABLE 1 Advantages and limitations of available biomarkers.

Biomarker	Advantages	Limitations
WBC count (bandemia > 10%)	• Simple and rapid test • Inexpensive	• Cannot differentiate infection from inflammation • SIRS can be associated with WBC < 4000 • May be falsely low in elderly and immunocompromised
CRP	• Rapid test • Relatively inexpensive	• Cannot differentiate infection from inflammation • Questionable role of prognostication in sepsis
Procalcitonin (PCT)	• Levels rise in 4–12 hours after infection • Increase only transiently (12–24 hours) postsurgery (HLP < 24 hours) • Role in de-escalation of antibiotics if serial PCTs monitored	• Expensive • Not easily available • False positive in trauma, CKD, cardiogenic shock, GVHD, autoimmune disease, and paraneoplastic syndromes • Higher values in bacterial over viral/fungal sepsis
1,3-β-D-glucan	• Pan-fungal biomarker present in the cell wall of most fungi including *Candida* spp., *Aspergillus* spp., and *Pneumocystis jirovecii* • Can identify cases of invasive candidiasis days to weeks prior to positive blood cultures • Sensitivity and specificity for diagnosing invasive candidiasis were 75–80% and 80%, respectively • Excellent negative predictive value to rule out invasive fungal infection	• Cannot detect *Cryptococcus* spp. and zygomycetes • False-positive results are seen with concomitant gram-positive and gram-negative bacteremia, certain antibiotics, such as intravenous amoxicillin-clavulanate, some cephalosporins, carbapenems, and ampicillin-sulbactam, chemotherapeutics such as pegylated asparaginase hemodialysis, fungal colonization, receipt of albumin or immunoglobulin, use of surgical gauze or other material containing glucan, and mucositis or other disruptions of gastrointestinal mucosa

Contd...

Contd...

Biomarker	Advantages	Limitations
Galactomannan	• Produced by growing hyphae in the cell wall of most *Aspergillus* and *Penicillium* spp. • Useful marker for IA from BAL or serum of neutropenic patients	• Poor sensitivity in serum from non-neutropenics • False-negative results with concurrent mold-active antifungal therapy or prophylaxis • False-positive results have been reported with receipt of certain antibiotics like piperacillin-tazobactam (no longer considered to be cross-reactive), neonatal colonization with *Bifidobacterium*, Plasmalyte is used in BAL fluids, other invasive mycoses (including penicilliosis, fusariosis, histoplasmosis, and blastomycosis)

(BAL: bronchoalveolar lavage; CKD: chronic kidney disease; CRP: C-reactive protein; GVHD: graft-versus-host disease; HLP: half life procalcitonin; IA: invasive aspergillosis; SIRS: systemic inflammatory response syndrome; WBC: white blood cell)

■ SPECIFIC ORGAN-RELATED INFECTIONS

Urosepsis

Urine sample is obtained by adequate cleaning of perineal area prior to collection to minimize contamination by urethral and perineal organisms. Patients and staff should be clearly instructed regarding the procedure for urine collection, and the importance of sterile containers should be stressed. Urine samples should reach the laboratory within 30 minutes and should be cultured with minimal delay, ideally within an hour of collection. If there is a delay in transport, refrigeration of urine sample at 4°C is required.

Urine for routine and culture examinations should be sent prior to starting antibiotics in all patients with suspected urinary tract infection (UTI). Screening for asymptomatic bacteriuria is not recommended and not indicated even in catheterized patients.

When collecting urine from catheters, it is important to collect from the port and not the bag. The presence of >100,000 colonies/mL signifies true infection in symptomatic patients only [fulfill criteria for systemic inflammatory response syndrome (SIRS)]. In patients with indwelling catheters, urine culture is invariably positive due to catheter colonization; hence, unless the patient is bacteremic with the same organism isolated from the blood and urine, other causes of fever must be ruled out. Absence of localizing features such as obstruction, hematuria, or costovertebral angle tenderness warrant search for an alternate diagnosis. When catheter-associated UTI is strongly suspected, a urine sample sent from a freshly placed urinary catheter (within 24 hours of insertion) may overcome problems of isolation of catheter colonizers.

Asymptomatic candiduria is a frequent finding in critically ill patients in the ICU. Removal of the urinary catheter alone suffices in most cases. Treatment of candiduria is not recommended unless the patient is neutropenic or scheduled to undergo urological manipulation.

Respiratory Tract Infections

Sputum samples may contain large number of oral and upper respiratory flora. Early morning samples are advisable as they contain pooled overnight secretions likely to contain pathogenic organisms. When sputum production is not possible, induction with heated or ultrasonic nebulized saline may be effective. Invasive methods include transtracheal aspiration, bronchoscopy, and bronchoalveolar lavage. Quantitative cultures of endotracheal aspirate (EA) samples are done on different culture media using 10^5 colony-forming units per milliliter as a cutoff point for interpreting ICU patients suspected of having pneumonia. This quantitative culture of EA is a good predictive method of identifying the prevailing organism in ventilator-associated pneumonia (VAP).

In community-acquired pneumonia, antigen testing is useful in patients on treatment to establish the etiological agent.

- *Streptococcus pneumoniae*: The Alere BinaxNOW™ test is a rapid immunochromatographic test (ICT) assay for detection of *S. pneumoniae* antigen in urine of patients with pneumonia and in the CSF of patients with meningitis. Pneumococcal urinary antigen sensitivity surpasses that of the Gram stain. The clinical sensitivity and specificity are 86% and 94%, respectively. In children, the specificity is lower due to carriage of *S. pneumoniae*.
- *Legionella pneumophila*: Similarly, an in vitro rapid ICT assay is available with BinaxNOW™ for detection of *L. pneumophila* serogroup I antigen secreted in urine, with a clinical sensitivity and specificity of >95%.
- *Histoplasma capsulatum*: Histoplasma antigen detection in serum, urine, and CSF, is a useful indicator of systemic infection. ELISA tests can be performed on urine, CSF, serum, and BAL. Sensitivity of the test is around 92% in urine and 82% in serum of patients with disseminated disease. The test has low sensitivity in self-limited disease and chronic pulmonary histoplasmosis.

Upper Respiratory Pathogens

The FilmArray® Upper Respiratory Panel tests for 17 viruses and 3 bacteria which cause upper respiratory tract infections (URTIs) with an overall sensitivity and specificity of 95% and 99%, respectively. This FDA approved system simultaneously identifies 20 respiratory pathogens causing URTI from the throat swab or nasopharyngeal swab, and the result is available in 1 hour.

Lower Respiratory Pathogens

The FilmArray® Lower Respiratory Panel tests 33 targets at once, comprising 18 bacteria (11 gram-negative, 4 gram-positive, and 3 atypical), 7 antibiotic resistance markers, and 8 viruses that cause pneumonia and other lower respiratory tract infections (LRTIs). Overall sensitivity and specificity for BAL-like and sputum samples are around 96% and 97%, respectively.

Gastrointestinal Infections

Gastric aspirates are used for the diagnosis of TB in children. Endoscopic biopsies are used to detect *Helicobacter pylori*. Stool specimens are cultured for identification of diarrheal pathogens as *Vibrio cholerae, Shigella* as well as *Salmonella*, for diagnosis of typhoid fever. Rota virus diarrhea can be diagnosed by a stool antigen detection test. Stool samples are cultured on special media to prevent the colonic flora from overgrowing the pathogen.

The FilmArray® Gastrointestinal (GI) Panel tests for most common GI pathogens including viruses, bacteria, and parasites that cause infectious diarrhea and other GI infections. This FDA approved system identifies the pathogen's nuclear material directly from the stool sample and can detect 22 pathogens simultaneously within an hour.

Fecal Samples

Clostridium difficile antigen: Clostridium difficile associated diarrhea (CDAD) is an infectious diarrhea seen in hospital settings due to antibiotic usage. Toxins A and B can be detected by EIA with a specificity of around 100%. Direct testing of toxin in stool samples using immunoassay techniques has largely replaced culture methods. Strains, which produce either toxin A or B, are pathogenic, so tests that detect both toxins are preferable.

GeneXpert C. difficile: Cepheid diagnostics has introduced this novel cartridge-based PCR system which detects *C. difficile* toxin A and B as well as binary toxin, within 2-3 hours. Also, it detects 027/NAP/BI strain, which is responsible for hospital-acquired *C. difficile* infections.

Helicobacter pylori: HpSA- H. pylori stool antigen assay (meridian diagnostics) is a useful noninvasive test for diagnosis and follow-up of *H. pylori* infections. It detects fecal excretion of *H. pylori* antigens with a sensitivity of 96% and specificity of 95%.

Central Nervous System Infections

In Cerebrospinal Fluid

Bacterial latex agglutination: Latex agglutination techniques are used to demonstrate the soluble polysaccharide antigens of *Neisseria meningitidis,*

Haemophilus influenzae type B, and *S. pneumoniae* in patients of acute pyogenic meningitis. In neonatal meningitis, the latex agglutination method can be used for detection of *Escherichia coli* and group B streptococci. These tests offer good specificity >98%, but the sensitivity varies with each bacterium tested. For *N. meningitidis* A, C, Y, W135, and *N. meningitidis* B/*E. coli* K1 it is 71% and 65%, respectively. For *S. pneumoniae* it is 88% and for *H. influenzae* and group B streptococci, it is 67%. This assay can also be used for serum after appropriate treatment with ethylenediaminetetraacetic acid (EDTA).

The BiofireFilmArray® Meningitis/Encephalitis (ME) Panel tests CSF for the 14 most common pathogens responsible for community-acquired meningitis or encephalitis, including viruses, bacteria, and yeast. This commercially available system is FDA approved and takes only 1 hour to identify the pathogen directly from the CSF.

Cryptococcal antigen: Latex agglutination and ELISA are the preferred tests for detection of cryptococcal antigen. They can be used for diagnosis as well as therapeutic monitoring. The latex agglutination methods have a sensitivity of approximately 93% and specificity from 93 to 100% and are equivalent to ELISA in detecting antigen. *Trichosporon beigelii, Capnocytophaga* spp., and *Stomatococcus* have been shown to produce a cross reacting polysaccharide antigen. Treatment with pronase B reduces the false positive in serum tests in certain rheumatological disorders.

■ CAVEATS OF ANTIMICROBIAL SENSITIVITY TESTING

Other factors influence the outcome of antimicrobial therapy, which cannot be addressed by in vitro susceptibility tests. These are discussed here.

Factors Related to the Antimicrobial Agents

- *Pharmacokinetic factors*: The penetration of antibiotics at the site of infection is one issue that cannot be addressed by the in vitro tests. High levels of antibiotics are achieved at sites of excretion from the body, e.g., urine and bile, whereas low levels relative to serum are found in prostatic fluid, bone, CSF. For example, aminoglycosides are ineffective in the treatment of *Legionella* infections despite excellent in vitro activity, due to their poor penetration into macrophages, which are the site of bacterial growth.
- *Pharmacodynamic factors*: Interactions between the antimicrobial agent and the pathogen also affect the outcome of therapy.

Factors Related to the Patient

Immune function, site of infection, and the presence of prosthetic devices have to be considered while guiding the choice of antibiotic along with in vitro susceptibility tests. There are various reasons why antibiotics may not work despite correct susceptibility and these include:
- *Incorrect spectrum of antibiotic*: An antibiotic class is used for treatment but there is lack of clinical response. Inadequate antibiotic coverage results

from not covering pathogens in a given situation, e.g., intra-abdominal infection. Treatment of serious intra-abdominal infection should include coverage directed against both aerobic gram-negative bacilli as well as anaerobic bacteria, *Bacteroides fragilis*.
- *In vivo versus in vitro susceptibility*:
  - Susceptibility tests have been designed for monomicrobial infections, but in a polymicrobial infection when one tests the individual pathogens, it is difficult to truly ascertain its value in vivo.
  - Also, the level of expression of virulence factors is not considered in in vitro susceptibility testing.
  - We do not take into account the effect of white blood cells (WBCs), complement, cytokines, or antibodies on AST results.
  - The organism may harbor a resistance gene, which is inducible and may not be expressed in vitro, e.g., AmpC positive *Enterobacter* spp. appears susceptible to third-generation cephalosporins.
- *Inadequate blood/tissue levels*: In general, there is a difference in the achievable concentration between the blood and tissue levels with beta-lactam antibiotics. With cephalosporins, tissue levels are about one quarter of serum levels in most well vascularized organs (excluding special locations, e.g., the urinary tract, central nervous system, and prostate).
- *Antibiotic tissue penetration problems*:
  - Most antibiotics penetrate abscesses poorly. Thus, surgical drainage remains the cornerstone of the therapeutic approach in abscess treatment.
  - Infections involving foreign implant material usually have a glycocalyx around the foreign body, which forms a biofilm, and these cannot be eliminated by antimicrobial therapy. Such infections almost always required removal of the prosthetic device.
  - Infections involving certain anatomic sites in the body are protected from the effects of most antibiotics given in the usually recommended doses, e.g., the CSF and prostate.
- *Colonization versus infection*: The mere recovery of an organism from a particular site does not implicate its etiological role in the underlying infectious disease process if that site harbors colonizers. Treating colonization not only wastes vital resources but is almost always unsuccessful.
- *Drug fever*: Fever may result from the patient's reaction to a given medication, and often it may be the sole manifestation to a given drug.

SUGGESTED READING

1. Candel FJ, Sá MB, Belda S, Bou G, Del Pozo JL, Estrada O, et al. Current aspects in sepsis approach. Turning things around. Rev Esp Quimioter. 2018;31(4):298-315.
2. Cormican M, Whyte T, Hanahoe B. Antimicrobial susceptibility testing in Ireland: an introduction to the methods of the National Committee for Clinical Laboratory Standards (NCCLS). Ireland: National University of Ireland Galway: 2001.

3. Jorgensen JH, Turnidge JD. Susceptibility test methods: dilution and disc diffusion methods. In: Murray PR, Baron EJ, Jorgensen JH, Pfaller MA, Yolker RH (Eds). Manual of Clinical Microbiology, 9th edition. Washington, D.C.: ASM Press; 2003. pp. 1102-07.
4. Jorgensen JH. Laboratory issues in the detection and reporting of antibacterial resistance. Inf Dis Clin North Am. 1997;11:785-802.
5. Koneman EW, Allen SD, Janda WM, Schreckenberger PC, Cwinn W Jr. Colour Atlas and Textbook of Diagnostic Microbiology, 5th edition. New York: Lippincott, Philadelphia; 1997. pp. 785-856.
6. Livermore DM, Winstanley TG, Shannon KP. Interpretative reading: recognizing the unusual and inferring resistance mechanisms from resistance phenotypes. [online] Available from: http://bsac.org.uk/wp-content/uploads/2012/02/Chapter_11.pdf. [Last accessed September, 2021].
7. Louie M, Cokerill FR 3rd. Susceptibility testing: phenotypic and genotypic tests for bacteria and mycobacteria. Inf Dis Clin North Am. 2001;15:1205-26.
8. Rodrigues C, Shah A. Laboratory diagnosis of infections. In: Munjal YP (Ed). API Textbook of Medicine, 11th edition. New Delhi: Jaypee Brothers Medical Publishers; 2019. pp. 96-101.
9. Sinha M, Jupe J, Mack H, Coleman TP, Lawrence SM, Fraley SI. Emerging technologies for molecular diagnosis of sepsis. Clin Microbiol Rev. 2018;31:e00089-17.
10. Turnidge JD, Ferraro MJ, Jorgensen JH. Susceptibility test methods: general considerations. In: Murray PR, Baron EJ, Jorgensen JH, Pfaller MA, Yolker RH (Eds). Manual of Clinical Microbiology, 9th edition. Washington, D.C.: ASM Press; 2003. pp. 1102-07.

CHAPTER 14

Invasive Fungal Infections in the ICU: Diagnosis and Management

Rajeev Soman, Rakshita Eashwernath

■ INTRODUCTION

Invasive fungal infections (IFIs) are associated with high morbidity and mortality and have gained significant interest over the last decade. This is due to the increase in critically ill patients and immunocompromised hosts in the intensive care unit (ICU). Although all invasive fungi are often considered together, each fungal pathogen is associated with a characteristic syndrome **(Table 1)**. However, these syndromes could have alternative microbial or noninfective etiologies. Differentiating between colonization and infection is another challenge. Clinical awareness and a high level of suspicion coupled with better diagnostics are imperative for early diagnosis and therapy. IFIs are somewhat predictable, are difficult to diagnose, and have adverse consequences if there is a delay in treatment. Hence, therapeutic approaches include prophylactic, empirical, and preemptive strategies in such infections.

TABLE 1	Fungal pathogens—risk factors, clinical manifestations, and treatment.		
Risk factors	**Syndrome**	**Fungal pathogen**	**Treatment**
Neutropenia and long ICU stay	Sepsis	*Candida*	• Echinocandins in critically ill patients • Fluconazole in stable patients
Prolonged neutropenia, prolonged steroid use, SOT, and HSCT recipients	Pulmonary involvement	*Aspergillus*	Voriconazole
HIV	Chronic meningitis	*Cryptococcus*	Amphotericin B + 5-flucytosine
Uncontrolled diabetes, CKD, SOT, and HSCT recipients	Rhino-orbital cerebral involvement with blackish discharge or eschar	*Mucor*	Amphotericin B and isavuconazole
(CKD: chronic kidney disease; HIV: human immunodeficiency virus; HSCT: hematopoietic stem cell transplant; ICU: intensive care unit; SOT: solid organ transplant)			

CANDIDA

Host Factors

The major risk factors for developing invasive candidiasis include neutropenia, critically ill patients, long stay in the ICU, treatment with broad-spectrum antibiotics and steroids, gastrointestinal (GI) surgery for perforation, pancreatitis, hemodialysis, and total parenteral nutrition (TPN).

Spectrum of Disease

It can present as sepsis syndrome, endovascular infections, endophthalmitis (**Fig. 1**), osteomyelitis, and disseminated candidiasis involving the skin (**Fig. 2**), liver, spleen, and/or kidney.

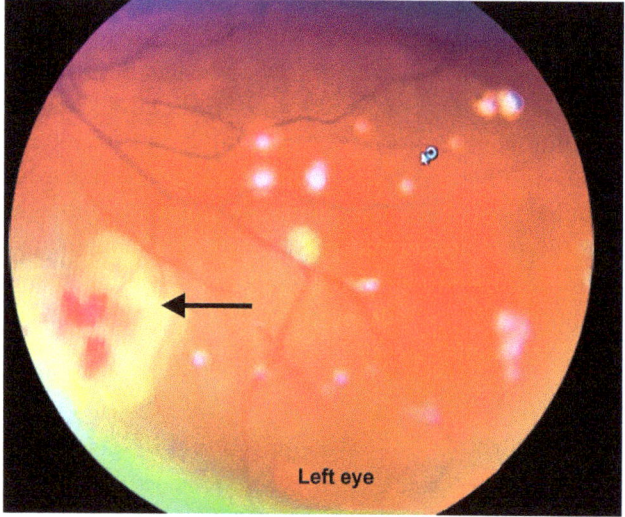

Fig. 1: *Candida* chorioretinitis (white spots are artifacts).

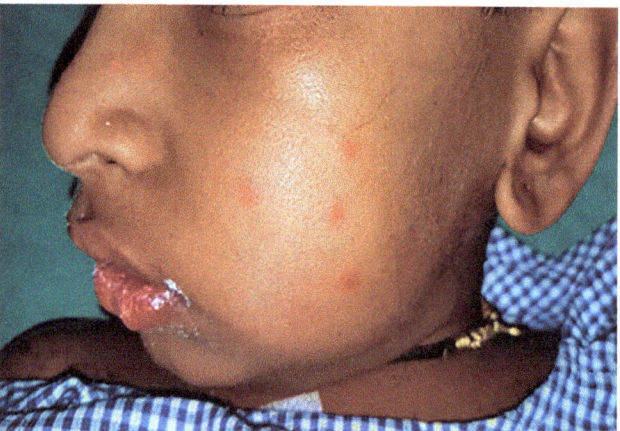

Fig. 2: Maculopapular skin lesions in an acute myeloid leukemia (AML) patient on chemotherapy.

Isolation of *Candida* from sputum, tracheal aspirate, and bronchoalveolar lavage (BAL) is exceedingly common, but pneumonia due to *Candida* is exceedingly rare. The decision to treat depends on evidence of dissemination and host factors like recent lung transplantation. Isolation of *Candida* from urine in critically ill patients is common and may not be treated, but rarely it may be the first sign of candidemia. Most patients can simply be managed by removing the indwelling catheter. Treatment of asymptomatic candiduria is advised when patients are neutropenic, in low-birth-weight neonates, or if urological procedures are planned. Positive *Candida* cultures from chest or abdominal drains placed >24 hours earlier require interpretation, and may not merit treatment due to colonization.

The incidence of candidemia in India ranges from 1 to 12 cases/1,000 admissions with a crude mortality rate of 46–75% and attributable mortality of 10–49% which can increase with treatment delay. The most common species of *Candida* in our country is *C. tropicalis* followed by *C. albicans*, and *C. parapsilosis*. About 10–15% of *C. albicans* and *C. tropicalis* are resistant to fluconazole. *C. krusei* is almost exclusively seen in hematological malignancy population on fluconazole prophylaxis.

The emergence of *C. auris* is a matter of concern as a considerable number of isolates are resistant to fluconazole and some are resistant to amphotericin B (AmB) and echinocandins. *C. auris* is spread mostly from the hands of healthcare workers (HCWs) and fomites, and therefore strict infection control practices, which include 2 hourly surface disinfection with sodium hypochlorite and terminal cleaning, should be followed in the ICU.

Diagnosis

It is based on risk factor assessment + colonization + culture/nonculture-based test/polymerase chain reaction (PCR).

- *Candida* colonization index and scoring systems have low sensitivity and poor positive predictive values as the risk of candidemia depends not simply on the sum of risk factors but whether other infections have been excluded, or are under control.
- Blood cultures have limitations for diagnosing invasive candidiasis due to poor sensitivity of 50% and slow turnaround time, with a time to positivity of about 2–3 days extending to 8 days. They also fail to detect deep tissue infections.
- *Nonculture-based tests*: β-D-Glucan (BDG) assay >80 pg/mL detected in two consecutive serum samples can be used to identify deep seated infections or candidemia when cultures are sterile.
- *Matrix-assisted laser desorption ionization time-of-flight mass spectrometry (MALDI-TOF MS)*: This test has a short turnaround time after the culture is positive, but its limitation is that it does not provide antifungal susceptibility testing (AFST) results, and is not available at all centers.

- Molecular methods like PCR can be done on the clinical specimen, but again does not yield susceptibility information.
- *Imaging*: Small target like abscesses in the liver or spleen in hematological malignancy patients are highly suggestive of deep-seated candidiasis.
- *Fundoscopy*: Look for chorioretinitis or endophthalmitis.

Management

The critical window of opportunity for initiating treatment appears to be within 12–24 hours following the drawing of the first ultimately positive blood culture. Antifungal agents used currently:
- *Echinocandins*: It is the first choice of drug in critically ill patients and in those who have had a recent exposure to azoles. It has a fungicidal action and good activity against biofilm but has poor penetration in the eye, central nervous system (CNS), and urine.
- Azoles are static drugs. Fluconazole is given in less severely ill patients with no previous azole exposure. Voriconazole is the drug of choice for *C. krusei* as it is intrinsically resistant to fluconazole. Voriconazole has a lesser role in ICU patients due to important interactions and toxicity.
- *AmB*: It is toxic but is an alternative in resource limited settings.

Transition from echinocandin to fluconazole is done if the patient is stable and if the susceptibility pattern is known.

Duration of Treatment

Blood cultures should be repeated every 48 hours and treatment is given for 14 days after the first negative blood culture, ruling out metastatic involvement, and recovery of neutropenia.

Adjuvant Treatment

- *Source control*: Removal of central venous catheter (CVC) in non-neutropenic patients is desirable. In neutropenic patients, CVC is removed if patient is unstable, with lack of resolution off ever in 2–3 days and/or persistent candidemia.
- *Metastatic infections should be ruled out*: Transthoracic echocardiogram (TTE) and ophthalmological evaluation should be done to rule out *Candida* retinitis/endophthalmitis. In neutropenic patients, fundoscopy is done after neutropenia resolves.

Approach to preemptive anti-*Candida* therapy is summarized in **Flowchart 1**.

ASPERGILLUS

Host Factors

The major risk factors for developing invasive aspergillosis (IA) include prolonged neutropenia [absolute neutrophil count (ANC) < 500 for >10 days],

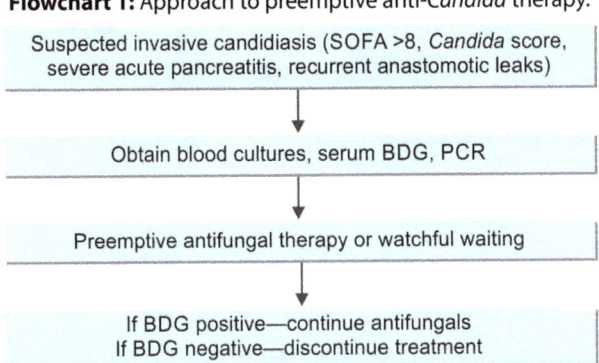

Flowchart 1: Approach to preemptive anti-*Candida* therapy.

(BDG: β-D-Glucan; PCR: polymerase chain reaction; SOFA: sequential organ failure assessment)

treatment with steroids >3 weeks or T-cell immunosuppressants, hematopoietic stem cell transplant (HSCT), solid organ transplant (SOT) recipients, and chronic granulomatous disease (CGD). The emerging risk factors are chronic obstructive pulmonary disease (COPD), chronic liver disease (CLD), chronic kidney disease (CKD), long ICU stay, human immunodeficiency virus (HIV) with CD4 <50 cells, influenza-associated pulmonary aspergillosis (IAPA), and coronavirus disease-2019 (COVID-19)-associated pulmonary aspergillosis (CAPA).

Spectrum of Disease

It can present as tracheobronchitis, pulmonary involvement, rhinosinusitis, or rarely disseminated disease involving the meninges, skin, and bones.

Invasive aspergillosis has a high mortality of about 80% in non-neutropenic patients as the symptoms are often nonspecific causing a delay in diagnosis. *A. fumigatus* is the most common organism responsible. Rarely indolent granulomatous sinusitis with intracranial and cerebral extension occurs, mostly caused by *A. flavus*.

Diagnosis

Radiological findings in invasive pulmonary aspergillosis (IPA) may sometimes be mistaken for tuberculosis (TB) and other lung diseases leading to diagnostic confusion. However, a combination of host factors, clinicoradiological syndrome and mycological criteria, help in establishing the diagnosis of IPA.

Bronchoalveolar lavage galactomannan (GM) antigen test is useful in non-neutropenic patients as the test sensitivity is 94.7%. However, serum GM has less sensitivity of only about 36.8% in non-neutropenic patients.

Clinical algorithm for the diagnosis of IA in non-neutropenic patients in the ICU could be:
- *Host factors*: At least one of the following:
  Glucocorticosteroid treatment, neutrophil abnormality, chronic airway abnormality, decompensated cirrhosis, treatment with recognized T-cell

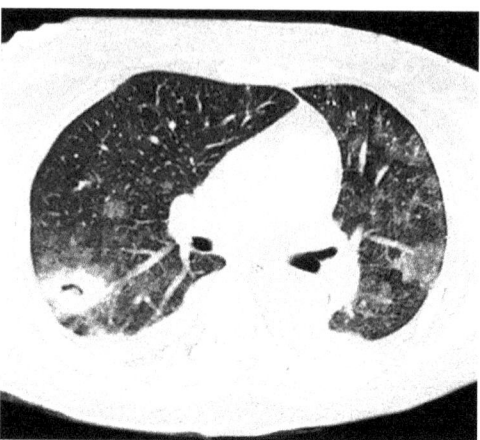

Fig. 3: Nodule with a ground glass halo and central air crescent sign.

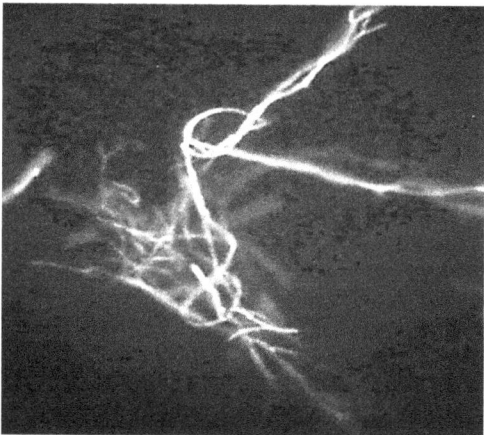

Fig. 4: Calcofluor stain showing thin septate hyphae with acute angle branching.

immunosuppressant, hematological malignancies/HSCT, SOT, HIV, and severe influenza.
- Clinical or radiological abnormalities consistent with a pulmonary infectious disease process that are otherwise unexplained. CT lungs showing dense, well-circumscribed lesions with or without halo sign, air crescent sign **(Fig. 3)**, cavity, and wedge-shaped and segmental or lobar consolidation.
- At least one of the following nondefinitive tests:
  – Cytology, direct microscopy, and/or culture showing *Aspergillus* species in a lower respiratory tract specimen **(Fig. 4)**.
  – GM in serum ≥0.5 and/or in BAL ≥0.8.

Management

Voriconazole is the drug of choice. Isavuconazole and posaconazole are alternative options. The second choice is AmB. Echinocandins are not clearly cidal, hence they are not used as primary therapy but can be used in combination for salvage or when the patient is unable to tolerate voriconazole and when there are unavoidable drug interactions.

Duration
Three weeks to 6 months or longer, depending on the site of infection, clinical, and radiological and microbiological improvement.

■ CRYPTOCOCCUS
Host Factors
The major risk factors for developing *Cryptococcus* infection are HIV patients with CD4 < 100 cells/μL, SOT recipients, and idiopathic CD4 lymphocytopenia. The emerging risk factors are sarcoidosis, systemic lupus erythematosus (SLE), CLD, uncontrolled diabetes mellitus (DM), CGD, hyperimmunoglobulin M (IgM) syndromes, treatment with steroids and monoclonal antibodies. It can rarely occur without an apparent underlying disease. Hence, it should be suspected in a case of subacute lymphocytic meningitis when TB is ruled out.

Spectrum of Disease
It can present as chronic meningitis **(Fig. 5)**, pulmonary nodules, infiltrates or cavities, and disseminated disease involving the skin and musculoskeletal system.

Diagnosis
- Cerebrospinal fluid (CSF) shows lymphocytic pleocytosis with high protein and low to normal glucose. CSF opening pressure >25 cmH$_2$O occurs in 60–80% of patients.

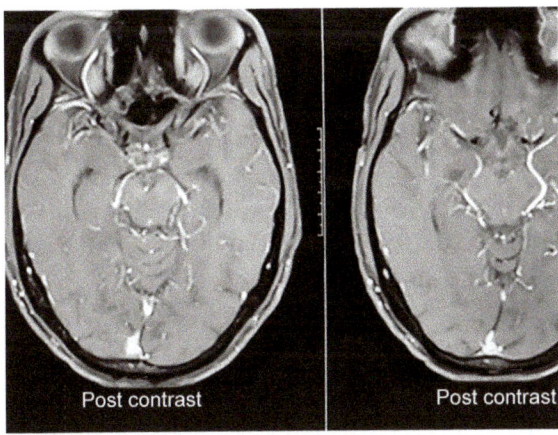

Fig. 5: Leptomeningeal enhancement in cryptococcal meningitis.

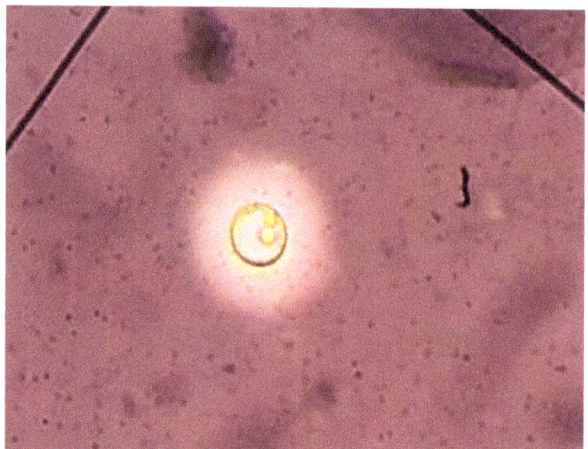

Fig. 6: Cerebrospinal fluid (CSF) India ink showing encapsulated yeast.

- India ink on CSF has a sensitivity of 50–80%. It detects capsulated yeasts **(Fig. 6)**.
- Detection of cryptococcal antigen (CrAg) in the serum, CSF, or urine by enzyme immunoassay has a sensitivity of 95%. A high titer > 1:1,024 is suggestive of high burden with poor response and likely failure. Latex agglutination or lateral flow assay methods can also be used for rapid screening of patients with CD4 < 100 cells/µL and can aid in early diagnosis of cryptococcal meningoencephalitis since cryptococcal antigenemia can precede the onset of neurological symptoms by up to 3 weeks.
- CSF culture has a 70% sensitivity rate but has to be incubated for a prolonged period of up to 21 days.
- Multiplex PCR like FilmArray®/meningitis panel includes *Cryptococcus* and can be helpful when not suspected and appropriate cryptococcal tests have not been asked for.

Management
- *Induction phase*: Given for 2 weeks:
  - AmB + 5 flucytosine or
  - AmB + fluconazole (high dose)
- *Consolidation phase*: 8 weeks with fluconazole
- *Maintenance phase*: >6 months to 1 year with fluconazole.

Regimens differ based on the host characteristics, disease extent, fungal burden, availability of drugs, and intolerance.

Duration

To continue till CD4 >100 cells/µL with undetectable HIV viral load for >3 months on potent antiretroviral therapy (ART) and minimal antifungal treatment for 1 year.

Therapeutic CSF drainage is required during the induction phase to lower intracranial pressure and is a very important part of treatment.

Highly active antiretroviral therapy (HAART) is initiated after a delay of 2–10 weeks of treatment to prevent immune reconstitution inflammatory syndrome (IRIS).

■ MUCOR

Host Factors

The major risk factors favoring development of mucormycosis are uncontrolled DM, diabetic ketoacidosis, HSCT, SOT recipients, penetrating trauma, CKD, burns, malnutrition, premature infants, steroid use, deferoxamine therapy, and illicit use of intravenous (IV) drugs. An emerging risk factor is COVID-19.

Spectrum of Disease

It presents as sinusitis with blackish discharge or eschar and/or orbital and cerebral involvement. Rhino-orbito-cerebral (ROC) form is the most common clinical presentation **(Figs. 7A and B)**. Isolated renal mucormycosis is a new clinical entity seen in India and China, affecting young immunocompetent individuals and has a high mortality rate. GI *Mucor* is difficult to diagnose without biopsy and is associated with high mortality.

Cases of necrotizing fasciitis due to Mucorales, occurring via contaminated intramuscular injections have been reported.

Diagnosis

Tissue from the necrotic area is the specimen of choice and swabs are unsatisfactory.
- Microscopy with either calcofluor stain or KOH mount showing broad aseptate hyphae with wide angle branching **(Fig. 8)**.

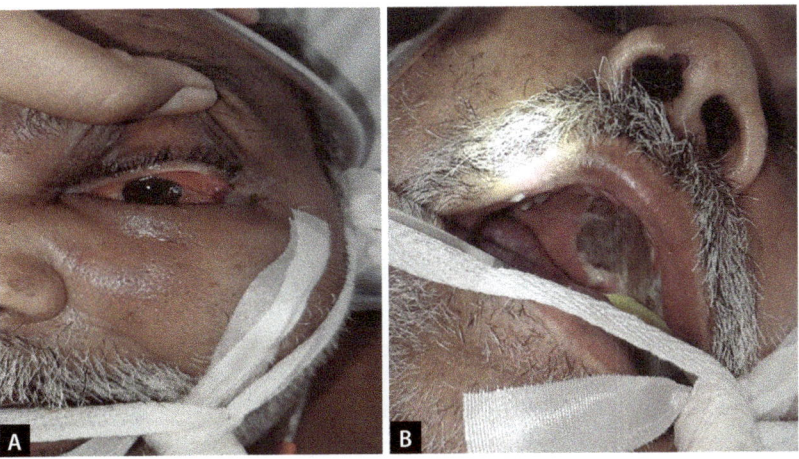

Figs. 7A and B: Orbital cellulitis with palate involvement.

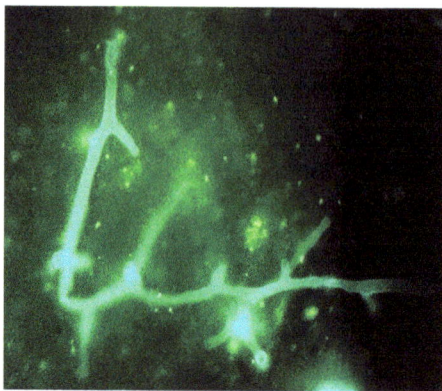

Fig. 8: Calcofluor stain showing broad aseptate hyphae with wide-angle branching.

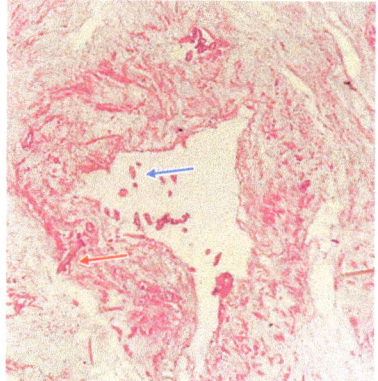

Fig. 9: Red arrow: Broad aseptate hyphae in the wall of a blood vessel. Blue arrow: Fungal elements in the lumen of the blood vessel.

- *Culture*: It is difficult to culture *Mucor* from homogenized tissue. Therefore, the laboratory should always be instructed not to mince or grind the tissue to prevent damage to *Mucor* and to improve culture yield.
- *Histopathology*: It is the gold standard diagnostic test. Evidence of aseptate hyphae with angioinvasion or tissue invasion on periodic acid–Schiff (PAS) (**Fig. 9**) or Grocott methenamine silver (GMS) stains.
- Negative GM and BDG tests point to *Mucor* when the differential diagnosis involves *Aspergillus* or certain other molds.
- *Radiological*:
  - Pulmonary >10 nodules, consolidation, pleural effusion, and reverse halo sign (**Fig. 10**) to differentiate from *Aspergillosis*.
  - *Peripheral nervous system (PNS)*: Showing inflammation and edema of the maxillary, ethmoid, and frontal sinuses. Involvement of the orbit, extraocular muscles, or cribriform plate.
  - *Brain*: Vascular invasion is a common finding of occlusion or thrombus of the cavernous sinus, carotid artery, and cerebral arteries (**Fig. 11**).

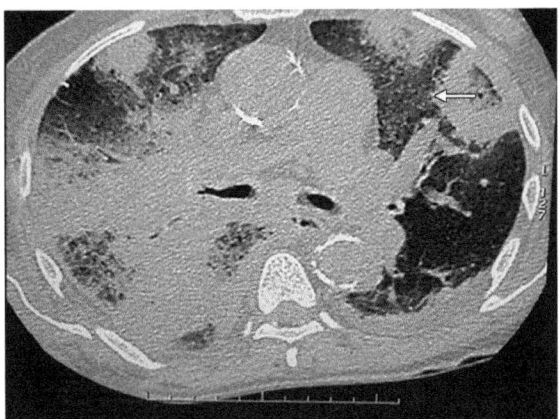

Fig. 10: Nodules with reverse halo in the left upper lobe (white arrow).

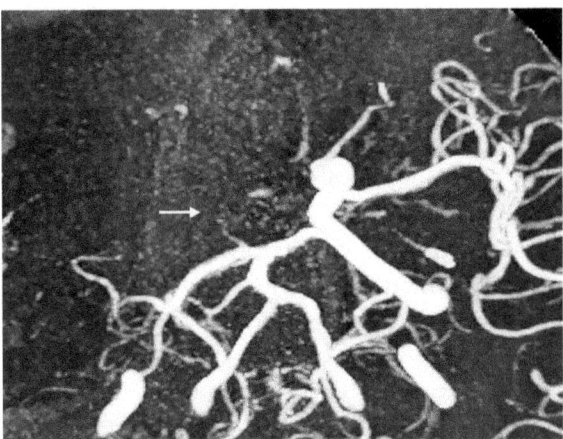

Fig. 11: Complete occlusion of right middle cerebral artery (MCA) and right posterior inferior cerebral artery (white arrow).

Management

Principles of management include:
- Timely diagnosis
- Reversal of underlying predisposing factors
- Surgical debridement
- Early initiation of antifungal therapy
- Adjuvant treatment.

Drugs of Choice

Amphotericin B and isavuconazole are drugs of choice. Poor penetration of AmB at the site of infection can be due to thrombosis. Even nonviable hyphae adhere to blood vessels and precipitate thrombosis. Therefore, repeated debridement is needed. Liposomal AmB is preferred and doses up to 10 mg/kg have to be used occasionally.

Alternative agent: Posaconazole.

Adjuvant Treatment
- Hyperbaric O_2
- Caspofungin
- Interferon γ (IFNγ) and granulocyte-colony-stimulating factor (G-CSF)
- Chelating agents—deferasirox.

Duration

Depends on clinical, radiological, microbiological improvement, and recovery from immunosuppression.

BIOMARKERS

Serological tests such as GM and BDG are used as markers for starting treatment preemptively in high-risk patients. These nonculture methods were developed due to limitations of conventional diagnostic procedures and lack of specific signs and symptoms. Biomarkers can be easily detected in small amounts in serum, BAL or CSF and can be quantified, which helps in monitoring the course of the disease.

Galactomannan is an antigen, which is released from the fungal cell wall during growth. The optimum cutoff values depend on the patient, specimen, and purpose of testing. However, this test may show false positivity with generic piperacillin/tazobactam and crossreactivity with non-*Aspergillus* molds such as *Fusarium, Penicillium, Acremonium, Alternaria* and *Histoplasma*. This assay does not detect Mucorales and *Cryptococcus*.

β-D-Glucan is a component of the cell wall of many pathogenic fungi except Mucorales and *Cryptococcus*. It has a good sensitivity and negative predictive value of 80%, making it a potentially useful tool to prevent unnecessary use of antifungals. The cutoff value of a single test is >80 pg/mL. False-positive results may occur because of glucan contaminated tubes/gauzes, cellulose-containing dialysis membranes/filters, contaminated intravenous immunoglobulin (IVIg)/albumin, gram-positive infections, gut inflammation, and some antibiotics like amoxicillin-clavulanic acid. Therefore, this test is recommended as an adjunct to culture.

DRUG INTERACTIONS

Voriconazole is metabolized by CYP2C19 isoenzyme. It has a narrow therapeutic window and major interaction with other drugs. As IPA can mimic TB, empiric antituberculosis treatment (ATT) leads to a problem. Rifampicin is an enzyme inducer, which reduces the action of voriconazole by 95%. This reaction persists for 2 weeks or longer even after the withdrawal of rifampicin, thus reducing the efficacy of voriconazole.

Voriconazole and posaconazole are inhibitors of CYP3A4. This leads to a significant increase in cyclosporine and tacrolimus serum concentrations, which requires downward adjustment and frequent monitoring of levels of

TABLE 2 Drug interactions with azoles.

Drug metabolite levels increased by azoles	Drugs which reduce the levels of azoles	Drugs which increase the levels of azoles
• Sirolimus and tacrolimus • Cyclosporine • Statins • Warfarin • Protease inhibitors • Calcium channel blockers	• Rifampicin • Carbamazepine • Phenytoin • Nevirapine	• Erythromycin • Azithromycin • Clarithromycin

these drugs. Voriconazole causes QT prolongation. Therefore, administration with other QT prolonging drugs should be monitored closely or avoided.

Also as IFIs occur in HIV patients, ART also has many drug interactions with azoles **(Table 2)**.

■ THERAPEUTIC DRUG MONITORING

Therapeutic drug monitoring (TDM) is extremely useful in clinical management of patients with life-threatening IFIs, especially with azole antifungal therapy. It helps clinicians to optimize the dose and avoid toxicities.

■ SUMMARY

Invasive fungal infections need to be viewed with a high degree of suspicion; various diagnostic and therapeutic strategies need to be implemented. This helps in early initiation of appropriate antifungal therapy. It is crucial to differentiate colonization from invasion while managing fungal infections. On the other hand, prophylaxis, preemptive, and empirical strategies are also useful. The choice of antifungal is based on the type of fungus, extent, and site, coupled with adjuvant treatment strategies. These are all essential for a successful outcome in these difficult to treat infections.

■ SUGGESTED READING

1. Bassetti M, Bouza E. Invasive mould infections in the ICU setting: complexities and solutions. J Antimicrob Chemother. 2017;72(1):39-47.
2. Cornely OA, Alastruey-Izquierdo A, Arenz D, Chen CA, Dannaoui E, Hochhegger B, et al. Global guideline for the diagnosis and management of mucormycosis: an initiative of the European Confederation of Medical Mycology in cooperation with the Mycoses Study Group Education and Research Consortium. Lancet Infect Dis. 2019;19(12):e405-e421.
3. Pappas PG, Kauffman CA, Andes DR, Clancy CJ, Marr KA, Ostrosky-Zeichner L, et al. Clinical practice guideline for the management of candidiasis: 2016 update by the Infectious Diseases Society of America. Clin Infect Dis. 2016;62(4):1-50.
4. Patterson TF, Thompson GR, Denning DW, Fishman JA, Hadley S, Herbrecht R, et al. Practice guidelines for the diagnosis and management of aspergillosis: 2016 update by the Infectious Diseases Society of America. Clin Infect Dis. 2016;63(4):e1-60.
5. Perfect JR, Dismukes WE, Dromer F, Goldman DL, Graybill JR, Hamill RJ, et al. Clinical practice guidelines for the management of cryptococcal disease: 2010 update by the Infectious Diseases Society of America. Clin Infect Dis. 2010;50(3):291-322.

CHAPTER 15

Ventilator-associated Pneumonia

Joanne Mascarenhas

■ INTRODUCTION

Hospital-acquired pneumonia (HAP) and ventilator-associated pneumonia (VAP) are the most common among the healthcare-associated infections. One of the preventable complications of intubation and mechanical ventilation is VAP. As with any hospital-associated infection, VAP has an adverse effect on duration of stay in intensive care unit (ICU) and hospital, cost, morbidity as well as mortality. It also has implications on infection control, surveillance, and quality of care. This is a brief overview of VAP, to identify, treat appropriately, and most importantly prevent it.

■ VENTILATOR-ASSOCIATED PNEUMONIA

There is no one clear objective definition of VAP. The best way to understand this is a stepwise derivation starting with pneumonia. Pneumonia is an inflammation and consolidation of the lungs due to an infective etiology. This infection of the lower respiratory tract is characterized by infiltrative shadows on imaging along with fever, purulent expectoration and leukocytosis with or without a change in the oxygen saturation.

Hospital-acquired pneumonia is a pneumonia that develops after 48 hours of admission. It is neither present nor incubating at the time of admission. Under this form of nosocomial infections, comes VAP, which is a pneumonia that occurs after 48 hours of endotracheal intubation. For surveillance purposes, VAP is described under the umbrella term of ventilator-associated conditions (**Box 1**). The infection-related conditions include tracheitis, tracheobronchitis, and VAP.

BOX 1 Ventilator-associated conditions.

Ventilator-associated condition (VAC):
- Increased requirement of fraction of inspired oxygen (FiO_2) by 0.2, or in positive end-expiratory pressure (PEEP) by 3 cm H_2O after 48 hours of stability or improvement

Infection-related ventilator-associated complication (IVAC):
- VAC associated with temperature <36°C or >38°C, leukocyte count <4,000/mm^3 or >11.000/mm^3 and change in antibiotic for ≥ 96 hours

Pneumonia—probable or possible:
- IVAC with purulent sputum/bronchoalveolar lavage (BAL) >25 neutrophils/hpf and/or positive culture of respiratory pathogens

Ventilator-associated pneumonia is characterized by new or increasing radiological shadows with the presence of systemic signs of infection (fever with no other cause, leukocytosis, or leukopenia) and respiratory signs (change in the quantity/nature of the tracheal secretions, dyspnea, bronchial breath sounds, increase in oxygen requirement, and positive cultures of tracheal secretion). In the absence of radiological findings, these same clinical features describe tracheobronchitis. This infective process occurs between colonization and VAP.

■ CAUSES OF VENTILATOR-ASSOCIATED PNEUMONIA

The onset of VAP begins with the transition of the colonizing flora in the upper and lower airways to hospital-acquired ones. This, followed by the use of antibiotics (as little as two doses), further promotes the proliferation of nosocomial pathogens. The risk of developing VAP is related to host, endotracheal tube, and hospital.

The *host factors* for VAP are the same as those that determine the risk for a drug-resistant infection. The most important being the antibiotic history, immune status of the patient, and the presence of underlying lung disease.

The *endotracheal tube* itself is another culprit. Firstly, it interferes with the natural anatomic defense mechanisms by keeping the epiglottis open, impairing the cough reflex, interfering with the mucociliary clearance, and permits pooling of oropharyngeal secretions above the cuff.

Secondly, it alters the microbial environment by aiding the translocation of oropharyngeal bacteria into the lower airways, changing the natural flora to pathogenic.

Thirdly, being a foreign body, the tube has the potential for biofilm formation on the inner lumen as well as the outer surface. This biofilm is formed by microorganisms, bacterial and fungal, that adhere to each other as well as to the surfaces of the tube. The microorganisms produce a polymer matrix coating that forms a protective layer that prevents the penetration of antimicrobial agents.

Hospital factors that determine VAP include the infection prevention practices, antibiogram, antibiotic policies, staff awareness and compliance with these.

The etiology of VAP is polymicrobial. The organisms can be gram positive or gram negative, drug resistant, or non-multidrug-resistant bacteria (MDR). They may differ from patient to patient or could be in concordance with the local/hospital antibiogram. The risk of an organism being *multidrug resistant* is determined by several factors. These are enumerated in **Box 2**.

■ CAUSATIVE ORGANISM DIAGNOSIS

The final diagnosis of VAP is on the basis of positive cultures. The following test reports help guide further treatment.

> **BOX 2** Risk factors for MDR VAP.
> - Antibiotic use in the preceding 90 days
> - Hospital stay of >5 days
> - Airway colonization: Both upper and lower
> - Septic shock
> - ARDS
> - Immunosuppressed state
> - Acute kidney injury needing renal replacement therapy
> - Underlying structural lung disease
>
> (ARDS: acute respiratory distress syndrome; MDR: multidrug-resistant bacteria; VAP: ventilator-associated pneumonia)

- *Blood cultures*: 15% of patients with VAP may have bacteremia. Therefore, blood cultures are part of the workup.
- *Endotracheal secretions*: More important are the respiratory secretion samples for culture. A noninvasive sample collection, i.e., of the endotracheal aspirate, is usually adequate. It will give a semiquantitative result. These samples are easier to collect, with less complications, require less resources, as well as more rapid to put for culture.
- *Invasive samples* [from bronchoalveolar lavage (BAL), mini-BAL, or protected specimen brushing (PSB) yield quantitative results on culture (10^4 CFU/mL for BAL and 10^3 CFU/mL for PSB)]. They are collected from the lower respiratory tract and need to be processed for culture within 2 hours of collection or need to be preserved at 4°C if processed later. There is no added advantage for these collections except when there is no growth from the noninvasive sample or there is persistence of the pneumonia and/or infection with no clinical improvement (having ruled out any other source). There may be a role for the quantitative cultures to guide antibiotic cessation when they are below the diagnostic threshold. Traditional cultures will give results within 3–5 days.
- *Polymerase chain reaction (PCR)-based tests*: From the same sample that is sent for culture, newer multiplex real-time PCR-based tests can also be performed. These give results within 1 hour. By nucleic acid amplification, they identify viruses, bacteria, and atypical bacteria. They are able to differentiate between colonizers and potential pathogens as well as some antimicrobial resistance genes. They work well when combined with the conventional culture sensitivity tests. The PCR test will give a species identification, sometimes for organisms that do not grow in culture. This guides initial antimicrobial treatment, which can be further modified according to the final drug sensitivity pattern obtained from the traditional test. If negative, the PCR-based tests also help in de-escalation of antibiotic therapy.
- Tests to rule out any other focus of infection.

■ TREATMENT

Treatment is guided by the culture report as well as the local antibiogram of the hospital; however, the initial treatment is empiric and based on the antibiogram of the hospital. This should include cover against gram-positive organisms (*Staphylococcus aureus*), *Pseudomonas aeruginosa*, and other gram-negative organisms. If the incidence of drug resistance is low in the unit or hospital or the risk of a drug-resistant organism is low for the patient, the choice includes a cover against methicillin-sensitive *S. aureus* (MSSA) and one antipseudomonal drug.

Empiric treatment for this scenario includes a β-lactam/β-lactamase inhibitor (BL/BLI) (like piperacillin-tazobactam), or a third- or fourth-generation cephalosporin (like ceftazidime or cefepime), or a carbapenem. Respiratory quinolones like levofloxacin, though advocated in Western guidelines and protocols, are preserved for the antituberculous regimens in our country. If *drug-resistant organisms* are anticipated, drug choice should be against methicillin-resistant *Staphylococcus aureus* (MRSA) (based on local antibiogram) and the antipseudomonal cover should be from two different groups. The additional antipseudomonal or gram-negative cover could be a monobactam (aztreonam) or aminoglycosides or colistin or polymyxin B. The MRSA cover advocated is vancomycin or linezolid.

Patients with structural lung disease like bronchiectasis or cystic fibrosis are prone to gram-negative infections. Hence, it is advisable to use two antipseudomonal drugs for this group of patients as well.

The *PCR-based* initial report will help guide the choice of antimicrobials. And the final culture sensitivity report will define the specific treatment. The choice of drugs is crucial in the presence of multi- or pandrug-resistant organisms.

The antibiotic history of the patient also plays a role in the choice and cycling of antibiotics.

Further, optimization of therapy includes de-escalation, appropriate dosing taking into consideration pharmacokinetics, pharmacodynamics, the drug side effect profile, the extent of organ dysfunction, and the patient's response to treatment.

The addition of *inhaled antibiotics* to systemic therapy may be considered for gram-negative organisms that are sensitive to aminoglycosides or polymyxins.

In addition to antimicrobial therapy, physiotherapy and postural drainage play an important role in helping with the clearing of respiratory secretions. This can be advised to the patients depending on the clinical scenario, severity of respiratory failure, and the ventilatory parameters.

Duration of Therapy

Usually, 7 to 8 days of appropriate drugs should be adequate for the treatment of VAP. This has shown to be as effective as an extended duration of 8 to 15 days of therapy.

The duration of therapy, de-escalation, or cessation of therapy can be guided by the clinical response, improvement or resolution of altered parameters (laboratory and radiological), decreasing trend of procalcitonin, and a decreasing value on quantitative cultures. Do keep in mind that there is a *lag in radiological recovery* as compared to clinical improvement. A longer duration is sometimes indicated depending on the severity of the disease as well as the nature of the organism. The prolonged use of antimicrobials increases the risk of drug resistance, adverse effects of the drugs, *Clostridium difficile* infection, and cost.

■ PREVENTION OF VENTILATOR-ASSOCIATED PNEUMONIA

Depending on the organism as well as the infection control practices there is always a risk of horizontal transfer of the organism and infection from one patient to another as well as a risk of an outbreak. As with any infection, more so with the hospital-acquired ones, prevention is one of the main factors in the treatment. The use of *bundles* in clinical practice has shown to help decrease device-associated infections. Over and above the VAP bundle **(Box 3)**, there are other measures that can be followed as given in **Box 4**.

- *Hand hygiene* continues to remain the backbone of infection prevention. This is to be followed during patient handling as well as during management of the airway.
- *Avoid the CULPRIT*: The main cause of VAP is the endotracheal tube and/or mechanical ventilation. Therefore, to start with, avoiding unnecessary intubations and reintubations is essential. Depending on the clinical condition of the patient, if possible, noninvasive ventilation is preferred. *Endotracheal tubes are preferred to nasotracheal tubes.*
- *Ventilator interventions:* If intubation is required, then certain interventions while on the ventilator have been found to help reduce VAP. These include the ventilator care bundle as well as:
  - The use of lung protective ventilation strategies
  - Daily sedation breaks
  - Assessment of weaning and spontaneous breathing trials, when appropriate and safe, should be done at the earliest
  - If a prolonged need for the endotracheal tube is anticipated, then an early tracheostomy is advocated. This will help both in tracheal toileting as well as ventilation and weaning.

BOX 3 Ventilator-associated pneumonia (VAP) bundle.

- Elevation of the head end 30–45°
- Daily sedation break and spontaneous breathing trial with assessment of readiness to wean
- Stress ulcer prophylaxis
- Deep vein thrombosis prophylaxis
- Selective decontamination of the oropharynx with chlorhexidine

> **BOX 4** Prevention of ventilator-associated pneumonia (VAP).
>
> *Avoid*:
> - Unnecessary intubation and mechanical ventilation
> - Instilling saline or sterile water for suctioning
> - Prolonged used of endotracheal tube (ET). If anticipated, then early tracheostomy to be considered
> - Reintubation
> - Frequent disconnection of ventilator circuit
> - Unnecessary use of antibiotic
> - Continuous sedation (daily sedation break to be given)
>
> *Implement specific care*:
> - Ventilator bundles (*See Box 3*)
> - Antibiotic stewardship
> - Lung protective ventilator strategies
> - Early weaning trials
> - Use of cuffed ETs with subglottic suction port
>
> *Implement general care*:
> - Hand and oral hygiene
> - Universal infection control practice
> - Physiotherapy
> - Nursing care
> - Education of healthcare workers
> - Surveillance

- Avoid reintubations
  Each procedure of reintubation increases the risk of VAP, other complications related to the procedure and has an adverse effect on the overall outcome.
- The use of tubes with subglottic suction ports: The use of cuffed endotracheal and tracheostomy tubes with subglottic suction ports is useful for maintaining oropharyngeal hygiene.
- Maintaining endotracheal and oropharyngeal hygiene: The use of chlorhexidine for oral hygiene. Some units use tooth brushes with a suction port.
- Avoid instilling sterile water or saline into the endotracheal tube prior to suctioning.
- Monitor and maintain the cuff pressure at <20 cm H_2O. This causes less trauma to the trachea.
- Minimal disconnections of the ventilator circuit.
- The use of bacterial and viral filters in the circuit.
- Chest physiotherapy
- Appropriate antimicrobial therapy along with an antibiotic stewardship program is another vital part of VAP prevention. This includes:
  - Appropriate drug, route, dosage, and duration of therapy
  - Avoiding unnecessary use of antimicrobials
  - Following the local antibiogram

- Surveillance and audits cast useful insights into the severity of the problem
- Maintain the nutritional status of the patient:
  - Enteral feeds with protein and caloric supplementation as required by the individual patient
  - The use of prokinetics to avoid aspiration of gastric contents as well as promote gastric emptying
- Looking after the patient as a whole including supportive care and maintenance of the other organ systems.
- Education and awareness among healthcare workers about infection prevention also helps in better outcomes.

SUGGESTED READING

1. Diaconu O, Siriopol I, Poloşanu L, Grigoraş I. Endotracheal Tube Biofilm and its Impact on the Pathogenesis of Ventilator-Associated Pneumonia. J Crit Care Med (Targu Mures). 2018;4(2):50-5.
2. Kalil AC, Metersky ML, Klompas M, Muscedere J, Sweeney DA, Palmer LB, et al. Management of Adults with Hospital-acquired and Ventilator-associated Pneumonia: 2016 Clinical Practice Guidelines by the Infectious Diseases Society of America and the American Thoracic Society. Clin Infect Dis. 20106;63(5):e61-e111.

CHAPTER
16

Case Studies in ICU Infections

Rajeev Soman, Rakshita Eashwernath

■ INTRODUCTION

This chapter concentrates on bacterial infections presented in form of case studies. Six case studies are illustrated, beginning with a brief clinical history and findings, followed by detailed discussion. The cases cover a wide spectrum of infections such as skin and soft tissue infection, deep seated infections, pneumonia, complicated intra-abdominal infections and infections associated with vasculitis. Discussion stresses on the right interpretation of microbiological data, use of antibiotics in complex cases such as Carbapenem-resistant Enterobacteriaceae (CRE), MRSA bacteremia and in choosing an appropriate empirical antibiotic. These case descriptions are about patients we had cared for in our hospital and discussed at the bedside during our morning rounds. The six cases illustrated here, tries to give the right approach to the complexity of the problem vis-a-vis the diagnosis and management. Ultimately, the idea of case discussion is to ignite interest in a subject which embraces all medical and surgical specialties.

■ CASE 1

A 40-year-old male, with uncontrolled diabetes mellitus (DM) and alcohol abuse, presented with bilateral lower limb swelling and redness for 1 week. There was no history of fever or trauma. On examination, lower limb cellulitis (R > L), discoloration, and blisters were present **(Fig. 1)**. The raw area of the ruptured blister was swabbed and sent for culture.

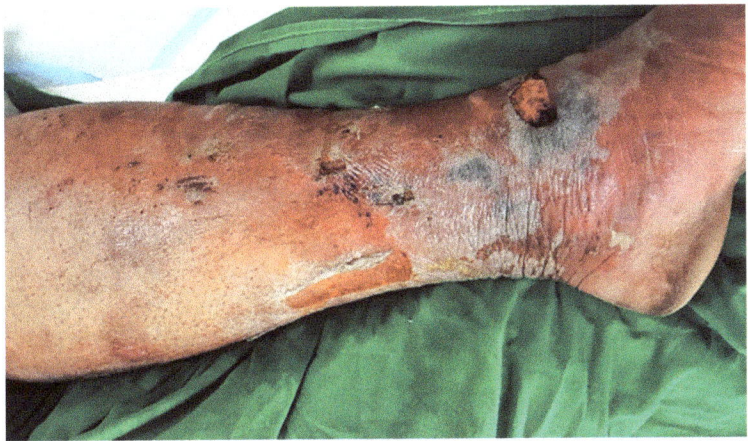

Fig. 1: Necrotizing fasciitis of right lower limb with blisters and discoloration.

Discussion

How to differentiate between cellulitis and necrotizing fasciitis (NF)?

Cellulitis: Involves the subcutaneous plane and deeper dermis with a more indolent course. Discharge could be purulent or nonpurulent and symptoms are localized to the involved area.

Necrotizing fasciitis: (1) The skin overlying a necrotizing infection is often edematous beyond the borders of erythema and may demonstrate blistering or bullae formation; (2) The pain is out of proportion to the degree of local signs and mental obtundation may be present; (3) There is decreased sensation overlying the area; (4) Direct palpation may demonstrate extreme tenderness and crepitus; (5) Easy passage of a probe; (6) Dishwater-like discharge may be present.

How to diagnose NF with laboratory parameters?

A Laboratory Risk Indicator for Necrotizing Fasciitis (LRINEC) score was developed to discriminate between necrotizing and non-necrotizing soft tissue infections. It has a positive predictive value (PPV) of 92% and negative predictive value (NPV) of 96%.

Value	Score	This patient
CRP		409
<150	0	
>150	+4	+4
WBC count		24,000
<15,000	0	
15,000–25,000	+1	
>25,000	+2	+1
Hemoglobin		14
>13.5	0	
11–13.5	+1	
<11	+2	0
Sodium		115
>135	0	
<135	+2	+2
Creatinine		1.93
<1.6	0	
>1.6	+2	+2
Glucose		160
<180	0	
>180	+1	0
Total score		9

(CRP: C-reactive protein; WBC: white blood cell)

Risk category: Low <5 (<50% chance of NF), intermediate 6–7 (50–75% chance of NF), and high 8 (>75% chance of NF).

A score of 9 indicates 93.4% PPV for NF. Therefore, surgical debridement + fasciotomy was advised.

The wound swab culture done earlier grew carbapenem-resistant *Acinetobacter baumannii* (CRAB).

Is *A. baumannii* a colonizer, a true pathogen, or the only pathogen involved?

Wound swab cultures often pick up skin colonies and may not be representative of the true pathogen(s), which are better appreciated on intraoperative deep tissue specimens.

There are two types of NF:
1. *Type 1 NF*: It is polymicrobial in nature. It occurs in diabetics, immunocompromised hosts, or patients with peripheral vascular disease. It is caused by Enterobacteriaceae, *Pseudomonas*, and β-hemolytic streptococci or anaerobes.
2. *Type 2 NF*: It is monomicrobial in nature.

β-hemolytic streptococci—seen in apparently healthy individuals, minor trauma or surgery or methicillin-resistant *Staphylococcus aureus* (MRSA)—seen in intravenous (IV) drug abusers and previous hospitalizations.

Since the patient had DM, with history of alcohol abuse, it was likely to be type 1 NF.

What will be the empirical choice of antibiotics?
- Gram-negative (GN) coverage with either meropenem and tigecycline (both have additional anaerobic coverage)
- Polymyxin B (no anaerobic cover)
- Streptococci—ampicillin, amoxicillin, and amoxiclav
- Methicillin-susceptible *Staphylococcus aureus* (MSSA)—cloxacillin
- MRSA—glycopeptides and linezolid
- Toxin inhibitors like clindamycin, linezolid, and tigecycline

In this patient, meropenem + teicoplanin + clindamycin were given empirically. However, after the wound swab report, treatment was changed to polymyxin B (*Acinetobacter*) + tigecycline (anaerobes) + linezolid [gram-positive (GP) coverage].

What are the various treatment strategies for NF apart from medical management?
- Surgery—debridement with fasciotomy **(Fig. 2)**
- Intravenous immunoglobulin (IVIG)—additional option in hemodynamically unstable and critically ill patients. It neutralizes bacterial antigen and toxin.

Intraoperative tissue specimen grew CRAB and β-hemolytic streptococci showing a polymicrobial culture. Additionally IVIG three doses were given. Treatment with polymyxin B and amoxiclav was given for a total of 14 days after which the wound look healthy **(Fig 3)**.

The patient was taken up for skin grafting later.

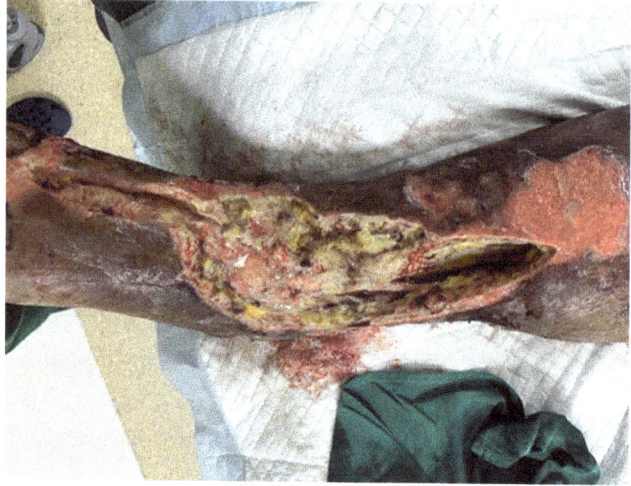

Fig. 2: Surgical debridement with fasciotomy.

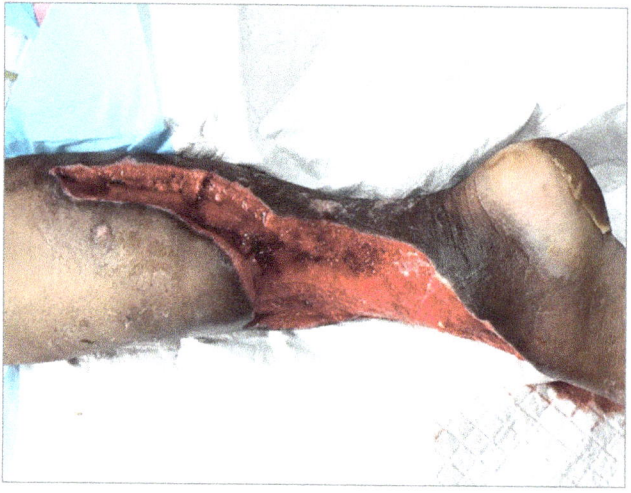

Fig. 3: Healthy granulation tissue.

■ CASE 2

A 68-year-old male, a case of carcinoma pancreas, underwent Whipple's procedure in 2018. Two years later, he developed metastatic lesions in the liver for which he underwent radiofrequency ablation. 15 days later, he developed fever and abdominal pain for which he was hospitalized many times and treated with antibiotics. Positron emission tomography–computed tomography (PET CT) showed peripherally enhancing lesions in the right lobe of the liver with air fluid level within **(Fig. 4)**, indicative of abscesses. Pig tail drainage grew carbapenem-resistant Enterobacteriaceae (CRE) sensitive to colistin, tigecycline, gentamicin, amikacin, trimethoprim-sulfamethoxazole (TMP-SMX), and fosfomycin.

Colistin susceptibility confirmed by broth microdilution method.

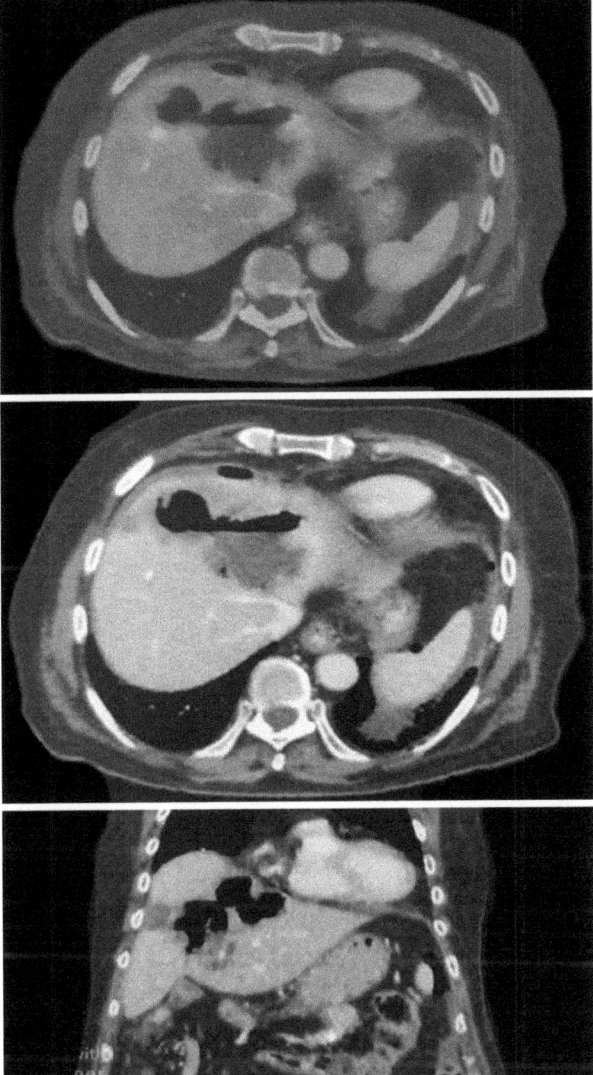

Fig. 4: Ruptured abscess with air fluid levels.

Discussion

When intra-abdominal infection is diagnosed, what is the empirical choice of antibiotics?

As the gut flora are commonly involved in intra-abdominal sepsis, organisms such as *Escherichia coli, Klebsiella, Enterobacter, Citrobacter,* and anaerobes should be kept in mind. In selected situations, GP cocci like *Enterococcus* spp. as well as *Candida* spp. should also be considered.

Hence, antimicrobials covering both GN and anaerobes should be given and should be defined according to the most frequently isolated microbes, taking into consideration the local trend of antimicrobial resistance. If there is a previous history of hospitalization and treatment, determine whether nonextended-spectrum β-lactamase (ESBL), ESBL, CRE, or colistin-resistant organisms are expected. In India, ESBL is found to be >50%, therefore empiric third-generation cephalosporins have no role in empiric therapy. Empirically, β-lactam/β-lactamase inhibitors (BL/BLIs) like piperacillin tazobactam or cefoperazone sulbactam could be used if patient has not been previously treated, is not immunocompromised, and source control is optimal.

Meropenem was advised in this patient as it has a good coverage against GN organisms as well as anaerobes. It was combined with teicoplanin to cover *Enterococcus* spp. and fluconazole for *Candida* spp., although this is not always needed.

How was the treatment tailored after the CRE report?

As the organism isolated was carbapenem-resistant *E. coli*, treatment with meropenem minimum inhibitory concentration (MIC) >16, would remain ineffective. Teicoplanin and fluconazole were discontinued as there was no isolation of GP organisms or *Candida*. Treatment was changed to high-dose tigecycline which has high concentrations in the liver, gallbladder, and colon. Since this drug covers anaerobes as well, there was no need to add metronidazole.

However, the patient had severe nausea and vomiting and did not tolerate tigecycline.

What are the other drug options?

Tigecycline and polymyxins are not BLs and have different mechanisms of resistance which are not related to β-lactamases. Use of polymyxin alone has limitations. For GN, it is most commonly given as a combination therapy with tigecycline or fosfomycin and has no role against GP and anaerobes and also has nephrotoxicity. In general, it has a suboptimal efficacy in clinical trials. The next option is the new BL/BLIs like ceftazidime-avibactam (CAZ-AVI) along with aztreonam (ATM), but it is important to know the genotypic profile of carbapenemases. Xpert CARBA-R is a rapid polymerase chain reaction (PCR) that detects and differentiates the most prevalent carbapenemase gene families such as VIM, IMP, NDM, and/or OXA-48. This organism was a found to be a NDM + OXA-48 producer.

	ESBL	AmpC	KPC	OXA-48	MBL (NDM, IMP, and VIM)	Remarks
Ceftazidime-avibactam	+	+	+	+	-	Avibactam is not stable against MBLs. Therefore, MBL will destroy ceftazidime
Ceftazidime-avibactam + aztreonam	+	+	+	+	+	Aztreonam is stable against MBL but is destroyed by other β-lactamases. However avibactam is able to inhibit ESBL, AmpC, KPC and OXA-48 and protects aztreonam

(ESBL: extended-spectrum β-lactamase; KPC: *Klebsiella pneumoniae* carbapenemase; MBL: metallo-β-lactamase)

CAZ-AVI ATM is ineffective for anaerobes and so additional metronidazole is needed in this patient.

What is the role of antifungals in intra-abdominal infections?
Cultures are often sterile in deep-seated infections due to its poor sensitivity. Empirically, antifungal treatment is given when suspecting a delayed perforation, pancreatitis, biliary leak, or if patient has undergone previous abdominal procedures. Echinocandins is preferred over fluconazole in critically ill patients and in those with recent azole exposure.

Nonculture-based tests like β-D-glucan (BDG) should be done. As BDG has a high NPV, antifungals can be discontinued if BDG is negative. False-positive BDG values may be noted in patients receiving blood products, IV albumin, IVIG, or exposure to high amount of glucan containing gauze during surgery. BDG values normalize approximately in 3–4 days following the above exposures.

What is the duration of treatment?
If appropriate source control is done, a duration of 7 days of antimicrobial therapy is enough. But in complicated intra-abdominal infections when source control is inadequate, a longer duration of 2–3 weeks may have to be given.

■ CASE 3
A 63-year-old male, with DM, hypertension (HTN), and chronic kidney disease (CKD), was on maintenance hemodialysis (MHD) through HD catheter for 5 months. Later he underwent dialysis through arteriovenous (AV) fistula. 2 months later, he presented with severe pain in right hip with inability to walk along with fever and chills. MRI pelvis was suggestive of right hip joint effusion and right iliopsoas bursitis **(Fig. 5)**. Pus aspirated from right hip **(Fig. 6)** showed

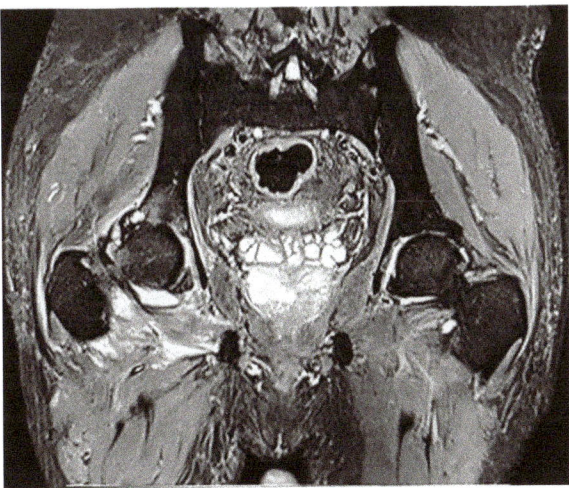

Fig. 5: Iliopsoas bursitis with right hip joint effusion.

gram-positive cocci (GPC) in clusters. Infectious Diseases (ID) reference was given. On examination, it was noted that the patient had a systolic murmur and blood cultures (two sets drawn 1 hour apart) GPC in clusters. Transthoracic echocardiography (TTE) showed a small vegetation in right atrium (RA) at the junction of superior vena cava (SVC) **(Fig. 7)**.

Discussion

What is the diagnosis?

Transthoracic echocardiography showed a vegetation indicating that the patient had infective endocarditis (IE). According to the Duke criteria, patient had two major criteria (multiple blood culture sets positive showing continuous

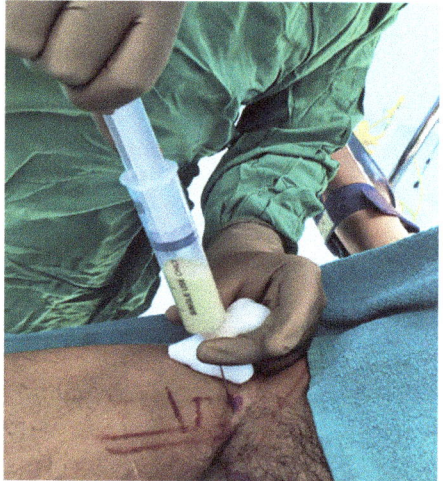

Fig. 6: Joint aspiration showing turbid fluid.

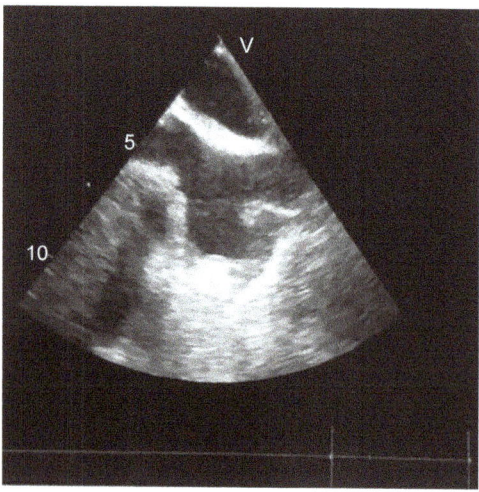

Fig. 7: Vegetation in right atrium (RA) at junction of superior vena cava (SVC).

bacteremia and TTE showing a vegetation), two minor criteria (fever and septic embolic lesion in the hip causing septic arthritis). Hence, it is a case of definite endocarditis.

In India, the common organisms to keep in mind when patient is on MHD and develops fever are *S. aureus, Candida,* and gram-negative bacteria (GNB) (e.g., *Pseudomonas, Stenotrophomonas, Burkholderia cepacia,* etc., and *Klebsiella*).

What do GPC in clusters signify and how does this impact the choice of antimicrobials?

Gram-positive cocci in clusters usually indicate *Staphylococcus* spp.—MSSA, MRSA, coagulase-negative staphylococci (CoNS), or methicillin-resistant CoNS (MRCoNS). Treatment covering MRSA and MSSA should be started when smear shows GPC in clusters and this is later modified according to the susceptibility report. Vancomycin is less effective for MSSA bacteremia and cloxacillin or cefazolin is ineffective for MRSA. Hence, cefazolin plus vancomycin in a renal modified dose, was given in this case.

Staphylococcus aureus bacteremia, IE, and septic arthritis are serious diseases associated with high morbidity, and mortality rates are 30–37% for MRSA endocarditis. The source, extent, and metastatic foci should be determined by careful history, physical examination, and imaging, as treatment failure and relapse can occur if source control is not done.

Pus and blood culture showed MRSA sensitive to tigecycline, vancomycin, teicoplanin, daptomycin, linezolid, and tetracycline.

What should be done if the patient is diagnosed with MRSA bacteremia?

It is important to consider whether the bacteremia is uncomplicated or complicated. Uncomplicated MRSA bacteremia is defined as positive blood cultures with no evidence of metastatic foci, exclusion of endocarditis and implants, sterile follow-up blood cultures after 2–4 days, and defervescence of fever within 72 hours of therapy. Vancomycin 15–20 mg/kg/day, 8–12 hourly is the drug of choice. Alternative agent is daptomycin 10 mg/kg/day. In case of uncomplicated MRSA bacteremia, the duration of treatment is 14 days.

This patient had complicated MRSA bacteremia as there was evidence of endocarditis with metastatic foci in the hip joint due to septic emboli or hematogenous seeding of the organism. Echocardiography, transesophageal echocardiogram (TEE) over TTE, is recommended for all patients with *S. aureus* bacteremia. Blood cultures should be repeated 2–4 days later to document clearance of bacteremia.

A crucial step is control of the metastatic focus. A thorough debridement and joint wash was done with local placement of vancomycin impregnated beads.

What is the antimicrobial approach in this patient?

Choice of drugs depends on the site and extent of the disease.

Drug	Bacteremia	Infective endocarditis	Septic arthritis/osteomyelitis
Vancomycin	+	+	+
Teicoplanin	+	–	+
Daptomycin	+	+ Right sided	+
Linezolid	+/–	–	– (Long duration of treatment may be associated with toxicity)
Clindamycin	–	–	+
TMP-SMX	–	+/–	+ But in combination
Doxycycline	–	–	+ But in combination

(TMP-SMX: trimethoprim-sulfamethoxazole)

The effectiveness of vancomycin depends on the level achieved in the site of infection and MIC of the organism. Although vancomycin MIC <2 is considered susceptible, MIC >1 is frequently associated with treatment failure. Therefore, just the identification of the organism is not enough; vancomycin MIC is important for successful outcome.

A loading dose of vancomycin of 25–30 mg/kg can be considered to achieve target trough concentrations, followed by 15–20 mg/kg/day 8–12 hourly, not exceeding 2 g/dose. Doses will have to be modified in CKD and in dialysis patients and it is given post HD. A target trough concentration of 15–20 μg/mL should be achieved for optimal efficacy.

Alternatively high-dose daptomycin 10 mg/kg/day can be given, which has a rapid bactericidal activity and good penetration in joints. Daptomycin has equal efficacy against MSSA and MRSA isolates. TMP-SMX is also cidal, but is inferior to vancomycin and can be given with doxycycline. Linezolid is static and when given alone has limited success. Teicoplanin has good bone and joint penetration but has suboptimal penetration in the vegetations of IE.

What is the duration of treatment of IE?
Duration of treatment is for 6–8 weeks. Blood cultures should be repeated to check for clearance of bacteremia. Follow-up TTE should be done.

CASE 4

A 51-year-old female, a case of carcinoma cervix on chemotherapy through chemoport, underwent double J (DJ) stenting for obstructive uropathy, 4 months ago. She was now admitted with complaints of fever with chills and dysuria for 2 days. Urine and blood cultures from chemoport and peripheral venipuncture grew carbapenem-resistant *E. coli* sensitive to colistin, tigecycline, amikacin, and fosfomycin.

Discussion

Is this a central line-associated bloodstream infection (CRBSI)?

A definitive diagnosis of CRBSI requires that the same organism grows from blood drawn from the catheter hub as well as the peripheral site and the differential time to positivity (DTP) is >2 hours. For DTP, growth of microbes from a blood sample drawn from a catheter hub is detected at least 2 hours before the growth detected in a blood sample obtained from a peripheral vein. Besides, there should not be an alternative cause of bacteremia. In this case, the DTP was <2 hours, suggesting that the source of infection was arising elsewhere and the patient did have features of urinary tract infection (UTI).

It is important to differentiate between the two because the line of management differs.

What is the treatment of choice?

Antibiotics should be decided based on the site, extent of infection, and action on biofilm.

Antibiotic	Urine	Blood	Activity on biofilm (DJ stent) in the urine
CAZ-AVI + ATM	+	+	+
Colistin	+	+	+
Polymyxin B	-	+	-
Fosfomycin	+	+	+
Aminoglycosides	+	+	+/-
Tigecycline	-	-	-
Nitrofurantoin	+	-	-

(ATM: aztreonam; CAZ-AVI: ceftazidime-avibactam; DJ: double J)

CAZ-AVI + ATM, colistin, and fosfomycin were the ideal options. However, CAZ-AVI + ATM is expensive, colistin is nephrotoxic, which will require regular monitoring of creatinine levels and fosfomycin can sometimes cause hypokalemia and K^+ levels will have to be monitored. But fosfomycin has a potential for oral treatment on follow-up. Hence, fosfomycin was advised. Since blood culture was positive, treatment for systemic infection was required with parenteral fosfomycin at a dose of 16–20 g in four divided doses.

Since resistance to fosfomycin monotherapy develops quickly, this should be avoided as far as possible and a companion drug like colistin may be needed.

■ CASE 5

A 83-year-old male, with DM and HTN, came with fever, cough, and dyspnea for 5 days. Chest X-ray (CXR) was suggestive of left lower lobe (LL) pneumonia. Sputum sent for BioFire [lower respiratory tract infection (LRTI) panel] showed a high bin value 10^5 for *Acinetobacter baumannii, Klebsiella pneumoniae,* and *Streptococcus agalactiae*. Sputum culture did not reveal any significant respiratory pathogen.

Discussion

How do you interpret this report?
Streptococcus agalactiae is very unusual organism causing community-acquired pneumonia (CAP). *A. baumannii* and *Klebsiella* causing CAP is very unlikely, considering he was a nonalcoholic and a nonsmoker. Also, the culture did not grow either of the two organisms. Three organisms with 10^5 bin value which is a semiquantitative estimation, suggests that this was genetic material from the organisms colonizing the respiratory tract and none of them may be the true pathogens causing CAP.

However the patient worsened, was intubated and developed fever with a new consolidation in the right upper lobe.

How to differentiate between ventilator-associated pneumonia (VAP) and colonization?
Ventilator-associated pneumonia is diagnosed if the radiograph exhibits a new or persistent pulmonary infiltrate, and two or more of the following criteria are met: temperature >38°C or <36°C, leukocytosis (peripheral blood leukocyte count >10 × 10^9/L) or leukopenia (peripheral blood leukocyte count <4 × 10^9/L), and the presence of purulent bronchial secretions. Pneumonia is considered to be ventilator-associated when the onset occurs 48 hours after the initiation of mechanical ventilation. Colonization is considered if patients have no clinical symptoms or radiological evidence for infiltrate, but only positive microbiological cultures.

What is the empirical choice of antibiotics to treat VAP?
This depends on the hospital antibiogram and the epidemiology of organisms causing VAP in each hospital.

In this patient endotracheal culture grew *A. baumannii* > 10^5 CFU/mL which was carbapenem resistant.

What are the various treatment options for CRAB?
- Although parenteral polymyxins are considered less effective due to inadequate penetration into the lung parenchyma, one of them has to be used along with nebulized colistin.
- Tigecycline is not preferred alone, but can be used as a combination therapy in high doses.
- Minocycline is another effective option if susceptibility is shown.
- The new BL/BLI like CAZ-AVI alone or with ATM has no role against *A. baumannii*, as it produces OXA-23 and 51 which are not inhibited by avibactam.

Therefore, polymyxin B + nebulized colistin + tigecycline/minocycline, may be preferred.

However, CAZ-AVI + ATM can be given in carbapenem-resistant *Klebsiella* as it may produce OXA-48 ± metallo-β-lactamase (MBL) which can be treated with this combination.

What is the duration of therapy?
The usual duration of treatment is 7 days for VAP when there is clinical improvement. But a 10–14 days course of antimicrobial therapy is recommended in pneumonia due to nonlactose fermenters like *Acinetobacter*. However, the exact duration depends upon the rate of improvement of clinical, radiologic, and laboratory parameters.

■ CASE 6

A 55-year-old male, with DM and HTN, complains of acute onset of petechial rash without fever and reduced urine output for 2 days and was admitted. On examination, he had nonblanching palpable purpuric rash involving both lower limbs, anterior abdominal wall and both eyelids suggestive of vasculitis **(Figs. 8A and B)**. He also had a nonhealing ulcer and impending gangrene of the left toe **(Fig. 9)**. His baseline investigations showed a WBC of 14,000,

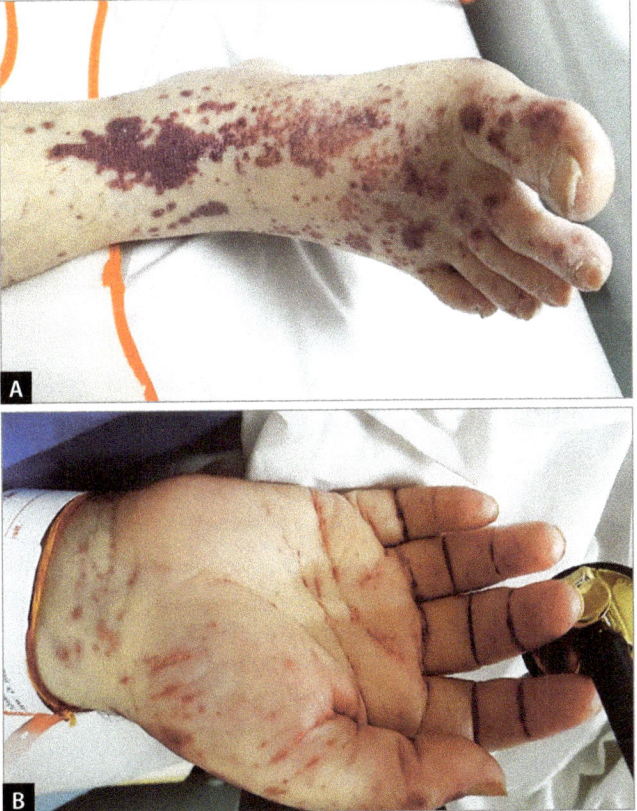

Figs. 8A and B: Purpuric rash on lower limb and hand.

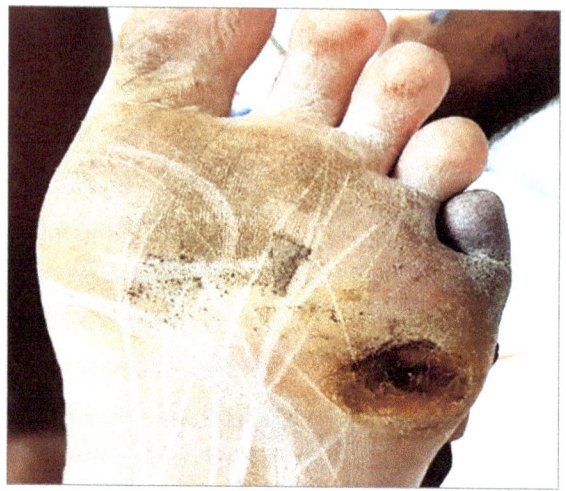

Fig. 9: Nonhealing ulcer with impending gangrene of little toe.

normal platelets, high C-reactive protein (CRP) and procalcitonin (PCT). Urine routine showed proteinuria and hematuria. CXR was normal.

Discussion

What are the various types and causes for vasculitis?
Vasculitis is classified based on (1) size of the blood vessel involved and (2) whether it is infectious/noninfectious.
- *Size of vessel:* Large vessel—Takayasu and giant cell arteritis; medium vessel—polyarteritis nodosa and Kawasaki disease; and small vessel—leukocytoclastic vasculitis.

Since the patient had palpable purpura with renal manifestations, it was thought to be small vessel vasculitis.

Noninfectious causes of leukocytoclastic vasculitis include:
- Immune complex mediated—rheumatoid arthritis, systemic lupus erythematosus (SLE), Henoch-Schönlein purpura, cryoglobulinemia, and hypersensitivity vasculitis;
- Drug induced—antihypertensives, antithyroid drugs, antibiotics, opioids, etc.
- Neoplasia—non-Hodgkin's lymphoma, solid tumors, etc.

Infectious causes are:
- *Viruses:* Hepatitis A, hepatitis B virus (HBV), cytomegalovirus (CMV), Epstein-Barr virus (EBV), varicella, and parvovirus B19
- *Bacteria:* Meningococcemia, rickettsia, β-hemolytic *Streptococcus*, *S. aureus*, pneumococci (endocarditis—septic emboli), *Mycoplasma*, *Klebsiella*, *Pseudomonas*, and *Capnocytophaga*.
- *Fungi:* Molds such as *Aspergillus and Fusarium*

The patient gave no history of any rheumatological condition, recent intake of any drugs, and no evidence of neoplasia was found clinically. With high

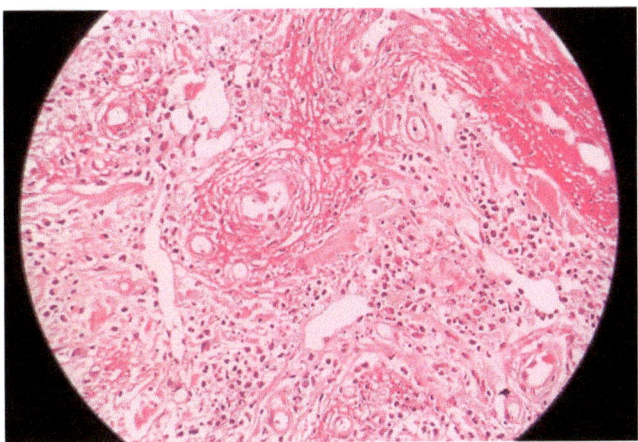

Fig. 10: Skin biopsy shows leukocytoclastic vasculitis of the small vessels.

WBC, CRP, PCT, and diabetic foot with early gangrene, an infectious cause due to *Staphylococcus*, *Klebsiella*, or *Pseudomonas* was most likely.

Rash and renal involvement could point to cholesterol embolism, which occurs in the lower limbs. However, the distribution of lesions in this patient included eyelids and anterior abdominal wall as well. As the patient had not undergone any recent endovascular procedure nor received thrombolytic therapy or anticoagulants, hence cholesterol embolism was unlikely.

What investigations should be obtained?
Antineutrophil cytoplasmic antibody (ANCA), cryoglobulin, antinuclear antibody (ANA), antiphospholipid antibody (APLA), complement levels, blood cultures, human immunodeficiency virus (HIV), hepatitis A and B, echocardiography, and skin and kidney biopsy.

Autoimmune workup was normal. Skin biopsy on histology showed small vessel leukocytoclastic vasculitis **(Fig. 10)**, blood culture was sterile and culture of the skin tissue grew ESBL *Klebsiella pneumoniae* sensitive to imipenem, meropenem, colistin, ertapenem, and amikacin. Patient was treated with meropenem and showed improvement.

■ SUGGESTED READING
1. Jason P. Burnham JP, Kirby JP, Kollef MH. Diagnosis and management of skin and soft tissue infections in the intensive care unit: a review. Intensive Care Med. 2016; 42(12): 1899-1911.
2. Montravers P, Snauwaert A, Welsch C. Current guidelines and recommendations for the management of skin and soft tissue infections. Curr Opin Infect Dis. 2016;29(2):131-8.
3. Perrone G, Sartelli M, Mario G et al. Management of intra-abdominal-infections: 2017 World Society of Emergency Surgery guidelines summary focused on remote areas and low-income nations. International Journal of Infectious Disease. 2020;99:140-8.

SECTION 5

Supports

- **Indications of Mechanical Ventilation**
  Jamshed Sunavala

- **Basics of Mechanical Ventilation**
  Jamshed Sunavala

- **Advanced Modes of Mechanical Ventilator**
  Joanne Mascarenhas

- **Weaning from Mechanical Ventilator**
  Jamshed Sunavala

- **Extracorporeal Membrane Oxygenator**
  Jamshed Sunavala

- **Mechanical Circulatory Supports**
  Jamshed Sunavala

- **Approach to Nutritional Support**
  Jamshed Sunavala

CHAPTER 17

Indications of Mechanical Ventilation

Jamshed Sunavala

■ INTRODUCTION

To gauge the appropriate moment to intubate and initiate ventilator support, requires judgment to decide, between initiating timely support or adopting the "wait and watch" approach. An astute physician, more often than not, relies on clinical findings indicating early signs of respiratory distress or fatigue **(Box 1)**, which would lead to respiratory failure, if left uncorrected.

■ INDICATIONS OF MECHANICAL VENTILATION

Respiratory arrest, shock, and respiratory failure are obvious indications for immediate intubation and ventilator support. However, critically ill patients who display early signs of respiratory distress or fatigue may rapidly deteriorate, resulting in hemodynamic decompensation or serious arrhythmias. This group of patients would seriously benefit with prompt respiratory support, but whether they should be immediately intubated and ventilated, or supported on noninvasive ventilation (NIV) alone, would depend on the clinician's judgment.

There is another subset of critically ill patients who are *hypoventilating* because of a depressed respiratory center, spinal cord lesions, myasthenia gravis, Guillain-Barré syndrome, etc. who may not necessarily, be in type II respiratory failure with a high arterial partial pressure of carbon dioxide ($PaCO_2$) **(Table 1)**. However, these patients have a slow and shallow respiration

---

BOX 1 Physical signs of acute respiratory distress.

Hypoxemic respiratory failure:
- Tachypnea, hypertension, and at times hypotension
- Use of accessory muscles of respiration—intercostals, abdominal, and sternomastoid muscles
- Tracheal tug
- Exaggerated retraction of the intercostals space
- Facial signs—nasal flaring, open mouth breathing, and pursed lips with labored breathing, as in chronic obstructive pulmonary disease (COPD)
- Moaning and grunting during exhalation
- Profuse sweating
- Diminished mentation or vacant gaze

Hypercapnic respiratory failure:
- Mostly similar to above
- Greater neurological manifestations
- Tremors of outstretched hands and asterixis
- Myoclonic jerks, irritability, behavioral changes, decreased sensorium, and seizures

TABLE 1 Indications for mechanical ventilation.

Absolute indications	Clinical judgment/ assessment	Supporting parameters
Cardiorespiratory arrest	-	-
Severe shock	Severity of hypotension, respiratory distress, and sensorium	*Elevated serum lactate, SvO_2 < 60% in cardiogenic shock*
Type I ARF	-	*PaO_2 < 60 mm Hg or SaO_2 < 90% despite supplemental O_2*
Type II ARF	Declining mental status	*$PaCO_2 \geq$ 50 mm Hg or acute increase from baseline in $PaCO_2$, pH < 7.25*
Potential indications		
Hypoventilation with inadequate lung expansion	Shallow and rapid breathing	*$V_T \leq$ 5 mL/kg, VC < 15 mL/kg, RR $\geq$ 35 breaths per minute*
Respiratory muscle weakness	Underlying clinical problem causing hypoventilation	*VC < 20 mL/kg*
Acute decompensated heart failure	Sign of heart failure	*Clinical judgment*
Increased work of breathing	Respiratory distress, use of accessory muscles, and paradoxical respiration	*Minute ventilation > 15 L/min, dead space > 50%*
Postoperative pulmonary complications (NIV*/IMV)	Mainly post-upper abdominal and cardiac surgery	*Abnormal blood gas values*
Acute exacerbation of COPD (NIV*/IMV)	Progressively decreasing sensorium, degree of respiratory distress, and air hunger	*Acute increase from baseline $PaCO_2$ pH < 7.25*
*Contraindications to NIV	*Impaired sensorium, poor respiratory drive, risk of aspiration, excessive secretions, head-neck and facial injuries, flail chest, upper airways obstruction, severe ARDS PaO_2/FiO_2 < 150*	

(ARDS: acute respiratory distress syndrome; ARF: acute respiratory failure; COPD: chronic obstructive pulmonary disease; FiO_2: fraction of inspired oxygen; IMV: invasive mechanical ventilation; NIV: noninvasive ventilation; $PaCO_2$: arterial partial pressure of carbon dioxide; PaO_2: partial pressure of arterial oxygen; RR: respiratory rate; SaO_2: oxygen saturation; SvO_2: mixed venous oxygen saturation; VC: vital capacity; V_T: tidal volume) with poor lung expansion and should be closely monitored. The bigger risk in these patients is the poor forced vital capacity (FVC) and an ineffective cough effort with pooling of secretions in the upper airways. We have seen patients of this group who continue to maintain their normal gas exchange despite hypoventilation but have had a catastrophic experience of choking on their secretions and arresting. Here, a planned tracheostomy serves best both for maintaining a clear airway and providing a ready access to ventilator support.

Patients with *decompensated heart failure and pulmonary edema* would benefit from positive pressure ventilation. Here NIV may help initially but intubation and ventilator support may become necessary, depending on the severity, of the clinical status and blood gas abnormalities.

Patients with *acute exacerbation of chronic obstructive pulmonary disease (COPD)* are very difficult to manage on mechanical ventilation. Once intubated and taken over by the ventilator, weaning and extubation can pose problems and almost one-third of COPD patients fail weaning trials, though they may meet the accepted weaning and extubation criteria. Several studies have shown the superiority of NIV over invasive ventilatory support, and should be the first choice, if assisted ventilation is indicated. NIV should be definitely initiated if the patient is seriously hypercapnic with a pH of <7.32. Both the degree of hypercapnia and pH are good early predictors of initiating NIV. There are of course relative and absolute contraindications to the use of NIV (*see* **Table 1**). Absolute contraindications such as cardiorespiratory arrest, impaired sensorium, poor respiratory drive, risk of aspiration, or excessive secretions would prompt the need for tracheal intubation and mechanical ventilation. The reason for initial preference of NIV over intubation and ventilation in COPD patients include ventilation asynchrony requiring paralytic agents, risks of barotrauma and circulatory collapse due to high mean airway pressure (MAwP), difficult weaning, plus extubation and problems associated with dynamic hyperinflation. Most importantly, studies have shown that patients who respond to NIV have better result and outcome than those on invasive ventilator support. However, it must be stressed that failure of NIV or marked oxygen desaturation should immediately prompt one to intubate and mechanically ventilate.

High-flow nasal oxygen (HFNO) has recently also been shown to be as effective as NIV and benefits both hypoxia and hypercapnia occurring in respiratory failure in COPD patients. In addition, in the postextubation period, HFNO has shown to decrease the reintubation rates in comparison to NIV.

In patients with severe *hypoxic respiratory failure* as in severe acute respiratory distress syndrome (ARDS), tracheal intubation with mechanical ventilation should be implemented without delay. Most of these patients have increased shunt and hence high concentration nonrebreathing mask or NIV will not correct the refractory hypoxia. However in mild-to-moderate ARDS, [partial pressure of arterial oxygen/fraction of inspired oxygen (PaO_2/FiO_2) > 150),

NIV may be tried initially but prompt intubation and ventilatory support should be expedited at the earliest evidence of oxygen desaturation, before any serious cardiorespiratory compromise occurs.

Postoperative pulmonary complications have a high morbidity and mortality and may require reintubation. Atelectasis is a common cause for respiratory failure after upper abdominal surgery. Other causes include aspiration pneumonia, severe bronchospasm in patients with previous history of asthma or COPD, pulmonary embolism, and diaphragmatic dysfunction following phrenic nerve injury. It is important to anticipate postoperative pulmonary complications in certain high-risk patients, especially in the elderly bed-ridden group, with poor cough effort, or patients with Parkinson's disease, or with any cause of neuromuscular weakness. These patients should be assessed preoperatively along with the anesthetist with regards to continuation of ventilator support postoperatively. Weaning should be attempted at an appropriate time in the intensive care unit (ICU). Often, postcardiac surgery patients are weaned prematurely, in the recovery room and need to be reintubated in the ICU, as some of them, are prone to develop mild left ventricular dysfunction despite NIV backup.

Finally, this is one of the few situations where the physician will have to make a judgment call based on his astute clinical skill and experience. The clinical information available at the bedside is often more helpful than guidelines or protocols in taking prompt decisions regarding initiation of ventilator support. Gas exchange abnormalities are vital in decision-making, but it would be unwise to depend on a predefined value of PaO_2 or $PaCO_2$ as the sole basis of initiating ventilator support. **Box 1** gives some of the physical signs of acute respiratory distress on clinical examination.

■ SUGGESTED READING

1. Cinel I, Dellinger RP. General principles of mechanical ventilation. In: Parrillo J, Dellinger RP (Eds). Critical Care Medicine—Principles of Diagnosis and Management in Adults, 5th edition. Amsterdam, Netherlands: Elsevier; 2019.
2. Laghi F, Tobin MJ. Indications for mechanical ventilation. In: Tobin MJ (Ed). Principles and Practice of Mechanical Ventilation, 3rd edition. New York: McGraw Hill publication; 2013.

CHAPTER 18

Basics of Mechanical Ventilation

Jamshed Sunavala

■ INTRODUCTION

During the polio epidemic of the 1930s and 1940s in Europe, there was a high demand for ventilators, and the first-generation negative pressure ventilators designed to create a pressure gradient between the airway opening and the alveoli by applying negative pressure around the torso were widely used. Negative pressure ventilators created a pressure gradient by decreasing the alveolar pressure to a level below the airway opening pressures at the mouth. This was enabled by using the *"iron lung"* or the *"chest cuirass"* which applied negative pressure around the chest to expand the lungs by encasing the patient, neck downwards. However, negative pressure ventilators had many limitations and in the 1950s, the *Emerson Company in Boston* made available a basic prototype positive pressure ventilator at the Massachusetts General Hospital, which was a success and was instantly accepted by the medical community; this was the birth of our modern mechanical ventilators and also probably of the concept of critical care medicine. Over the years, this worked into more efficient machines with better understanding of various respiratory variables of flow, volume, and pressure. The first reporting of acute respiratory distress syndrome (ARDS) by Ashley Ashbaugh and Petti in 1968 made our understanding of lung-ventilator interaction even better, and by understanding the concepts of lung compliance (C_L) and airway resistance, it made way for safer modes of ventilation. Technological advances and newer modes enabled better lung recruitment and improved oxygenation with less likelihood of ventilation-induced lung injury (VILI).

■ THE BASICS

In spontaneous breathing, a negative pleural pressure (Ppl) causes the thoracic cage to expand, thus decreasing the intra-alveolar pressure below the atmospheric pressure, thereby creating a pressure gradient whereby the ambient air enters the lungs. Reversely during expiration, the intra-alveolar pressure increases following the elastic recoil of the lungs and the pressure gradient now reverses with air exiting the lungs. Interestingly, at rest (i.e., between the expiratory and inspiratory phases), to prevent the lungs from collapsing secondary to the elastic recoil, the intrapleural pressure always remains subatmospheric; however, if the thoracic cage is punctured and air gushes into the pleural spaces (pneumothorax), it will cause the lungs to collapse. *In case of patients mechanically ventilated on positive pressure ventilation,* the opposite happens, as the higher pressures delivered by the ventilator pushes air into the lungs creating a positive alveolar pressure during inspiration and a negative alveolar pressure during expiration.

Pressure and Volume Control Ventilation (Fig. 1)

The main purpose of positive pressure ventilation is to move a volume of gas into the lungs by the machine, creating a positive pressure gradient towards the alveoli. This is done by either a *volume-controlled ventilation (VCV) or a pressure-controlled ventilation (PCV)* and therefore, understanding the ventilator-lung interaction and the advantages and disadvantages of these two very basic modes, is critical in comprehending the essentials of mechanical ventilation (MV).

Volume-controlled ventilation delivers a preset tidal volume (V_T) and the ventilator automatically adjusts the inflation pressure, whereas in PCV the pressure is preset to deliver the desired volume. Hence, in VCV the V_T is always constant despite the changing compliance of the lung; thus in patients with stiff lungs and poor compliance (e.g., ARDS), the pressure delivered may increase disproportionately and there is always a risk of barotrauma, whereas in PCV mode there is little risk of barotrauma as the airway pressure (Paw) remains steady and within set limits, but the V_T can vary.

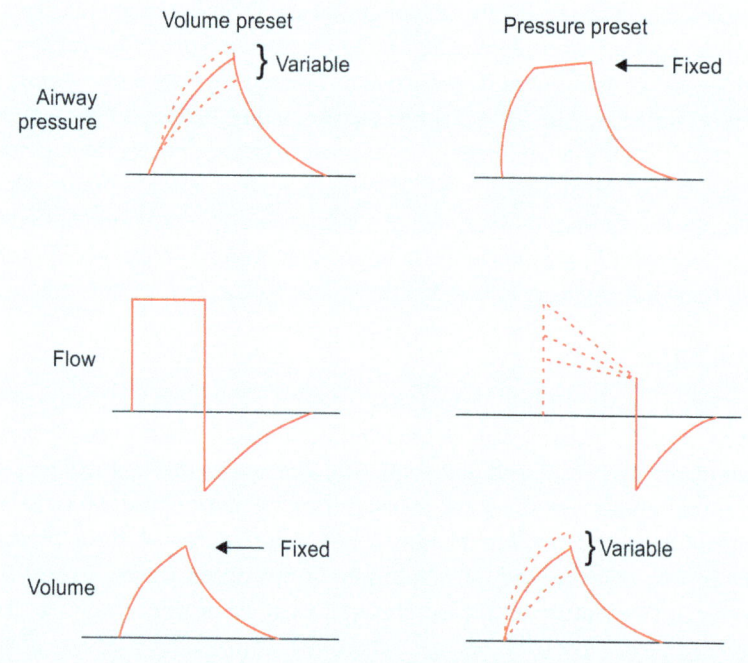

Fig. 1: Volume preset versus pressure preset ventilation.

Eventually, the main purpose of MV is either to act as replacement for failing respiratory muscles by providing an external source of ventilatory pressure or to counter the escalating elastic forces and airway resistance, which may oppose normal breathing. This is best illustrated in the *equation of motion.*

Equation of Motion

Ventilator pressure + Muscle pressure = Resistance to flow + Elastance volume

Where elastance is inverse of compliance which will be discussed soon, compliance is change in volume upon change in pressure (C = $\Delta V/\Delta P$).

Therefore, rewriting the equation:

$$\Delta P = R \times F + \frac{\Delta V}{Cst}$$

Where ΔP is change in pressure, ΔV is change in volume, R = resistance, F is flow, and Cst is static compliance.

Translating this into "ventilator control" as we discussed earlier:
- In VCV with fixed volume; the pressure will have to change to keep the equation of motion balanced.
- In PCV with fixed pressure; the volume will change to keep the equation balanced. Of course this is provided the R, F, and Cst remain unchanged.

Lung Compliance and Airway Resistance

It is important to understand that C_L plays an important role, especially when ventilating stiff lungs such as in patients with ARDS. C_L by simple definition is change in V_T per change in unit pressure, and as the equation shows (C_L = $\Delta V/\Delta P$) a poorly compliant lung will need increasing positive pressure to inflate it. However, when we talk of Paw at end-inspiration, it implies peak airway pressure (Ppeak) and this is the pressure generated by the ventilator to overcome both resistance to the flow of air provided by the airway pressure (Pr), and the elastic forces of the lungs and chest wall (P_{CL}); therefore Ppeak = Pr + P_{CL}. In brief, the latter gives you an idea of the stiffness of the lung as in ARDS, and the former tells you if there is any airways obstruction as in chronic obstructive pulmonary disease (COPD). **Figure 2** is a graphic of a mechanically ventilated pressure curve of volume-controlled (VC) breath showing Ppeak and plateau pressure (Pplateau). This curve is obtained by occluding the expiratory circuit at the end of lung inflation i.e. end-inspiration (Ppeak) and holding it for a second, during which time the airway pressure decreases initially and then plateaus till the occlusion is released and exhalation is completed. This maneuver, called *"inspiratory hold",* is best done during volume-cycled rather than pressure-cycled mode, because pressure is variable in volume-cycled mode and best reflects the changing compliance.

In modern ventilators the graphics are displayed continuously on the monitor and hence the maneuver of manually performing an "inspiratory hold" is not necessary. The plateau pressure represents the maximum pressure

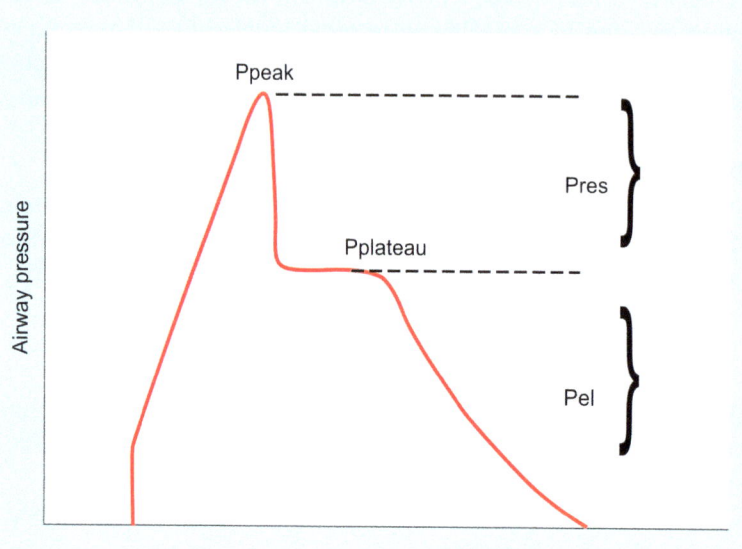

Fig. 2: Graph of a mechanically ventilated pressure curve of volume-controlled (VC) breath showing peak airway pressure (Ppeak) and plateau pressure (Pplateau). (Pres - pressure needed to overcome airway resistance; Pel - pressure required to overcome the forces of elastic recoil).

in the alveoli at end-inspiration pressure (EIP) and this level of pressure from the baseline [i.e., end-expiratory pressure (EEP)] is the pressure required to overcome the forces of elastic recoil and represents the C_L. *The difference between the peak and plateau pressures represents the pressure needed to overcome the airway resistance* (**Fig. 2**). The graph on the pressure-controlled (PC) mode will not give this information as the end-inspiratory pressure here is in fact the peak alveolar pressure, as there is no airflow at end-inspiration; hence on PC mode the difference between the peak at end-inspiration and the baseline will represent compliance, but will not be able to assess the airway pressures.

With the above explanation one should be able to interpret the basics of "ventilator graphics", which will be useful to understand the changing lung physiology at the bedside.

Positive End-expiratory Pressure

Unlike the EIP which is the airway pressure at the peak of each lung inflation, the EEP is the pressure in the alveoli and not in the airways, during the end of expiration. Hence, during spontaneous ventilation or on normal ventilatory settings, there is no airflow at end-expiration and hence the alveolar pressure is the same as the atmospheric pressure and is reflected on the pressure waveform on the graph as zero baseline. However, one can get a positive pressure in the

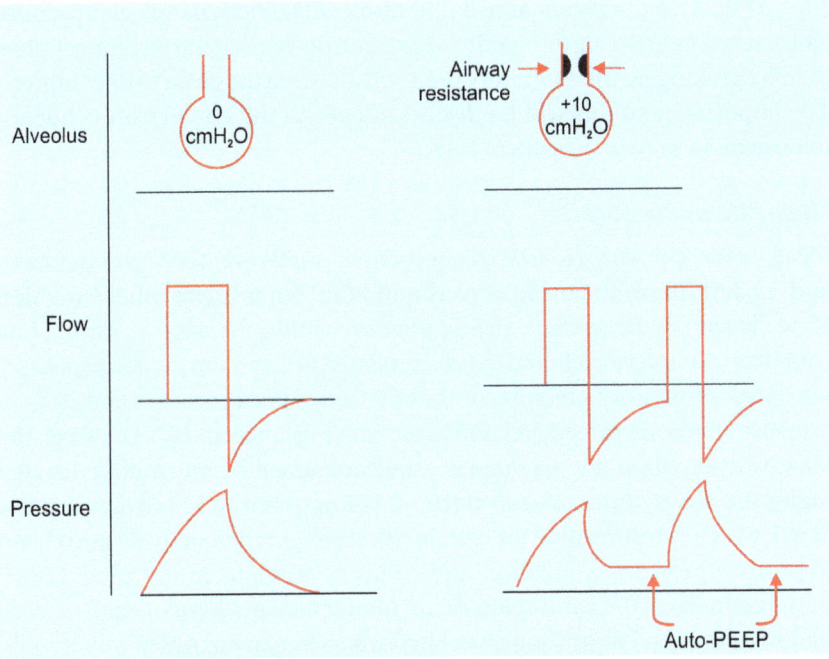

Fig. 3: Auto-positive end-expiratory pressure (Auto PEEP).

alveoli above the atmospheric pressure by selecting a mode on the ventilator called positive end-expiratory pressure (PEEP).

The normal physiological PEEP of 0–5 cmH$_2$O is commonly applied during initiation of ventilation but higher therapeutic PEEP is now a routine practice to improve oxygenation. High levels of PEEP prevent collapse of distal alveoli during expiration, hence, decreases atelectasis and improves ventilation/perfusion (V/Q) mismatch in patients with hypoxic respiratory failure. Details of application of PEEP are discussed in Chapter 19, Advanced Modes of Mechanical Ventilator.

Note that PEEP can also occur without applying the PEEP mode on the ventilator; this happens when lungs are not capable of completely emptying the air during end-expiration and this is called auto-*PEEP or intrinsic-PEEP* **(Fig. 3)**. This may occur as a result of dynamic hyperinflation in asthmatics or in COPD patients as a result of airflow limitation during a prolonged expiration, and is also commonly called "air trapping". This happens because the "time constant" of a lung unit, which is the length of time required for inflation and deflation at a set respiratory rate, is directly proportional to the airflow resistance in the airways. As a result of this, the time for the lung to deflate increases, leaving the alveoli partially inflated during the expiratory phase. This is particularly important in patients with emphysema, where pressures can build within various lung units; this phenomenon is called auto- or intrinsic-PEEP and is graphically reflected on the expiratory flow curve (**Fig. 3**). A persistent auto-PEEP results in hemodynamic compromise which requires lowering the ventilator rate and decreasing the inspiratory time, thereby prolonging the expiratory time and allowing the chest to decompress. The importance of this will be discussed later in the chapter on ventilator management in patients with COPD.

Mean Airway Pressure

Mean airway pressure (MawP) is another parameter we need to understand and it is not simply the mean of peak and PEEP but involves other variables. MawP is simply the average airway pressure within the airways during one complete respiratory cycle and is directly related to inspiratory time, respiratory rate, peak inspiratory pressure, and PEEP, unlike peak pressure and plateau pressure which are directly related to airway resistance and C_L. However, the MawP displayed on the machine is usually obtained by integrating the area under the airway pressure waveform. It is important to know that it is the MawP which is responsible for certain adverse hemodynamic effects related to positive pressure ventilation and needs continuous monitoring. MawP thus, best reflects the cardiopulmonary interaction and hence requires close monitoring, especially during severe hypoxia secondary to ARDS which could result in pulmonary hypertension and right ventricular overload. To prevent cardiac decompensation as well as volutrauma or barotrauma to the lungs, especially in ventilating ARDS patients, the MawP should be maintained below 30 cmH_2O at all times.

It is best to be conversant with some physiological variables and their terminologies and abbreviations commonly used whilst ventilating a patient. We are now somewhat familiar with EIP, EEP, VC mode, PC mode, C_L, Ppl, Ppeak, Palv, PEEP (extrinsic and intrinsic), and MawP.

Gas Exchange Alterations with Mechanical Ventilation

We have briefly covered the mechanics of volume, flow, and pressure, as applied to the ventilator and the effects of elastic resistance and airway impedance offered by the lungs. However, the end result of this ventilator-lung interaction is reflected on gas exchange and hemodynamic alterations. V/Q mismatch occurs either due to nonuniform ventilation but uniform perfusion (low V/Q <1 or shunt) or uniform ventilation but nonuniform perfusion (high V/Q ≥ 1 or dead space effect). A low V/Q or shunt will result in venous admixture. MV by itself can increase the venous admixture to around 10% as compared to normal of 2–5% because of a mild alveolar redistribution of air, but in cases such as ARDS, it decreases venous admixture by improving the distribution of ventilation in the collapsed underventilated lung area. However, if overdistention of alveoli occurs due to the high positive pressures, pulmonary blood flow would be redistributed to the poorly ventilated lung units causing V/Q mismatch resulting in hypoxemia. A modest elevation of arterial partial pressure of carbon dioxide ($PaCO_2$) may also be observed due to an increase in dead space, which is of little consequence. This may occur because of a few overventilated alveoli in relation to the perfusion or due to a mechanical dead space occurring because of the rebreathed volume in the ventilator circuit. If on the other hand, the dead space fraction is seriously increased due to poor pulmonary perfusion following pulmonary embolism or shock; it can result in a marked disparity between minute ventilation and $PaCO_2$ which could at times be a subtle expression of pulmonary embolism.

Cardiac Consequences

One of the serious consequences of MV is the adverse effects on cardiac output, O_2 delivery, and right-sided pressures which are all compromised. These are the direct consequences from increased intrathoracic pressure resulting in decreased venous return. However, during routine respiratory support with minimal PEEP, it would have no significant clinical impact but when high levels of MawP and PEEP are applied for recruiting the lungs in patients with refractory hypoxia or in ARDS, it can cause serious hemodynamic compromise. In these situations hemodynamic monitoring may become necessary.

BASIC MODES

Basic modes imply those settings which are used for initiation of ventilation and enabling lung-ventilator synchrony. Hence, this is best described as part of this chapter, unlike the strategic modes described in the next chapter, which are innovations to overcome mainly life-threatening physiological complications following progressively worsening lung pathology.

A mechanical ventilator's role is to replace one's normal spontaneous breathing with positive pressure mechanical breaths; however, it could still allow the patient to spontaneously trigger a breath before delivering a V_T by using the a*ssist mode ventilation [adaptive support ventilation (ASV)]*. Mechanical ventilator could also be set on a mode which allows the patient to spontaneously breathe on his own, but takes over at fixed intervals or earlier if required, like a demand pacemaker and is called *intermittent mandatory ventilation (IMV)*; and these mandatory breaths when synchronized with the patient's own efforts to breathe in order to avoid asynchrony, is called *synchronized IMV (SIMV)*. **Figure 4** *displays the various waveforms—ASV showing an initial small negative wave induced by the patient trigger and SIMV showing mandatory synchronized breaths interspaced with normal patient breaths.*

Assist control ventilation (ACV) is probably the most common mode used in an intensive care unit (ICU), especially when initiating patients who are in acute respiratory failure, on ventilator support. Over two-thirds of patients requiring invasive ventilation, including those ventilated for ARDS, initially receive ACV. On volume-assist control ventilation (V-ACV), the ventilator

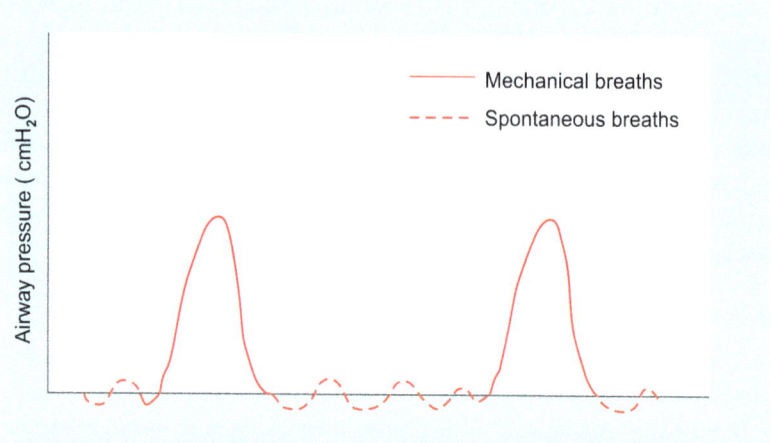

Fig. 4: Synchronized intermittent mandatory ventilation (SIMV).

delivers a steady V_T regardless of the respiratory effort or airway impedance. V_T also remains unchanged for both the ventilator-triggered or patient-triggered breath. If after a certain lapse, the patient defaults in initiating an inspiratory effort whilst breathing spontaneously, the machine triggers the breath and takes over at a preset rate. However as long as the patient triggers the ventilator, the machine senses the change in airway pressure and inhibits its triggering mechanism.

The patient's effort can trigger the ventilator either by generating a negative airway pressure of 2–3 cmH_2O, or it can be triggered with less effort using the "inspiratory flow rate" generated by the ventilator. As the latter involves less respiratory effort and work load, most modern ventilators have adopted this form of triggering signal.

The main advantage of ACV is in preventing respiratory muscle disuse as a result of spontaneous triggering effort and it also helps to rest the respiratory muscles when the ventilator takes over. The other advantage is that it allows the patient to control the respiratory frequency and therefore the minute ventilation which is required to keep the $PaCO_2$ within acceptable limits. The main disadvantage of ACV is the alveolar hyperventilation and respiratory alkalosis that can occur if the patient's respiratory drive is inordinately high, leading to an excessive assist frequency. In such a case it is best to change to another mode such as SIMV.

Intermittent mandatory ventilation (IMV), as described earlier, facilitates spontaneous breathing between ventilator breaths. The mandatory breath could be either VC or PC and when mandatory breaths are delivered in synchrony with the patient's breath, it is termed as SIMV. The main indication of IMV is to replace ACV in the event of rapid breathing resulting in incomplete exhalation during ACV. IMV also reduces the risk of intrinsic-PEEP during spontaneous breathing by emptying the alveoli. However, IMV has two major adverse effects. It can decrease cardiac output in patients with compromised cardiac function due to increased work of breathing and hence should be avoided in patients with left ventricular failure (LVF). IMV further increases the work of breathing when the spontaneous breathing is rapid. This is attributed to the resistance built up in the ventilator circuit, and this can be overcome by using pressure support ventilation (PSV) during the periods of spontaneous breathing in IMV. The modes discussed so far help during initiation of ventilation and overcoming the lung/ventilator interaction.

■ CLASSIFICATION OF MODES

Chetburn RL proposed a decent classification published in Resp Care 2007, based on three components: (1) breathing patterns and control variable within breath; (2) control used within and between breaths; and (3) operational variable. However, over the years, with the advance in ventilator technology and newer modes of ventilation with unique characteristics, the classification becomes more complicated. I have simplified the classification which would be useful for clinical applications **(Boxes 1 and 2)**.

Breath pattern describes the breath as either ventilator-assisted breath or a spontaneous breath by the patient without any assistance from the ventilator. If the breath is assisted, is it VC or PC? Once this is ascertained, a *breath sequence* needs to be recognized. It could be continuous, intermittent, or spontaneous

---

BOX 1 General classification of ventilation modes.

Basic Modes as per Breath Pattern

- **Breath pattern within the breaths:**
  - Volume-controlled ventilation (VCV)
  - Pressure-controlled ventilation (PCV)
- **Breath sequence between breaths:**
  - Continuous mandatory ventilation (CMV)
  - Intermittent mandatory ventilation (IMV)
  - Continuous spontaneous ventilation (CSV)

Strategic Modes

- **Mainly for lung recruitment:**
  - Positive end-expiratory pressure (PEEP)
  - Inverse ratio ventilation (IRV)
  - High frequency oscillation ventilation (HFOV)
  - Pressure release volume control (PRVC)
  - Prone position ventilation
- **Facilitate difficult weaning:**
  - Pressure support ventilation (PSV)
- **Lung protection ventilation (LPV):**
  - Low tidal volume ventilation (LTV)
  - Permissive hypercapnia
- **Noninvasive ventilation (NIV)**

> **BOX 2** Basic modes of ventilation.
>
> VC-CMV = Volume-controlled continuous mandatory ventilation
> VC-IMV = Volume-controlled intermittent mandatory ventilation
> ACV = Assist control ventilation which could deliver tidal volume (V_T) as per volume or pressure
> PC-CMV = Pressure-controlled continuous mandatory ventilation
> PC-IMV = Pressure-controlled intermittent mandatory ventilation
> PC-CSV = Pressure-controlled continuous spontaneous ventilation

throughout. If we combine the above variables we will derive six basic modes of ventilation **(Box 2)**.

As you note, volume-controlled continuous spontaneous ventilation (VC-CSV) is not feasible as this would be incompatible with this definition of spontaneous breath, as ventilation determines the V_T in VC, whereas in spontaneous breath the patient totally dictates the V_T.

SUGGESTED READING

1. Cinel I, Dellinger RP. General principles of mechanical ventilation. In: Parrillo J, Dellinger RP (Eds). Critical Care Medicine—Principles of Diagnosis and Management in Adults, 5th edition. Amsterdam: Elsevier; 2019.
2. Tobin MJ. Principles and Practice of Mechanical Ventilation, 3rd Edition. McGraw Hill publication, 2014.

CHAPTER 19

Advanced Modes of Mechanical Ventilator

Joanne Mascarenhas

■ INTRODUCTION

Beyond the basic features of mechanical ventilation, as described in the previous chapter, are the advanced modes of ventilation and ventilatory strategies that help in improving oxygenation and ventilation. A combination of the two is usually used depending on the patient **(Box 1)**.

■ STRATEGIES IN MECHANICAL VENTILATION

These are used to improve oxygenation in refractory hypoxia.

The modes (i.e., controlled mode, with either volume or pressure limits) as well as the principles of lung protective ventilation remain the same. When using these, patients need to be deeply sedated and paralyzed.

Positive End-expiratory Pressure

Positive end-expiratory pressure (PEEP) is the positive alveolar pressure above atmospheric pressure that remains at the end of exhalation. The normal physiological PEEP of 0–5 cm H_2O is used in normal ventilation as seen in the immediate perioperative period. Though it is a basic setting on the mechanical ventilator, a higher extrinsic PEEP is applied therapeutically during mechanical ventilation to improve oxygenation, ventilation, and decrease the work of breathing (WOB). After the adjustment of the fraction of inspired oxygen (FiO_2), PEEP is the next setting that is usually titrated along with the tidal volume (V_T).

BOX 1 Strategies for improving oxygenation and advanced modes of mechanical ventilator.

Strategies in ventilation:
- Positive end-expiratory pressure (PEEP)
- Prone position ventilation
- Inverse ratio ventilation (IRV)

Advanced modes of ventilation:
- Controlled
  - Pressure-regulated volume control (PRVC)
- Assisted
  - Airway pressure release ventilation (APRV) or bilevel ventilation
  - Pressure support ventilation (PSV)
  - Adaptive supportive ventilation (ASV)

It acts by preventing the collapse of the distal alveoli during expiration, decreases atelectasis, improves oxygenation as well as the ventilation/perfusion mismatch. There are different methods followed to titrate the level of PEEP. Some follow the table suggested by the ARDSNet (FiO_2/PEEP chart), while others adjust it according to the lower inflection point, lung compliance, driving pressure, gas exchange, oxygen saturation (SpO_2), and hemodynamic stability; aiming for the targets of a plateau pressure (Pplat) < 30 cm H_2O, partial pressure of oxygen (PaO_2) > 55 mm Hg, SpO_2 > 88%, V_T 4–6 mL/kg, and decreasing the FiO_2. The approach depends on the individual.

- *Incremental PEEP*: Usually, a controlled mode like volume control (VC) or pressure control (PC) is chosen with the V_T at 6 mL/kg, and the PEEP set at 5 cm H_2O. The PEEP is then gradually increased by two provided the SpO_2 improves, the driving pressure remains <15, and the Pplat remains < 30 cm H_2O. Should there be a drop in SpO_2 or blood pressure, or a rise in the Pplat, the PEEP is reduced to the previous level where the target parameters are stable.
- *Decremental PEEP*: Some prefer the use of decremental PEEP, where the setting starts at a higher level of PEEP and then decreased depending on either the transpulmonary pressure or the pressure-volume curve. This method works on the principle that at the higher level of PEEP there is maximum recruitment and as the PEEP is decreased there is no further loss of recruitment of alveolar units. This method excludes the changes in compliance contributed by the chest wall thickness.

Though it has its benefits, PEEP is to be used judiciously, as it has the side effects of hemodynamic instability and barotrauma. In the event that with the application of PEEP and adjusting of the basic modes of ventilation, the goals of mechanical ventilation are not met, the next step would be to use advanced techniques.

Prone Position Ventilation

Here again, it is the position of the patient that is changed from the traditional supine or lateral to prone. The mode of ventilation remains the same, that is controlled, either VC or PC.

The prone position improves ventilation of the dorsal lung and recruitment of the dependent portions of the lung. The compliance improves and there is a reduction in the oxygen and PEEP requirement. Early proning has improved mortality in severe acute respiratory distress syndrome (ARDS).

Usually, the patient is kept prone for at least 16–18 hours daily. Again, sedation and paralysis are essential. There is a risk of displacement of lines and tubes as well as development of pressure sores. Precautions are to be taken to fix all devices securely. Some of the contraindications to prone ventilation include hemodynamic instability, trauma, or surgery involving the face, chest, or abdomen.

Inverse Ratio Ventilation

The normal respiratory pattern has the expiratory phase longer than the inspiratory. The usual inspiration:expiration (I:E) ratio is 1:2. This mode reverses this, and the ratios are set from 1:1 and higher.

The easiest way of setting this is to directly change the I:E ratio in the ongoing mode of ventilation, preferably PC. As the I:E is not physiological, patients need to be well sedated and paralyzed for this.

Some of the other modes with spontaneous breathing [e.g., airway pressure release ventilation (APRV)] indirectly have an inverse ventilation.

At the optimum PEEP, the longer inspiratory time and increased mean airway pressure improve alveolar recruitment thereby improving oxygenation without affecting the PIP. But with the shorter and incomplete expiration, there is a risk of hypercarbia, increasing auto-PEEP, hypoventilation, lung injury (initially barotrauma, but later volutrauma as well), and hemodynamic instability. This is therefore contraindicated in patients who are hemodynamically unstable, patients with chronic lung disease, and those with a tendency to retain carbon dioxide.

■ ADVANCED MODES OF MECHANICAL VENTILATION

The conventional modes have fixed parameters as per the settings without being able to adapt to the patient-lung parameter feedback. Therefore, these "open loop" modes may not always be suitable for all patients. As the patient and lung dynamics vary, there is a need for different modes and ventilation strategies.

With the advances in technology and better understanding of patient and ventilator dynamics, there are some newer adaptive modes of ventilation, where some of the conventional mode settings are regulated depending on certain patient parameters. There is also the integration of artificial intelligence to enhance this "closed loop" feedback of ventilator-patient interaction and decrease the ventilator associated lung injuries. These modes are useful in patients who are difficult to ventilate, those with refractory hypoxia, or during the weaning process. These include controlled and assisted that help in synchrony as well as weaning.

Controlled Ventilation

Pressure-regulated Volume Control

This adaptive pressure-controlled mode of ventilation is chosen in patients with a varying lung compliance where the traditional PC mode does not deliver a required minute ventilation due to changing compliance and effort. These are usually hypoxic patients, those with ARDS, who need a consistent V_T delivered.

The settings to be fixed include the V_T, respiratory rate, PEEP, FiO_2, I:E, inspiratory time, and trigger.

It is a combination of VC and PC modes. The initial breath is in VC, where the Pplat is assessed. The subsequent ones are PC with the previous Pplat as the maximum pressure. The machine assesses the pressures required to deliver the preset V_T, and thereafter it adjusts the peak inspiratory pressures accordingly. The pressure limit is initially set at 30–35 cm H_2O to prevent barotrauma. Depending upon the lung compliance and airway mechanics, the pressures change from breath to breath and the V_T is delivered at the lowest level possible within the Paw limit. As the compliance improves the V_T is delivered at a lower pressure, but if the compliance worsens then the pressure required increases and this will set off the alarm for regulation pressure.

Though there is a risk of worsening auto-PEEP, this mode works well in delivering a fixed V_T, at the lowest peak airway pressure (PIP) and with low WOB.

Assisted Ventilation

Airway Pressure Release Ventilation or Bilevel Ventilation (Fig. 1)

This is a bilevel mode of open lung ventilation used in patients with ARDS, refractory hypoxia, with collapsed alveoli or atelectasis. Depending on the ventilator used, the mode may be called by either name. It is time cycled and pressure limited.

This mode has two levels of continuous PEEP (P high and P low) that are maintained for a long (inspiratory) and short (expiratory) duration (T high and T low), respectively. Thus, it maintains an inverse ratio ventilation (IRV). The V_T generated depends on the driving pressure (which is the difference between the P high and P low) and the lung compliance. The longer P high

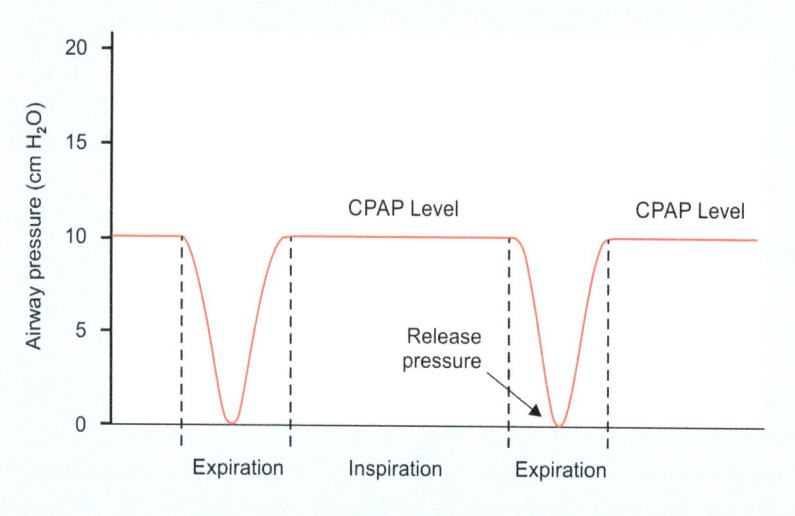

Fig. 1: Airway pressure release ventilation (APRV). (CPAP: continuous positive airway pressure)

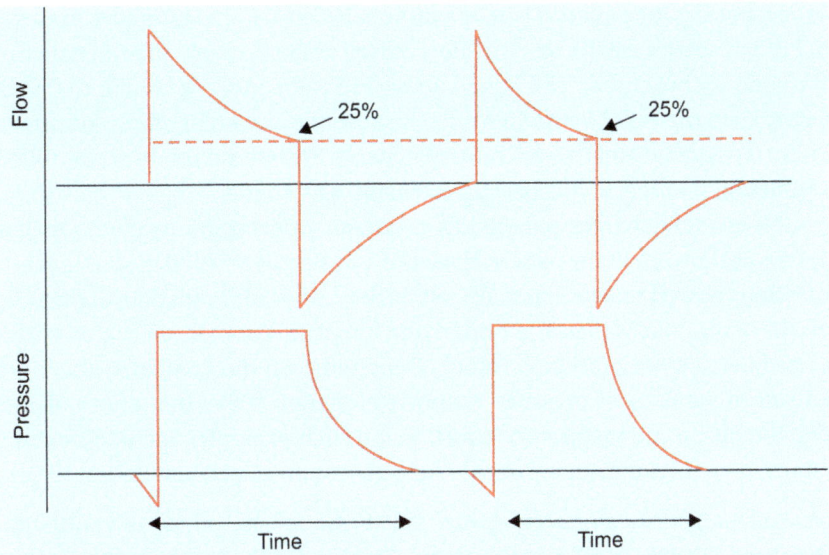

Fig. 2: Pressure and flow waveforms of pressure support ventilation (PSV).
- Pressure support remains constant as long as the inspiratory flow continues and ends when the inspiratory flow reach as 25% of the peak inspiratory flow.
- Inspiratory flow and time are dependent on the patients spontaneous breathing.

phase prevents alveolar collapse, improves lung recruitment, and ultimately oxygenation; while the P low phase is associated with lower PIP. In this mode, spontaneous breathing is possible during any phase of the cycle. Therefore, the need for sedation and paralysis is less. Hence, as opposed to PC-IRV, this is better tolerated hemodynamically.

Since the inspiratory time is prolonged, there is a tendency for dynamic hyperinflation, which in turn will increase the alveolar pressure and increase the risk of barotrauma. Hence, it is to be avoided in chronic obstructive pulmonary disease (COPD) patients.

Pressure Support Ventilation (Fig. 2)

The use of this bilevel mode in the noninvasive setting has been discussed in the chapter 30, Management of Exacerbation of COPD. Similar to that, this is a mode used in intubated patients with spontaneous breathing. The parameters to be set include the PEEP [which acts as continuous positive airway pressure (CPAP)], pressure support (PS), trigger, FiO_2, rise time, and a backup mode of invasive ventilation. The PS is the mechanical support given by the machine above the constant PEEP. The initial PS is set higher, to ease the effort of breathing. Just as in the noninvasive form, the PS is adjusted according to the effort of the patient, the V_T target as well the degree of hypercarbia, while the PEEP is set according to the degree of hypoxia. As the patient improves, the levels are decreased. The ultimate aim is to set the lowest PS and PEEP possible as accepted by the patient. Usually a minimal PS of 4–6 cm H_2O above the level of PEEP is set to ease the patient effort as well as to overcome the resistance of the endotracheal tube. If PS is zero above PEEP, the mode is similar to that of CPAP. Here the PEEP is the CPAP. In the absence of patient effort, the apnea alarm is triggered and the machine switches to the backup mode of controlled ventilation that is set. This backup is usually a PC mode.

It is essential that the patient has a spontaneous respiratory effort and it is always preferred that the patient be awake and alert. It is useful in spontaneous breathing as well as weaning trials. As with any mode of ventilation, depending on the settings as well as the underlying lung condition, there is always risk of ventilator associated lung injury. Depending on the ventilator, there are advanced versions of pressure support ventilation (PSV) that are available, dependent on the inspiratory effort. Some such examples include neurally adjusted ventilatory assist (NAVA) and proportional assist ventilation (PAV).

Neurally adjusted ventilatory assist: This is an assisted mode of ventilation that uses the electrical activity of the diaphragm as the trigger to initiate the assisted ventilation with PSV. The diaphragmatic activity is measured transoesophageally by a special catheter. This catheter is a special gastric feeding tube mounted with electrodes and placed at the level of the diaphragm crura. The pressure signals from diaphragmatic activity are detected and amplified and according to the Paw and V_T, the ventilator PS is adjusted. It promotes synchrony between the neural path of the patient's respiratory cycle and the ventilator flow, thereby reducing the sedation requirement. It senses both the inspiratory and expiratory time of the patient quicker than the usual pressure trigger of the ventilator and is supposed to be the best with regard to patient-ventilator synchrony.

Proportional assist ventilation: This mode measures the inspiratory effort and pressure trigger of the patient, and the respiratory mechanics (elastance and resistance) are calculated. The flow and volume are then adjusted on the bases of these readings, i.e., the degree of support is in proportion to the patient effort, with only safety limits set for volume and pressure. This mode encourages spontaneous ventilation, improves patient-ventilator synchrony, and decreases the WOB and the need for sedation. But there remains the risk of developing auto-PEEP.

Adaptive Supportive Ventilation

With the advances in technology, there are now automated integrated modes in the ventilators, where the ventilator parameters are adjusted according to the patient respiratory dynamics and demand to maintain the target minute ventilation. Depending on the patients drive and effort, the modes can change from VC or PC to PSV to suit the set parameters of ideal body weight, minute ventilation and PEEP. This is useful in conditions where there are fluctuations in compliance and resistance as in ARDS and asthma, respectively. But, since it cannot adjust ventilation for shunts or dead space, it is not of use in pulmonary embolism and COPD, as there is a risk of developing auto-PEEP.

■ CONCLUSION

Irrespective of the mode or strategy the basic principles of *lung protective strategy* remain the core of ventilation, be it a normal lung or a diseased one. These include low V_T (4–8 mL/kg predicted or ideal body weight) to target a plateau pressure <30 cm H_2O.

The advantage of this low volume-low pressure strategy is that it reduces ventilator-associated lung injury (volutrauma, barotrauma, and biotrauma) and the associated mortality and morbidity.

In this process there is a tendency for hypoventilation which leads to respiratory acidosis and a rise in partial pressure of carbon dioxide (PCO_2) above the normal range of 35–45 mm Hg. This was initially described by Darioli and Perret in patients with status asthmaticus. Later, Hickling et al studied it in ARDS and termed it *"permissible hypercapnia".* The higher PCO_2 is accepted, monitoring the pH (target > 7.2) and the hemodynamic condition. As the lung improves, the oxygenation as well as the hypercapnia reduces.

The adverse effects of hypercapnia include pulmonary vasoconstriction, impaired cardiac function (initially right ventricular dysfunction and cor pulmonale but eventually with worsening acidosis left ventricular dysfunction too), arrhythmias, and raised intracranial pressure. It is therefore contraindicated in patients with cerebral edema and intracranial hypertension.

The choice of mode of ventilation or the ventilation strategy is modified according to the physician's preference, each patient's physiology, and clinical condition. These modes improve patient-ventilator synchrony and help in refractory hypoxia and weaning. Some may have features of endotracheal tube resistance compensation, pressure-targeted inspiratory slope adjustment as well as closed-loop modification. With the advances in technology, the use of integrated modes and artificial intelligence further enhance this patient-ventilator feedback cycle. The name and technology differ from company to company.

■ SUGGESTED READING

1. Darioli R, Perret C. Mechanical controlled hypoventilation in status asthmaticus. Am Rev Respir Dis. 1984;129(3):385-7.
2. Guérin C, Reignier J, Richard J-C, Beuret P, Gacouin A, Boulain T, et al. Prone positioning in severe acute respiratory distress syndrome. N Engl J Med. 2013;368(23):2159-68.
3. Hasan A. Understanding Mechanical Ventilation: A Practical Handbook, 2nd edition. New York: Springer; 2010.
4. Hickling KG, Joyce C. Permissive hypercapnia in ARDS and its effect on tissue oxygenation. Acta Anaesthesiol Scand Suppl. 1995;107:201-8.
5. Tobin MJ. Principles and Practice of Mechanical Ventilation, 3rd Edition. McGraw Hill publication, 2014.

CHAPTER 20

Weaning from Mechanical Ventilator

Jamshed Sunavala

■ INTRODUCTION

Liberating the patient from mechanical ventilator factually means freeing the patient from invasive ventilation totally, by allowing the patient to breathe spontaneously and this entails a process which is termed "weaning". However after weaning, the patient may or may not require the need for an artificial airway [endotracheal tube (ET) or tracheostomy], hence the next step in successful liberation from mechanical ventilator is extubation and we shall consider both the processes—weaning and extubation, separately.

■ CAUSES OF WEANING FAILURE

To begin with, a smooth weaning process depends on the resolution of the underlying disease. It also requires adequate recovery of the respiratory muscles and patent airways to maintain normal tidal volume (V_T) and gas exchange using minimum effort during spontaneous breathing. When this fails to happen, we suspect weaning failure and in physiological terms it manifests as (1) increasing demand (work of breathing); (2) poor respiratory drive or effort, and (3) respiratory muscle fatigue.

1. *Increased work of breathing can occur either due to increased metabolic demand, increased airflow resistance, or decreased compliance.*

    Increased metabolic demand can occur if the underlying disease is still active and the patient remains hypermetabolic (sepsis), or complications such as metabolic acidosis, remain uncorrected. It is also seen, though rarely, in patients receiving parenteral nutrition with a high carbohydrate load. Carbohydrates have a higher respiratory quotient (R) than other nutritional substrates, which increase CO_2 production (VCO_2), and so require increasing minute ventilation to wash out the CO_2.

    It is always necessary to monitor for expired CO_2 [end-tidal CO_2 ($ETCO_2$)]. If it is significantly lower than the partial pressure of arterial carbon dioxide ($PaCO_2$) level, one would be right to suspect a dead space (V_D) effect as in pulmonary embolism and poor cardiac output. V_D to V_T ratio > 0.3 indicates significant dead space ventilation, which will require an increased respiratory effort to maintain adequate alveolar ventilation, consequently increasing the work of breathing.

    Increased airflow resistance most commonly occurs following kinking or blockage of the ET which needs to be immediately corrected; if necessary, the tube has to be replaced. Reappearance of bronchospasm and lower airways obstruction is common in chronic obstructive pulmonary disease (COPD) or asthmatic patients. COPD patients are notorious for weaning failure and it is wise to support them on noninvasive ventilation (NIV) and avoid intubation as far as possible. Bilateral pleural effusions or increased intra-abdominal pressure can also restrict lung expansion and cause weaning failure.

Decreased compliance can increase the work of breathing by impairing the patient's ability to maintain efficient gas exchange. The most common cause of poor compliance during weaning is unresolved acute respiratory distress syndrome (ARDS) or cardiac failure, leading to a noncardiogenic or cardiogenic pulmonary edema. The alveolar leak in both instances may be clinically subtle, to an extent that it could be easily overlooked as a cause of weaning failure. In fact, repeated failure of weaning trials in a postcardiac surgery patient should raise suspicion of early left ventricular failure (LVF) which may not be apparent clinically or on imaging. Brain natriuretic peptide (BNP) as a marker of silent left ventricular (LV) dysfunction as a preweaning predictor is discussed later in this chapter.

2. *Decreased respiratory drive*: The causes for the decreased respiratory drive are synonymous with causes for type II respiratory failure. These include the lingering effects of earlier sedative drugs or increased somnolence due to partially recovered sensorium, residual respiratory muscle weakness due to critical care neuropathy electrolyte and metabolic abnormalities, malnutrition or prolonged use of steroids. Poor respiratory effort could also result from chest wall pain following trauma. Two clinical problems, which are very difficult to overcome, are flail chest and paralysis of the diaphragm due to accidental injury to the phrenic nerve. Patients have been known to be dependent on some form of ventilator support for months, especially when the diaphragm, which is the peripheral center of the respiratory drive, is paralyzed.

3. *Respiratory muscle fatigue* usually manifests after a protracted period (few hours) *of spontaneous breathing.* Here the increased work of breathing overtime may affect the patient's ability to sustain adequate spontaneous ventilation. The work of breathing gradually escalates above the tolerated threshold value due to the increased transpulmonary pressure. This occurs due to persistently low or worsening compliance or due to an unremitting high airway resistance. Both poor compliance and increased airway resistance fall in the earlier two categories (1) and (2), but the difference here is that the patient maintains normal breathing for a short period before respiratory fatigue sets in, or the underlying physiology may not have completely resolved.

Lastly, respiratory muscle disuse due to prolonged ventilator support can lead to respiratory muscle dysfunction and diaphragmatic atrophy. This may require patience and retraining of the disused muscles by prolonging the period of spontaneous breathing trials (SBTs), at times extending over 2-5 days.

INDICATORS OF WEANING FAILURE

- Evidence of hemodynamic instability which includes sudden rise or fall in blood pressure (BP) or heart rate (HR).
- A rising $PaCO_2$ above 50 mm Hg, or fall in atrial oxygen saturation (SaO_2) below 90% during the trial.
- Decreasing force or rate of breathing as evidenced by a fall in V_T below 4 mL/kg, or a gradually rising respiratory rate (RR) above 30 breaths per minute.
- Increased dead space effect evidenced by disparity between $PaCO_2$ and $ETCO_2$, as discussed earlier.

All of the above factors should be monitored closely and detected early before respiratory distress or fatigue set in.

WEANING PROCEDURE

Weaning from mechanical ventilator is generally classified as (1) simple to wean; (2) difficult to wean; and (3) prolonged weaning. Majority of intensive care unit (ICU) patients are simple to wean—these include uncomplicated postoperative patients or those with ailments that require mechanical ventilator for a short period of a day or two, as the deranged physiology has responded promptly to treatment. These are a group of patients who are weaned and extubated at the first attempt and have a low mortality. An astute physician or an intensivist should be able to sense this and initiate weaning at the earliest opportune time, as needless delay invites trouble in form of ventilator-associated complications.

A smaller group of patients fall in either *"difficult to wean"*, who require up to three attempts or 7 days from the onset of weaning, or *"prolonged weaning"* who require >7 days. "Difficult to wean" patients usually have an underlying reversible problem, but once this is corrected, they can be weaned within a short time. Patients on prolonged ventilation comprise those who have a more serious inherent lung damage from a chronic disease such as advanced COPD, neurological disorder, or cachexia causing muscle wasting. These patients have a higher morbidity and mortality and may be a challenge to liberate them from the mechanical ventilator. To discuss the weaning process in both these groups of patients, I would like to elaborate on the *four stages of weaning* (**Box 1**).

Stage I: Unresolved Lung Pathology

No attempt at weaning should be contemplated at this stage as the patient's ventilation and oxygenation are totally supported by the mechanical ventilator and also because the underlying disease and lung pathology remain unresolved.

> **BOX 1** Four stages of weaning.
> 1. *Unresolved stage:* At this stage any attempt to wean is undesirable as the underlying pathology and physiology is not adequately resolved
> 2. *Resolving stage:* This is a stage where early signs of resolving pathology or physiology may prompt weaning-clinical judgment, followed by screening tests
> 3. *Screening tests:* This stage consist of pretest probability and preweaning tests
> 4. Weaning trials

Stage II: Resolving Pathology

During this phase the physician contemplates the possibility that the patient may be able to breathe spontaneously and maintain a reasonable gas exchange. This is purely judgmental, hinging on the physician's clinical expertise and experience and no guidelines or protocol can help to make this call—there are no explicit rules, only an unexplained reasoning from experience can perceive the probability of the outcome and any hesitation at this point can unnecessarily delay the weaning process. Of course, this needs to be followed by screening tests which serve as predictors of successful weaning.

Stage III: Screening Tests

Unfortunately, we still do not have a predictive test to guarantee a cent percent weaning success without need for reintubation. More importantly, before attempting a weaning test, a *pretest probability* of weaning outcome should be screened and this would entail a proper clinical assessment of the patient's vitals, underlying disease, and cardiopulmonary status including parameters of gas exchange **(Table 1)**. *Preweaning tests* are useful to ensure safe and rapid liberation from ventilator with the least risk of reintubation. However as mentioned earlier, these tests are not perfect and have their own limitations. Minute ventilation (V_E) and maximum inspiratory pressure (MIP) as a measure of muscle strength have not shown acceptable positive or negative predictive values. However, rapid shallow breathing index (RSBI) measuring RR to tidal volume (f/V_T) over 1 minute of spontaneous breathing, has demonstrated a sensitivity of over 90% and a moderate specificity of 60-70% in predicting a successful weaning. It has proved to be superior in comparison to other tests and is regularly used in many ICUs and the cutoff point of 105 or rounded to 100, above which the possibility of unsuccessful weaning is high. However, I am more comfortable with values below 90, provided it correlates well with the pretest probability described earlier **(Table 1)**. The method of measuring (f/V_T) index is given in **Box 2**. To obtain a more accurate prediction and reproducibility from this test, it is vital that a steady state of spontaneous breathing can be achieved by waiting for at least a minute before measuring (f/V_T), because the first 30 seconds may be unrepresentative of an accurate reproducible value. I would again emphasize that the clinician's estimate of the likelihood of weaning (pretest probability), determines the reliability of any weaning predictor test.

TABLE 1	Pretest probability (physicians' estimate of weaning outcome). Used also as checklist after a failed SBT trial.
A	*Awake and aware:* Patient should be conscious enough to be awake and aware to follow commands
B	*Breathing:* RSBI (f/V_T) <100, normal pattern of breathing (without the use of accessory muscles of breathing)
C	Cardiac stability
D	*Drugs:* No recent sedatives or long-term steroids *Disease:* Resolution of underlying disease
E	*Electrolyte balance:* Na^+/K^+/Ca^+ (should be within normal limits)
F	*Fluid imbalance:* No significant volume overload or hypovolemia
G	*Gases:* PaO_2/FiO_2 ratio >150 mm Hg; $PaCO_2$< 50 mm Hg with normal pH Metabolic acidosis or severe alkalosis (should be corrected)
H	*Hb:* Rule out recent blood loss and anemia
I	*Infection:* Rule out sepsis or low grade fever with smouldering infection

(FiO_2: fraction of inspired oxygen; Hb: hemoglobin; $PaCO_2$: partial pressure of arterial carbon dioxide; PaO_2: partial pressure of arterial oxygen; RSBI: rapid shallow breathing index; SBT: spontaneous breathing trial)

BOX 2 Procedure for measuring rapid shallow breathing index (RSBI).

1. Disconnect the ventilator circuit from the endotracheal tube (ET)
2. Wait for a minute or till the patient has established a regular breathing pattern
3. Measure the minute expired volume (V_E) and the respiratory frequency (f) in 1 minute, using the Wright spirometer
4. Divide "V_E" by "f" to obtain the average V_T in (L)
5. Divide "f" by "V_T" (f/V_T index) = RSBI in breath/min/L (<100 acceptable)
6. *Example:* f = 30/minutes; average V_T = 250 mL or 0.25 L; f/V_T = 30/0.25 = 120 = unfit for weaning

Stage IV: Weaning Trials

In stable patients, including routine postoperative cases, requiring ventilator support for a short period, a one-step approach to immediate extubation may be justified based on routine variables such as vitals, chest auscultation, and peripheral oxygen saturation (SpO_2) levels. However, all other patients with significant lung pathology such as ARDS, sepsis, shock, following prolonged major surgery and prolonged periods of ventilator (>48 hours), and also in patients whose pretest probability to wean is suspect, will require a two-step weaning trial. This would include a *preweaning trial* followed by an attempt at weaning. RSBI (f/V_T) as a preweaning test has been repeatedly shown to have a very high sensitivity but a low specificity, hence it should be followed by a more specific test (one of the weaning trials which is assumed to be more specific).

The usual weaning trials described, include T-tube trials, intermittent mandatory ventilation (IMV), and pressure support ventilation (PSV). SBT was always considered synonymous with T-tube trial and used interchangeably. Later the term SBT was extended to patients breathing spontaneously without

> **BOX 3** Spontaneous breathing trial (SBT) procedure.
> 1. Disconnect the circuit from the ventilator
> 2. Use T-tube and let the patient breathe spontaneously on 6L of oxygen
> 3. Assess the patient continuously for vitals, arrhythmias and signs of respiratory distress, hypoventilation, and O_2 desaturation [peripheral oxygen saturation (SpO_2)]
> 4. If the patient tolerates step 3 for 30 minutes, consider extubation. At times a longer observation period of 3 hours or more may be warranted in patients with previously failed SBT; frequent SBT trials may be tried in a day

disconnecting the ventilator. Here, both positive pressure and inspiratory assistance are bypassed using the *"flow-by"* facility incorporated in the newer generation of ventilators. The term SBT has been erroneously used to include PSV, which is in no way an unassisted ventilation as its name suggests, whereas SBT is entirely an unassisted weaning technique.

T-tube trials and SBT **(Box 3)** are probably the most commonly used techniques for weaning and at times they become necessary even after a PSV trial. After disconnection, the patient is allowed to breathe spontaneously with 6 L of oxygen through the ET or tracheostomy tube (TT). One continues the trial under close monitoring of the vitals, and if the patient does not develop distress during a 30-minute trial, he may be safely extubated. However some intensivists continue the trial up to 2 hours provided the patient can tolerate the ET that long, surprisingly many patients do. If the patient fails the trial, one would consider a new trial after 24 hours as the respiratory muscles take 24 hours to recover from stress; meanwhile it is best to reinstitute full assistance through volume control ventilation (VCV) in order to rest the muscles.

In patients on prolonged ventilatory support following a slow resolving lung pathology or an unexplained derangement of physiology, weaning attempts may repeatedly fail after a few hours of ventilator support. These are patients who are otherwise very stable on minimum ventilator support maintaining normal gas exchange and hemodynamics, but cannot maintain the same stability when breathing on their own. In this group of patients, we have been successful by patiently weaning them over a few days. Here we alternate their periods on ventilator with spontaneous breaths, done gradually with overnight rest for 8 hours on VCV. Trials are conducted from 6 AM to 10 PM in 4 hourly slots, and as most of these patients are known to tolerate spontaneous breathing for over 1 hour, we begin with the first 4 hourly slot with an hour of SBT followed by 3 hours of VCV, and slowly lengthen the SBT by half an hour in each slot of 4 hours; this may need to continue over 2–3 days. We have found good results towards successful weaning using this method. It is however important that the support should be on VCV in order to rest the respiratory muscles intermittently.

Intermittent mandatory ventilation provides ventilated breaths at a preset volume and rate, with the patient breathing spontaneously between the mandatory breaths. During weaning the mandatory breathes are reduced in steps until three to four mandatory positive pressure breaths/minute can achieve acceptable blood gas values. It was a popular mode of weaning once, but now it is not regularly used for weaning as it may actually contribute to respiratory muscle fatigue from excessive work of breathing. Theoretically, it was believed that the respiratory muscles would rest during the mandatory breaths, but studies have revealed otherwise, in that, both assisted and unassisted breaths equally increased the work of breathing.

Pressure support ventilation with gradual decrements of pressure till the patient can breathe comfortably at minimum pressure of 5–10 cmH$_2$O is considered acceptable for weaning. Though PSV is now used commonly as a weaning trial, it is often observed that patients titrated to low levels are comfortable as long as they are on PSV but develop distress when unassisted during spontaneous breathing. This is because it is difficult to judge the minimal pressure at which work of breathing is acceptable for successful weaning. In practice, the intensivist arbitrarily accepts 5–10 cmH$_2$O on PSV as being good enough to disconnect the ventilator because they attribute the low pressure of PSV as compensation for the workload imposed by the ET hence this may be ignored, though this is not entirely valid. However, in the event the patient continues to have mild respiratory distress one can step down to NIV, as otherwise a stable and conscious patients may not tolerate ET for long.

Pro-BNP or its inactive fragment NT-pro BNP is used as a preweaning predictor in patients with suspected cardiac dysfunction, especially in patients who fail SBT. Particularly, patients with moderate-to-severe diastolic dysfunction with high BNP levels are "difficult to wean" candidates. A significant change in BNP levels between the beginning and end of weaning attempts has been used to evaluate the cardiac causes of weaning failure. Most studies found change in BNP to be superior to change in NT-pro BNP in predicting cardiac failure, probably because of the superior and more specific performance of BNP with its shorter circulating half-life.

In conclusion majority of patients can be weaned on T-tube or PSV; however, the most difficult patients to wean are those requiring prolonged ventilation, or critically ill COPD patients who eventually require tracheostomy. Most of these patients continue on PSV and many of them eventually require protracted breathing trials, perhaps stretching over 1–4 days as described earlier. If they still continue to have some degree of respiratory distress, NIV support may be necessary after removal of ET or closure of tracheostomy.

■ EXTUBATION

Ordinarily extubation becomes a part of one-step weaning. However, there is always an uncertainty of maintaining a patent airway after extubation in a subgroup of patients, especially in those who have been on ventilator support for long periods. I have intentionally avoided merging weaning with extubation as one subject, as there cannot be a bigger mistake than relying on preweaning predictors for successful extubation. It would be wrong to assume that patients

> **BOX 4** Prerequisites before extubation.
>
> *Sensorium:* Patient conscious enough to make coughing effort on demand
> *Secretions:* Absence of copious, thick secretions which can block the upper airways
> *Strength:* Adequate strength of respiratory muscles to produce effective cough for expectoration (testing of FVC > 10 mL/kg)
> *Stamina:* Maintain spontaneous breathing without fatigue; RSBI to be <100
>
> (FVC: forced vital capacity; RSBI: rapid shallow breathing index)

after a successful weaning trial will be able to maintain a patent airway and normal breathing. I have coined four easy to remember prerequisites to be checked before extubation **(Box 4)**. The two most important prerequisites are secretions and strength, as many patients postweaning still have copious secretions and they require adequate strength to expectorate, which was not anticipated earlier. Despite good respiratory effort, patients very often may be slightly drowsy or lapse into a drowsy state, causing thick secretions to pool in the upper airways; hence it is important to ascertain the patient's sensorium. One subset of problematic patients are those with neuromuscular weakness, who have otherwise adequate respiratory strength to maintain normal breathing and gas exchange, but their respiratory muscles are not strong enough to produce an effective effort to expectorate. These are the most deceptive group of patients who could abruptly choke on their secretions and may require emergency intubation.

The last prerequisite for extubation is stamina—a patient may have good forced vital capacity (FVC) but may not be able to sustain spontaneous breathing for long. This of course, should be anticipated during the preweaning tests and weaning trials. More importantly, it requires an experienced and astute clinician to foresee such an event but despite satisfying all above criteria a few patients may require reintubation within 24 hours or at times even after few days as they experience respiratory distress. However, in most patients reintubation can be avoided and they can be tided over by using NIV after extubation, or as and when they are in distress. It is important to rule out any of the local causes in the upper airways which may be responsible for the distress. Edema of the subglottic areas or the vocal cords, laryngospasm, tracheomalacia, mechanical trauma to the larynx, and mucosal ulcerations from prolonged intubation are some of the causes. Laryngeal edema is often manifested by stridor, but is usually self-limiting and resolves within a week and may not require reintubation.

Cuff leak test gives an estimated idea regarding upper airways injury or obstruction, as direct visualization in the presence of ET is not possible. The test works on the premise that the amount of air leaking from around the ET after the balloon cuff is deflated is inversely proportional to laryngeal edema causing obstruction. The leak is calculated indirectly by measuring the loss of V_T during expiration with a deflated cuff. As per most studies, if the difference in expiratory volume is >110 mL or >12% of V_T, it is assumed that adequate air is leaking from around the tube and the cuff leak test is considered negative. However, if the difference in expired V_T is <110 mL or <12% of V_T, the cuff leak test is considered positive suggesting laryngeal edema. The test is performed on VCV using V_T of 10 mL/kg. The test by itself is not very sensitive or specific in predicting the possibility of reintubation. However, the predictability of reintubation increases when done in patients who have a higher pretest probability of reintubation, and hence the test should be ideally restricted to high-risk patients.

One study has suggested doing the test by measuring the V_T, a few seconds after the peak inspiratory pause to eliminate the inspiratory flow leak. At high flow and volume, especially in patients with lower airways obstruction, the inspiratory flow leak will give a wrong interpretation of the cuff leak test. Finally, for high-risk patients with a cuff leak test suggesting laryngeal edema, one should give a trial of steroids and extubate after 48 hours.

■ SUMMARY

All possible causes that lead to increased work of breathing, poor respiratory drive, or increased respiratory muscle fatigue can result in weaning failure. Often the earliest indicator of weaning failure could be a gradual worsening of hemodynamic parameters or gas exchange values, even before clinical signs of respiratory distress become apparent. Patients who can be weaned earlier and at the first attempt, have a lower mortality than those who require multiple weaning trials and the most difficult patients to wean are those requiring prolonged ventilator support and those with an acute exacerbation of COPD. Pretest probability of weaning should be properly assessed before considering a weaning trial.

The diagnostic accuracy of weaning trials will not necessarily predict postextubation outcome, and here too, an astute clinical evaluation is the best pretest probability. The four checks mentioned in **Box 4** are mandatory before contemplating extubation. Severe respiratory distress after extubation, which is serious enough to require reintubation, is associated with a high mortality. One should bear in mind that difficult extubation can become a demanding exercise and perhaps even more problematic than "difficult weaning"; hence it should be dealt as a separate discipline from weaning.

■ SUGGESTED READING

1. Boles JM, Bion J, Connors A, Herridge M, Marsh B, Melot C, et al. Weaning from mechanical ventilation. Eur Respir J. 2007;29(5):1033-56.
2. Munshi L, Ferguson ND. Weaning From Mechanical Ventilation: What Should Be Done When a Patient's Spontaneous Breathing Trial Fails? JAMA. 2018;320(18):1865-67.
3. Thille AW, Cortés-Puch I, Esteban A. Weaning from the ventilator and extubation in ICU. Curr Opin Crit Care. 2013;19(1):57-64.
4. Tobin MJ. Weaning from mechanical ventilation. In: Parrillo JE, Dellinger PR (Eds). Critical Care Medicine—Principles of Diagnosis and Management in Adults, 5th edition. Amsterdam, Netherlands: Elsevier; 2019.

CHAPTER 21

Extracorporeal Membrane Oxygenator

Jamshed Sunavala

■ INTRODUCTION

Extracorporeal membrane oxygenator (ECMO) was first introduced by Hill and Bartlett in 1970, as a device to support patients having severe respiratory failure with refractory hypoxia, which cannot be corrected by mechanical ventilation. The first ever attempt at using ECMO in India was in a patient with refractory hypoxia at the Breach Candy Hospital in 1979. Here a prototype of an ECMO device was applied on young jockey who fell and was trampled under the hoof of a running horse during a racing event. He had bilateral injury to his lungs resulting in a serious lung contusion with intrapulmonary bleeding and bilateral pneumothoraces.

■ PRINCIPLE

The basic principle of ECMO is to drain deoxygenated blood and return oxygenated blood (after removal of CO_2), back into the circulation. This is enabled by using an external circuit through which the blood is pumped back into the bloodstream with the help of a rotadynamic centrifugal pump. The whole system is composed of inflow and outflow cannulas, connecting tubings, a rotary pump generating forward flow, an oxygenator, and a heat generator.

■ CONFIGURATION

Depending on the clinical scenario, either a venovenous ECMO (VV-ECMO) **(Fig. 1)** or a venoarterial ECMO (VA-ECMO) **(Fig. 2)** configuration can be applied. Various other configurations are possible as per the demands made by many diverse and complex clinical exigencies. In VV-ECMO, the deoxygenated venous blood is returned as oxygenated blood back into the venous circulation, whereas in VA-ECMO, the venous blood is pumped via the motor placed in the external circuit into the arterial system, to augment the mean arterial pressure (MAP) and cardiac output (CO). **Figures 1 and 2** show the placements of both inflow and outflow cannulas in both types of configurations.

■ INDICATIONS

- *Respiratory support*: VV-ECMO setup is primarily used for respiratory failure with refractory hypoxemia which cannot be corrected by mechanical ventilation [e.g., in severe acute respiratory distress syndrome (ARDS)] but without any cardiac decompensation.

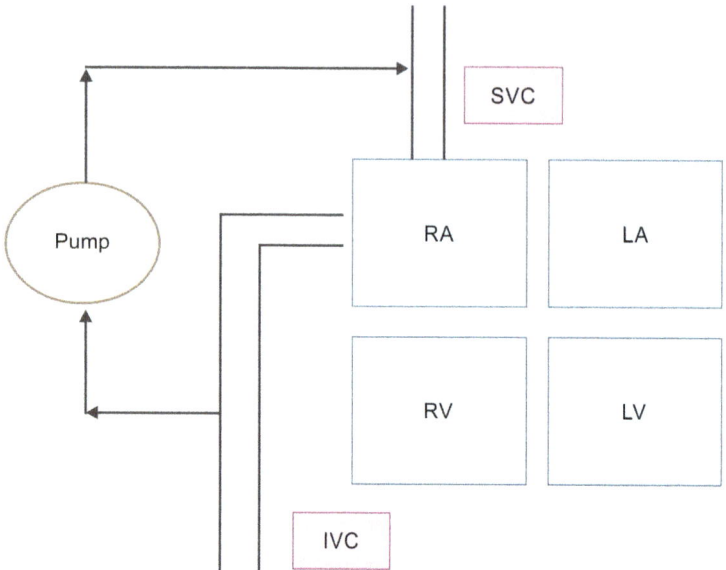

Fig. 1: VV-ECMO configuration. (IVC: inferior vena cava; LA: left atrium; LV: left ventricle; RA: right atrium; RV: right ventricle; SVC: superior vena cava; VV-ECMO: venovenous extracorporeal membrane oxygenator)

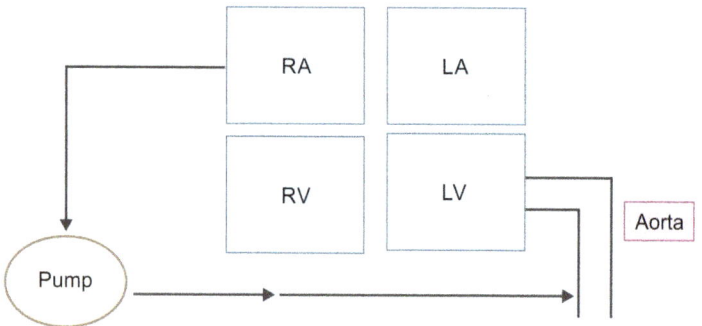

Fig. 2: VA-ECMO configuration. (LA: left atrium; LV: left ventricle; RA: right atrium; RV: right ventricle; VA-ECMO: venoarterial extracorporeal membrane oxygenator)

- *Severe cardiogenic shock*: The main indication of VA-ECMO is to support patients with severe cardiogenic shock and marked oxygen desaturation. Here the venous blood is withdrawn from right atrium/inferior vena cava/superior vena cava (RA/IVC/SVC) and drained into the arterial circulation (femoral or subclavian artery), thus increasing the systemic blood pressure (BP) and oxygenation.
- *Severe cardiogenic shock requiring added support*: Here, in addition to VA-ECMO, a left ventricle (LV) venting strategy is used. This is done by combining VA-ECMO with a ventricular assist device such as Impella, and is termed as ECPELLA. This device will help to further augment MAP and

CO and in addition to increasing coronary flow, it also improves myocardial perfusion gradient (MPG). It may also reduce pulmonary capillary wedge pressure (PCWP) and pulmonary vascular resistance (PVR).
- *Pulmonary embolism (PE)*: Patients with refractory hypoxemia due to severe PE without cardiovascular collapse would benefit with VV-ECMO. In massive PE with severe right-sided heart failure refractory to inotropes, an inflow from RA to pulmonary artery (PA) or left atrium (LA) via the ECMO circuit, would be helpful for RV support. Severe PE with cardiogenic shock can benefit through VA-ECMO configuration with LV venting such as an ECPELLA device.
- *Biventricular failure*: In severe biventricular heart failure using dual inflow from RA and LA, the latter through atrial septal puncture with an outflow in the arterial circulation, would help to reduce both LV and RV preload and simultaneously maintain CO and MAP.
- *Severe cardiopulmonary failure*: Here one needs to augment CO and simultaneously relieve right-sided failure and venous congestion. This can be achieved by placing two venous inflow cannulas (spliced together), making it a configuration of veno-veno-arterial ECMO (VVA-ECMO) which would enhance venous drainage into the centrifugation pump, leading to a greater reduction of pulmonary blood flow.
- *Refractory ventricular arrhythmias*: Life-threatening refractory ventricular arrhythmias in patients with heart failure following myocarditis have been shown to benefit using VA-ECMO.

It is to be noted that all of the above indications are temporary, either as bridging to interventions or anticipated recovery. Ideally, use of the device should not exceed 4–6 days at the most, because of serious adverse events with little benefit.

ADVERSE EVENTS

- *Catheter related*: Local complications such as vascular injury, limb ischemia, infection from insertion sites, bleeding, deep vein thrombosis (DVT), and air embolism are all dreadful events but could be avoided by close monitoring and use of prophylactic strategies such as anticoagulation to prevent DVT and limb ischemia. Strict asepsis should be maintained using proper cannulation techniques and limiting the duration of ECMO.
- *ECMO configuration related:* Use of VA-ECMO may help in reducing the RV filling pressure from an increased venous reservoir, but can unduly pressurize the arterial circulation and rapidly increase the BP and the afterload. This may not cause any adverse hemodynamic effect as long as the LV function is somewhat preserved; however, if LV function is seriously compromised, a sudden LV back pressure could lead to gross pulmonary edema and rarely pulmonary hemorrhage. Hence, the use of VA-ECMO in patients with LV decompensation should be hemodynamically monitored

with the help of pulmonary artery catheter (PAC). If pulmonary capillary wedge (PCW) is elevated sharply, one may employ an LV venting facility in addition to VA-ECMO.
- *North–South syndrome*: In patients with severe hypoxemia as in ARDS on VA-ECMO, oxygenated blood via the femoral artery may compete with the deoxygenated blood in the arch of aorta. The great vessels from the aortic arch will distribute less oxygen to the brain and upper extremities leading to a discordance of oxygenation between the upper and lower parts of the body and this is termed as the North–South syndrome.

RELATIVE CONTRAINDICATIONS TO EXTRACORPOREAL MEMBRANE OXYGENATOR IN GENERAL

- End stage lung disease or potentially irreversible lung pathology;
- Limited vascular access;
- Inability to accept blood products;
- Severe coagulopathy;
- Additional organ dysfunction that would limit the benefit of ECMO, e.g., severe brain injury and untreatable cancer;
- Age >65 years (clinical judgment required, based on overall health of the patient and anticipated outcome).

RELATIVE CONTRAINDICATIONS TO VENOARTERIAL EXTRACORPOREAL MEMBRANE OXYGENATOR

- Severe anoxic brain damage;
- Irreversible cardiac failure and if transplant is not considered;
- Severe aortic insufficiency;
- Aortic dissection.

SUGGESTED READING

1. Mosier JM, Kelsey M, Raz Y, Gunnerson KJ, Meyer R, Hypes CD, et al. Extracorporeal membrane oxygenation (ECMO) for critically ill adults in the emergency department: history, current applications, and future directions. Crit Care. 2015;19:431.
2. Napp LC, Kühn C, Hoeper MM, Vogel-Claussen J, Haverich A, Schäfer A, et al. Cannulation strategies for percutaneous extracorporeal membrane oxygenation in adults. Clin Res Cardiol. 2016;105:283-96.
3. Udwadia FE, Dastur KN, Sunavala JD, Gudibanda CK, Udwadia TE, Mehta RR, et al. Use of extracorporeal membrane oxygenation (membrane lung) in acute respiratory failure. Indian J Chest Dis Allied Sci. 1980;22:59-68.

CHAPTER 22

Mechanical Circulatory Supports

Jamshed Sunavala

■ INTRODUCTION

Mechanical circulatory supports (MCS) devices vary from simple to more complex devices and are used for temporary support. The two commonly used devices in our settings are intra-aortic balloon pump (IABP) which works on the principle of counter pulsation and Impella device based on the mechanism of axial flow.

■ INTRA-AORTIC BALLOON PUMP

Intra-aortic balloon pump is the only accepted method of mechanical circulatory assistance available at present. It is now being increasingly used for sustaining patients with potentially reversible cardiac problems affecting the pumping function of the left ventricle (LV), when pharmacological therapy has failed to restore adequate coronary artery and systemic perfusion. The goal of balloon assistance is to provide temporary support to the LV when corrective surgery is planned in the near future or spontaneous ventricular recovery is anticipated.

Intra-aortic balloon pump works on the principle that a balloon catheter inserted in the thoracic aorta inflates during diastole and deflates during systole. The inflation improves diastolic-dependent coronary perfusion and myocardial oxygen consumption, whereas the sudden deflation occurring in systole decreases the aortic end-diastolic pressure and lessens the workload on the LV, thereby decreasing the myocardial oxygen demand **(Fig.1)**. *Common indications for the use of IABP are:*

- Immediate postoperative support for unstable cardiac surgery patients.
- Inpatients with unstable angina or impending infarction who are refractory to medical therapy and are awaiting bypass surgery.
- In acute myocardial infarction (AMI) with cardiogenic shock.
- In patients with mechanical complications of AMI which warrant surgical intervention, e.g., acute ventricular septal rupture and papillary muscle dysfunction or rupture.
- In unstable patients with high risk for percutaneous transluminal coronary angioplasty (PTCA).
- In hemodynamically unstable patients who are awaiting surgery after a failed angioplasty.

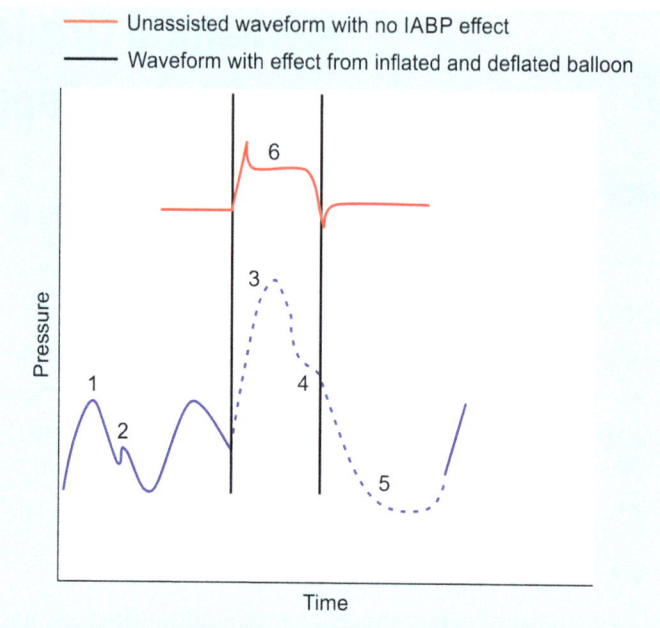

Fig. 1: Aortic pressure waveform during IABP

Key:
1. Unassisted systole
2. Diaortic notch
3. Diastolic augmentation on inflated balloon, responsible for increased coronary perfusion
4. Aortic pressure plateaus due to expansion of aortic wall
5. Aortic EDP with sudden deflation of balloon, responsible for decreased SVR and improved CO
6. Inflated balloon effect as seen on the screen of IABP machine

- *Absolute contraindications* for the use of IABP are dissecting aortic aneurysms, aortic regurgitation (AR), irreversible brain damage, and end-stage heart disease.

■ EQUIPMENT AND PROCEDURE

The two basic equipments required for this procedure are: (1) a drive unit and (2) intra-aortic balloon catheters. The operation of a drive unit is based on recognition of the variability of the interval between the electrical and mechanical events of the cardiac cycle. Hence, the precise timing of both inflation and deflation in relation to the events of the cardiac cycle becomes the most important function of the drive unit. The large-bore catheter has a 30 cm long polyurethane balloon wrapped tightly around its intra-aortic end, and has two concentric lumens running through its length. The central lumen leads to the catheter tip allowing a J-tip safety guidewire, which helps to introduce the balloon. This central lumen also allows recording of critical arterial pressure in the proximity of the balloon tip, thus eliminating the need of a separate arterial pressure line to obtain waveforms required for balloon pump timing. Concentric to the central lumen is the helium channel, through which the balloon is inflated with helium to a capacity of 30–40 mL.

Before selecting the groin through which the balloon catheter is to be inserted, all the pulses in both lower extremities are compared and graded, and the leg with the greater pulse velocity is selected. A Swan-Ganz thermodilution catheter and an intra-arterial line to record arterial waveforms should also be inserted. However, separate arterial lines may not be necessary in most catheters, as it allows intra-aortic waveform recording through their central lumen. The entire balloon device is inserted into the femoral artery at the groin, either percutaneously, or by performing an arteriotomy. The balloon is then advanced up the aorta until the tip lies 1 cm below the origin of the left subclavian artery. Fluoroscopic guidance should be used whenever available, as it assures more precise placement. The display graphs on the monitor show both the augmented blood pressure (BP) and the intrinsic BP.

COMPLICATIONS

The most commonly encountered complications in order of frequency are vascular (limb ischemia), infections, failure to place the balloon catheter, and bleeding.

WEANING

The balloon assistance should be withdrawn gradually by either decreasing the frequency of balloon inflations per cardiac cycle or by stepwise reduction in the volume of the balloon. Weaning can usually be completed within 60 minutes provided the patient remains hemodynamically stable. If the patient's condition deteriorates, full volume IABP is resumed and weaning may be reattempted after 6–24 hours.

IMPELLA DEVICE

Impella devices are peripherally inserted heart pumps used as a temporary ventricular assist device (VAD) in patients with severe ventricular failure and cardiogenic shock and also as a prophylactic support during a high-risk percutaneous coronary intervention (PCI). It differs from IABP in that it is less bulky, more compact, and does not require to be timed to the cardiac cycle. Further, its main benefit is ventricular unloading, meaning the active removal of blood from the LV cavity, thereby achieving reduction in left ventricular end-diastolic volume (LVEDV) and left ventricular end-diastolic pressure (LVEDP) resulting in an augmented peak coronary blood flow.

The family of Impella devices includes Impella 2.5, CP, 5, RP, and LD. Impella 2.5 and 5 devices provide a blood flow of 2.5 L/min and 5 L/min, respectively. CP stands for "cardiac power" and provides a blood flow of 3.5 L/min, but in all other respects its functions are the same as a 2.5, with similar configuration of the cannula and its connection to the Impella catheter and the connecting cable. These are all left-sided devices used for cardiogenic shock with LV dysfunction and are introduced retrogradely across the aortic valve into the LV cavity. In contrast, the "RP" device is used for right ventricular shock and is introduced antegradely via the femoral vein across the tricuspid and pulmonary valves, with the "inlet" placed in the RA and the "outlet" in the main pulmonary artery. However, the most commonly used types in the intensive care unit (ICU) are the 2.5 and CP devices for cardiogenic shock due to LV dysfunction and hence, the rest of the discussion will be mainly pertaining to these two devices. It is important to note that before operating either the left- or right-sided device, one should ensure that the contralateral ventricular functions are preserved (explained later).

Principle and How it Works

Impella 2.5 or CP is used to bridge patients of cardiogenic shock to recovery or high-risk PCI. These are less bulky, compact, and fully implantable continuous flow (CF) pumps that generate a minimally pulsatile blood flow through an indwelling motor in the cannula. Hence, the blood from the LV is pulled via the inlets in the distal end of the cannula, by the rotary dynamic microaxial flow pumps situated within the cannula compartment, and empties in the aorta via the outlet. Physiologically, this device now increases the systemic blood flow because of the additional emptying of the otherwise poorly pumping LV through the cannula inlets, thereby increasing the cardiac output (CO) and also optimizing the mean artery pressure (MAP). In the process of ventricular unloading, it simultaneously reduces LVEDV and LVEDP, which in turn decreases the wall tension and microvascular resistance, thereby not only increasing the coronary flow, but also improving the myocardial perfusion gradient. Hence, it achieves an overall benefit of increasing the CO, optimizing the MAP, and augmenting myocardial perfusion **(Flowchart 1)**.

Indications

- *High-risk PCI*: The Impella 2.5 or CP can be used to prevent hemodynamic instability. This instability occurs during the transient period of total occlusion following balloon inflation causing reversible ischemia, which can result in procedure-induced adverse events. This is more common with high-risk PTCA in patients with complex coronary artery disease and can also occur in high-risk patients undergoing ablation therapy.
- *Cardiogenic shock*: Ongoing cardiogenic shock occurring within 48 hours of acute myocardial infarction or open heart surgery. Impella device 2.5 and CP are intended for short-term use (48 hours).
- *Bridging*: Patients with AMI and cardiogenic shock awaiting PCI or surgery.

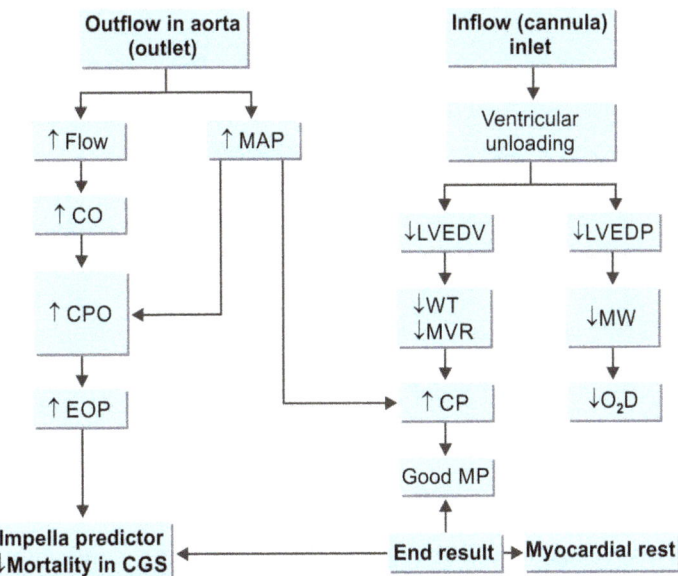

Flowchart 1: Physiological effect of Impella device.

CPO is measured as an index (cardiac index × MAP/451).
Normal CPO is 0.5–0.7 W/m². It is the best index of mortality in a patient with CGS.
(CGS: cardiogenic shock; CP: coronary perfusion; CPO: cardiac power output; EOP: end-organ perfusion; MAP: mean arterial pressure; MP: myocardial perfusion; MPG: myocardial perfusion gradient; MVR: microvascular resistance; MW: myocardial work; O_2D: oxygen demand; WT: wall tension)

Contraindications (For Impella 2.5 and CP)

- Severe RV failure
- Combined cardiorespiratory failure with significantly low partial pressure of oxygen (PaO_2) (may require EC-PELLA)
- Moderate-to-severe AR
- Mechanical aortic valve or severe aortic stenosis AS (<0.6 cm)
- Aortic dissection
- Atrial septal defect/ventricular septal defect (ASD/VSD)
- LV thrombus
- Uncontrolled sepsis
- Severe peripheral vascular disease.

Procedure

Device Components (For 2.5 and CP) (Fig. 2)

- *Cannula (12 Fr for 2.5 and 14 Fr for CP)*: It has a spiral-shaped body which is angled and made of nitinol and covered in polyurethane.
- *Inlet area*: It is located at the distal end of the cannula and has four openings that allow blood to be sucked in, channeled through the cannula, and exit from outlet area at the proximal end of the cannula.

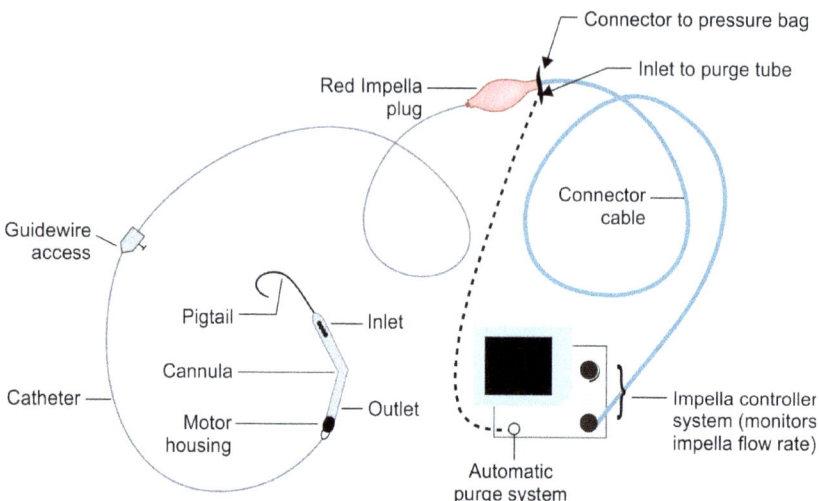

Fig. 2: Impella device.

- *Motor housing*: It is encapsulated at the proximal end of the cannula.
- *Pigtail (6 Fr)*: It is attached to the cannula at the distal end and it helps in stabilizing the catheter in the correct position directed towards the LV apex.
- *Catheter shaft (9 FR)*: It is located between the motor housing and the red Impella plug. It has longitudinal and horizontal markings for correct positioning. Through the lumen of the shaft run two other fine lumens for purge and pressure measurements; in addition, a nitinol wire and an electrical cable also run through the main lumen.
- *Red Impella plug*: It connects the proximal lead of the catheter shaft to a connector cable from the main controller unit.
- *Two side arms:* One red and one clear, branch from the Impella catheter shaft. The red arm is connected to the pressure bag and the white clear arm to the purge cassette tubing. *Check valve* ensures that the purge fluid does not flow in reverse direction.
- *The Impella controller system*: It monitors the Impella flow rate, motor current in milliampere (mA), purge flow, and gives a signal to ensure proper system placement in the LV.

Catheter and Cannula Placement (Fig. 2)

Impella 2.5 and CP devices are implanted by percutaneous technique via the femoral artery and at times via the axillary artery. Proper placement of the system is best confirmed by a transthoracic echo where the pigtail should be directed towards the LV apex, but should stay clear of the mitral valve and papillary muscles and the end of the visualized catheter should be 3.5 cm past the aortic valve. The pigtail should be able to stabilize the catheter in the correct position.

The connection of the cannula to the catheter and the connector cable with proper placement of the outlet near the aortic root should all be done stepwise as per the instructions in the *Abiomed* Impella procedural and operating manual.

Impella Controller

After the placement of the lines, the Impella device should be placed in auto mode where the flow is maximized by an integral algorithm. However, the flow can be changed by increasing the power setting and the calculated flow in L/min is displayed at the bottom left of the controller screen and this is in addition to whatever is the native flow from the LV. *The Impella flow depends on the motor speed, which is adjusted as per the performance (P) and the P level corresponds to the rotations of the motor per minute. Higher the P, higher is the flow and less is the stroke work for the native heart.*

Potential Adverse Events

During the procedure, the main complications are aortic valve injury, bleeding, arrhythmias, or vascular injury. However, during, or postprocedure, patients can develop acute renal dysfunction, cerebrovascular accident, hemolysis, thrombocytopenia, and the dreaded problem of limb ischemia and gangrene, the latter being a common complication in all cases of prolonged proximal arterial cannulations.

■ EC-PELLA

This is a use of concomitant venoarterial extracorporeal membrane oxygenation (VA-ECMO) with Impella device for patients in cardiogenic shock who also require VA-ECMO because of refractory hypoxia. Studies have also shown that compared to VA-ECMO used alone, the EC-PELLA group had significant improvement in hospital mortality and higher success rates in bridging to recovery or intervention.

■ IMPELLA VERSUS INTRA-AORTIC BALLOON PUMP

Impella has the advantage of being less bulky, compact, and having a fully implantable CF pump; however, it is prohibitively more expensive than IABP and requires superior expertise.

Comparison studies have shown superiority of Impella devices over IABP in cases of high-risk PCI, by evidencing fewer major adverse cardiac and central events at both 30 and 90 days after PCI. Further Impella 2.5 and CP devices maintain a longer time of hemodynamic stability, enabling the operator to perform a more thorough high-risk procedure without intervening adverse events. Though the IMPRESS trial showed no difference in 30 days mortality between the two devices, it however revealed a significant improvement in hemodynamic and renal functions and faster lactate clearance with the Impella device as compared to IABP.

SUGGESTED READING

1. Dangas GD, Kini AS, Sharma SK, Henriques JPS, Claessen BE, Dixon SR, et al. Impact of hemodynamic support with Impella 2.5 versus intra-aortic balloon pump on prognostically important clinical outcomes in patients undergoing high-risk percutaneous coronary intervention (from the PROTECT II randomized trial). Am J Cardiol. 2014;113(2):222-8.
2. Kantrowitz A, Cardona RR, Freed PS. (1992). Percutaneous intra-aortic balloon counterpulsation. Crit Care Clin. 1992;8(4):819-37.
3. Ouweneel DM, Eriksen E, Sjauw KD, van Dongen IM, Hirsch A, Packer EJS, et al. Percutaneous mechanical circulatory support versus intra-aortic balloon pump in cardiogenic shock after acute myocardial infarction. J Am Coll Cardiol. 2017;69(3):278-87.
4. Thiele H, Jobs A, Ouweneel DM, Henriques JPS, Seyfarth M, Desch S, et al. Percutaneous short-term active mechanical support devices in cardiogenic shock: a systematic review and collaborative meta-analysis of randomized trials. Eur Heart J. 2017;38(47):3523-31.
5. Wernly B, Seelmaier C, Leistner D, Stähli BE, Pretsch I, Lichtenauer M, et al. Mechanical circulatory support with Impella versus intra-aortic balloon pump or medical treatment in cardiogenic shock-a critical appraisal of current data. Clin Res Cardiol. 2019;108(11):1249-57.

CHAPTER 23

Approach to Nutritional Support

Jamshed Sunavala

■ INTRODUCTION

In recent years nutritional support (NS) has become a very important part of critical care management. Critically ill malnourished patients, particularly during the hypercatabolic phase of the illness are at a high risk of succumbing to serious complications. There is adequate evidence to show that poor nutritional support in critically ill patients is responsible for delayed recovery, prolonged time on the ventilator, delayed healing of surgical wounds and generally poor outcome. These group of patients have an increased caloric and protein requirements, during the very critical phase of the illness and are in negative nitrogen balance resulting in hypoalbuminemia which can cause extravasation of fluids and electrolytes and hemodynamic instability. Hence, nutritional support with adequate caloric and protein intake is mandatory for these patients, at the same time, recent studies have shown that over-feeding should be avoided as they also lead to poor outcome. There are many aspects of nutritional support in critically ill patients which are still debatable with studies showing contradicting evidence mainly regards the quantum of nutrition requirement, routes and timing of feeds and the indications of immunonutrition. NS for critically ill patients is no more a supportive therapy alone and is considered an active therapeutic intervention.

■ MALNUTRITION

The present classification of malnutrition encompasses both undernutrition and overnutrition (obesity) (**Flowchart 1**). However, in this chapter we will deal with those nutritional syndromes that are relevant to critically ill patients. Malnutrition is common among critically ill patients causing deficiency of both macronutrients and micronutrients and as a consequence, there is reduced body mass, protein loss, and an immunodeficiency state. The end result is a poor clinical outcome due to pulmonary complications and an increased tendency towards infection and sepsis, which finally contributes to organ dysfunction. Malnutrition in the intensive care unit (ICU) can manifest as acute disease-related malnutrition (ADM) in hypercatabolic patients and in those due to acute mechanical obstruction to enteral feeds (MOEF), as in acute intestinal obstruction, ileus, and gastric stasis. It is also seen in critically ill patients, associated with their inability to take food, reduced appetite, or due to preexisting malnutrition. ICU patients with extensive burns or serious

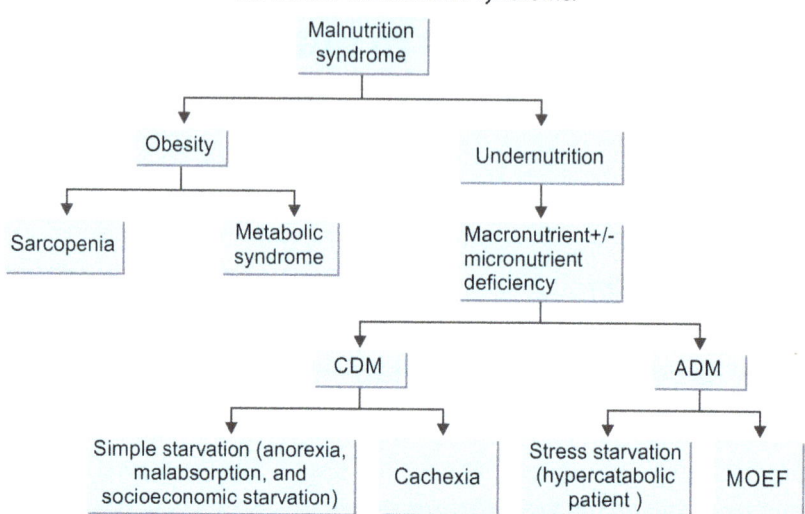

Flowchart 1: Nutritional syndrome.

(ADM: acute disease-related malnutrition; CDM: chronic disease-related malnutrition; MOEF: mechanical obstruction to enteral feeds)

wounds can have increased protein loss, whereas a group of seriously ill patients with liver failure may have decreased protein synthesis. Patients most likely to succumb to severe systemic complications associated with malnutrition are the elderly and immunocompromised patients and those who are markedly hypercatabolic. Though nutritional support (NS) plays a very important role in the overall care of critically ill patients, the guidelines on nutritional management have changed over the last two decades. Previously, most critically ill patients were infused with parenteral nutrition (PN) at the onset, till the initial critical phase was resolved and the patient had reasonably recovered to tolerate enteral feeds [enteral nutrition (EN)]. Current guidelines emphasize more on EN even in the early phase of critical illness, though partial parenteral nutrition (PPN) is used as an additional supplement when the required caloric target cannot be met through EN.

■ PHYSIOLOGICAL IMPACT OF MALNUTRITION IN CRITICALLY ILL PATIENTS

Simple starvation, also termed as simple marasmic starvation (SMS), results from a partial or total cessation of caloric intake in otherwise healthy individuals and is commonly associated with patients suffering from anorexia nervosa or malabsorption. However, this does not usually result in any life-threatening complication as the body is able to provide adequate fuel to vital organs by means of glycogenolysis and lipolysis in cases of short-term starvation (<48 hours). However, with prolonged starvation (>72 hours) with depleted glycogen levels, since fatty acids cannot be converted to glucose, essential glucose is now derived from gluconeogenesis. Here the structural body proteins breakdown to provide amino acids as a substrate for gluconeogenesis, but soon this process of protein breakdown is halted by adaptive processes whereby the brain uses ketones for its metabolic fuel and the lipid stores supply basal metabolic requirements for the body. It is only when the fat stores are depleted does further protein breakdown and gluconeogenesis become significant.

In contrast to simple starvation, *stress starvation* in hypercatabolic critically ill patients, who have reduced ability to utilize fat as an energy source, results in skeletal muscles becoming a major source of fuel and this leads to marked wasting of lean body mass within a few days. Stress starvation is usually seen in major postoperative states, polytrauma, extensive burns, shock, severe infection, sepsis, and its sequelae. This condition is also called hypoalbuminemic malnutrition because of its characteristic clinical manifestation of hypoalbuminemia and negative nitrogen balance (NB) due to both breakdown of proteins and protein losses. In addition, the intense inflammatory response mediated by cytokine-induced vascular permeability leads to protein extravasation, along with extracellular water accumulation and electrolyte losses, resulting in hypovolemia and serious hemodynamic instability **(Flowchart 2)**. This catabolic state is also responsible for insulin resistance and hyperglycemia. The protein breakdown from the muscles during the catabolic phase of the illness continues unchanged and this results in a significant negative nitrogen balance (NB) which is the hallmark of stress starvation.

The main laboratory and clinical parameters that distinguish stress from simple starvation are presence of hypoalbuminemia, water retention with edema, marked negative NB, increased energy expenditure, and severely decreased prealbumin and transferrin levels **(Table 1)**.

■ NUTRITIONAL PLANNING

A physician who orders NS for the patient should consider the six "Rs" whilst planning the nutritional prescription **(Table 2)**.

■ INDICATIONS OF NUTRITIONAL SUPPORT

List of indications for NS are given in **Box 1**, but hypercatabolic patients with negative NB and those with inability to take enteral or oral feeds, remain the main indications in clinical practice for NS in the ICU.

Flowchart 2: Increased inflammatory response and its consequences.

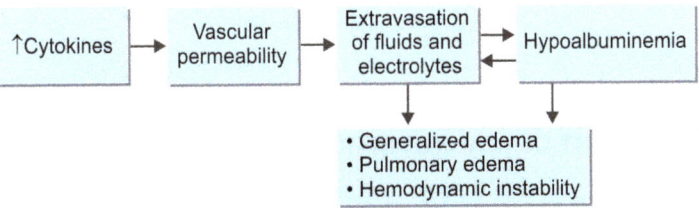

(*Source:* JD Sunavala. Nutritional Support in Critically Ill patient. Publisher Fresenius Kabi Private Limited)

TABLE 1 Physiological impact of starvation versus stress.

Category	Starvation	Stress
Catabolism	+	+++
Glycogenolysis	+	+++
Gluconeogenesis	+	+++
Lipolysis and ketosis	+++	++
Energy expenditure	Decreased	Increased
Serum albumin	No change	Decreased
Urine urea nitrogen	<5 g/day	≥ 5 g/day
Nitrogen balance	Normal or mildly negative	Strongly negative
Extra cellular water	Mild increase	Marked increase
Disease states	Anorexia nervosa and malabsorption	Severe inflammation, sepsis, burns, and head injury

(*Source:* JD Sunavala. Nutritional Support in Critically Ill patient. Publisher Fresenius Kabi Private Limited)

TABLE 2 Consideration in planning a prescription for nutritional support (NS).

Reason (indications)	• Simple starvation • Stress starvation (hypercatabolic) • Inability to take oral feeds • Inability to feed by enteral route
Requirements	• Total caloric and protein requirements • Individualized allocation of substrates • Disease-related requirements
Restrictions	• Caloric or specific substrates • Electrolyte restrictions • Fluid restriction • Restrictions due to pre-existing comorbidities
Route of delivery	• Oral • Enteral—nasogastric, nasojejunal, and percutaneous endoscopic gastrostomy (PEG) • Parenteral nutrition
Rate of delivery	• Speed of achieving target calories (within 2 or 3 days or begin with trophic feeds) • Speed of fluid volume delivery • Risk of refeeding syndrome
Responsibility	• Mandatory to monitor patients receiving NS

ASSESSMENT OF MALNUTRITION

In the setting of social and economic malnutrition (SEM), chronic disease-related malnutrition (CDM) and for malnutrition in children, certain standard tests for nutritional assessment are commonly used. These

Chapter 23 | Approach to Nutritional Support

BOX 1 Indications of nutritional support in critically ill patients.

- Inability to take oral feeds
  - Loss of appetite
  - Severe stomatitis
  - Trauma or burns involving the face
  - Lower cranial nerve palsy with poor gag reflex and risk of aspiration
  - Inhalation injury
- Failure to enteral feeding
  - Gastric stasis
  - Ileus
  - Intestinal obstruction
- Intolerance/complications of enteral feeding
  - Diarrhea
  - Gastrointestinal (GI) bleeds
- Hypercatabolic patients with negative nitrogen balance
  - Severe sepsis
  - Polytrauma
  - Extensive burns
- Pre-existing malnutrition
- Pre-existing comorbidities requiring special nutritional support—renal, cardiac, hepatic, and diabetes mellitus
- *Increased protein loss:* Extensive burns

include anthropometry, body mass index (BMI), creatinine height index, serum albumin, prealbumin, transferrin, Harris–Benedict equation, and indirect calorimetry (IC). However, these tests may not be appropriate in the critical care setting, as most of these tests can be falsely influenced by drugs, disease states and fluctuations in body water, including use of diuretics, leading to nonreliable anthropometric data, weight, BMI, and other measurements.

Indirect calorimetry is probably the most reliable test and is considered a gold standard to determine energy expenditure. This is a method which estimates substrate utilization and energy expenditure using gas exchange measurements of both CO_2 production and O_2 consumption during rest and steady state exercise. The modified Weir equation which was developed in 1949, remains the basis of measuring the metabolic rate. Most of these are stand-alone dedicated apparatus, which are impractical and cumbersome and have technical drawbacks for use in the ICU. However, newer devices incorporated in the mechanical ventilator circuit are more convenient and reliable for ICU use. Further, using newer infrared CO_2 and electrochemical O_2 sensors combined with mass flow sensors, make gas analysis more accurate and simplified at the bedside. Vmax™ Encore 29n calorimeter is presently considered very accurate, showing least variance for resting energy expenditure (REE) measurement. Special canopies/face masks to trap gas exchange are also available for spontaneously breathing patients, but their accuracy could be suspect if a proper resting state cannot be maintained.

Some small, hand-held devices are available, but not yet validated. Many situations in a critically ill patient can influence a patient's steady state, such as agitation, hyper- or hypothermia, fluctuating feeds, certain drugs like beta-blockers or sedatives, muscle relaxants, and extremes of inflammatory response or serious metabolic abnormalities. The influence of extracorporeal membrane oxygenation (ECMO) and continuous renal replacement therapy (CRRT) in altering the VO_2 and VCO_2 measurements is controversial but many studies show that alteration in the IC measurements may be insignificant. However, it is rarely used in adult ECMO settings because of technical challenges of the two simultaneous gas exchange sites viz. the native and the artificial lung. This however, could be bypassed using two separate estimations of gas exchange at the two sites and finally the data is combined and introduced in the modified weir equation. However, this novel method still needs validation.

The *subjective global assessment* (SGA) is a comprehensive nutritional assessment mode described in the 1980s. This method of assessment has been validated and commonly used by most ICUs and includes history of pre-existing malnutrition and also incorporates the metabolic stress of disease component and physical examination **(Box 2)**.

Subjective global assessment is also useful to classify individuals between well-nourished and mildly, moderately, or severely malnourished. It can be universally applied for all categories of disease states and particularly is useful where other tools of assessment mentioned earlier are not effective in critically ill patients. Due to the global perspective it can distinguish body composition changes due to poor dietary intake, cachexia, or sarcopenia. In clinical practice

---

BOX 2 Subjective global assessment (SGA).

- History of pre-existing malnutrition
  - History of estimated weight loss
  - Time since last normal feed
  - Cause of malnutrition (malabsorption, cachexia, anorexia, etc.)
  - Functional loss
- Physical examination
  - Muscle wasting, body composition, edema, signs of micronutrient and vitamin deficiencies
  - Signs of organ dysfunction
- Stress level
  - Estimation of stress level according to the severity of the disease or hypercatabolic state
- Calculation of nitrogen balance **(Box 3)**
- Clinician's perception
  - Is the patient at increased risk of medical complications without nutritional support?
  - Does the nutrition have effect on organ function?
  - What is the anticipated time delay before the patient can resume normal feed?

> **BOX 3** Nitrogen balance calculation.
>
> The overall metabolism of protein in the body is summarized by nitrogen (N) balance
> This represents the difference between N intake and N output
> (A) NB = NI − (U + F + S)
> Where, NB = nitrogen balance, NI = nitrogen intake, and U, F, S = nitrogen loss from urine, feces, and skin, respectively.
> For every 6.25 g of dietary protein consumed, 1 g of nitrogen is available
> (B) NB = (protein intake/6.25) − (urinary urea nitrogen + 4*)
> *Constant factor of 4 is added to urinary N to account for nonurea nitrogen loss
>
> (*Source:* JD Sunavala. Nutritional Support in Critically Ill patient. Publisher Fresenius Kabi Private Limited)

for rapid appraisal of bed-ridden critically ill patients, the SGA format includes the following:

- *History*: Here, the patient or close relatives are questioned regards approximate weight loss, dietary changes, and gastrointestinal symptoms that have persisted for >2 weeks. *Weight loss* of 10% or more, compared to a weight measured prior to the recent illness is associated with a higher postoperative morbidity and mortality, especially after a major abdominal surgery. Often the weight prior to the illness may have to be an intelligent guess, or one may have to accept a standard weight of an average Indian male or female.
- *Time since the last normal feed*: If there is a history of an inadequate intake (enteral or parenteral) for 7 days, it would be appropriate to commence NS pre- or postoperatively, or soon after admission for all critically ill patients.
- *Anticipated time delay*: Estimation of the anticipated time delay before the patient can resume a near normal feed is based on the nature of the primary illness or postoperative complications.
- *Physical examination*: Muscle wasting and body composition, especially with abnormal fat distribution over the abdomen and pelvic region with thin and wasted upper body, are very suggestive of malnutrition. Peripheral and sacral edema may confound weight measurements but give a good indication of reduced visceral proteins. Edema may also be observed with thiamine deficiency.
- *Functional loss* can be assessed by assessing simple physical performance by measuring the hand grip strength, gait, and ability to climb steps. However, this may not be possible in critically ill patients, and one may have to depend on the recent history of malnutrition. More important is to check whether malnutrition has affected organ function.
- *Level of hypercatabolic state* is assessed by the degree of stress as mild, moderate, or severe. Major surgeries, high fever, and mild degree of burns may all result in mild-to-moderate stress levels, but sepsis, polytrauma, and extensive burns result in severe stress and need specific NS.

- *Visceral protein levels*: Serum albumin is useful in predicting surgical morbidity and mortality and long-term monitoring of nutritional status, but is not useful in assessment of nutritional status in complicated critically ill patients. Transferrin levels are influenced by the same complications common in most critically ill patients, such as dehydration or sudden volume expansion, hepatic failure, enteritis, and renal dysfunction. Hence, both serum albumin and transferrin levels do not correctly reflect the nutritional status in critically ill patients and neither are they prognostic indicators in predicting morbidity or mortality.
- *Nitrogen balance (NB)* is one nutritional parameter most consistently associated with patient outcome in those who are critically ill. Determining the NB is useful to determine the degree of catabolism and accordingly prescribe NS to keep the patient in a positive NB. However, maintaining a positive balance may not be a realistic goal, considering the fact that protein breakdown continuously exceeds protein synthesis in all severely hypercatabolic patients. Calculation of NB is shown in **Box 3**.

Finally the decision to implement NS is based on the clinician's (1) ability to detect or suspect malnutrition; (2) judgment to predict good clinical outcome by offering NS; and (3) experience to decide on the proper mode of delivery and the choice of feeds.

CALORIC REQUIREMENTS

The daily energy requirements are usually calculated as per various equations **(Table 3)**, though hypercatabolic patients will require modification of the Harris–Benedict equation with corrective stress factor. However, these incremental stress factors often overestimate the caloric requirements; hence to simplify matters, one can evaluate the caloric needs ranging from 25 to 35 kcal/kg/day according to the appropriate stress level, taking the severity of the disease into consideration and similarly protein intake can be tailored to the degree of stress **(Table 4)**.

The current practice is to avoid overfeeding most critically ill patients and to restrict their caloric intake to 1,500 kcal per day. This is contrary to earlier thinking where hypercatabolic patients often received 2,000–3,000 kcal per day, or at times, even more with the intent to meet the metabolic demands. Overzealous feeding may contribute to complications such as hyperglycemia, pulmonary edema, and excess of CO_2 production resulting in ventilator dependence. However, in exceptional cases, as in extensive burns or polytrauma with sepsis, higher energy requirements may be justified and certain dedicated equations may be used.

The major substrates contributing to caloric intake are carbohydrates, proteins, and fats in an approximate proportion of 50%, 20%, and 30%, respectively. In order to achieve a total caloric intake of 25 kcal/kg/day with increments for stress level one may have to give 2–4 g/kg/day of carbohydrates, 1–2 g/kg/day of proteins, and 2 g/kg/day of fats.

TABLE 3 Predicted formulae to estimate energy requirements of critically ill adult patients.

Curreri formula	Age 16–59: 25 (weight in kg) + 40 (BSA burned) Age >60: 20 (weight in kg) + 65 (BSA burned)
Harris–Benedict equation	Men: BEE (kcal) = 66.5 + 13.8 (weight in kg) + 5 (height in cm) – 6.76 (age in years) Women: BEE (kcal) = 655 + 9.6 (weight in kg) + 1.85 (height in cm) – 4.68 (age in years)
Corrective stress factors	Sepsis/major surgery: 1.3 × BEE Severe sepsis: 1.5 × BEE Extensive burns (>20% of BSA): 2 × BEE BEE: As calculated by Harris–Benedict equation
Ireton–Jones equation (for ventilator-dependent patients)	(kcal) = 1784 – 11(A) + 5(W) + 244G + 239T + 804B
Toronto formula for burns	BEE (kcal) = –4,343 + (10.5 × % TBSA burned) + (0.23 × kcals) + (0.84 × HB) + (114 × T) – (4.5 × postburn days)

(A: age in years; BSA: body surface area; BEE: basal energy expenditure; G: gender; H: height in cm; HB: Harris–Benedict equation with no stress or activity factor; kcal: calorie taken in past 24 hours; T: body temperature in degree Celsius; TBSA: total body surface area; W: weight in kg)

TABLE 4 Protein and energy requirements according to stress levels.

Stress level	Proteins (g/kg/day)	Energy (kcal/kg/day)
Unstressed	1.0	25
Mild	1.2	25–30
Moderate	1.5	30–35
Severe	2.0	35–40
Burns	2.0	25 kcal/kg/day + 20 kcal per% BSA burns

(BSA: body surface area)
(Source: JD Sunavala. Nutritional Support in Critically Ill patient. Publisher Fresenius Kabi Private Limited)

ENTERAL NUTRITION (EN)

Here we will discuss (1) indications and contraindications of EN; (2) route of delivery; (3) choice of feeds; (4) advantages of EN; and (5) complications and monitoring of patients on EN.

Enteral nutrition is most commonly *indicated* in patients with impaired consciousness, severe dysphagia, upper gastrointestinal dysfunction, and patients on mechanical ventilation where oral fees are not possible. Very often, one resorts to EN when a patient's oral feeds are curtailed by problems such as anorexia, nausea and vomiting, delirium, severe oral thrush, or painful stomatitis, or chewing difficulties.

The main *contraindications* to EN are intestinal obstruction, ileus, gastric stasis, severe diarrhea, gastrointestinal bleeds, or any complications that hinder achieving the nutritional goal.

As per present guidelines, EN is the preferred route of delivery and should be commenced at the earliest opportune time—best within 24-48 hours, provided there are no contraindications to EN. Further, EN should be continued throughout the catabolic phase, regardless of the quantity of food intake tolerated and this is particularly important as it is responsible for maintaining gut integrity and preventing translocation of bacteria.

Routes of EN include feeding via nasogastric tubes (NG tubes), jejunal tubes (J tubes), and percutaneous endoscopic gastrostomy (PEG). NG tubes are the most common and practical route of feeding, provided that the stomach is functioning with regards to gastric contractility and this can be confirmed by aspirating the tube and checking for gastric residue. On an average, one should expect a patient to tolerate delivery of at least 1,500 mL of feeds per day. Softer and less traumatic tubes are available (Freka tube) which are better tolerated by most of the patients.

If however the stomach is not functional, a *nasojejunal tube* (NJ tube) can be placed, past the stomach, into the jejunum. The insertion can be done using a special tube as a blind procedure at the bedside, by a skilled intensivist, but difficult cases may require radiological or endoscopic assistance for proper placement. However, one should be aware that the small intestine does not tolerate intermittent feeding; hence, a continuous delivery of nutrients through a feeding pump may be necessary. Feeding tubes can also be inserted directly into the stomach surgically (gastrostomy) or less invasively by PEG. This procedure is indicated for patients requiring long-term feeding, especially in those with swallowing impairment secondary to neurological deficits. Contrary to common belief; this procedure, though it reduces the risk of aspiration, does not entirely obviate the problem of aspiration pneumonia, especially in critically ill patients or in those with partial or complete pyloric stenosis. PEG can be extended to jejunal feeding (PEG J) system, but it is yet to be proven whether this can completely obviate the risk of pulmonary aspiration. Apart from oropharyngeal secretions, poor positioning of the tube is usually responsible for aspiration in these patients. *Jejunostomy* is another procedure requiring open surgery which facilitates a larger tube to be directly placed in the jejunum by a purse-string controlled enterotomy (Witzel technique), but it is best done at the end of an emergency laparotomy or major surgery, as opposed to doing it later in the ICU.

Choice of Feed

In general, most patients with a normally functioning gastrointestinal tract and with no other encumbrances should be able to tolerate a standard *whole protein feed containing* soluble fiber, though constipated patients may benefit with feeds containing insoluble fiber. However, one should bear in mind that nonsoluble particles and very viscous feeds tend to block most feeding tubes. All feeds should contain both macro- and micronutrients and currently a wide variety of ready-to-use commercial feeds are available in the market which meet the requirements. Exclusive home-made blenderized diets, or in combination with commercial feeds, are still preferred by many doctors as they are less expensive, though more often the preference is for freshly prepared unprocessed natural food. Though blenderized diets are relatively safe and have certain nutritional benefits, they may have serious disadvantages, as they cannot ensure full caloric and protein needs of the patients. Strict vegetarians are deprived of sufficient proteins and may fail to achieve the positive NB in the hypercatabolic phase. In patients with lesser injury or those in the rehabilitation phase, such homemade feeds may suffice and probably benefit the patient psychologically. Blenderized feeds usually require extra water intake to flush the tubes frequently as they are more likely to clog.

Commercial feeding formulae are available in the market ranging from densities of 1 kcal/mL to 2 kcal/mL and with protein contents of 35 g/L as in standard formula, to high protein formula providing 60–70 g/L. Feeds providing 2 kcal/mL are useful when fluid restriction is a priority but being hyperosmolar, these are prone to diarrhea, though the risk is small when delivered directly into the stomach where large volumes of gastric secretions attenuate the osmolality of the feed. It is worth noting that feeding formulae are not solely responsible for diarrhea but certain liquid drug preparations delivered through the feeding tubes can be extremely hyperosmolar and some preparations may contain sorbitol that may act as a laxative, hence, all such preparations should be discontinued before stopping the essential feeds **(Table 5)**.

Most enteral formulae are polymeric where intact proteins are broken into amino acids in the upper GI tract **(Table 6)**. Semi-elemental formulae

TABLE 5	Diarrhea checklist.	
D	Drugs to be avoided	Inappropriate use of antibiotics, laxatives, and prokinetics
I	Infection	Contamination of food and feeding system
A	Allergy	Intolerance to certain foods
R	Rectal examination	For impaction and overflow diarrhea
R	Reduce the rate	Do not immediately stop
H	Hypoalbuminemia	Correct it
O	Osmolality	Shift to iso-osmolar feeds
E	Excess	Fluid intake, glucose polymer, or medium chain triglycerides (MCT)
A	Assess further	Colonoscopy

TABLE 6 Source of nutrients in standard polymeric commercial formulae.

Nutrient	Polymeric formulae
Protein content	40–80 g/L
Source of protein	Caseinate, soy protein isolate, delactosed lactalbumin, beef, egg albumin, egg white, and low fat milk
Carbohydrate content	100–200 g/L
Source of carbohydrate	Maltodextrin, glucose polymers, sucrose, glucose, and fructose
Fat content	20–90 g/L
Source of fat	Soybean oil (LCT), corn oil, canola oil, sunflower oil, safflower oil, and coconut oil (MCT)
Caloric density	1–2 kcal/L

(LCT: long chain triglycerides; MCT: medium chain triglycerides)

containing small peptides or elemental formulae containing individual amino acids are more readily absorbed than intact proteins and also promote water reabsorption from the intestines, which is helpful in patients intolerant to certain feeds causing diarrhea. Largely, most commercial feeds available are polymeric in composition as they are tolerated well by the majority of patients. Elemental feeds are expensive and usually prescribed for patients having impaired digestive and absorptive capacity as in patients with malabsorption syndrome, short gut syndrome, and in patients with pancreatitis, by decreasing exocrine pancreatic stimulation. Certain feeding formulae are enriched with immunonutrients such as omega-3 fatty acids, selenium, beta-carotenes, vitamins C and E, and arginine. The large array of feeding formulae available in the market can be confusing; however, there is no convincing evidence that one is superior to the other except in very specific conditions. Hence, it will be best to use less expensive and standard polymeric formulae tailored appropriately to the patient's caloric and protein needs.

A standard polymeric formula (1 kcal/mL) is infused initially at a rate of 50 mL/h for the first 3 hours and checked for residual volume. If tolerated well, it may be continued at the same rate or increased by 10–15 mL/h every 8 hours, until the target caloric goal is achieved. However, one should avoid increasing the rate >100 mL/h. Elemental formulae should commence at a much slower rate and be progressively increased, but very slowly.

The *main advantage of EN* in critically ill patients, other than meeting the nutrient requirement, is to maintain a normal intestinal integrity. Even small amount of feeds should be initiated at the earliest as these help to sustain a normal intestinal barrier and immunological function during the severe phase of systemic inflammatory response. Current guidelines support *trophic feeds* (discussed later in the chapter), beginning with an initial caloric intake of 10–20 kcal/h (250–500 kcal/day) and 25 g of protein per day. Slowly, the rate of delivery is increased to meet the caloric goal over 5–7 days. However, in case of poor tolerance to enteral feeds, one may not be able to achieve the caloric target and more often the necessary protein provision falls short significantly, despite giving high protein enriched products. This protein calorie deficit is unacceptable in critically ill patients who are seriously hypercatabolic and supplemental PN may be required to achieve the protein caloric target.

The *main complications of EN* are diarrhea, gastrointestinal intolerance, aspiration pneumonia, metabolic and electrolyte abnormalities, malposition and occlusion of the tube, nasopharyngeal irritation, and rarely, sinusitis and esophagitis. However, the prolonged delay or failure to reach the nutritional goals in hypercatabolic patients remains a serious concern. Details of the causes, prevention, and management of these complications are given in **Table 7**. Finally, it is mandatory to observe the standard protocol for tube

TABLE 7 Enteral nutrition-related complications.

Complication	Causes	Prevention and cure
Gastrointestinal: • Diarrhea, nausea, vomiting, and abdominal cramps • Constipation • *Others*: GI bleeding, ileus, malabsorption, distension, and esophageal reflux	• Infective feed and rapid infusion • Dehydration and recumbency • GI-related causes	• Symptomatic treatment, review diet and drug regimen and modify, do not immediately stop feeding • Review diet regimen and modify, suppositories, and avoid dehydration • Withhold feeds and review
Mechanical: • Tube malposition and tube displacement • Tube occlusion • *Others*: Esophageal erosions, perforation, and pulmonary aspiration	• Accident and failure of fixation • Viscous diet, failure to flush tube, feed stasis, pill fragments, and tube kinking	• Monitor insertion protocol, confirm placement before infusion, X-ray for checking, and regular observation • Flushing regularly with water and replacement of the tube • Withhold feeds
Metabolic: Disorders of calcium, magnesium, phosphate metabolism, and hyperglycemia	• Refeeding and concurrent disease	• Regular monitoring for the first 10–12 days, adjust diet or supplement IV as appropriate
Infectious: Rhinitis, otitis, parotitis, pharyngitis, and esophagitis	• Use softer tubes • Microbial contamination of the feed and colonization of the tube	• Regular monitoring, cleaning of the tube, and antibiotics

(GI: gastrointestinal; IV: intravenous)

> **BOX 4** Standing instructions for enteral nutrition (tube feeding).
>
> - Physician to place feeding tube
> - Elevate head of bed >30° during enteral feeding
> - Aspirate if symptomatic (distension)
>   - If aspirate <150 mL, return aspirate and continue feeding
>   - If aspirate is >150 mL but <500 mL, reduce feeding rate, notify physician, and consider prokinetics
>   - If aspirate >500 mL, hold feeding, notify physician, and assess the cause Physician may consider use of prokinetics or nasojejunal feeding or partial parenteral nutrition or reduce feeding rate by 50% depending on the residual volume
> - Irrigate tube 4 hourly with 30 mL water and 12 hourly with 10 mL soda bicarbonate and after each medication
> - Enteral pump to be used for continuous feeding and do not let formula hang for longer than 8 hours
> - Administration—set to be changed every 24 hours
> - Hemoglucotest (HGT) to be done every 6 hours
> - Weigh the patient on alternate days
> - Renal and liver function tests—check once a week or as required for the underlying disease severity

feeding during EN, as given in **Box 4** and follow the tube feeding algorithm as in **Flowchart 3**.

■ PARENTERAL NUTRITION

Total parenteral nutrition (TPN) was the standard line of treatment till the early nineties for all critically ill patients with the prevailing perception that enteral feeds were not tolerated during the early phases of critical illness or in the immediate postoperative period. It was assumed that hypercatabolic patients needed to achieve maximum caloric and protein intake within 2 or 3 days and this could not be managed by EN alone. Further, it was believed that feeding through the gastrointestinal tract this early was fraught with serious adverse effects. Current practice is to start EN even in the early catabolic phase and to continue for a week, despite the fact that only 70–80% of the caloric target can be achieved. Hence, as per current guidelines, TPN has been replaced by EN as the first route of NS in critically ill patients. PN is however indicted in a selective group of patients who have a total or partial mechanical obstruction or a nonfunctioning alimentary tract. TPN or supplemental PN is also indicated when EN alone is unable to meet appropriate nutritional needs of the patients. In general, the composition of PN is amino acids as a protein source and glucose with lipids to provide nonprotein energy. Trace elements and electrolytes are often incorporated in the solutions, but may not be sufficient to cover the daily requirements of critically ill patients; hence vitamins and trace elements may have to supplemented.

It is preferable to commence PN after the patient has been resuscitated from shock and is reasonably stable; it is also imperative to correct any gross

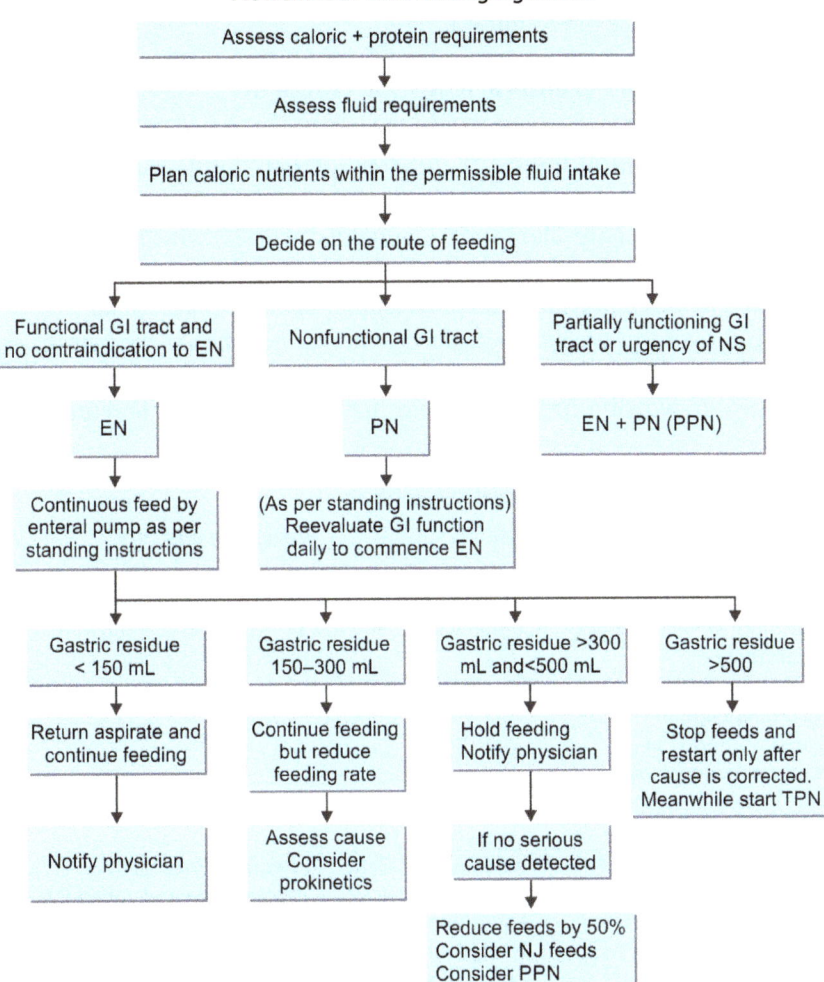

Flowchart 3: Tube feeding algorithm.

(EN: enteral nutrition; GI: gastrointestinal; NJ: nasojejunal; PN: parenteral nutrition; PPN: partial parenteral nutrition; TPN: total parenteral nutrition)

abnormalities of arterial blood gas (ABG), fluid electrolyte balance, and blood sugar levels before administering PN. The initial dose of glucose should not exceed 200 g/day to avoid hyperglycemia and in susceptible patients with preexisting and prolonged starvation both glucose and caloric intake should be restricted in the first few days to avoid refeeding syndrome. Full requirement of amino acids (equivalent to 1–1.5 g/kg of protein/day) can be administered from the first day, provided there are no specific contraindications. Lipids are by and large safe and well tolerated by most critically ill patients; however, serum triglycerides levels should be monitored. Hypertriglyceridemia occurs when lipid infusion far exceeds plasma triglyceride clearance, which can be affected in patients with renal failure and in those receiving excessive glucose, which stimulates lipogenesis. Soya-based lipid emulsions are best avoided during the first week of PN infusion.

Complications of Parenteral Nutrition (Table 8)

The main drawbacks of PN include (1) mechanical and technical complications related to the central lines; (2) catheter-related bloodstream infection (CRBSI); and (3) metabolic complications. Of all these, the *catheter-related infection* is the most prevalent and if unattended, will lead to sepsis and septic shock. Unexplained fever in a patient with a central venous catheter must be attributed to the central line until proven otherwise. Fever accompanied with chills and rigors, or unexplained glucose intolerance should raise suspicion of an underlying CRBSI. Final confirmation of CRBSI is isolation of the same organism drawn simultaneously from the central line and percutaneous

TABLE 8 Parenteral nutrition-related complications.

Complication	Cause	Prevention and cure
Insertion related: Arterial puncture, arrhythmias, chylothorax, hemothorax, hydrothorax, hemopericardium, hydropericardium, pneumothorax, air-embolism, nerve injury, and catheter malposition	Lack of expertise and insertion protocol not followed	Insertion followed by radiological confirmation of CVC. Insertion training to the concerned
Not related to insertion: • Late displacement of CVC • Thrombosis of CVC	• Inadequate/failed fixation • Long-term total parenteral nutrition and hypercoagulability	• Regular observation of fixation site and cuffed CVCs • Streptokinase/urokinase infusion or 70% ethanol infusion. Polyurethane CVC, radiological monitoring, prophylactic addition of 3,000 IU/L heparin to infusate
Metabolic: Disorders of calcium, magnesium, phosphate metabolism, hyperglycemia, and hypoglycemia	Monitoring failure	Monitoring protocol for short- and long-term total parenteral nutrition
Septic: CVC infection or CVC-related sepsis	Unsterile handling of CVC	Aseptic precautions in insertion and manipulations, replacement of CVC on confirmation of sepsis, and new CVC insertion site

(CVC: central venous catheter)
(*Source:* JD Sunavala. Nutritional Support in Critically Ill patient. Publisher Fresenius Kabi Private Limited)

collection. The most common pathogens isolated are coagulase-negative *Staphylococcus, Staphylococcus aureus,* and *Candida* species. Multilumen catheters and those introduced via femoral or jugular sites are more prone to infections. Regular dressings, use of single lumen catheters, dedicated central lines, and using fresh sites for patients needing replacement of infected catheters will help in reducing the incidence of CRBSI. Empirical antibiotics started whilst awaiting blood cultures should cover gram-negative and gram-positive organisms. Catheters should be immediately replaced preferably at a newer site in case of confirmed CRBSI and the practice of changing an infected catheter over a guidewire is not recommended. A protocol for catheter care should be stringently observed as it will go a long way in preventing CRBSI.

Technical complications are mainly related to catheter placement and include pneumothorax, hemothorax, hydrothorax, arterial injury, cardiac arrhythmias, and venous thrombosis. Use of the subclavian route is usually associated with a higher rate of technical complications as compared to the jugular route; however, it is strongly recommended to do the procedure under ultrasound guidance irrespective of the route (subclavian or jugular). However, for long-term use, the subclavian route of delivery is preferable for maintaining better asepsis.

The most common metabolic complication is hyperglycemia. Maintaining a well-controlled glucose level is important, but the earlier practice of very tight control of blood sugar levels below 110 mg% is not encouraged by the current guidelines, because of the risk of precipitating hypoglycemia which can be detrimental with dire consequences in critically ill patients as it can attenuate humoral and clinical response resulting in autonomic dysfunction. Further, there are studies that propagate "permissive hyperglycemia" to avoid the possibility of *"relative hypoglycemia."* The concept of relative hypoglycemia suggests that the counter regulatory release of epinephrine, norepinephrine, and cortisol preventing autonomic dysfunction occurs at a higher glucose level of 120–150 mg% in poorly controlled diabetics, than in well controlled or nondiabetic patients where hypoglycemia occurs at levels below 70 mg%. Consequently autonomic dysfunction associated with hypoglycemia can occur even at normal blood sugar levels, which could be detrimental to critically ill patients with poorly controlled diabetes. Of course this is a newer concept, but it would be worth pursuing, especially as there is enough supportive evidence to show that hyperglycemia at levels of 150–180 mg% does not harm critically ill patients. The current guidelines recommend glucose levels between 150 and 180 mg% at all times during the critical phase of the illness. However, many ICUs dealing with polytrauma and extensive burns prefer a tighter control of blood sugar between 130 and 150 mg% with close monitoring to avoid hypoglycemia. For critically ill patients, continuous insulin is infused through a syringe pump to maintain blood sugar within the acceptable range, using a dilution of 50 units of regular insulin in 50 mL of normal saline, giving a calculation of 1 unit of insulin in 1 mL of normal saline. Current guidelines consider a sliding scale or correction algorithm outdated, as it tries to correct the blood sugar of the previous few hours rather than the next few hours, and hence recommend bolus insulin initially, followed by a scheduled basal insulin to continue intravenously in order to maintain a desired blood sugar level. The bolus dose depends on the normogram set by the respective ICUs and commonly the same dose is continued as basal insulin. Many ICUs still follow the sliding scale method; however, it is inconsequential which method one uses to control blood sugar during PN, as the levels will remain practically the same, because the infusion of the total substrates will be uniformly delivered and remain unchanged throughout the day.

Serious hepatic dysfunction with TPN is rare in adults; mildly elevated levels of liver enzymes usually return to normal and do not warrant discontinuation of TPN. Intrahepatic cholestasis may occur, though rarely, on continuation of TPN for prolonged periods, but more often it is multifactorial. Protein intake will have to be reduced to 0.5 g/kg/day in patients with encephalopathy, but in severely hypercatabolic patients requiring high protein intake, branch chain amino acids can be used.

Peripheral parenteral nutrition is readily available in the market and is recommended when one wants to avoid using central venous access. Peripheral veins by and large, tolerate low osmolar solutions (<800 mOsmol/L) without the risk of developing thrombophlebitis; hence the osmolality of this solution is reduced by decreasing the glucose component and substituting with lipid solutions which have lower osmolality, but can provide adequate calories.

■ MONITORING OF NUTRITIONAL SUPPORT

The monitoring protocol for both EN and PN are given in **Table 9**. Other than the clinical and laboratory parameters, it is also essential to maintain the daily caloric substrates and micronutrient delivery, fluid volume assessment, and NB. The latter is important in severely hypercatabolic patients and in those with sarcopenia where excessive protein loss can result in severe negative balance, loss of lean body mass, and poor outcomes. Further, monitoring of the specific parameters affecting the underlying disease process, such as sepsis, etc., should not be overlooked. Frequency of all these tests is primarily dictated by the severity of illness, complexity of the NS, and the facilities available.

■ TROPHIC FEEDS AND AUTOPHAGIA

As this topic has recently received considerable attention, it would be appropriate to discuss it briefly. Trophic feeds (permissive hypocaloric feeds) have been advocated in many guidelines based on certain studies and observations. The reason behind trophic feeds is the concept of "autophagia", which is supposed to have a protective mechanism for cells which are under stress or inflammation, and works best during periods of fast and is suppressed

TABLE 9: Monitoring of patients on NS.

	PN or EN	EN—specific	PN—specific
Frequent assessment	Changing calorie, protein, and nutrient requirement from the catabolic phase to rehabilitation		
Tolerance to feeds		Regular measurement of resting gastric residue	Strict maintenance of fluid balance to avoid volume overload
Metabolic derangements	• Blood sugar • Serum electrolytes • Serum triglycerides • CBC • Serum creatinine • Serum calcium • Serum magnesium • Liver functions • PT • Serum albumin • Serum prealbumin		
Catheter with tubes		Position and patency of feeding tubes	Standard care of central venous catheters and prevention of inherent catheter-related complications and maintenance of asepsis
Nitrogen balance	Common to all hypercatabolic patients		

(CBC: complete blood count; EN: enteral nutrition; NS: nutritional support; PN: parenteral nutrition; PT: prothrombin time)

during forced feeding. This concept of autophagia is essentially a process used by the eukaryotic cells to recycle old or damaged cellular components in response to cellular stress and damage and was first conceived by the Noble Laureate Yoshinori Ohsumi.

However, one can counter this view by questioning whether lean body mass is better preserved during the peak catabolic phase by a starvation diet of hypocaloric feeds of <500 kcal/day or by delivering adequate calories and by maintaining a positive NB. The answer to this lies in the fact that though trophic feeding had shown benefits in some studies, but when later analyzed, showed that the patients who benefited were less complicated and less critical.

Further Heylands Nutrition Risk in Critically Ill (NUTRIC) scoring showed that patients with higher NUTRIC score (≥6) benefited with early and adequate caloric feeding and not with trophic feeds. Hence, as a guideline, all critically ill patients such as those with extensive burns, severe pancreatitis, and polytrauma, who have a high NUTRIC score, should not receive trophic feeds during this very hypercatabolic phase.

■ DISEASE MODIFIED NUTRITIONAL SUPPORT IN CRITICALLY ILL PATIENTS

Nutritional support is often required to be tailored to specific diseases. These include patients having concomitant comorbidities such as hepatic, respiratory, or renal failure and patients with severe pancreatitis or morbid obesity. In these conditions, certain aspects of NS may need to be appropriately adjusted. The main changes would include assessment of caloric and protein requirements, route of administration, substrate alterations, and use of pharmaconutrients **(Box 5 and Table 10)**.

■ IMMUNONUTRITION

The link between malnutrition and impaired immune function has been well documented. "Immunosuppression" caused by malnutrition is so predictable that reduced lymphocyte count and impaired response to antigens have traditionally been used as components of nutrition screening. Hence, the conventional role of nutrition support vis-à-vis immune function has been aimed at preventing or reversing immunosuppression related to malnutrition. However, today, there is an ongoing research into specific nutritional components which favorably affect immune function. This has stimulated the development of commercial enteral and parenteral products designed to improve the outcomes of hospitalized patients.

The capacity for nutrients to modulate the actions of the immune system and to affect clinical outcome has become an important issue in clinical practice and public health. The application of nutrients for this purpose is referred to as "immunonutrition". A working definition of "immunonutrition" might be "modulation of the activities of the immune system and the consequences on the patient of immune activation by nutrients or specific food items fed in amounts above those normally encountered in the diet". These nutrients are called as "immunonutrients" and include the amino acids (arginine and glutamine), omega-3 fatty acids, nucleotides, and antioxidants—vitamins and minerals.

Polyunsaturated fatty acids (PUFAs), omega-6 fatty acids and omega-3 fatty acids, cannot be synthesized in the body and hence are obtained from the food we eat. PUFAs which are predominant in our normal diet today are obtained from vegetable oils and from depot fat of mammals and these are mainly linoleic acids (omega-6 fatty acids). In contrast, those societies whose food

BOX 5 | Disease modified NS in ICU patients.

Mechanical ventilated patients:
- Adequate calories and proteins needed to improve respiratory muscle strength and endurance and take care of pre-existing undernutrition
- Avoid excess calories from glucose source as it may lead to increased CO_2 production and increased ventilator demands

Liver failure:
- In presence of encephalopathy, the total protein will need to be restricted to as low as 0.5 g/kg/day; however, larger amounts of modified amino acids (branch/chain amino acids) may be given to ensure positive nitrogen balance without worsening the encephalopathy

Renal dysfunction:
- Fluid restriction
- Calories compromised because of fluid restriction and lipids become an important source of energy
- Monitor for electrolyte imbalance, hyperkalemia, and hypermagnesemia
- To restrict protein or consider RRT in severely catabolic patients and allow liberal use of fluids and electrolytes

Pancreatitis:
- Determine disease severity
- Confirm volume resuscitation
- Achieve enteral access (gastric/jejunal tube)
- Tolerance during SNIP improved mainly during jejunal feeds and changes in feeding formula
- Small peptide medium chain triglyceride and semi-elemental formula reduces endocrine secretion
- An immune modulating formula (fish oil, glutamine, and arginine)
- Avoid probiotic
- Monitor of tolerance, 1—enzyme secretion, 2—gut mobility, 3—triglycerides <400 mg/dL
- PN worsens outcomes, (if started <24 hours) should be given after 5 days if EN <60% of goal

(EN: enteral nutrition; ICU: intensive care unit; NS: nutritional support; PN: parenteral nutrition; RRT: renal replacement therapy; SNIP: severe necrotizing infective pancreatitis)

TABLE 10 | Critically ill obese patients (BMI > 30 kg/m²).

Respiratory risks	Management
• Decreased ventilator capacity • Decreased work of breathing • Hypoalbuminemia and increased risk of pulmonary edema • Overfeeding and increased CO_2 production causing weaning failure	• Correction of malnutrition • Increased protein intake • Avoiding high carbohydrate intake • May require ventilator support
Metabolic risks	Management
• Nitrogen balance does not depend on energy balance • Energy expenditure is difficult to predict • Overfeeding detrimental	• Maintain positive nitrogen balance • Correlate energy expenditure on IBW or AdBW • Hypocaloric high protein feed

(AdBW: adjusted body weight; BMI: body mass index; IBW: ideal body weight) mainly contains a major intake of 'deep sea fish' incorporate larger quantities of alpha-linolenic acid (omega-3 fatty acids). Once consumed, these fatty acids are converted to larger chains of more unsaturated derivatives. Linoleic acid is converted to arachidonic acid (ARA) and alpha-linolenic acid is converted to eicosapentaenoic acid (EPA) and docosahexaenoic acid (DHA). Both EPA and DHA are produced in algae and plankton; hence, fish oils extracted from deep sea fish (e.g., herring, salmon, mackerel, tuna, and sardines) which live on plankton, provide the main source of omega-3 fatty acids for humans. Both omega-3 and omega-6 fatty acids are important "essential fatty acids (EFAs)" and their deficiency can lead to a wide array of clinical disorders.

In critically ill patients (especially those with severe sepsis), ARA (omega-6 fatty acids) products are thought to be proinflammatory mediators whereas EPA (omega-3 fatty acids) products act as anti-inflammatory, or rather, less proinflammatory, thereby making their interaction critical, considering they are both competitive substrates. It is therefore essential to have optimal ratio of omega-6 and omega-3 fatty acids in critical care settings. If systemic inflammatory response syndrome (SIRS) is left unchecked without a proper balance of this ratio, the consequences may be worsening of sepsis and organ failure.

The lipids commonly used in parenteral feeds have been traditionally based on soya bean oil which is rich in omega-6 fatty acids. Hence, adding omega-3 fatty acids as a separate lipid emulsion that is now commercially available may help in attaining the balanced ratio of omega-6 and omega-3 fatty acids in critically ill patients. Omega-3 fatty acids can be given as a supplement in a relatively small proportion of 10–20% of the total lipids given. This can effectively adjust the fatty acid profile of a PN regimen. Prospective studies in critically ill patients reveal encouraging results so far; however, due to limited experience, one should refrain from using the product in grossly unstable patients or in patients with severe renal or liver failure and in pregnant women.

Glutamine is considered a nonessential amino acid; however, during hypercatabolic states when skeletal muscles stores and plasma levels become depleted in glutamine, it may become a conditionally essential amino acid. Glutamine depletion can result in decreased gut integrity and immunity; IV glutamine probably improves both and hence decreases bacterial translocation. It is difficult to mix glutamine in TPN and it is more stable as dipeptides. Meta-analysis of 14 randomized trials of *glutamine supplemental PN in surgical patients* when compared with standard nutrition showed reduced incidence of infection and morbidity. Addition of glutamine in enterally fed patients has not shown a similar benefit and is currently not recommended.

Conflicting data from many studies in the last two decades has created an uncertainty regarding the benefit of glutamine in critically ill patients. However, a significant meta-analysis of 843 articles and 18 randomized

control trials published in Critical Care in 2014 by Chen et al. concluded the following:
- There was no overall mortality benefit or reduction in length of hospital stay
- There was reduction in the nosocomial infection rate mainly in the surgical patients
- Patients who received a higher dose than the recommended dose (0.3–0.5 g/kg/day) had a higher mortality rate.

Arginine is a nonessential amino acid and has beneficial and deleterious effects. Arginine deficiency develops after trauma or major surgery and can impair wound healing and arginine supplements may benefit these groups of surgical patients. However, arginine is a precursor for the synthesis of nitric oxide which may benefit in certain specific conditions by producing vasodilation, but it can adversely affect patients of severe sepsis, resulting in marked hypotension and hemodynamic collapse. For this reason and also the fact that its potent oxidizing and nitrating action may increase the gut barrier permeability, arginine is contraindicated in critically ill patients, particularly in the setting of severe sepsis.

Antioxidants supplements include selenium, zinc, copper, and vitamins B, C, and E. Selenium may have potential benefits if given in appropriate doses, though it has not shown any significant reduction in mortality. Zinc, copper, and vitamins, though important for long-term NS, have shown no definite benefit as supplements in NS in critically patients, as there are no major trials conducted. However, it is important to note that trace elements can be potentially harmful in large quantities; zinc given in doses >50 mg/day may cause immunosuppression and progressive cholestasis, while copper may lead to liver damage and hemolytic anemia.

In conclusion, one can say that despite the extensive studies and meta-analyses, there is still no definitive evidence to suggest that immunonutrition improves survival in critically ill patients. However, there is an overall impression that it significantly lowers the rate of infections, particularly in critically ill surgical patients. It is unlikely that mere substituting one form of nutrition for another will change the course of prognosis in cases of overwhelming sepsis. Hence, the current thinking is to avoid immunonutrition in life-threatening septic patients with the Acute Physiology and Chronic Health Evaluation (APACHE) scores >20, where such radical changes in nutrients may perhaps adversely affect the outcome. Instead, it may be used in less serious patients of sepsis or in early sepsis, and in surgical patients where it may help in wound healing and reduction of infection rate, where it is more likely to be of benefit. The 2016 guidelines [Society of Critical Care Medicine (SCCM) and American Society for Parenteral and Enteral Nutrition (ASPEN)] from the Journal of Parenteral and Enteral Nutrition (JPEN) recommend that immune modulating enteral formulae should not be used in the medical ICU but such formulae may be appropriate for surgical patients. The majority of studies have shown that immune nutrition has potential benefits for elective surgery patients, but not for critically ill medical patients. Almost all studies have shown no benefit in term of mortality, hospital stay, or ventilator days.

SUGGESTED READING

1. Chen Q-H, Yang Y, He H-L, Xie J-F, Cai S-X, Liu A-R, et al. The effect of glutamine therapy on outcomes in critically ill patients: a meta-analysis of randomized controlled trials. Crit Care. 2014;18(1):R8.
2. Elke G, Zanten AR, Lemieux M, McCall M, Jeejeebhoy KN, Kott M, et al. Enteral versus parenteral nutrition in critically ill patients: an updated systematic review and meta-analysis of randomized controlled trials. Crit Care. 2016;20(1):117.
3. Gunst J, Van den Berghe G. Parenteral nutrition in the critically ill. Current Opin Crit Care. 2017;23(2):149-58.
4. Marik PE, Hooper MH. Normocaloric versus hypocaloric feeding on the outcomes of ICU patients: a systematic review and meta-analysis. Intensive Care Med. 2016;42(3):316-23.
5. McClave SA, Heyland DK. The physiologic response and associated clinical benefits from provision of early enteral nutrition. Nutr Clin Pract. 2009;24(3):305-15.
6. McClave SA, Taylor BE, Martindale RG, Warren MM, Johnson DR, Braunschweig C, et al. Guidelines for the Provision and Assessment of Nutrition Support Therapy in the Adult Critically Ill Patient: Society of Critical Care Medicine (SCCM) and American Society for Parenteral and Enteral Nutrition (A.S.P.E.N.). JPEN J Parenter Enteral Nutr. 2016;40(2):159-211.
7. Mizock BA. Immunonutrition and critical illness: an update. Nutrition. 2010;26(7-8):701-7.
8. Singer P. Nutrition in Intensive Care Medicine: Beyond Physiology. World Rev Nutr Diet. 2016;105:I-XI.

SECTION 6

Monitoring

- **Hemodynamic Monitoring**
  Jamshed Sunavala

- **Arterial Blood Gases and Acid-base Abnormalities**
  Jamshed Sunavala

- **Echocardiography in Critical Care**
  Nitin Burkule, Bomi B Ichaporia

CHAPTER 24

Hemodynamic Monitoring

Jamshed Sunavala

■ INTRODUCTION

Any physician interacting with an intensivist should have a background understanding of the principles of hemodynamic monitoring (HM) in order to comprehend the justification of doing these invasive and minimally invasive procedures. More importantly, one should be competent in the interpretation and application of the measurements obtained from the respective monitoring devices. Hence this chapter will briefly touch on the following aspects of HM.
- Physiological basis of HM
- Monitoring devices:
    - Type of devices
    - Techniques
    - Indications
    - Procedural complications
    - Pitfalls in measurements and interpretations

■ PHYSIOLOGICAL BASIS OF HEMODYNAMIC MONITORING

The three main aims of HM are to assess and monitor the determinants of:
1. Cardiac performance
2. Tissue oxygenation
3. Fluid responsiveness

Determination of Cardiac Performance (Flowchart 1)

Cardiac performance is influenced by a wide spectrum of physiological variables but the three main factors that determine cardiac performance are (1) preload; (2) contractility; and (3) afterload.

Preload, by definition of Brunwald and Ross, "is the force acting to stretch the left ventricular (LV) muscle fibers at end-diastole and determining the resting length of the sarcomeres". This stretch of the myofibrils increases the strength of muscle contraction and is one of the main determinants of cardiac performance. Hence, in essence, it is the returning venous blood that fills the ventricle and which is responsible in exerting the ventricular force by stretching the heart muscle; in other words, preload is end-diastolic volume (EDV). This relationship between preload and the strength of ventricular contraction was discovered independently by Otto Frank and Ernest Starling and is referred to as the *Frank-Starling relationship of the heart*. In brief, therefore, the force

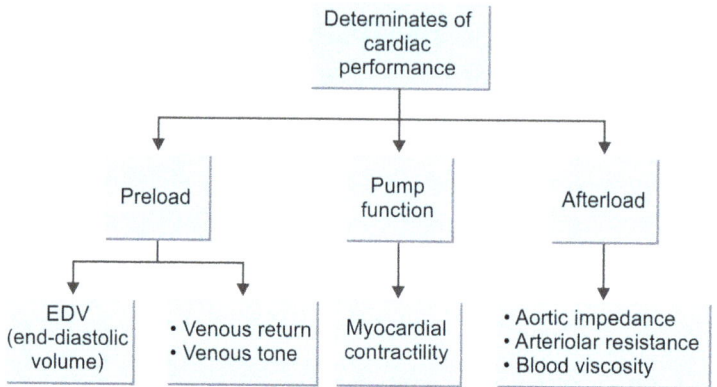

Flowchart 1: Determinants of cardiac performance.

created by the EDV (preload) governs the strength of ventricular contraction. However, as the left ventricular end-diastolic volume (LVEDV) is not easily measured at the bedside, the left ventricular end-diastolic pressure (LVEDP) is used as a surrogate for LVEDV to measure the preload.

Central venous pressure (CVP) is equivalent to right atrial pressure (RAP) and in the absence of tricuspid valve dysfunction, RAP reflects the right ventricular end-diastolic pressure (RVEDP). In a normal heart with an uninterrupted conduit between the right ventricular (RV) and left atrium (LA), and in the absence of mitral valve dysfunction, the RVEDP/CVP correlate well with LVEDP provided the LV compliance is normal. Hence CVP monitoring, which is more practical at the bedside, can be used to guide fluid resuscitation in emergencies such as severe diarrhea or blood loss, in young healthy individuals with a normal heart.

Pulmonary capillary wedge pressure (PCWP) on the other hand, directly measures the left atrial pressure (LAP) and in the presence of a normal "mitral outflow tract", it is equivalent to LVEDP. However, this concept of LVEDP being a surrogate for LVEDV or a measure of cardiac performance to guide fluid therapy is not entirely correct for the following reasons:

- *Studies have shown* that there is a poor relationship between end-diastolic pressure (EDP) and EDV for both ventricles and as stated earlier, it is the force exerted by LVEDV (preload) which determines the LV contraction. Hence CVP or PCWP are not the most reliable measures of ventricular filling and have failed to predict either preload or fluid responsiveness.
- The PCWP in the absence of LV inflow obstruction may give an indication of the relative changes in preload. However, this is true only if the ventricular compliance is normal; in a diseased heart, the LVEDP does not correlate with LVEDV, as the *ventricular compliance is altered*. For instance, in dilated cardiomyopathy, the ventricular compliance increases, and a large increase in ventricular filling volume is accompanied by only a small change in the filling pressure. On the other hand, in a stiff noncompliant

ventricle, as in ischemic heart disease, the ventricular filling pressure needs to be high to maintain an adequate ventricular filling volume. Hence the clinical importance of maintaining a *slightly* high LVEDP in cases of acute myocardial infarction, in order to achieve an adequate cardiac output (CO).
- LVEDP may also rise without any significant increase in the true transmural filling pressures, thereby producing little increase in preload or stroke volume (SV), as it may be falsely influenced by the surrounding pressure. One important situation where the surrounding pressures produce significant external constraints is the use of a mechanical ventilator and high positive end-expiratory pressure (PEEP), here the PCWP may overestimate the effective distending (transmural) pressure.

However, despite its limitations the filling pressures are still important to assist decision-making at the bedside, in patients with heart failure or volume overload. A therapeutic reduction in LVEDP is always correlated with improved outcome in heart failure patients, hence unloading the LV by reducing the LVEDP is a physiologically accepted therapeutic maneuver to improve outcome.

Contractility is defined as the inherent capacity of the myocardium to contract independently, regardless of the alterations in pre- and afterload. This capacity of "intrinsic force" is the *inotropic state* of the cardiac muscle. Presently, we have no bedside method of monitoring contractility alone; however, if two of the fundamental determinants of SV (pre- and afterload) can be kept constant then obviously the changes in *stroke work* performed by the ventricle becomes the determinant of ventricular function solely affected by the inotropic state of the heart.

Stroke work for the two ventricles is calculated as follows:
- LVSWI = SI × (MAP − PCWP) × 0.0136 g/min/m^2
- RVSWI = SI × (MPAP − CVP) × 0.0136 g/min/m^2

Where LVSWI is the LV stroke work index, RVSWI is RV stroke work index, MAP is the mean arterial pressure, MPAP is mean pulmonary artery pressure and SI is the stroke index.

Echocardiographic measure of ejection fraction (EF) is frequently used as a parameter to assess LV function and which is interpreted not infrequently as a measure of contractility. This is far from the truth, as EF is also influenced by alterations in pre- and afterload; however, despite this limitation and having no other alternative, EF is perhaps the most practical parameter to assess contractility at the bedside, as compared to others.

More specific markers of contractility such as dp/dt or speckle tracking and strain rate imaging have limitations—the former requires the presence of mitral regurgitation and the latter is currently not widely available on portable echo machines used in the intensive care unit (ICU) settings.

Afterload is defined as the impedance to blood flow from the ventricle. Whilst preload determines the force of the ventricular contraction, afterload denotes the tension developed by the cardiac muscle during systole as a result of systemic vascular resistance (SVR). Resistance is typically calculated as a pressure gradient divided by mean flow. Hence the resistance to the two ventricles [indexed to the body surface area (BSA)] is derived by the following equations:

$$SVRI = \frac{\text{Mean arterial blood pressure} - CVP}{\text{Cardiac index}} \times 80$$

$$PVRI = \frac{\text{Mean pulmonary artery pressure} - PCWP}{\text{Cardiac index}} \times 80$$

The above equations are based on the "fundamental equation of circulation" [MAP = CO × systemic vascular resistance]. This correlation between the afterload, CO, and MAP is useful in clinical practice, because the interdependence between these three variables strongly suggests that mild lowering of the peripheral resistance (SVRI) in patients with acute heart failure will increase the SV and without the MAP falling precipitously. However, if MAP falls markedly one may have to consider the following possibilities: (1) severe mitral regurgitation; (2) inadequate preload due to relative hypovolemia; (3) severe myocardial damage with extremely poor contractility; or (4) leftward shift of the septum because of increased RV pressure and volume overload causing diastolic ventricular interaction (DVI) and resulting inadequate filling of the LV. The normal range of hemodynamic values are given in **Table 1**.

The SVRI is usually raised in cardiogenic and hypovolemic shock, in systemic hypertension, and with the use of vasoconstrictor drugs. It is

TABLE 1 Normal hemodynamic values.

Variables	Abbreviations	Units	Normal range
Right atrial pressure	RAP	mm Hg	2–6
Mean pulmonary artery pressure	MPAP	mm Hg	11–15
Pulmonary capillary wedge pressure	PCWP	mm Hg	3–15
Cardiac index	CI	L/min/m²	2.8–3.6
Left ventricular stroke work index	LVSWI	g/min/m²	44–68
Right ventricular stroke work index	RVSWI	g/min/m²	4–8
Systemic vascular resistance index	SVRI	Dynes/sec/cm⁵/m²	1,700–2,600
Pulmonary vascular resistance index	PVRI	Dynes/sec/cm⁵/m²	255–285
Oxygen delivery index	DO_2I	mL/min/m²	500–650
Oxygen consumption index	VO_2I	mL/min/m²	110–150

(*Source:* Sunavala JD. Cardiac monitoring in adults. In: Udwadia FE (Ed). Principles of Critical Care, 3rd edition. New Delhi: Jaypee Brothers Medical Publishers (P) Ltd.; 2014.)

TABLE 2	Hemodynamic changes caused by some commonly used IV drugs.				
Drug	HR	MAP	PCWP	CO	SVR
Nitroprusside	↑	↓	NC or ↓	↑	↓
Nitroglycerin	↑	↓	↓	↑	↓
Norepinephrine	NC or ↑	↑	↑↓	↑ or NC	↑
Dopamine	NC or ↑	NC or ↑	NC or ↑	↑	↑
Dobutamine	NC or ↑	NC or ↑	NC	↑	NC
Amrinone	NC	↓	↓	↑	↓

(CO: cardiac output; HR: heart rate; IV: intravenous; MAP: mean arterial pressure; NC: no change; PCWP: pulmonary capillary wedge pressure; SVR: systemic vascular resistance ↑: increased; ↓: decreased)
(*Source:* Sunavala JD. Cardiac Monitoring in Adults. In: Principles of Critical Care Medicine by Dr F. E. Udwadia, 3rd edition. New Delhi, Jaypee Brothers Medical Publishers (P) Ltd.; 2014.)

characteristically low in septic shock, thyrotoxicosis, anemia, cirrhosis, and with vasodilator therapy. The pulmonary vascular resistance index (PVRI) is primarily raised in pulmonary edema, following pulmonary embolism, and in some valvular or congenital heart diseases. It is also raised in hypoxemia, due to pulmonary vasoconstriction.

Hemodynamic parameters can be markedly influenced by certain drugs which may rapidly change the hemodynamic status in critically ill patients. Hence it is important to know the pharmacological influence of the drugs commonly used in the ICU on the hemodynamic variables (**Table 2**).

Tissue Oxygenation

Tissue oxygenation depends on two important determinants—oxygen delivery (DO_2) from the systemic circulation to the capillaries and oxygen uptake (VO_2) by the tissues from the capillaries. In normal healthy subjects, the DO_2 is approximately 1,000 mL/min and the VO_2 is 250 mL/min. This fractional uptake of O_2 into the tissue determines the oxygen extraction ratio (O_2ER); as the VO_2 is normally 25% of the DO_2, the normal O_2ER is 0.25. This means that in normal conditions, 25% of O_2 delivered to the capillaries is taken up by the tissues (i.e., 250 mL/min).

Oxygen delivery is a function of CO and O_2 content of arterial blood (CaO_2). Hence $DO_2 = CO \times CaO_2$ where $CaO_2 = (1.34 \times Hb \times SaO_2) + 0.0031 \times PaO_2$, showing that CaO_2 is a function of both oxyhemoglobin and ventilation. VO_2 is a product of CO and the difference between arterial and venous O_2 content ($CaO_2 - CvO_2$) and O_2ER, is the ratio of O_2 uptake (VO_2) to DO_2. Hence $O_2ER = VO_2/DO_2$. The equations for determinants of tissue perfusion (oxygenation) are given in **Box 1** and the normal values of DO_2 and VO_2 are given in **Table 1**.

A reasonably good bedside marker of tissue oxygenation is the *saturation of mixed venous oxygen (SvO_2)*, which varies inversely with the changes in oxygen extraction. Hence in low CO states where O_2ER is increased, the SvO_2 will fall

> **BOX 1** Determinants of tissue perfusion (oxygenation).
> - Mean arterial pressure (MAP) = CO × SVR
> - Arterial O_2 content (CaO_2) = (1.34 × Hb × SaO_2) + 0.0031 × PaO_2
> - O_2 delivery (DO_2) = CO × CaO_2
> - O_2 uptake (VO_2) = CO × (CaO_2 − CvO_2)
> - O_2 extraction ratio (O_2ER) = VO_2/DO_2 = CaO_2 − CvO_2/CaO_2
>
> (CO: cardiac output; Hb: hemoglobin; PaO_2: partial pressure of arterial oxygen; SaO_2: arterial oxygen saturation; SVR: systemic vascular resistance)

below the normal of 75% to improve tissue oxygenation. However, in a state of severe sepsis and shock, one may find the SvO_2 to be normal or even slightly higher. This is because of the tissues' inability to extract O_2 from the capillaries as a result of the severe mitochondrial damage at the cellular level. At the bedside, O_2 saturation measured from the central venous line placed in the superior vena cava ($ScvO_2$) is a good surrogate for SvO_2 and prevents the need for pulmonary artery (PA) catheterization. It is however important to note that the $ScvO_2$ is usually 5–10% higher than the SvO_2 and this difference may be still higher in patients with cardiac failure, shock, or sepsis. Despite this discrepancy, the changing trends in $ScvO_2$ run parallel to that of SvO_2.

Serum lactate is a clinical marker of tissue oxygenation, used frequently in the ICU in all patients who are critically ill with shock. Lactate is an end product of anaerobic glycolysis and is a readily available measurement which can be estimated either from the venous or arterial blood with no discordance in values. The normal blood lactate level is <2 mmol/L.

Serum lactate is now an accepted marker of both diagnostic and prognostic values in patients with severe sepsis, all types of shock, severe hypoxic respiratory failure, and during and after cardiorespiratory resuscitation. As a prognostic marker, studies have shown that early recovery of lactate levels to normal (within 24 hours after onset of treatment) have shown good outcome, but if it remains persistently high (>4 mmol/L), it indicates a higher possibility of ICU mortality. This relationship between *lactate clearance* and mortality is more apparent in patients with severe sepsis. The diagnostic and prognostic aspects of serum lactate and lactate clearance mentioned here pertain only to those conditions where elevated lactate levels are associated with abnormalities of DO_2 and VO_2. There are many other causes of hyperlactatemia like thiamine deficiency and drugs (metformin, antiretroviral agents, etc.), which may have different prognostic implications. In conclusion, a raised serum lactate level (>2 mmol/L) and a decreased SvO_2 (<60%) with a suggestive clinical picture, may help in supporting an earlier diagnosis of tissue hypoxia.

Organ-specific Tissue Perfusion

The earlier discussion of overall (global) tissue perfusion may not be entirely correct when applied to specific organ perfusion. The autoregulation of most organs maintains a constant organ specific blood flow over a broad range of fluctuating blood pressure (BP) and changes in metabolic rates. However, hypotension (defined as systolic BP < 90 mm Hg and MAP of < 60 mm Hg) is pathological and impairs autoregulated blood flow to the organs. In hypertensive patients, autoregulation may be impaired even at MAP < 85 mm Hg. Renal blood flow is maintained by autoregulation above 80 mm Hg, though a minimum of 70 mm Hg is required to prevent acute kidney injury (AKI). The brain requires an adequate cerebral perfusion pressure (CPP) during critical illnesses. CPP = MAP − (intracerebral pressure + CVP) and this should be at least 60–70 mm Hg. Similarly, a coronary perfusion pressure (CPP = diastolic BP − LVEDP) of at least 50 mm Hg or more is essential for myocardial perfusion.

A normal BP by itself may not necessarily reflect hemodynamic stability or adequate organ perfusion, however maintaining a MAP of 70 mm Hg or more by continuous bedside monitoring is the best support that one can provide to ensure tissue perfusion.

Determinants of Fluid Responsiveness

The main purpose of giving fluid challenge to a patient in shock is to improve the CO by increasing the LVEDV, thereby restoring adequate tissue perfusion. Achieving objective end points through fluid resuscitation has improved clinical outcomes; but overzealous attempts at resuscitation without proper monitoring leads to volume overload and increases both morbidity and mortality. This concept is referred to as fluid responsiveness, where the fluid response to CO remains on the ascending portion of the Frank-Starling curve **(Fig. 1)**.

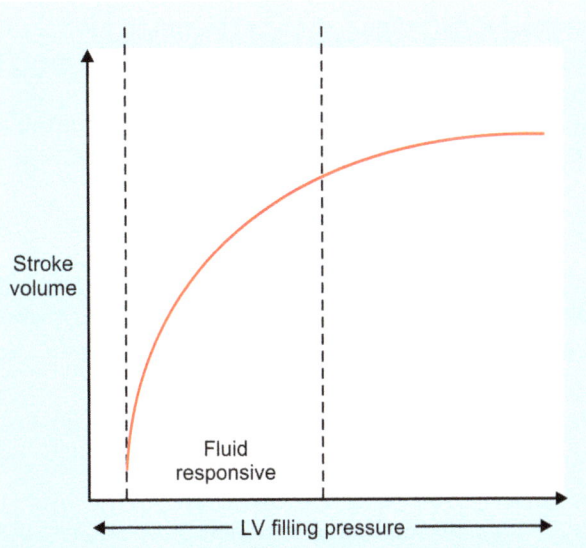

Fig. 1: Fluid responsiveness correlates with preload responsiveness part of the Frank–Starling curve. (LV: left ventricular)
(*Source:* Sunavala JD. Cardiac Monitoring in Adults. In: Principles of Critical Care Medicine by Dr F. E. Udwadia, 3rd edition. New Delhi, Jaypee Brothers Medical Publishers (P) Ltd.; 2014.)

Determination of fluid responsiveness for many years relied on the static estimates of preload measured by CVP or PCWP. However, as discussed earlier, static pressure-based measurements have failed to predict fluid responsiveness and neither the direct or indirect measurements of LVEDV have been showed to predict fluid responsiveness. In essence, preload is not preload responsiveness, because the interplay between venous return and CO is also dependent on other factors such as the afterload and the contractility of the heart. Hence, in critically ill patients with pathological alterations in cardiac contractility, one could risk volume overloading without improvement in CO, by increasing the fluid challenge albeit within the normal acceptable range of CVP or PCWP.

In contrast to the static pressure measurements which provide limited information regarding fluid responsiveness, the less invasive monitoring by stroke volume variation (SVV) and pulse pressure variation (PPV) measure dynamic changes in CO as a function of filling pressure. Here the indices of venous return, cardiac filling pressure, and CO are based on heart lung interaction causing changes with increasing or decreasing intrathoracic pressure during the respiratory cycle. However, the reproducibility of these monitoring devices (SVV and PPV) is limited to patients who are sedated and on mechanical ventilation (MV), whereby their tidal volumes and changes in the intrathoracic pressures are maintained constant. Equations for determinants of fluid responsiveness are given in **Table 3**.

Spontaneously breathing patients may respond to simple provocation tests such as passive leg raising (PLR). Here the fluid challenge is intrinsic in the form of increasing the venous return by elevating the lower extremities by 30°-50° for 1-5 minutes and measuring the CO. Increasing the CO by 10-15% after PLR is predictive of fluid responsiveness.

Measurement of inferior vena cava (IVC) collapsibility on echo or ultrasound by calculating the difference in diameter of IVC on inspiration

TABLE 3 Determinants of fluid responsiveness.

Methodology	Equation	Suggestive of fluid responsiveness
IVC–distensibility index (dIVC)	$dIVC = \frac{ID - ED}{ID}$	>18%
Pulse pressure variation (PPV)	$PPV\% = 100 \times \frac{(PP\ max - PP\ min)}{PP\ max + PP\ min/2}$	>13%*
Stroke volume variation (SVV)	SV variation over respiratory cycle on mechanical ventilation	>10%#

*Implies 85% probability of benefit from fluid challenge
#Predicts increase in CO of ≥15% for bolus of 500 mL of fluid
(ED: expiratory diameter; ID: inspiratory diameter; IVC: inferior vena cava; SV: stroke volume)

and expiration is a useful and noninvasive bedside test to assess a patient's filling pressure. IVC collapsibility correlates well with the CVP measurements.

■ HEMODYNAMIC DEVICES

Arterial Pressure Monitoring

The usual cuff method of recording BP is likely to be inaccurate, as Korotkoff sounds are less audible at low flow rates. Intra-arterial pressure monitoring is indicated in all hemodynamically compromised patients who are on vasopressor or inotropic support and need careful titration of dosage to avoid precipitous changes in BP.

The radial artery is always the preferred site for placement of an arterial catheter, provided the collateral flow in the ulnar artery is present. Hence, Allen's test should be performed before radial artery cannulation in order to determine the adequacy of blood flow in the ulnar artery. The brachial and femoral arteries are alternative sites when radial artery cannulation is unsuccessful. However, these sites should never be the first choice as they have many disadvantages and serious complications can ensue, the worst complication being ischemia of the lower extremity, leading to gangrene of the toes and feet following prolonged femoral catheterization.

An additional advantage of intra-arterial pressure monitoring is in the study of its characteristic waveform, particularly in assessing fluid responsiveness through observation of systolic pressure variations (SPVs) occurring during positive pressure ventilation, which is discussed in more details later in the chapter.

Central Venous Pressure Monitoring

The actual measurement can be done by using a simple water manometer or attaching the central line to a transducer. *Water manometer technique* is a simple bedside procedure which does not require any sophisticated equipment. The central venous catheter is connected to a three-way stopcock via an extension tubing, which in turn is connected to a precalibrated manometer placed on a stand. The level of CVP is read by observing the descent of the fluid column in the manometer, which is in direct continuity with the blood in the central veins. The descent eventually stabilizes and the reading at this level is the CVP measurement (in cmH_2O). However, most ICUs today use a *transducer monitoring technique*, whereby the proximal end of the CVP line is connected directly to a pressure transducer and a continuous digital recording and a waveform of RAP are obtained on the monitor.

Clinical Application

The mean pressure in the right atrium (RA) is 0-6 mm Hg (using a transducer monitoring system), and 3-8 cmH_2O (when using a simple water manometer), the conversion being 1 mm Hg = 1.36 cmH_2O. The CVP catheter may be placed in the superior vena cava instead of the RA because it accurately reflects the RAP and waveforms. Placing the catheter tip in the right atrial cavity may inadvertently cause the tip to negotiate the tricuspid valve and momentarily record the higher RV pressure; this may also result in ventricular premature contractions (VPCs). However in the case of a PAC, the proximal port would automatically lie in the RA.

The CVP or RA pressure reflects the RVEDP. Ordinarily in healthy individuals the RVEDP and the LVEDP correlate rather well. Therefore in a young person with normal cardiac function, the CVP correlates well with the LV filling pressure, and can be used as a guideline for monitoring the LV preload during fluid therapy. *However in clinical practice, it is fallacious to assume that the CVP is a good guide to LV filling pressure in all cases;* in fact, there may be a disparity between the right and LV functions in critically ill patients for more than one reason. This disparity can occur in patients with isolated RV dysfunction caused by tricuspid or pulmonary valve defects, RV infarcts or pulmonary hypertension. In all these conditions, the CVP will be high and will not correctly reflect the LV preload. Disparity can also occur in patients with isolated LV dysfunction in which case the CVP will remain within normal limits and will not reflect the high LVEDP. Because of this frequent disparity between RV and LV functions in critically ill patients, CVP readings should be interpreted with circumspection.

A CVP reading can be most misleading if it is interpreted as an isolated reading. In order to obtain maximum benefits, serial measurements over a period of time should be studied and correlated with the patient's clinical state. This is most important when considering fluid replacement in elderly patients suspected of having cardiac dysfunction. In such patients, small amounts of fluid challenge should be given whilst closely monitoring the rise in CVP. If there is a sharp rise, further fluid challenge should be withheld or given very cautiously. Also, in such patients, a CVP value even at the lower limit of normal should be accepted as the end point, provided there is a significant clinical improvement in perfusion. If this is practiced meticulously, CVP monitoring can be a safe alternative in the absence of a PAC.

There are several other limitations to the use of CVP, for instance, if the venous tone is increased in severe hypovolemia, the CVP may not fall in proportion to the fluid loss. Similarly, patients on mechanical ventilator support may show falsely elevated CVP values due to raised intrathoracic pressure. Falsely raised CVP values may also occur with external compression of the vena cava because of a tumor mass or due to increased intra-abdominal pressure.

Pulmonary Artery Pressure Monitoring

Measurement of the LV filling pressure (or LVEDP) without actually entering the left side of the heart was first made possible by the discovery of a flow-directed PAC by Swan and Ganz in 1970. Here the catheter tip with an inflated balloon just proximal to it was floated far into one of the branches of the PA and wedged so that the catheter tip was in direct continuity with the LA via the pulmonary veins, and hence reflected the LA pressure which was the same as LVEDP, provided there was no LV inflow obstruction. In addition, the PAC could measure the RA pressure through its proximal lumen and the CO could also be measured by the thermodilution technique. Further, mixed venous blood could be collected from the distal lumen of the catheter for assessment of pressure of mixed venous oxygen (PvO_2) and SvO_2.

Indications

It is clear that PAC provides data that can be used to make therapeutic decisions. However, the critical question is whether these therapeutic decisions improve outcomes. Some studies have suggested that the use of PAC actually worsens outcome. This rekindled the strong debate regarding the efficacy and safety of PAC.

Recent studies have consistently shown that PAC monitoring has not demonstrated improved survival or reduced ICU or length of hospital stay compared with control groups. However, it remains possible that there is a subgroup of the patient population for whom PAC, as a guide to hemodynamic management, may be helpful. Though in the final analysis, it is worth stressing that diagnostic tests and monitoring devices do not alter clinical outcome, treatment does. If PAC does not alter treatment decisions it can have no positive effect on the clinical outcome, but may unnecessarily add to potential complications. Hence, to benefit patients, the PAC must provide information that is not otherwise available and the information so provided should be useful in selecting a treatment plan that has proven clinical benefit. **Box 2** gives a broad list of guidelines where PAC monitoring may give useful information in certain subsets of critically ill patients. The four subsets being unstable hemodynamics, uncertain diagnosis, complicated cases of fluid management, and in those patients where high risk of hemodynamic decompensation is anticipated.

Catheter Design (Fig. 2)

A wide range of catheters (from the adult to the pediatric size) are available for various clinical applications. They range from 60 to 110 cm in length, 4–7.5 Fr in caliber, with balloon inflation volumes ranging from 0.5 to 1.5 mL. The catheter material is polyvinyl chloride which is pliable at room temperature, and softens further at body temperature. The simplest type of catheter contains only two lumens, one to transmit PAP and the other for balloon inflation; however, the most commonly used one is the sophisticated triple-lumen thermodilution catheter. In fact, there are various types of catheters available and their use depends on the clinician's choice.

> **BOX 2** Indications for pulmonary artery pressure monitoring.
>
> - In critically ill, hemodynamically unstable patients:
>   - Shock (of any etiology)
> - In cases where the diagnosis is uncertain:
>   - Cardiogenic versus noncardiogenic pulmonary edema
>   - Acute respiratory failure with uncertain cardiac status
>   - Acute myocardial infarction with a new loud murmur indicating
>   - Acute rupture of the interventricular septum or of a papillary muscle
>   - In patients with acute myocardial infarction and shock, in whom hypovolemia has to be differentiated from pump failure
> - As a therapeutic guideline under the following conditions:
>   - Massive fluid replacement in patients with severe fluid loss, especially in elderly patients or in those with a history of ischemic heart disease
>   - Fluid management in patients with noncardiogenic pulmonary edema [acute respiratory distress syndrome (ARDS)]
>   - In acute hemorrhage necessitating massive transfusions, particularly in patients with associated cardiac or renal problems
>   - Management of patients with shock or other critically ill patients on inotropic and/or vasodilator drugs
>   - In patients with pump failure who respond unsatisfactorily to initial therapy
> - Patients at risk of hemodynamic decompensation:
>   - Preoperative monitoring in all seriously ill patients (cardiac or noncardiac surgery)
>   - Patients with underlying cardiac disease on mechanical ventilator
>
> *All the above are only a broad list of guidelines, to be used with judgment, so that the information available will alter treatment plan towards clinical benefit.*
> (*Source:* Sunavala JD. Cardiac monitoring in adults. In: Udwadia FE (Ed). Principles of Critical Care, 3rd edition. New Delhi: Jaypee Brothers Medical Publishers (P) Ltd.; 2014.

Insertion Technique

Balloon catheters float easily from the vena cava to the pulmonary wedge pressure position, and knowledge of the various intracardiac waveforms is generally sufficient to be able to insert the catheter. Bedside fluoroscopy is not mandatory, and fluoroscopic equipment can be very cumbersome in an already small and cluttered ICU room. Percutaneously, a Seldinger technique is usually employed, which leaves an introducer catheter in situ through which the PA catheter is easily passed. Before insertion of the PAC, the pressure monitoring system should be setup and kept ready

After ascertaining the integrity of the balloon, the catheter is advanced into the RA. Once in the RA, inflate the balloon with air or carbon dioxide to the recommended volume (printed on the catheter). In the presence of intracardiac shunts, CO_2 should be used instead of air for inflation of the balloon, in order to avoid systemic air embolization in case of accidental balloon rupture. Further passage of the catheter from the RA to the pulmonary wedge position should normally not take longer than 30–40 seconds, provided there is no abnormal flow pattern in the heart or markedly elevated RV pressures. The shape of the waveform and RV, PA, and PCWP pressure readings are used as a guide in advancing the catheter **(Fig. 3)**.

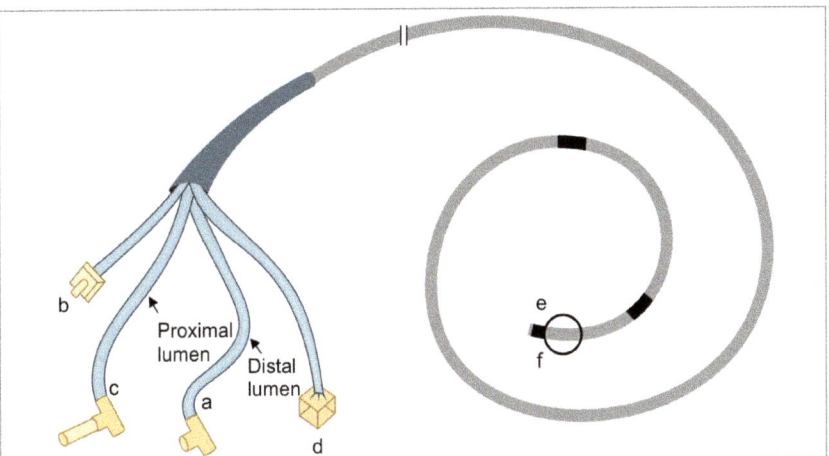

Fig. 2: Triple-lumen pulmonary catheter. a = distal pulmonary artery (PA) port, b = balloon inflation port, c = proximal right atrium (RA) port, d = thermistor hub, e = balloon, f = thermistor.
(*Source*: Sunavala JD. Cardiac Monitoring in Adults. In: Principles of Critical Care Medicine by Dr F. E. Udwadia, 3rd edition. New Delhi, Jaypee Brothers Medical Publishers (P) Ltd.; 2014.)

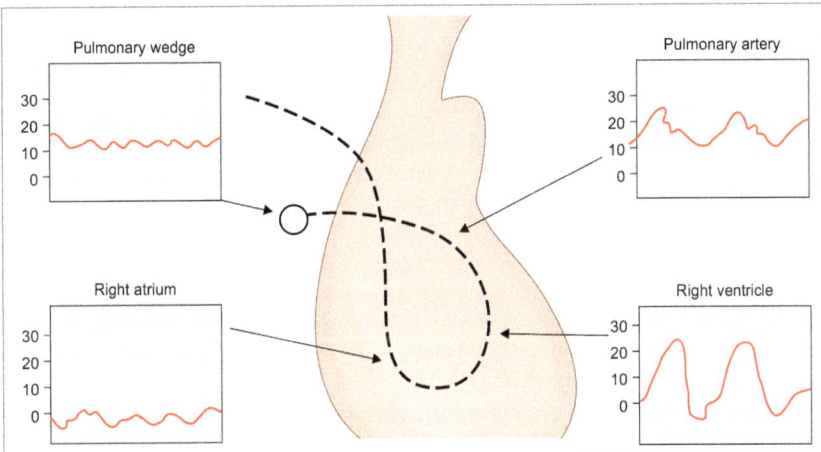

Fig. 3: Pressure waveform configuration as seen during the passage of the pulmonary artery catheter through the various chambers of the heart and in wedge position. The position of the catheter shown here is as seen in fluoroscopy.
(*Source*: Sunavala JD. Cardiac Monitoring in Adults. In: Principles of Critical Care Medicine by Dr F. E. Udwadia, 3rd edition. New Delhi, Jaypee Brothers Medical Publishers (P) Ltd.; 2014.)

Correct Wedging Procedure

The balloon should not be allowed to remain inflated in the occluded position beyond 10–15 seconds. Inflation beyond this period can lead to pulmonary infarction. In addition, artifactually elevated pressures may result due to prolonged wedging. Note that the PCWP when measured should never be higher than the pulmonary artery diastolic pressure (PADP) and if so, it represents an artifact. Further, the blood sample withdrawn from the catheter which is truly wedged should represent and be equal to the oxygen saturation of arterial blood, whereas blood drawn from the PA with the balloon deflated gives the oxygen saturation of mixed venous blood, averaging 75%.

Normally, if there is a good correlation between PADP and PCWP, the PADP should be used to estimate the LAPs instead of rewedging the catheter frequently. This reduces the risk of pulmonary vascular damage and pulmonary infarction, and also prolongs the balloon life.

Complications of Pulmonary Artery Catheterization

Complications directly attributable to PA catheterization and their prevention are discussed in **Table 4**. Briefly, arrhythmias and an increased incidence of

TABLE 4 Complications directly attributable to PAC.

Complications	Action/prevention
Arrhythmias	• Decrease insertion time • Use fluoroscopic guidance in high-risk groups so that less maneuvering of catheter is necessary • Promptly remove catheter if arrhythmias persist
Infection	• Meticulous, sterile technique with all aseptic precautions during insertion and after care • Avoid repeated manipulations • Catheter to be removed at the earliest
Balloon rupture	Inflation of balloon is typically associated with a feeling of resistance, the absence of resistance and failure to wedge suggest balloon rupture
Knotting	• Knots may be resolved by insertion of suitable guidewires and manipulation under fluoroscopy • If knot does not include any intracardiac structure, apply gentle traction to tighten the knot and then withdraw slowly • Only in worst cases, a thoracotomy and cardiotomy may be required
Clotting and thromboembolic complications in RA or systemic veins	• Intermittent flushing of catheters with heparinized saline • Avoid long-standing catheter placements • Heparin-coated catheters may reduce catheter • Thrombogenicity
Pulmonary infarction and PA rupture	• Avoid prolonged or overinflation of the balloon in the wedge position • Avoid repeated inflation of balloon for PCWP measurements; instead use PADP for continuous monitoring as PADP equals PCWP • Avoid inserting the catheter too far peripherally into a branch of PA. If catheter is seen beyond the hilum there is increased chance of infarction or rupture

(PA: pulmonary artery; PAC: pulmonary artery catheter; PCWP: pulmonary capillary wedge pressure; PADP: pulmonary artery diastolic pressure; RA: right atrium)
(*Source*: Sunavala JD. Cardiac Monitoring in Adults. In: Principles of Critical Care Medicine by Dr F. E. Udwadia, 3rd edition. New Delhi, Jaypee Brothers Medical Publishers; 2014.)

infection are the most common complications. The occurrence of *arrhythmias* and of ventricular ectopics in particular is common during insertion of the catheter. Further, critically ill patients are commonly immunocompromised and are frequently at a higher risk for *catheter-induced infections*. Some less common complications are balloon rupture, knotting of the catheter, pulmonary thromboembolic complications, and PA rupture.

Persistent or repeated wedging of PAC, inadvertent migration of the catheter tip into the smaller branches of the PA, or prolonged balloon inflation can lead to *pulmonary infarction*. *PA infarction*, though rare, is the most dreaded of all complications with a high mortality rate. It may clinically present as mild hemoptysis to begin with, but if ignored, may progress to massive hemorrhage. For details of "problem solving" and steps taken to prevent complications secondary to PA catheterization, refer to **Table 4**.

Pitfalls in Pulmonary Artery Pressure Measurement and Artifacts

Several practical factors may be crucial in obtaining meaningful information whilst performing hemodynamic studies. Problems related to pressure lines, transducers, and monitors, which commonly manifest as overdamped or underdamped waveforms are common to both arterial and venous catheterizations. Similarly, improper "zero leveling" and whip artifacts may be seen. In addition to all these problems, PA waveforms in particular are affected by cardiac dysfunction and by changes in intrathoracic pressures and effects of gravity, and more importantly, the artifacts due to the effects of MV and PEEP.

The two important artifacts which can be responsible for inaccurate reading of the PAC measurement are those due to changes in intrathoracic pressure and those influenced by gravity. Ventilatory movements of inspiration and expiration cause cyclical changes in the intrathoracic pressure, which are transmitted to the intravascular pressure tracings, creating a minimally wandering baseline, with expiration producing positive deflections, and inspiration producing negative deflections during spontaneous breathing. These pressure changes are insignificant and minimally affect the mean PCWP. However, in case of marked labored breathing, as in patients with acute lung injury or chronic obstructive pulmonary disease (COPD), greater swings in pleural pressures are required to move air in and out of the lungs. As a result, there is a wide fluctuation in the pressure waveform baseline, leading to inconsistent and inaccurate recordings. In such a situation, it is best to disregard the digital display and record a long tracing of the PAP or PCWP waveforms, and read that portion of the waveform that corresponds with end-expiration. *It should however be noted that in patients on MV, the end-expiration is reflected by the negative deflection of the wandering pressure baseline.*

In case of an *artifact produced by gravity,* the PAP increases progressively as the blood flows in the lower part of the lung due to gravity. However, the alveolar pressures remain equal throughout. West divided the lung model conceptually

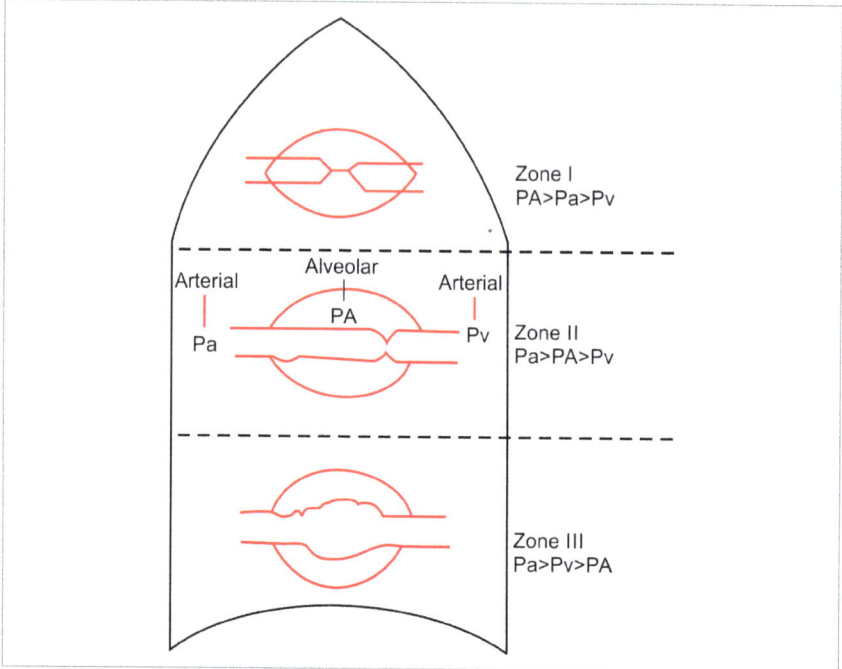

Fig. 4: Interrelationship between the alveolar and vascular in the three West Zones. PA = alveolar pressure; Pa = pulmonary artery pressure; Pv = pulmonary venous pressure (see text for details).
(*Source:* Sunavala JD. Cardiac Monitoring in Adults. In: Principles of Critical Care Medicine by Dr F. E. Udwadia, 3rd edition. New Delhi, Jaypee Brothers Medical Publishers; 2014.)

into three zones, called the *West Zones* (**Fig. 4**), which illustrated the interrelationship between the alveolar and vascular pressures and the effect of gravity.

It is vital that for the PCWP to correctly reflect the LAP, a continuous uninterrupted conduit needs to be maintained between the catheter tip and the LA. For that, the pressure in the PA should be constantly more than both the alveolar (P_A) and pulmonary venous (Pv) pressures, which is only possible in Zone 3, as shown in **Figure 4**, where the PCWP best reflects the LA pressure in all phases of respiration.

To confirm the Zone 3 catheter position, one should constantly be able to identify the wedge waveform. A damp tracing in absence of other problems suggests a Zone 1 or Zone 2 position. Lastly, in patients on PEEP, the PCWP should not be influenced by sudden increase or decrease in PEEP levels if the catheter is properly positioned in Zone 3.

The three zones described here hold true for an individual in an erect position, and as measurements are so often made with the patient supine or semi-inclined, it is important to place the catheter tip at or below the left atrial level, confirming the Zone 3 position. However, in the supine position, most of the alveolar capillary units fall in the gravity-dependent area of the lung having the characteristics of Zone 3 condition, and as most of the blood flows in this area, the PA catheter invariably floats into Zone 3.

Artifacts due to Effects of Mechanical Ventilation and Positive End-expiratory Pressure

Positive changes in the airway pressures produced by MV reflect on the heart and vascular structures of the thorax. This can lead to inaccurate measurements and wrong interpretation of hemodynamic parameters, showing increase in PAP and PCWP.

Mechanical ventilation also has the potential to decrease CO by increasing the intrathoracic pressure and thus reducing the venous return to the heart. In addition, the positive pressure surrounding the heart may produce a tamponade effect, further interfering with the diastolic filling. Though the CO may fall, the CVP, PAP, and PCWP may rise because of perivascular compression distorting the volume-pressure relationship. In other words, pressures that appear to be normal may be insufficient to ensure adequate preload and CO.

All these effects of MV will be exaggerated in patients on either PEEP or continuous positive airway pressure (CPAP). Generally PEEP levels <10 cmH$_2$O do not compromise the measurements of PCWP or CO very significantly. However, PEEP levels >10–15 cmH$_2$O certainly increase the disparity between the PCWP and LA pressure relationship, and also compromise cardiovascular function.

Many clinicians prefer to disconnect the patient from the mechanical ventilator during PCWP measurements; this practice should however be discouraged. As long as the pressure tracings show the characteristic PCWP waveforms and one-half of PEEP is approximately subtracted from the PCWP, it seems reasonable to measure the pressures that apply to the patient during therapy, rather than during a brief interval without it. Also, on discontinuing MV or PEEP, a sudden change in hemodynamics occurs because of an increase in venous return and the measured parameters may be different from those that exist when the patient is on ventilator support.

Cardiac Output Measurement

Thermodilution Technique

The Fick oxygen consumption method described by Adolph Fick in 1870 is usually considered to be the gold standard to which other methods are compared, because of its extreme accuracy in measuring the CO. However, this method is not practical for day-to-day use in the ICU as it is time consuming and requires the patient to be in a steady metabolic state.

The *thermodilution technique* is currently the most widely used method in clinical practice. Though first introduced by Fegler in 1954, its first reported use in humans was published by Margaret Branthwaite and Ronald Bradley in 1968. The basic principle underlying this method is the detection of the change in temperature of blood over a period of time; this can be accomplished by injecting cold saline in the RA from a proximal port of the PA catheter, whilst the thermistor on the catheter tip detects the temperature change in the PA. This change is inversely proportional to the blood flow or CO. The CO computer calculates the temperature difference between the injectate solution and the blood, and displays the temperature-time curve. The area under the curve is inversely proportional to the flow rate in the PA, which is representative of the CO.

It is important that serial measurements should be obtained, after discarding the first trial which is often unreliable. The average value of three measurements is taken as the CO, provided that they do not differ from each other by >15%. The injections should be always timed during end-expiration to avoid unacceptable variations in CO which may occur during different phases of the respiratory cycle. This is particularly important for patients on mechanical ventilator support.

Pitfalls in Cardiac Output Monitoring by Thermodilution Technique

Erroneous CO readings may be produced by conditions such as tricuspid regurgitation, by a clot partially blocking the catheter lumen, or due to intracardiac shunts.

Besides other technical points, the temperature and volume of the injectate solution must be precisely determined to avoid errors in CO measurements. A larger volume will produce a greater temperature change in the pulmonary circulation, which is interpreted by the monitor as a low CO. Conversely, a lesser volume will produce a smaller temperature change, which will be interpreted as a high CO.

If the injectate solution is at room temperature, producing very minor temperature changes the serial CO readings will be less reproducible. This is therefore the practical disadvantage of using a room temperature injectate instead of an ice cold solution. Similarly the reproducibility of the measurements may be affected despite using iced injectate, if there is a significant temperature change between the time the solution is drawn and the time it is injected. However, several systems are available today that measure the injectate temperature at the time it enters the proximal port of the PAC. This minimizes injectate temperature errors and improves the reproducibility of the measurements.

Continuous Cardiac Output Monitoring

Continuous CO measurements using thermodilution techniques are also available. Instead of cold water, a small heating filament at the end of the catheter warms the pulmonary blood and a downstream sensor records changes in temperature. These measurements are found to lag behind by a few minutes, but they are reliable and able to provide near real-time COs.

TABLE 5 Conditions affecting saturation of mixed venous oxygen (SvO_2).

Decrease in SvO_2	Increase in SvO_2
Poor O_2 supply • Decreased CO • Anemia • Hypoxic hypoxia	*Impaired O_2 utilization* • Sepsis • Cyanide poisoning
Excessive O_2 demand • Fever • Seizures • Increased metabolic rate • Increased physical activity	*Decrease in O_2 demand* • Hypothermia • Prolonged anesthesia

(*Source:* Sunavala JD. Cardiac monitoring in adults. In: Udwadia FE (Ed). Principles of Critical Care, 3rd edition. New Delhi: Jaypee Brothers Medical Publishers (P) Ltd.; 2014.)

Most minimally invasive and noninvasive methods, including continuous monitoring of SvO_2 or its surrogate central venous oxygen saturation ($ScVO_2$), described next, also enable continuous CO monitoring. For the physiological explanation pertaining to the relationship between SvO_2, $ScVO_2$, and CO refer to the earlier section on physiological aspects of hemodynamics and for the conditions affecting SvO_2, refer to **Table 5**.

Minimally Invasive Cardiac Output Monitoring

Systems requiring calibration: The pulse-induced contour cardiac output (PiCCO) requires calibration by transpulmonary thermodilution to obtain accurate CO measurements. It therefore requires a central venous line placement with a temperature sensor on the distal lumen and a thermodilution sensor at the arterial catheter end. Calibration is required to measure the aortic impedance and needs to be repeated at least every 8 hours in a hemodynamically stable patient and at shorter intervals under certain conditions. Once calibrated, the system computes left ventricular stroke volume (LVSV) by measuring the area under the systolic part of the arterial waveform, from end-diastole to the end of the ejection phase and then divides this area by the aortic impedance; the SV is thereby continuously monitored.

Self-calibrated devices: Methods like PiCCO, described earlier, require regular manual calibration from time to time, as they cannot automatically correct the patient's changing vascular tone. Therefore, the accuracy of these techniques is highly dependent on the delay between two normal calibrations and on the hemodynamic stability of the patient. A self-calibrated method (*FloTrac*/Vigileo, Edwards Life Sciences) has been in use since 2005 and the latest third-generation version is able to update the self-calibrated CO every 20 seconds. This is an improvement over the earlier generation software. The monitoring device consists of a transducer (FloTrac) that is connected to a standard radial or femoral arterial catheter and to a Vigileo monitor. It is important to keep the FloTrac sensor level to the phlebostatic axis at all times to ensure accuracy of CO.

Transesophageal doppler monitoring devices: Doppler ultrasound can provide a relatively noninvasive and continuous real-time quantification of CO. It involves inserting a flexible probe into the midthoracic esophagus where it lies in close proximity to the aorta, without any signal interference from other anatomical structures. A pulse wave Doppler transducer placed in the probe tip calculates the changes in blood flow velocity in the descending aorta. Aortic diameter is estimated by using a normogram after entering age, gender, height, and weight of the patient. The aortic diameter can also be assessed by M-mode echocardiography which allows for the actual measurement of the aortic diameter, eliminating the possible errors associated with normogram-based estimates. Once the cross-sectional area of the aorta is known, SV can be derived from the blood flow velocity (i.e., multiplying cross-sectional area of the aorta by blood flow velocity). As the measurements are made in the descending aorta, they represent only 70% of the total CO, since coronary and brachiocephalic flows are not measured, creating a partition between caudal and cephalic blood supply areas. Clinical validation studies initially had shown conflicting results; however, a recent meta-analysis reviewing all validation studies, confirms the reliability of CO measurement in clinical practice.

Transesophageal echocardiography (TOE): In this method, one uses a combined two-dimensional (2D) echo and Doppler approach to measure the CO. The 2D echo measures the diameter of the aortic annulus in midsystole which allows the calculation of the flow cross-sectional area; this, when multiplied by the velocity of blood flow across the aortic valve, measured by the aid of Doppler, gives the CO. It is necessary to ensure that blood flow is parallel to the path of the pulse wave Doppler ultrasound. In experienced hands, TOE can give valuable hemodynamic information and in addition can identify the presence of vegetations in infective endocarditis or pericardial effusion. The 2D echo measurement of aortic valve diameter is clinically well established and of proven accuracy; however, it is challenging, time-consuming, and requires training and skill. For instance, a wrongly measured diameter can be magnified when squared (as required in the equation) or if the angle between the Doppler beam and blood flow is not exact, it will lead to an underestimation of velocity.

Minimally Invasive Devices to Predict Preload Responsiveness
Stroke Volume Variation (SVV)

Earlier in this chapter we discussed the role of invasive PA catheterization in assessing the LVEDP by measuring the PCWP. However, filling pressures such as CVP/PCWP cannot predict preload (fluid) responsiveness. Hence parameters other than pressures need to be measured. Studies have shown that SVV in patients on MV is highly predictive of preload responsiveness. However, dynamic indicators lose their validity during spontaneous nonuniform breathing. Hence monitoring of SVV requires the patient to be on MV and properly sedated to attain uniform ventilation. Similarly, these parameters will lose their predictive value in presence of irregular R-R intervals, as in atrial fibrillation. SVV ≥10%, predicts an increase in CO of ≥15% for a bolus of 500 mL of fluid. SVV can be assessed directly by the esophageal Doppler or by pulse pressure analysis using devices such as PiCCO, LIDCO, or FloTrac systems described earlier in this chapter.

Arterial Pulse Pressure Variation (PPV)

Pulse pressure variation is a fairly reliable alternative, being more practical and showing reasonable accuracy. Arterial pulse pressure, defined as the difference between systolic and diastolic pressures, is directly proportional to LV SV and inversely related to arterial compliance. Hence the respiratory variations in the pulse pressures reflect the changes in LV SV and become a marker for preload dependence. PPV is calculated as a percentage, i.e., PPV% = (Ppmax – Ppmin)/ [(Ppmax – Ppmim)/2] × 100, where Ppmax is the difference between maximum systolic and maximum diastolic pressures and Ppmin is the difference between the minimum systolic and minimum diastolic pressures. A PPV of >13% implies 85% probability that the patient will benefit by fluid administration. Once again here, the parameters will lose their predictive value and accuracy under conditions of varying RR intervals (atrial fibrillation) or varying tidal volumes; hence the patient has to be sedated and on MV during the measurements.

Entirely noninvasive methods that predict the response of the ventricles to fluid loading is the measurement of the IVC diameter during respiratory variations by an M-mode echocardiography. This method is best applicable to the patient with a good window which may not be always possible in critically ill patients.

Passive Leg Raising (PLR)

Passive leg raising is a test that predicts whether CO increases with volume expansion without external fluid infusion, as mentioned earlier in this chapter. PLR mimics fluid challenge by transfusing approximately 250 ± 50 mL of venous blood from the lower body towards the RA. This test is reasonably reliable and should be used when indices of fluid responsiveness using dynamic measurements such as SVV and PPV cannot be used in patients who are spontaneously breathing or in those who have serious arrhythmias or low tidal volumes. The methodology of PLR is of utmost important and should be followed as under:

- PLR should always start from a semirecumbent position (45°) and not supine position.
- Leg raising is done along with lowering of the trunk flat on the bed. Leg elevation should be 30–45°. This maneuver should be preferably performed by bed adjustment.

- Assess PLR by directly measuring the CO and not the BP. Use a real-time measurement of CO.
- Reassessment of CO should be done in the original semirecumbent position which should return to baseline.
- Increase in CO by 10–15% during PLR, gives a reliable prediction of central hypovolemia and is a reliable assessment of fluid responsiveness.

SUMMARY

The indications to do HM will always rest on the clinician's judgment regards the application of the measurements: (1) Would these measurements change or affect therapeutic decisions? (2) Is the intensivist well trained to obtain accurate and reliable measurements and competent to interpret them vis-a-vis the clinical setting?

In most centers in India, CVP monitoring is common and may be applied where sophisticated hemodynamic devices are not available, *provided its limitations are fully understood.*

Catheter-induced sepsis is one of the most common long-term complications of invasive monitoring devices; hence strict asepsis is to be maintained. Further, one should be very circumspect and judicious before application of any invasive monitoring.

One of the most common applications of HM in ICU today is to ensure appropriate fluid resuscitation and obtain optimal level of preload to improve SV. Static measurements like CVP or PCWP have their limitations and pressure measurements like LVEDP do not express preload responsiveness. Dynamic measurements such as PPV/SVV are more reliable in demonstrating response towards SV following a fluid challenge, but they too have certain limitations. The clinical response of the patient to a volume challenge, even today, is the sheet anchor to gauge the presence or absence of ventricular responsiveness to an increase in preload.

SUGGESTED READING

1. Allsager CM, Swanevelder J. Measuring cardiac output. Br J Anaesth. 2003;3:15-9.
2. Bongard FS, Sue DY. Critical Care Monitoring. In: Bongard FS, Sue DY (Eds). Current Critical Care Diagnosis and Treatment. USA: Appleton and Lange; 1994. pp. 170-90.
3. Brain F, Dellinger P. Lactate as a hemodynamic marker in the critically ill. Curr Opinion Crit Care. 2012;18(3):267-72.
4. Carsetti A, Cecconi M, Rhodes A. Fluid bolus therapy: monitoring and predicting fluid responsiveness. Curr Opin Crit Care. 2015;21(5):388-94.
5. Cavallaro F, Sandroni C, Marano C, Torre GL, Mannocci A, Waure CD, et al. Diagnostic accuracy of passive leg raising for prediction of fluid responsiveness in adults: systematic review and meta-analysis of clinical studies. Intensive Care Med. 2010;26:1475-83.
6. Dalen JE, Bone RC. Is it time to pull the pulmonary catheter? JAMA. 1996;276:916-8.
7. Dalen JE. The pulmonary artery catheter: friend, foe or accomplice? JAMA. 2001;286(3):348-50.
8. Kumar A, Anel R, Bunnell E, Habet K, Zanotti S, Marshall S, et al. Pulmonary artery occlusion pressure and CVP fail to predict ventricular filling volume, cardiac

performance or the response to volume infusion in normal subjects. Crit Care Med. 2004;32(3):691-9.
9. Leone M, Asfar P, Radermacher P, Vincent J-L, Martin C. Optimizing mean arterial pressure in septic shock: a critical reappraisal of the literature. Crit Care. 2015;19(1):101.
10. Mayer J, Boldt J, Poland R, Peterson A, Manecke GR Jr. Continuous arterial pressure waveform-based cardiac output using the FloTrac/Vigileo: a review an meta-analysis. J Cardiothorac Vasc Anesth. 2009;23:401-6.
11. Monnet X, Marik P, Teboul J. Prediction of fluid responsiveness: an update. Ann Intensive Care. 2016;6(1):111.
12. Oren-Grinberg A. The PiCCO monitor. Int Anesthesiol Clin. 210;48:57-85.
13. Parienti J, Mongardon N, Mégarbane B, Mira J-P, Kalfon P, Gros A, et al. Intravascular complications of central venous catheterization by insertion site. N Engl J Med. 2015;373(13):1220-9.
14. Pinsky MR. Hemodynamic evaluation and monitoring in the ICU. Chest. 2007;132:2020-9.
15. Pulmonary Artery Catheter Conference: Consensus Statement. Crit Care Med. 1997;25:910-25.
16. Rivers E, Nguyen B, Havstad S, Ressler J, Muzzin A, Knoblich B, et al. Early goal-directed therapy in the treatment of severe sepsis and septic shock. N Engl J Med. 2001;345(19):1368-77.
17. Roche AM, Miller TE, Gan TJ. Goal-directed fluid management with transoesophageal Doppler. Best Pract Res Clin Anaesthesiol. 2009;23:327-34.
18. Sunavala JD. Cardiac monitoring in adults. In: Udwadia FE (Ed). Principles of Critical Care, 3rd edition. New Delhi: Jaypeee Brothers Medical Publishers (P) Ltd.; 2014.
19. Sunavala JD. Procedures in the Intensive Care Unit. In: Udwadia FE (Ed). Principles of Critical Care, 3rd edition. New Delhi: Jaypeee Brothers Medical Publishers (P) Ltd.; 2014.
20. Teboul J, Saugel B, Cecconi M. Less invasive hemodynamic monitoring in critically ill patients. Intensive Care Med. 2016;42(9):1350-9.
21. Vincent J, Rhodes A, Perel A, Martin GS, Rocca GD, Vallet B, et al. Clinical review: Update on hemodynamic monitoring—a consensus of 16. Crit Care. 2011;15(4):229.

CHAPTER 25

Arterial Blood Gases and Acid-base Abnormalities

Jamshed Sunavala

■ INTRODUCTION

Acid-base imbalance can occur in any serious disease state where the body's regulatory mechanism fails to maintain a normal pH of our body fluids. Acid-base disorder is common in critically ill patients and needs to be identified immediately and promptly corrected. To keep the pH in the optimal range of 7.35–7.45, the body employs compensatory mechanisms like the buffer systems. The term metabolic or respiratory acidosis refers to a pH <7.35 secondary to a metabolic or respiratory disorder respectively and likewise, metabolic and respiratory alkalosis refer to a pH >7.45 secondary to metabolic or respiratory disorders respectively. Hence these four acid-base disturbances are classified as primary disorders. Each of the primary disturbances has a compensatory response which attempts to correct the pH towards the normal. Critically ill patients may manifest with more complex forms of acid-base disorders (mixed acid-base disorders). Respiratory acidosis is characterized by a primary increase in arterial partial pressure of carbon dioxide ($PaCO_2$) (above 45 mm Hg) secondary to hypoventilation, and type II or hypercapnic respiratory failure results when the $PaCO_2$ is increased >50 mm Hg. Respiratory alkalosis occurs when the patient hyperventilates and washes out the $PaCO_2$, which falls below 35 mm Hg (common causes and detailed discussion on the types of respiratory failure are given in the Chapter on Acute Respiratory Failure). The abnormalities of metabolic acid-base disturbances are reviewed in this chapter.

■ BASIC CONCEPT

It is the hydrogen ion (H^+) concentration in the body fluids that defines the acid-base balance, though, rightfully the (H^+) are protons which do not exist in isolation in the body fluids but react with water to form hydronium ions. Further, the absolute concentration of (H^+) in plasma is miniscule and is measured in nmole/L, which is difficult to manipulate and requires an extremely sensitive process in order to maintain it within the narrow limits of normality; hence the concept of pH was developed. The pH is the negative logarithm of (H^+) concentration [pH = –log(H^+)] and is not expressed as specific units. The normal value of pH is 7.4 and it represents 40 nmole/L of (H^+), the normal range being 7.35–7.45. As pH is a negative log of (H^+), the lower the pH in the arterial blood, the greater the (H^+), and greater the acidity; likewise, higher the pH, lower the (H^+), and greater the alkalinity.

The disorders of acid-base imbalance are governed by the equation of the bicarbonate-carbon dioxide buffer system:

$$H_2O + CO_2 \overset{\text{Lungs} \uparrow\uparrow}{\longleftrightarrow} H_2CO_3 \longleftrightarrow H^+ + HCO_3^- \downarrow \text{Kidneys}$$

This equation explains how the excessive acid accumulation in the body is prevented. There are two classes of acids—the carbonic acid (H_2CO_3) and the noncarbonic acid which are generated daily in the body. The H_2CO_3 is generated by the metabolism of carbohydrates and fats; in fact it is the large amount of CO_2 which is generated, which combines with H_2O to form H_2CO_3 and the excess CO_2 is washed out by alveolar ventilation. Hence, if alveolar hypoventilation occurs for any reason, there would be progressive accumulation of acid in the body. The noncarbonic acid is primarily generated by the metabolism of proteins and is eliminated initially by combining with bicarbonates, and subsequently excreted as (H^+) and HCO_3^- by the kidneys.

The buffer system which helps to maintain the normal pH in the blood acts by counteracting the effects of excessive acid or alkali to reestablish the acid-base equilibrium by correcting the primary imbalance. The primary respiratory imbalance (acidosis or alkalosis) is compensated by the metabolic component through the bicarbonate buffer system, and the primary metabolic imbalance (acidosis or alkalosis) is compensated by respiratory component by eliminating or retaining CO_2.

Respiratory compensation (by hyperventilation) in metabolic acidosis begins immediately (within 6 hours), although it may take up to 24 hours for full or near complete compensation to occur. However, in metabolic alkalosis, the compensatory respiratory response (hypoventilation) also begins immediately, but is not as vigorous as in metabolic acidosis. This is because the chemical chemoreceptors even in the normal state are easier to stimulate than suppress, and particularly so with underlying cardiopulmonary complications; this weak response is clinically evidenced by a borderline elevation of $PaCO_2$. In contrast, the renal compensation in chronic respiratory acid-base disorders develops slowly. Here the kidney compensates for the changes in the $PaCO_2$ by adjusting the excretion of bicarbonate and (H^+) accordingly. The near complete compensation may take up to 72 hours or more. In acute respiratory acid-base disorder the compensation is rapid but incomplete as there is a small effect on plasma HCO_3 **(Table 2)**. Hence normal or near normal HCO_3 indicates that the respiratory disorder is acute.

The Henderson–Hasselbalch equation explains the relationship between the blood pH and the acid-base balance determined by the main H_2CO_3/HCO_3 buffer system. The equation is best explained as:

$$pH = pK + \log \frac{[HCO_3^-]}{[H_2CO_3]}$$

As concentration of H_2CO_3 is difficult to measure because it is present in the blood in very small quantities as compared with the dissolved CO_2, and since H_2CO_3 is in equilibrium with dissolved CO_2 (measured as $PaCO_2$), the latter can be substituted for H_2CO_3. The equation can thus be rewritten as:

$$pH = pK + \log \frac{[HCO_3^-]}{[0.03 \, PaCO_2]}$$

Where pK is the negative log of the dissociation constant of carbonic acid, and has the value of 6.1. The constant 0.03 converts $PaCO_2$ from mm Hg to nmole/L. To intelligently integrate acid-base disorders, one simply needs to understand that the equation points to the fact that pH is a ratio of HCO_3^- to $PaCO_2$. Hence, for all practical purposes this can be simplified as:

$$pH = \frac{HCO_3^- (kidneys)}{PaCO_2 (lungs)}$$

Since the kidneys affect HCO_3 and change it slowly and the lung washes out $PaCO_2$ rapidly, the ratio can be viewed as slow over fast. This concept shows why pH corrects slowly in respiratory events where bicarbonates are involved as buffers, and rapidly when $PaCO_2$ is washed out by the lungs by hyperventilation in metabolic acidosis.

Metabolic alkalosis is mainly the rise in plasma bicarbonate concentration due to loss of hydrogen ions from the gastrointestinal tract (e.g., from vomiting) and from the urine (e.g., with diuretic therapy). It is reflected on arterial blood gas (ABG) reports with high pH and HCO_3 values. The major causes of metabolic alkalosis in intensive care unit (ICU) patients are given in **Table 1**.

Metabolic acidosis is a common primary acid-base disorder witnessed in the ICU setting. Here the ABG is manifested by a low pH and a low HCO_3^- value. However, the ABG alone will not be able to differentiate between the types of metabolic acidosis. Hence, it is useful to measure the anion gap (AG). An elevated AG discloses the unmeasured anions (UA) such as lactates or ketones; whereas a normal AG is seen in hyperchloremic acidosis where the loss of HCO_3^- is replaced by chlorides (further details are given in the section on interpretation of ABG).

TABLE 1 Causes of metabolic alkalosis.

Chloride responsive (urinary chloride < 15 mEq/L)	Chloride resistant (urinary chloride > 25 mEq/L)
H = Hypovolemia (contraction alkalosis)	C = **C**ushing syndrome
A = **A**ntacids (nonabsorbable)	R = **R**enovascular hypertension
N = **N**asogastric aspiration and vomiting	A = Primary **a**ldosteronism
D = **D**iuretics (thiazides and loop diuretics)	M = Severe hypo**m**agnesemia
	P = Severe **p**otassium depletion
	S = **S**teroids (exogenous glucocorticoids or mineralocorticoids)

Acid-base imbalance could be simple or complex. Simple acid-base disorders consist of the primary disorders and their secondary or compensatory responses. However, in the critical care setting, the acid-base imbalance can be more complex where we see mixed acid-base disorders. As per the rule of compensation, the direction of the compensation should be the same as of the primary disturbances; in short, the $PaCO_2$ and HCO_3 will always move in the same direction **(Table 2)**. However, when correlating pH and $PaCO_2$, both variables move in the same direction for metabolic events, and in the opposite direction for respiratory events **(Table 3)**. Remembering these correlations is useful for a rapid interpretation of acid-base imbalance.

TABLE 2 Primary acid-base disorders and their secondary response.

Primary acid-base disorder	Primary disturbance	Secondary response	Magnitude of response	Expected response (Ex)	Time to complete compensation
Metabolic acidosis	↓ HCO_3	⇓ $PaCO_2$	Δ $PaCO_2$ = 1.2 × Δ HCO_3	Ex $PaCO_2$ = 40 − [1.2 × (24−ms HCO_3)]	12–24 hours
Metabolic alkalosis	↑ HCO_3	⇑ $PaCO_2$	Δ $PaCO_2$ = 0.7 × Δ HCO_3	Ex $PaCO_2$ = 40 + [0.7 × (ms HCO_3−24)]	12–24 hours
Acute respiratory acidosis	↑ $PaCO_2$	⇑ HCO_3	Δ HCO_3 = 0.1 × Δ $PaCO_2$	Ex HCO_3 = 24 + [0.1 × (ms $PaCO_2$ − 40)]	<6 hours*
Acute respiratory alkalosis	↓ $PaCO_2$	⇓ HCO_3	Δ HCO_3 = 0.2 × Δ $PaCO_2$	Ex HCO_3 = 24 + [0.2 × (40 − ms $PaCO_2$)]	<6 hours*
Chronic respiratory acidosis	↑ $PaCO_2$	⇑ HCO_3	Δ HCO_3 = 0.4 × Δ $PaCO_2$	Ex HCO_3 = 24 + [0.4 × (ms $PaCO_2$ − 40)]	>5 days
Chronic respiratory alkalosis	↓ $PaCO_2$	⇓ HCO_3	Δ HCO_3 = 0.4 × Δ $PaCO_2$	Ex HCO_3 = 24 + [0.4 × (40 − ms $PaCO_2$)]	>7 days

Δ: Change from normal value (normal values of $PaCO_2$ and HCO_3 is taken as 40 mm Hg and 24 mEq/L in the above equation)
↓↑: Direction of primary disturbances
⇓⇑: Direction of secondary disturbance
ms: Measured value
$PaCO_2$: Arterial partial pressure of carbon dioxide
*Incomplete compensation with near normal HCO_3

TABLE 3: Groupwise, the eight possibilities of primary acid-base disorder (corrected pH vs. $PaCO_2$). See text for interpretation

Group	pH	$PaCO_2$	Acid-base disorders
Group 1	↓	↑	Respiratory acidosis
Group 1	↑	↓	Respiratory alkalosis
Group 1	↓	↓	Metabolic acidosis
Group 1	↑	↑	Metabolic alkalosis
Group 2	N/NN	↑	*Chronic respiratory acidosis or mixed disorders:* Respiratory acidosis and metabolic alkalosis
Group 2	N/NN	↓	*Chronic respiratory alkalosis or mixed disorders:* Metabolic acidosis and respiratory alkalosis
Group 3	↓↓	N/NN	*Mixed disorder:* Metabolic acidosis and respiratory acidosis
Group 3	↑↑	N/NN	*Mixed disorder:* Metabolic alkalosis and respiratory alkalosis

(N/NN: normal or near normal; $PaCO_2$: arterial partial pressure of carbon dioxide)

TABLE 4: Possible causes of mixed acid-base disorders in intensive care unit (ICU) setting.

Causes	Acid-base disorders
• Septic shock • Salicylate over dosage	High anion gap (AG) metabolic acidosis + respiratory alkalosis
Cardiorespiratory arrest	High AG metabolic acidosis + respiratory acidosis
Use of diuretics or vomiting in a patient with a chronic lung disease	Metabolic alkalosis + respiratory acidosis
Vomiting or use of diuretics in a patient with ketoacidosis or lactic acidosis	Metabolic alkalosis + high AG metabolic acidosis
Use of diuretic or vomiting in a patient of hepatic failure; pneumonia with vomiting	Metabolic alkalosis + respiratory alkalosis
Diarrhea in a patient with lactic acidosis	Hyperchloremic non-AG metabolic acidosis + high AG, metabolic acidosis

Mixed acid-base disorders are common in the critically ill patients and they generally manifest in patients with severe primary disorders. For instance, a severe respiratory acidosis with a $PaCO_2$ > 75 mm Hg is more likely to have an accompanying metabolic disorder than a $PaCO_2$ of 50 or 60 mm Hg; this is because these cases are more likely to have a concomitant cardiovascular event with hypotension and low cardiac output with lactic acidosis. The various mixed disorders are given in **Table 4**. A mixed acid-base disorder

> **BOX 1** Six steps to interpretation of ABG.
>
> 1. First look
>   - Is the ABG abnormal?
>   - Is the ABG physiologically correct? ($H^+ = 24$ ($PaCO_2/HCO_3$))
>   - Is it roughly compatible with clinical findings (e.g., shock and lactic acid acidosis; hyperventilation, and respiratory alkalosis)
>   - Does it suggest a critical condition?
> 2. Determine the type of acid-base disorder
> 3. Determine the degree of compensation (secondary response)
> 4. Assess mixed acid-base disorders
> 5. Calculate the gaps to assess the causes of metabolic acidosis
> 6. Analysis of metabolic alkalosis
>
> (ABG: arterial blood gas; $PaCO_2$: arterial partial pressure of carbon dioxide)

is usually recognized as having a normal or near normal pH in presence of an abnormal $PaCO_2$, or a normal or near normal $PaCO_2$ in presence of a pH which is out of range. Metabolic acidosis with metabolic alkalosis is possible as in a patient with vomiting and lactic acidosis or ketoacidosis; however, respiratory acidosis with alkalosis is not possible for obvious reasons, as one cannot hypoventilate and hyperventilate at the same time. Further details are discussed in the section on interpretation of ABG.

■ INTERPRETATION OF ARTERIAL BLOOD GASES

To unravel the cause of acid-base imbalance and the associated diagnosis, a stepwise approach as given in **Box 1** would be most appropriate. This is important because not all acid-base disturbances are straightforward in a critically ill patient and need to be analyzed with an astute understanding of the underlying correlation between the variables involved in leading to acid-base disorders. The following stepwise approach should begin with the "first look" of the ABG report.

Step 1: "First Look" (Box 1)

In the very "first look" one should establish if the ABG is abnormal and if so, is it physiologically correct, does it suggest a critical condition, and is the ABG report acceptable for the suggestive diagnosis. *If anyone variable of the Henderson–Hasselbalch equation is outside the normal limits, it should be accepted as abnormal and needs further scrutiny.*

The ABG report should not always be accepted at face value as it may not be physiologically correct and may misdiagnose an acid-base disorder. To ascertain the physiologically correct values of ABG one may refer to the following equation:

$$(H^+) = 24 \times \frac{PaCO_2}{HCO_3}$$

TABLE 5	Relationship of H⁺ ion concentration and pH (pH is log function of H⁺).								
pH	≤6	7	7.1	7.2	7.3	7.4	7.5	7.6	≥7.7
H^+ (mEq/L)	≥126	100	80	64	50	40	32	25	≤20

where pH is substituted by (H^+) (**Table 5**). *However, this equation will apply only to primary acid-base disorders with secondary response.*

Lastly, with a "first look" of the ABG report one should immediately be able to assess the underlying severity of the respiratory and metabolic derangements. This of course needs to be correlated with the clinical findings and other relevant variables. The most important variant that should raise a "red flag" is the pH. A pH < 7.25 would indicate an imminent emergency involving a critical situation usually encountered in the ICU, such as shock, organ failure, and other life-threatening cardiorespiratory and metabolic complications.

Step 2: Correlate pH and $PaCO_2$ to Determine the Type of Acid-base Disorder

Correlating these two variables will immediately give a clue to the following:
- Indicate type of primary disorder
- Indicate a possibility of a chronic disorder
- Indicate a possibility of a mixed disorder

All the above three entities could be divided into three groups for convenience of immediate diagnosis (*see* **Table 3**).

- *Group 1*: pH and $PaCO_2$ are both abnormal; helps to diagnose the four primary acid-base disorder
- *Group 2*: pH is normal or near normal, but $PaCO_2$ is abnormal; helps to indicate a possibility of mixed disorder or may also suggest a chronic disorder
- *Group 3*: $PaCO_2$ is normal or near normal, but pH is abnormal; helps to indicate a possibility of a mixed acid-acid or alkali-alkali disorder (**Table 3**)
- *Note how the pH and $PaCO_2$ change in opposite directions in respiratory disorders and change in the same direction in metabolic disorders.*
- Note that a possibility of a mixed metabolic acidosis + alkalosis exists. For example, lactic acidosis or ketoacidosis with vomiting; however, for obvious reasons, mixed respiratory acidosis + alkalosis is not possible as mentioned earlier.
- One may be curious to know the reason for correlating pH with $PaCO_2$ to identify all the four primary disorders and wonder why one cannot directly correlate pH with HCO_3 for metabolic disorders. The reason is the time lag; as unlike CO_2 which is a rapid buffer, HCO_3 is a slow buffer and may take long to change. Hence in the early period of the disorder, the HCO_3 may not show any significant compensatory change.

Step 3: Correlating PaCO₂ to HCO₃—for Assessing Compensation

Correlating $PaCO_2$ to HCO_3 helps to assess the magnitude of compensation. *As a rule, the $PaCO_2$ and HCO_3 always move in the same direction.* The equation to assess the compensation is given in **Table 2**.

Secondary response can be defined as the means of limiting the change of pH in the primary disorder by the buffer systems, so as to keep the pH more towards normal. The terms secondary and compensatory responses are used synonymously by most physicians, though the secondary response does not correct the change in pH completely, whereas compensation implies a complete shift of the pH towards normal or near normal values and this can be ascertained by the compensation equations shown in the **Table 2**. Secondary response to metabolic acidosis is hyperventilation, which is reflected by a decreasing $PaCO_2$ value which will begin within 6 hours, but may take even up to 24 hours to completely compensate (*see* **Table 2**) and the magnitude of the response is measured by the change in $PaCO_2$ from the accepted normal of 40 mm Hg. In metabolic acidosis, it is assessed by the equation $\Delta PaCO_2 = 1.2 \times \Delta HCO_3$. For example, if the expected final value of $PaCO_2$ (i.e., $40 - \Delta PaCO_2$) is 25 as full compensation for that degree of metabolic acidosis, then we have the following possibilities:

- $PaCO_2$ shows full compensation of 25 mm Hg and the pH returns to near normal—in that case, the diagnosis would a "completely compensated metabolic acidosis"
- $PaCO_2$ is >25 mm Hg (i.e., towards 40 mm Hg), but pH has still not returned to normal and remained below 7.35—in this case, the diagnosis then would be "partially corrected metabolic acidosis" and the incomplete $PaCO_2$ shift is termed as a secondary response
- $PaCO_2$ is >25 mm Hg (i.e., towards near normal value of 40 mm Hg) and the pH is markedly low. This could be a possible mixed disorder of metabolic acidosis with respiratory acidosis, mainly because the $PaCO_2$ is grossly undercorrected for the compensation of metabolic acidosis and the pH is markedly low because of the double impact on acidosis
- $PaCO_2$ is <25 mm Hg (i.e., towards 0) and the pH is normal or near normal. The possible diagnosis would be a mixed disorder of metabolic acidosis and respiratory alkalosis. This is because the $PaCO_2$ is overcorrected more than expected and the pH is neutralized. More examples of mixed disorders are given in step 4.

Similarly, it works for other primary disorders when the expected compensation is normal, overcorrected, or undercorrected.

For the calculation of the equations consider the reference value of $PaCO_2$ as 40 mm Hg and HCO_3 as 24 mEq/L.

Step 4: Assessing Mixed Acid-base Disorders (Table 6)

As a general rule, more severe the primary acid-base disorder, the higher the likelihood of a mixed disorder, hence critically ill patients often suffer from a

TABLE 6	Mixed disorders.	
pH	PaCO$_2$	Acid-base disorders
N/NN pH	↑ PaCO$_2$	Respiratory acidosis + Metabolic alkalosis
N/NN pH	↓ PaCO$_2$	Respiratory alkalosis + Metabolic acidosis
↓ pH	N/NN (PaCO$_2$)	Metabolic acidosis + Respiratory acidosis
↑ pH	N/NN (PaCO$_2$)	Metabolic alkalosis + Respiratory alkalosis

(N/NN: normal or near normal value; PaCO$_2$: arterial partial pressure of carbon dioxide; ↑: high value; ↓: low value)

mixed disorder. This is because a critically ill patient with a severe primary acid-base disorder will often be having an underlying severe hypoxemia or hemodynamic compromise.

Usually a combination of two acid-base disorders is seen, but at times a combination of three disorders may occur. The clinical settings in which these mixed disorders occur are given in **Table 4**.

A simple observation of the primary acid-base variables and their unexpected secondary responses will help you to suspect mixed disorders as in the following examples:

- *Metabolic acidosis*: If the level of PaCO$_2$ is higher (towards 40) than expected for a complete compensation (undercorrected), there is an associated respiratory acidosis and if it is lower than expected (overcorrected), there is an associated respiratory alkalosis.
- *Metabolic alkalosis*: If the level of PaCO$_2$ is higher than the limits of expected compensation (overcorrected), there is an associated respiratory acidosis and if the level of PaCO$_2$ is lower than the expected, there is an associated respiratory alkalosis.
- *Respiratory acidosis*: Here the level of expected compensation would be a mild increase in bicarbonate level in the acute phase (<2 days), and a further rise in bicarbonate is expected if the acidosis is chronic. If the level of bicarbonate is less than the expected, then associated metabolic acidosis is likely, and if it more than the expected there is a likelihood of an associated metabolic alkalosis. However, the allowance for the expected level would depend on the phase of respiratory acidosis.
- *Respiratory alkalosis*: Similar to respiratory acidosis, there is a mild or greater fall in the expected levels of bicarbonate depending on the mild or chronic phase of respiratory alkalosis, respectively. Again, after allowance for the phase of respiratory alkalosis, if the fall in bicarbonate level is more than expected, then there is an associated metabolic acidosis, and if the fall is less than expected, there is an associated metabolic alkalosis.

To diagnose mixed metabolic acidosis and metabolic alkalosis requires an understanding of the "AG—bicarbonate" relationship, which is discussed in the next step of diagnosing the causes of metabolic acidosis. This would happen, for example, if a patient with an increased AG acidosis following uremia were to develop concomitant alkalosis due to retention of HCO_3 due to loss of gastric HCl following vomiting. Here, one would expect a marked increase of AG and decreased HCO_3^-, but instead the magnitude of decrease in bicarbonate is less than expected and is more near normal. For obvious reasons, a similar picture for respiratory events is not possible as respiratory acidosis and alkalosis cannot coexist.

Triple acid-base disorders, though not commonly seen, may manifest in a patient with severe hepatic failure. They develop metabolic acidosis due to uremia, diarrhea, or lactic acidosis; metabolic alkalosis due to excessive vomiting or nasogastric aspiration or diuretics; and they may develop respiratory alkalosis due to hyperventilation which is centrally provoked secondary the high levels of ammonia. A clinical suspicion and correlation is essential to diagnose triple disorders.

Step 5: Calculate the Gaps to Know the Causes of Metabolic Acidosis

Anion Gap

The plasma AG helps to distinguish between the various causes of metabolic acidosis **(Table 7)**. AG is the difference between the serum cations and the anions as measured routinely in the laboratory; hence AG is a rough estimation of the unmeasured anions (UA). However, in actuality the concentration of all cations in plasma is equal to the sum of all anions in order to maintain an electrochemical neutrality. The anions that are not normally measured in the regular blood chemistry panel are mainly albumin, phosphates, and sulfates. AG is calculated as per the following equation:

$$AG = (Na^+ + K^+) - (Cl^- + HCO_3^-)$$

The normal AG is approximately 8–12 mEq/L, though this varies with different laboratories ranging from 8 to 16 mEq/L.

TABLE 7 Causes of metabolic acidosis.

Normal anion gap (AG)	High AG
D = **D**iarrhea	G = Ethylene **g**lycol ingestion
R = **R**enal	O = **O**xoproline
• Renal tubular acidosis (RTA)	L = **L**actic acidosis
• Early renal insufficiency	D = **D**-lactic acid
I = **I**atrogenic	M = **M**ethanol
• Rapid isotonic saline infusion	A = **A**spirin (salicylate toxicity)
• Calcium chloride	R = End-stage **R**enal failure
• Magnesium sulfate causing diarrhea	K = **K**etoacidosis
• Cholestyramine causing bile acid diarrhea	
• Ileal conduits	
P = **P**ancreatic fistula	

There is however one pitfall in the interpretation of the AG. The AG is proportional to the plasma albumin concentration; hence in severe hypoalbuminemia, the baseline normal value of AG is falsely lowered and may mask the presence of a high AG metabolic acidosis. This, of course can be corrected by using the following equation:

Corrected AG = measured AG + 2.5 (4.5 − measured albumin mg%)

Causes of high AG metabolic acidosis (Table 7): The causes of high AG metabolic acidosis in critically ill patients are limited and the most commonly encountered is lactic acid acidosis.

Lactic acid acidosis: Causes of lactic acid acidosis are divided into type A and type B. In ICU patients, type A is commonly seen in conditions like shock or severe oxygen desaturation depriving oxygen supply to the tissues; whereas type B is secondary to excessive lactate production (sepsis or thiamine deficiency), decreased lactate metabolism (liver failure), or impaired oxygen utilization by the tissues (metformin, acetaminophen, cyanide poisoning, and certain antiretroviral agents) and beta-agonist agents. "GOLDMARK" is a useful mnemonic to memorize the important causes of high AG metabolic acidosis **(Table 7)**, which was coined by Mehta et al. (Lancet 2008). *D-lactic acidosis* occurs in a subset of patients with high AG metabolic acidosis following accumulation of D-lactate. It usually does not show up in the blood on normal testing and if it does, it is only borderline high (2–3 mmol/L). This is because D-lactate cannot be sensed by the routine blood gas analyzer which measures only the L-lactate form. *L-lactate* form is the commonly seen lactic acidosis in clinical practice. D-lactate acidosis occurs in patients with small bowel resection or jejunoileal bypass where large amounts of carbohydrates are directly delivered to the colon, which otherwise would have been reabsorbed in the small intestine in patients with a normal gut. The high load of carbohydrates delivered to the colon is metabolized into D-lactate by the colonic bacteria and is absorbed in the circulation. Hence, following a heavy carbohydrate diet, these groups of patients may succumb to metabolic acidosis with neurological abnormalities such as confusion and ataxia.

Ketoacidosis: Ketoacidosis is the next most common cause of high AG metabolic acidosis in ICU practice. Accumulation of ketone bodies is responsible for diabetic ketoacidosis (DKA) and alcoholic ketoacidosis. Acetoacetate and beta-hydroxybutyrate (both acids) are the main ketone bodies in the plasma which are neutralized by the bicarbonates. As the bicarbonates are used up it leads to high AG metabolic acidosis in both these disorders. However, in patients with alcoholic ketoacidosis, beta-hydroxybutyrate is the primary ketoacid but it cannot be detected by using the nitroprusside test for ketonuria, because nitroprusside can estimate only the acetone and acetoacetate in DKA. In starvation ketoacidosis, there is excessive lipolysis leading to ketonuria as a result of increased ketone bodies excreted in the urine.

Advanced renal failure: Another important cause of high AG metabolic disorder is advanced renal failure where glomerular filtration rate (GFR) is <20 mL/minute. Here, the decreased ammonia production required for buffering the (H^+) in the urine along with the low excretion of phosphate, sulfates, and urates (as a result of the decreased GFR) are the main causes of high AG metabolic acidosis.

- In *liver failure,* the high AG metabolic acidosis is due to the impaired lactate clearance.
- Toxic alcohols

Methanol and ethylene glycol are toxic alcohols and can result in accumulation of toxic metabolites with associated high AG metabolic acidosis when ingested. Methanol leads to formation of an organic acid (formic) which can further lead to acidosis, blindness, and pancreatitis. Immediate administration of $NaHCO_3$ reverses the acidosis thereby lessening the tissue penetration of the toxins. Fomepizole (4 methylpyrazole) is a competitive inhibitor and serves to block the formation of formate, which is a toxic substance. In severe cases, hemodialysis is indicated to expel the toxic metabolites.

Ethyl alcohol after ingestion is metabolized to glycolic and oxalic acid, which can result in metabolic acidosis and kidney injury, respectively. Treatment is the same as for methanol toxicity.

Toxins: Isoniazid (INH) overdose can inhibit gamma-aminobutyric acid (GABA) synthesis, thereby lowering the threshold for seizures. Here high AG metabolic acidosis is a result of the interference of INH with nicotinamide dinucleotide, which is a cofactor in the conversion of lactate to pyruvate. Pyridoxine is the treatment for INH overdose as it is an essential cofactor for production of GABA.

Salicylate overdose can lead to fatal consequences. The hallmark of salicylate intoxication is a combined respiratory alkalosis with a high AG metabolic acidosis. Salicylate overdose can directly stimulate the respiratory center leading to hyperventilation and lowering of $PaCO_2$ resulting in respiratory alkalosis. However, it is also responsible for the increased production of lactic acid causing lactic acid acidosis. Primarily, it may present with respiratory alkalosis, following severe toxicity and increasing lactic acid production; however, the $PaCO_2$ may eventually start rising and this is a foreboding sign of a poor prognosis. Management includes general supportive measures such as fluid resuscitation and ventilator support; activated charcoal may help if given within 2–3 hours of the drug overdose. However, the most important aspect of management is alkalinization of urine with administration of $NaHCO_3$ which enhances the renal elimination of salicylates. Hemodialysis is indicated in severe cases as it is the most effective method of eliminating salicylates from the body.

Causes of nonanion gap acidosis (Table 7): Loss of alkali (HCO_3) can occur from the gastrointestinal tract as in diarrhea or from the kidney as in renal tubular acidosis (RTA). The loss of HCO_3 causes a reciprocal increase in chlorides in the blood, resulting in a *hyperchloremic* (non-AG metabolic) acidosis. The usual causes of non-AG metabolic acidosis are listed in **Table 7** and these are rarely life-threatening in comparison to the high AG metabolic acidosis and they resolve on correction of the underlying cause. A good mnemonic for the four common causes of non-AG metabolic acidosis seen in the ICU setting is "Diarrhea, Renal causes, Iatrogenic and Pancreatic fistula (DRIP)".

Gastrointestinal cause: The loss of bicarbonate-rich fluid in diarrhea, urethral diversions using ileal conduits and pancreatic fistulae are responsible for the acidosis. Loss of excessive fluid in diarrhea is corrected by replacement of appropriate fluids. In urethral diversions using ileal conduits, the chloride from the urine enters the colon and is reabsorbed in exchange for bicarbonate by the colonic mucosa, which leads to gastrointestinal loss of bicarbonate. Pancreatic fluid which is rich in bicarbonate is lost through the pancreatic fistula leading to hyperchloremic non-AG metabolic acidosis and this would persist till such time as the fistula is repaired.

Renal causes: Loss of bicarbonates due to impaired reabsorption from proximal tubules occurs in *early renal failure*. This is counterbalanced by gain in chlorides resulting in hyperchloremic non-AG metabolic acidosis. In RTA, the kidneys fail to adequately manage the body acids and this can occur due to impaired (H^+) secretion as in distal type 1 RTA which is commonly caused by autoimmune disorders such as lupus. In proximal type 2 RTA, there is an excessive loss of bicarbonate due to a defect in bicarbonate reabsorption; this is a rare disorder seen in conditions such as multiple myeloma, amyloidosis, heavy metal toxicity, and in patients with kidney transplant. The most common is type 4 RTA which occurs in the setting of hypoaldosteronism and characteristically presents with hyperkalemia.

Iatrogenic causes: Rapid infusion of large amounts of normal saline during volume resuscitation can result in non-AG metabolic acidosis. It could be prevented by using normal saline sparingly or replacing it with Ringer lactate or Ringer acetate, which have a more neutrally balanced pH.

Delta Gap or the Gap-gap Ratio

Delta gap (Δ gap) is the comparing of two gaps—the AG excess in the high AG acidosis versus the bicarbonate deficit. For every 1 mEq/L rise in the AG there should be a concomitant 1 mEq/L fall in the bicarbonate level. It is calculated by the following equation:

$$\Delta \text{Gap} = \frac{\text{Measured AG} - \text{Normal AG}}{\text{Normal HCO}_3 - \text{Measured HCO}_3}$$

The equation helps us to determine the presence of an additional (hidden) primary metabolic process (acidosis or alkalosis) in a patient with a pre-existing high AG metabolic acidosis (refer to **Box 2** for interpretation of the equation).

> **BOX 2** Delta gap to determine an additional hidden metabolic process in patients with high anion gap (AG) metabolic acidosis.
>
> $$\Delta\text{ Gap} = \frac{\text{Measured AG} - \text{Upper normal AG}}{\text{Normal HCO}_3 - \text{Measured HCO}_3}$$
>
> Upper normal AG = 15 mEq/L; normal HCO$_3$ = 24 mEq/L
>
> *Interpretation*
> - In coexisting non-AG metabolic acidosis, the ratio is <1 (e.g., diarrhea) because the HCO$_3$ deficit denominator here is greater than the increased AG numerator
> - In high AG metabolic acidosis, the ratio is 1 because for every unit rise in the AG there is equivalent fall in HCO$_3$ hence the numerator and denominator remain unchanged
> - If there is a hidden metabolic alkalosis, the ratio is >1 as the bicarbonate here is higher than expected, making the denominator lesser than the numerator

Urinary Anion Gap

$$UAG = Na^+ + K^+ - Cl^-$$

Determination of the urinary anion gap (UAG) is useful to distinguish between extrarenal causes of non-AG metabolic acidosis (e.g., diarrhea) from renal causes (e.g., RTA). In extrarenal causes such as severe diarrhea, UAG is a negative value, but it is a positive value in renal etiologies. To understand this let us go stepwise:

- The cations normally present in the urine are Na^+, K^+, NH_4^+, Ca^+, and Mg^+, and the anions are Cl^- and HCO_3^-, sulfate and phosphate.
- However, only Na^+, K^+, and Cl^- are commonly measured in the urine, so the rest of the charged ions are unmeasured cations (UC) and UA.
- For electroneutrality, the total anion charge always equals the total cation charge

$$\text{i.e., } Cl^- + UA = Na^+ + K^+ + UC$$

hence, rearranging the equation

$$UAG = UA - UC = Na^+ + K^+ - Cl^-$$

- Now in gastrointestinal causes of hyperchloremic non-AG metabolic acidosis, for instance in severe diarrhea, the acidosis is due to the loss of bicarbonates via the bowels and the kidneys respond appropriately by increasing the NH_4^+ excretion, thereby loss of (H^+) ions to avoid severe deviation of pH. Hence as the NH_4, i.e., the UC concentration in urine is increased; the UAG in the equation will be a negative value.
- In renal causes (e.g., RTA) the problem being the kidney, it is not able to excrete NH_4 and so the UC will be decreased and as per the equation the UA will be more than UC and the UAG will be a positive value.
- One should understand here that experimentally it has been found that measuring only Na^+, K^+, and Cl^- gives an approximate measure of UAG.

As a memory aid, remember the mnemonic negGUTive—as negative for UAG in gut disorders.
- There is however one important limitation in the ICU setting where UAG may be misleading. Patients with moderate-to-severe volume depletion and metabolic acidosis may have a false positive UAG suggesting RTA.

Step 6: Analysis of Metabolic Alkalosis

As described earlier, primary metabolic alkalosis is diagnosed on ABG sample showing elevated pH and HCO_3 values with an increase in $PaCO_2$ as a secondary response. Measurement of the delta AG may be needed at times to differentiate between primary metabolic alkalosis and metabolic compensation of respiratory acidosis. Refer to **Box 2** for determining the possibility of a hidden metabolic alkalosis.

Some of the clinical manifestations may indicate the causes of metabolic alkalosis such as loss of (H^+) due to vomiting or use of diuretics, particularly thiazides or loop diuretics, and the prolonged use of glucocorticoids. Metabolic alkalosis reduces ionized calcium and may present with tetany or Chvostek's sign. It is important to assess the volume status of the patient in order to identify the type of metabolic alkalosis. Chloride resistant alkalosis is accompanied by volume overload, whereas patients with chloride responsive alkalosis are usually volume depleted. Metabolic alkalosis is associated with hypertension as in hyperaldosteronism (Conn's syndrome), Cushing syndrome, renovascular hypertension, or exogenous use of mineralocorticosteroids or glucocorticosteroids.

Causes of Metabolic Alkalosis (Table 1)

Causes of metabolic alkalosis can be divided into *(1) chloride responsive and (2) chloride resistant.* The former is usually accompanied by volume depletion; hence it is responsive to intravenous infusion of normal saline. In addition, there is also an accompanying hypokalemia which needs to be replaced. If chloride responsive alkalosis occurs in presence of volume overload as in congestive cardiac failure, normal saline is to be avoided but potassium loss will need to be replaced and corrected along with strict fluid restriction and use of potassium-sparing diuretics such as spironolactone. *Three common causes of chloride resistant metabolic alkalosis seen in the ICU setting are hyperaldosteronism, hypokalemia, and an exogenous administration of alkali.* The treatment depends on the underlying condition. For primary hyperaldosteronism, spironolactone, or other potassium-sparing diuretics should be used if there is concurrent hypokalemia. Hypokalemia maintains metabolic alkalosis by a different mechanism but mostly hypokalemia influences the shift of (H^+) intracellularly and bicarbonate reabsorption in the collecting ducts. Large quantities of soda bicarbonate administered in excess of the kidneys' ability to excrete are the main exogenous cause of alkali overload causing metabolic alkalosis.

To diagnose the cause of metabolic alkalosis, firstly rule out the obvious causes such as excessive vomiting or continuous nasogastric suction, overuse of antacids, long-standing use of diuretics particularly thiazides or loop diuretics, accelerated hypertension, and hypokalemia. If metabolic alkalosis remains unexplained and sustained, estimate urinary chloride levels to differentiate between chloride responsive and chloride resistant causes and accordingly investigate. **Table 1** has listed the causes using a helpful mnemonic "HAND-CRAMPS"—incidentally, this is also one of the clinical manifestations and hence easy to remember.

In conclusion, the main reasons for the generation of alkalosis in critically ill patients are loss of (H^+) as in vomiting or gastric aspiration, intracellular shift of (H^+) due to hypokalemia, administration of excessive soda bicarbonate, and contraction alkalosis. Causes of maintenance of sustained metabolic alkalosis are volume loss (contraction alkalosis), hypokalemia, and mineralocorticoid excess. The term contraction alkalosis is perhaps misleading because here the underlying mechanism is chloride loss; hence the alkalosis is not rectified by volume replacement, but rather by chloride replacement even without correcting the volume deficit.

■ EXAMPLES OF ACID-BASE IMBALANCE IN THE CRITICALLY ILL PATIENTS (ALL ELECTROLYTES ARE MEASURED AS mEq/L)

Case 1

A 36-year-old female patient presented with history of diarrhea with four to five stools in last 24 hours, feeling very weak, and washed out and tachypneic [respiratory rate (RR) = 28 breaths/min) and blood pressure (BP) = 100/86 mm Hg].
ABG: pH = 7.26, PaO_2 = 108 mm Hg, $PaCO_2$ = 26 mm Hg, HCO_3^- = 14 mEq/L
Serum electrolytes: Na^+ = 134, K^+ = 3.4, Cl^- = 111

Interpretation

Arterial blood gas shows a non-AG metabolic acidosis which correlates with the clinical presentation of diarrhea. However, the markedly low pH is suggestive of severe diarrhea with gross dehydration which is somehow underestimated by the patient's history of only 4–5 moderate-sized loose stools and requires urgent volume replacement. On first look—tachypnea, the very low pH revealed that the patient was critical and required urgent volume replacement and monitoring.

Case 2

This is a hypothetical example, where we are given only the following ABG values. What is the probable ABG diagnosis?
ABG: pH = 7.35, AG = 10
Serum electrolytes: Na^+ = 131, K^+ = 4, Cl^- = 110

Interpretation

As the serum electrolytes values and the ABG are known—bicarbonate (HCO_3) can be calculated as follows:

$AG = (Na^+ + K^+) - (HCO_3 + Cl)$
$10 = (135) - (HCO_3 + 110)$

Hence, HCO_3 has to be 15

Now to calculate the $PaCO_2$ and as this seems with the low bicarbonate values to be a non-AG metabolic acidosis

$$\text{The } \Delta PaCO_2 = 1.2 \times \Delta HCO_3$$
$$= 1.2 \times 9 = 11$$
$$\text{Hence, the } PaCO_2 = 40 - 11 = 29$$

Final ABG diagnosis is a near compensated non-AG metabolic acidosis

Case 3

Clinical: A 67-year-old male, chronic smoker presents in the outpatient department for chronic and incessant coughing bouts with copious expectoration and dyspnea on climbing one flight of stairs.
ABG: pH = 7.37, $PaCO_2$ = 51, PaO_2 = 78, HCO_3 = 29
Serum electrolytes: Na^+ = 140, K^+ = 4, Cl^- = 102
Interpretation: Chronic respiratory acidosis due to chronic obstructive pulmonary disease (COPD)

After 1 Week

Clinical: Same patient is rushed to the emergency medical services (EMS) with severe breathlessness, high fever, and drowsiness. He is immediately given oxygen by mask
ABG: pH = 7.25, $PaCO_2$ = 76, PaO_2 = 140, HCO_3 = 32
Serum electrolytes: Na^+ = 146, K^+ = 4.5, Cl^- = 94
Interpretation: Presenting chronic respiratory acidosis is now showing a marked rise in $PaCO_2$ with a partial secondary response as expected for an acute exacerbation of COPD. High fever and drowsiness suggests acute infection which may have been responsible for the acute exacerbation. The increased AG reveals an underlying high AG metabolic acidosis probably due to lactic acid acidosis secondary to sepsis. The sharp rise in PaO_2 after the use of high flow oxygen by mask given in the EMS may also be partly responsible for the worsening of $PaCO_2$ by suppressing the respiratory drive.

Case 4

Clinical

A 49-year-old male, presents with vomiting, high fever, and is delirious on admission to the ICU.
ABG: pH = 7.41, $PaCO_2$ = 25, PaO_2 = 104, HCO_3 = 15
Serum electrolytes: Na^+ = 140, K^+ = 3.5, Cl^- = 100
Blood sugar: 37 mg%

Interpretation

The presence of normal pH with a low $PaCO_2$ suggests a mixed acid-base disorder. The increased AG reveals high AG metabolic acidosis along with the respiratory alkalosis.

Lactic acidosis and hyperventilation as in severe sepsis can explain this ABG, but this does not explain the low blood sugar. Here it is important to obtain history of diabetes as patients continue to receive hypoglycemic drugs in particular metformin with inadequate nutrition or a possibility of an underlying cirrhosis of the liver.

Case 5

Clinical

Patient of hepatocellular failure with hypotension and severe vomiting was transferred to ICU.
ABG: pH = 7.4, $PaCO_2$ = 35, PaO_2 = 88, HCO_3 = 22
Serum electrolytes: Na^+ = 139, K^+ = 3.6, Cl^- = 94
Blood sugar: 44 mg%

Interpretation

Though the ABG looks near normal, the AG when calculated is high (26) suggestive of a high AG metabolic acidosis. In a high AG metabolic acidosis one should look for any hidden metabolic process (i.e., Δ gap and gap-gap ratio).

$$\Delta \text{ gap} = \frac{26 - 12}{24 - 22} = \frac{14}{2} = 7$$

As the ratio is >1, there is an associated hidden metabolic alkalosis probably due to vomiting.

Case 6

Clinical

A 60-year-old male lands in Mumbai at late night after a long flight from New York. Next morning he is admitted to the ICU with severe breathlessness and tachycardia. There were no other symptoms or clinical signs. No relevant past medical history. His X-ray chest, electrocardiogram (ECG), and routine blood tests were normal.
ABG: pH = 7.48, $PaCO_2$ = 32, PaO_2 = 54, HCO_3 = 22
Vitals: Heart rate (HR) = 110 beats/min, BP = 150/80 mm Hg, RR = 36 breaths/min, V_T = 650 mL, V_E = 23.4 L

Interpretation

Hypoxic respiratory failure with a marked disparity between the minute ventilation of 23.4 L and the $PaCO_2$ of only 32 mm Hg (one would have expected a much lower $PaCO_2$ with such severe hyperventilation). This is suggestive of a ventilated but unperfused lung—physiological dead space. Correlating with history of recent long air flight the ABG seems to be appropriate for pulmonary embolism.

Case 7

Given the following ABG—what would be your interpretation?
ABG: pH = 7.50, $PaCO_2$ = 51, PaO_2 = 46, HCO_3 = 46

Interpretation

At times it is difficult to interpret an ABG report in isolation without knowing the underlying clinical problem. Hence, it can be interpreted differently depending on the presenting clinical scenarios as follows:

Primary metabolic alkalosis with $PaCO_2$ showing a secondary response in a patient vomiting excessively or following continuous nasogastric aspiration.

Chronic respiratory acidosis (COPD) with sudden hyperventilation following acute pneumonia where $PaCO_2$ falls but bicarbonate takes time to change.

Patients with COPD develop sudden cardiac failure with hyperventilation and worsen with overuse of diuretics leading to secondary metabolic alkalosis.

These examples are illustrated to stress on interpreting ABG with clinical correlation

■ SUGGESTED READING

1. Adrogué HJ, Madias NE. Management of life-threatening acid-base disorders. N Eng J Med. 1998;338:26-34.
2. Berend K, van Hulsteijn LH, Gans RO. Chloride: queen of electrolytes? Eur J Intern Med. 2012:23(3):203-11.
3. Brend K, de Vries APJ, Gans ROB. Physiological approach to assessment of acid-base disturbances. N Engl J Med. 2014;371(15):1434-45.
4. Charles JC, Heilman RL. Metabolic acidosis—clinical review. Hosp Physician. 2005;41(3):37-42.
5. Emmet M, Narins RG. Clinical use of the anion gap. Medicine. 1977;56(1):38-54.
6. Emmett M, Palmer BF. (2021). Urine anion and osmolal gap in metabolic acidosis. [online] Available from https://www.uptodate.com/contents/urine-anion-and-osmolal-gaps-in-metabolic-acidosis. [Last accessed October, 2021].
7. Gabow PA, Anderson RJ, Potts DE, Schrier RW. Acid-base disturbances in the salicylate-intoxicated adult. Arch Intern Med. 1978;138(10):1481-84.
8. Isenhour JL, Slovis CM. Arterial blood gas analysis: A simple three-step approach. J Resp Dis. 2008;29(2):74-82.
9. Kellum JA. Disorders of acid-base balance. Crit Care Med. 2007;35(11):2630-36.
10. Khanna A, Kurtzman NA. Metabolic alkalosis. Respir Care. 2001;46(4):354-65.
11. Lurke RG, Galla JH. It is chloride depletion alkalosis, not contraction alkalosis. J Am Soc Nephrol. 2012;23(3):2004-07.
12. Rose BD, Post T, Stokes J. Clinical Physiology of Acid base and Electrolyte Disorders, 6th edition. New York: McGraw Hill; 2013.
13. Wyckoff J, Abrahamson MJ. Diabetic Ketoacidosis and Hyperosmolar Hyperglycemic State. In: Kahn CR, Weir GC, King GL (Eds). Joslin's **Diabetes** Mellitus, 14th edition. Philadelphia, Lippincott Williams & Wilkins; 2005. pp. 887-99.

CHAPTER 26

Echocardiography in Critical Care

Nitin Burkule, Bomi B Ichaporia

■ PREAMBLE

This chapter is intended to give a working background knowledge of the important uses of echocardiography, in the critical care setting, to postgraduate students or practicing physicians who may be unfamiliar with its details.

■ "POINT OF CARE ECHOCARDIOGRAPHY" IN THE INTENSIVE CARE UNIT

Critical care demands quick diagnosis and rapid corrective intervention, often in hemodynamically unstable patients. Portable or "point of care echocardiography" (i.e., at the bedside) offers fast imaging with valuable diagnostic information in real time, at a relatively low cost, either within the intensive care unit (ICU) space or the emergency room.

■ ADVANTAGES OF BEDSIDE ECHOCARDIOGRAPHY

It offers noninvasive diagnostic and physiological information, in real time, about the cardiac status, e.g., estimation of the cardiac function and hemodynamics. Being fast it can often be done before invasive indwelling pressure lines can be established or laboratory data is received. There are no radiation or contrast agent hazards. The equipment, being compact and portable, can squeeze into the crowded bedside space of the ICU patient. It can be used for guiding invasive bedside procedures to improve safety and can also be used, in an expanding role for lung ultrasound, to scan the lung for evidence of pulmonary venous congestion. Being noninvasive, it can be reused in follow-up studies for feedback on the outcome of corrective interventions, or to look for possible causes of further deterioration. Finally, transesophageal echocardiography (TEE), though minimally invasive as a special probe is introduced into the esophagus, offers unparalleled high-resolution imaging of the cardiac structures.

■ LIMITATIONS OF BEDSIDE ECHOCARDIOGRAPHY

The data acquired is a snapshot at that point in time and continuous monitoring of hemodynamics is not feasible. The presence of dressings or chest drainage tubes may hinder positioning of the probe to acquire good images. Images may also be unsatisfactory due to a poor "echocardiography window", the patient's position, or hyperinflated lungs. Small, portable echocardiography machines may not have some of the advanced echocardiography modalities which are available on the large, high-end cart-based machines used in the department. Also, ultrasound being very operator-dependent, the intensivist or physician personally performing echocardiography is required to attain suitable levels of echocardiography training and experience to elicit reliable information from the study. Lastly, TEE is a semi-invasive procedure requiring sedation.

■ MODALITIES OF ECHOCARDIOGRAPHY

Two-dimensional Echocardiography

The echocardiography probe (transducer) both (1) emits ultrasound beams of 2.5–5 MHz frequency and (2) receives the signals reflected back from the anatomical structures. The location and signal strength (decibel level) of these reflected signals are used to form a two-dimensional (2D) gray scale image of the cardiac anatomy **(Figs. 1 to 4)**. As the images are formed very rapidly in real time, the motion of the cardiac structures (i.e., the walls and valves) can also be appreciated in real time.

Color Flow and Doppler

The shift in the frequency of ultrasound reflected from flowing red blood cells (i.e., the Doppler shift) can be usefully displayed in real time, in three different ways:

1. Color flow imaging, in which flow towards or away from the probe is color coded either red or blue, respectively, enabling detection of an abnormal flow, e.g., valvar regurgitation or a shunt **(Figs. 5 and 6)**.
2. Spectral Doppler, which is a gray scale map (graph) plotting the velocity of flow along the Y (vertical) axis, against time along the X (horizontal)

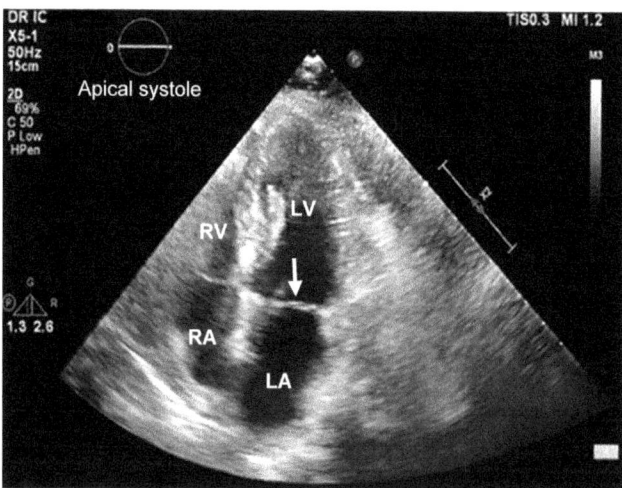

Fig. 1: Apical four-chamber view in systole. Arrow—closed (coapted) mitral leaflets. *Note*: the transducer is customarily positioned at the top of the image. As this view is from the apical position, the apex of the heart is shown at the top. (LA: left atrium; LV: left ventricle; RA: right atrium; RV: right ventricle)

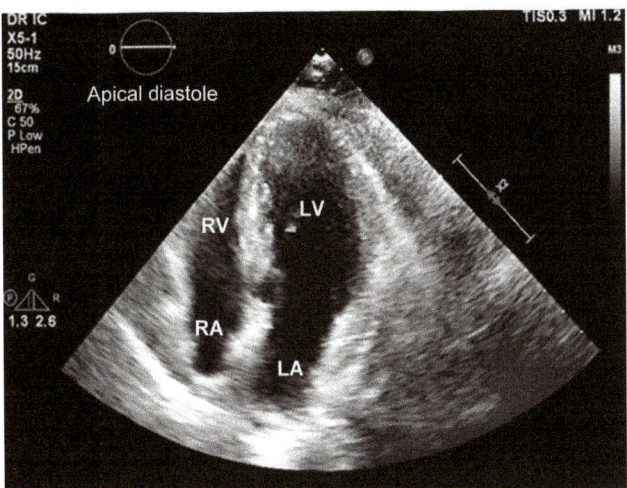

Fig 2: Apical four-chamber view in diastole. The mitral leaflets are open. (LA: left atrium; LV: left ventricle; RA: right atrium; RV: right ventricle)

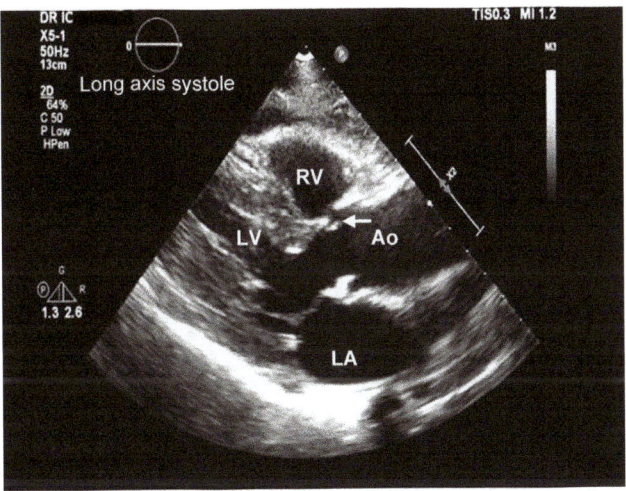

Fig. 3: Parasternal long axis view in systole. Arrow—open aortic valve leaflets. (Ao: aorta; LA: left atrium; LV: left ventricle; RV: right ventricle)

axis. There are two forms of spectral Doppler, continuous wave (CW) and pulse wave (PW). They can be used to give vital information about several hemodynamic parameters (see later).

3. *Tissue Doppler:* PW Doppler is also used to estimate myocardial wall motion velocities, at the mitral annulus, to give information on the diastolic function of the left ventricle (LV) and the LV filling pressure.

From the various echocardiography and Doppler modalities routinely used in the ICU, the following information is then obtainable for clinical correlation: (1) the size of the cardiac chambers, (2) the systolic and diastolic function of the left and right ventricles, (3) hemodynamic data such as estimations of the

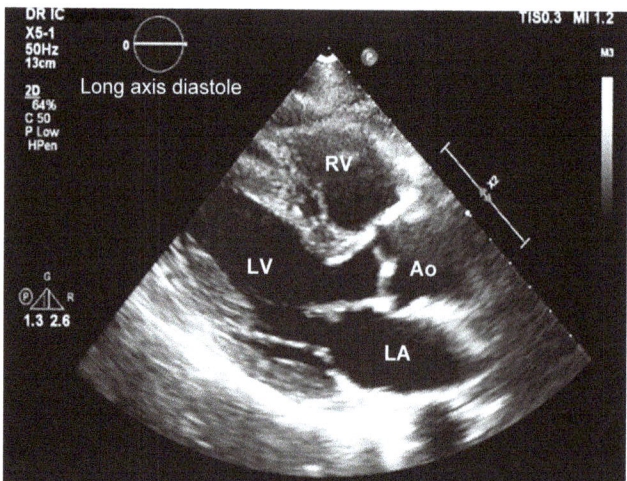

Fig. 4: Parasternal long axis view in diastole. Closure (coaptation) of the aortic valve leaflets. (Ao: aorta; LA: left atrium; LV: left ventricle; RV: right ventricle)

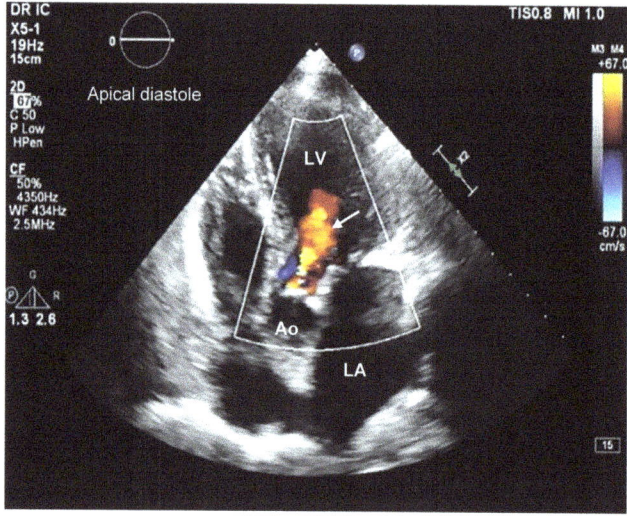

Fig. 5: Apical view in diastole. Arrow—aortic regurgitation. Color flow mapping shows flow in red, i.e., towards the probe [from aorta (Ao) to LV]. (LA: left atrium; LV: left ventricle)

pulmonary artery (PA) pressure, LV filling pressure and cardiac output, (4) the structure and functional status of the valves, (5) the presence and size of any pericardial effusion, or (6) the presence of any intracardiac clots, vegetations, or shunt. Examination of the great arteries reveals their size and the possible presence of a dissection of the aorta. Imaging of the inferior vena cava (IVC) (its diameter and respiratory variation) gives information on the preload status. A more detailed list of the pathophysiological information derived from them is shown in **Table 1** [three-dimensional (3D) echocardiography and myocardial

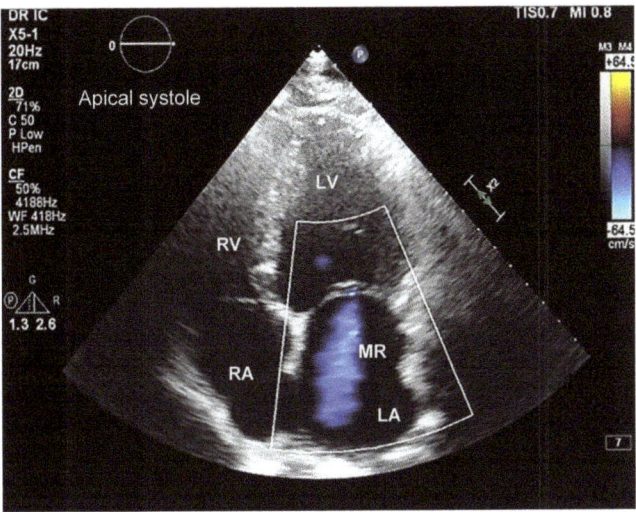

Fig. 6: Apical view in systole. Mitral regurgitation (MR). Color flow mapping of mitral regurgitation shows flow in blue, i.e., away from the probe (from LV to LA). (LA: left atrium; LV: left ventricle; RA: right atrium; RV: right ventricle)

strain imaging form a part of conventional comprehensive studies and are not discussed here].

■ COMMON CLINICAL PRESENTATIONS IN CRITICAL CARE AND THEIR DIFFERENTIATION BY ECHOCARDIOGRAPHY

The echocardiographic information to be rapidly acquired in the various clinical syndromes commonly seen in critical care is summarized below. It may be followed later by a comprehensive and quantitative examination performed by a cardiologist at an appropriate time.

Note: A more detailed discussion of how to actually obtain certain measurements and their interpretation is given later in this chapter.

Acute Chest Pain

The important causes of chest pain in the ICU setting include: (1) acute coronary syndrome (ACS), (2) pericarditis, (3) pulmonary embolism, (4) acute aortic dissection, and (5) ruptured sinus of Valsalva. All these entities carry a high risk of serious complications, with increased morbidity and mortality. Here echocardiography would offer a safe and immediate investigation leading towards the diagnosis.

For example, LV regional wall motion abnormalities would be diagnostic of an ACS, whereas a pericardial effusion would be strongly suggestive of pericarditis **(Fig. 7)**. Isolated dilatation and dysfunction of the right ventricle (RV) would not only indicate a probable pulmonary embolism **(Fig. 8)** but would, together with the identification of pulmonary hypertension, also help

TABLE 1 Echocardiography-Doppler modalities and pathophysiological information in critical care.

Modalities used in ICU	Cardiac structures	Pathophysiological information
Gray scale image	Valves	Structural integrity, coaptation, and vegetation
	Atria	Size, volume status, and clot
	Ventricles	Global and regional systolic function and volume status
	Great vessels	*Ao and MPA:* Dilatation, dissection, and clots *SVC/IVC:* Volume status and catheters
	Pericardial/pleural space	Effusion and tamponade
	Lungs	Fluid overload, comets and consolidation
PW and CW Doppler	LVOT and aorta	Stroke volume, AS and AR
	Mitral valve	LV diastolic function, left heart filling pressure, MS and MR
	Pulmonary vein	Left heart filling pressure
	Pulmonary valve	PR, PA diastolic pressure, PVR, stroke volume, and shunt
	Tricuspid valve	TR and PA systolic pressure
	IVC/SVC/HV	Right heart filling pressure
Tissue Doppler	Mitral annulus	LV diastolic function and left heart filling pressure
	Tricuspid annulus	RV systolic function and right heart filling pressure
Color Doppler	Valves, IAS, IVS, and great vessels	Detecting location of stenosis, regurgitation, and shunt
IV saline-bubble contrast	Left heart	Detecting right-to-left shunt via PFO or pulmonary AV shunt
Transesophageal echocardiography (TEE) (gray scale and Doppler)	All the above structures	In case of poor or limited transthoracic echocardiography window, TEE is performed to get high-resolution images of the posterior cardiac structures, valves, IAS, aorta, and arch
IV ultrasound contrast	Ventricles and atria	LV and RV global and regional systolic function, LV apical clot, and intracardiac mass

(Ao: aorta; AR: aortic regurgitation; AS: aortic stenosis; AV: arteriovenous; CW: continuous wave; HV: hepatic vein; IAS: interatrial septum; ICU: intensive care unit; IV: intravenous; IVC: inferior vena cava; LV: left ventricle; LVOT: left ventricular outflow tract; MPA: main pulmonary artery; MR: mitral regurgitation; MS: mitral stenosis; PA: pulmonary arterial; PFO: patent foramen ovale; PR: pulmonary regurgitation; PVR: pulmonary vascular resistance; PW: pulse wave; RV: right ventricle; SVC: superior vena cava; TR: tricuspid regurgitation)

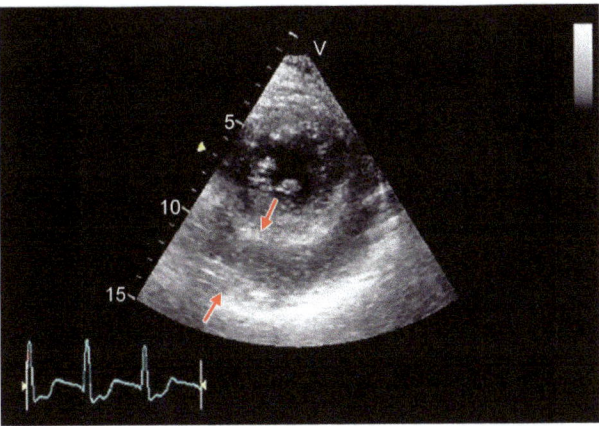

Fig. 7: Pericardial effusion (red arrows) seen posterior to left ventricle (LV) in short axis view.

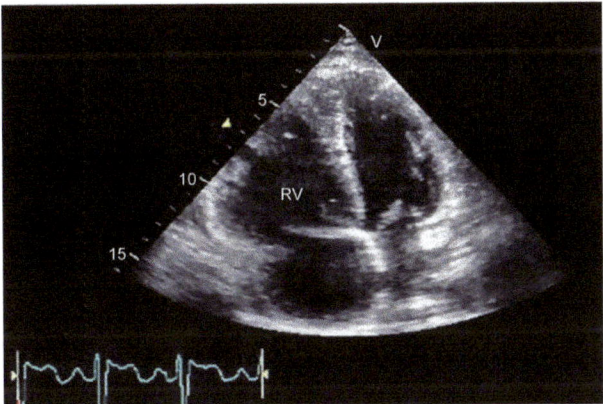

Fig. 8: Dilated and dysfunctional right ventricle (RV) due to subacute pulmonary embolism.

evaluate its severity, guiding clinical management as regards anticoagulation or thrombolysis. Aortic dissection is a life-threatening problem and can be picked up on scanning the ascending aorta, arch, or the descending aorta **(Fig. 9)**.

Though a ruptured sinus of Valsalva is a rare complication, it too can be detected on echocardiography by the presence of an aorta to right atrium (RA) or an aorta to RV shunt.

Hemodynamic Deterioration in ST Elevation Myocardial Infarction

The most common cause to look for on echocardiography would be a deterioration in either LV systolic or diastolic function, or the onset of new wall motion abnormalities. Often, unsuspected right ventricular myocardial infarction (RVMI) can be identified on echocardiography by the presence of RV dysfunction and dilatation. Carefully scanning for an acute mitral regurgitation (MR) can point towards a papillary muscle rupture. Importantly nowadays,

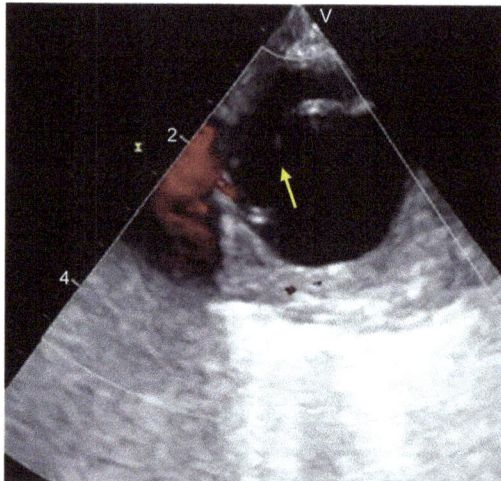

Fig. 9: Dissection flap (yellow arrow) in arch of aorta.

in postangioplasty patients the presence of a pericardial effusion can give a clue to coronary artery perforation; less commonly it may be a sign of free wall rupture. A rupture of the interventricular septum at the site of a regional septal wall motion abnormality can be identified by visualizing the defect and the associated shunt.

Shock/Hypotension/Heart Failure

Again, assess whether the left ventricular ejection fraction (LVEF) is normal or whether there is systolic dysfunction. Dysfunction may be global, i.e., present uniformly throughout the ventricle (as in cardiomyopathy) or it may be regional, i.e., present only in a part of the ventricle (ischemic). The stroke volume and cardiac output can be estimated by spectral Doppler. Also useful is an estimation of the LV filling pressure, from the mitral flow, mitral annular tissue Doppler, left atrium (LA) volume, and the pulmonary arterial systolic pressure (PASP).

The diameter of the IVC and its respiratory variation can give an estimate of the preload status (see later for details). A small and collapsing IVC and/or small and hypercontractile ventricles would indicate hypovolemia, suggesting dehydration, third spacing, or blood loss. Pulmonary embolism would be indicated by isolated RV dilatation and dysfunction, the presence of pulmonary hypertension, estimated from the tricuspid regurgitation (TR) jet, and the presence of any right heart thrombi **(Fig. 10)**.

Pericardial tamponade would of course be established by the presence of a pericardial effusion, and the presence of diastolic collapse of the RA and RV free walls. Ballooning of the LV apex is seen in Takotsubo syndrome, usually precipitated by physical or psychological stress.

The presence of severe aortic or mitral stenosis (MS) can be easily demonstrated by assessing the leaflet morphology and measurement of the Doppler gradients. Malfunction or thrombotic occlusion of prosthetic valves can likewise be detected by restricted movement of the valve disk/s and elevated Doppler gradients. Volume enlargement of any ventricular or atrial cavity can give an indication of chronicity of cardiac remodeling, dysfunction, or volume overload. Venous and pulmonary congestion is indicated by the presence of a pleural effusion and anterior lung field comets **(Fig. 11)**.

Color Doppler mapping can show the presence of acute aortic regurgitation (AR), raising the possibility of aortic dissection or infective endocarditis; it can also reveal the presence of acute MR **(Fig. 12)** or ventricular septal rupture.

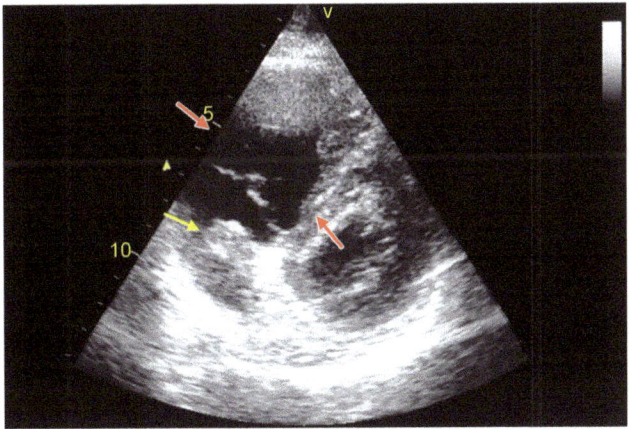

Fig. 10: Dilated right ventricle (RV) (red arrows) with intracavitary clot (yellow arrow) in a case of pulmonary venous thromboembolism.

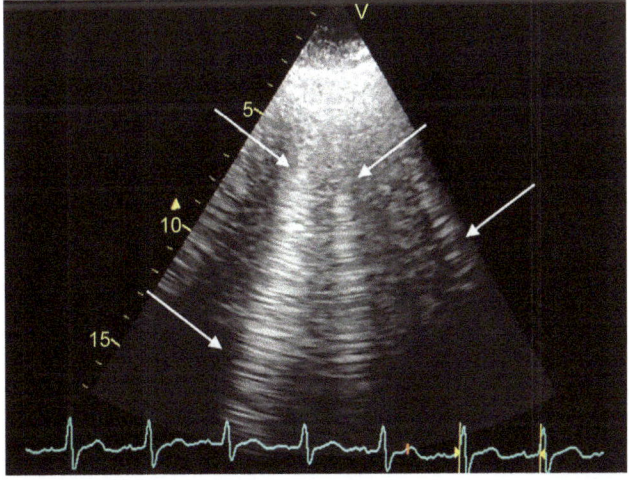

Fig. 11: Vertical comet like (white arrows) reverberations seen in lung fields suggestive of interstitial edema.

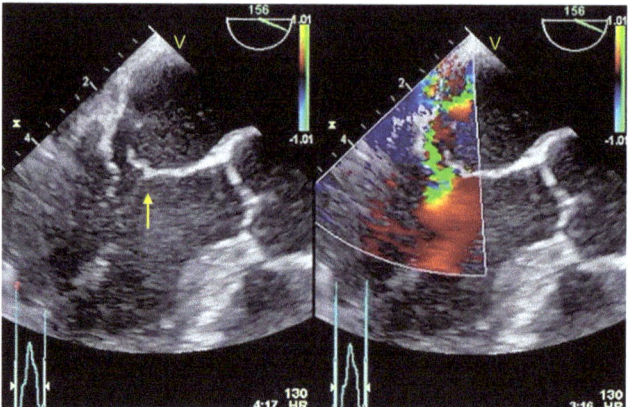

Fig. 12: Flail anterior mitral leaflet (yellow arrow) with mitral regurgitation (MR).

Acute Dyspnea

A very common clinical manifestation in critical care, its important causes, from the standpoint of echocardiography are: (1) significant LV dysfunction, systolic, or diastolic; (2) pulmonary edema; (3) pulmonary embolism; and (4) pericardial tamponade.

In this setting the points to evaluate on echocardiography are whether there is left ventricular systolic dysfunction, either global (e.g., cardiomyopathy) or regional (ischemic) and whether there is evidence of a raised LV filling pressure, as indicated by the mitral Doppler flow, the mitral annular tissue Doppler, and the LA volume. Pulmonary edema would be evidenced by the presence of a pleural effusion and anterior lung field comets, while a dilated IVC with reduced respiratory excursions would imply venous congestion. Dilated right heart chambers with evidence of pulmonary hypertension would raise the suspicion of pulmonary embolism, while the presence of a large pericardial effusion with diastolic collapse of the RV/RA free walls would reliably incriminate pericardial tamponade.

■ CALCULATION AND INTERPRETATION OF ECHOCARDIOGRAPHY/DOPPLER PARAMETERS

Spectral Doppler, coupled with 2D imaging, enables a number of useful hemodynamic calculations for the evaluation of LV systolic function (LVEF), LV diastolic function, LV filling pressure, estimation of the stroke volume, and cardiac output. On the right side, the mean RA pressure (RAP) from IVC diameter, the systolic/diastolic pressures of the PA and infrequently pulmonary vascular resistance (PVR) can be evaluated by 2D echo and Doppler. The velocity of flow, estimations of the pressure gradients, and the quantification of flow across any valve, vessel, or orifice can all be obtained.

Given below is a more detailed presentation of the actual calculations.

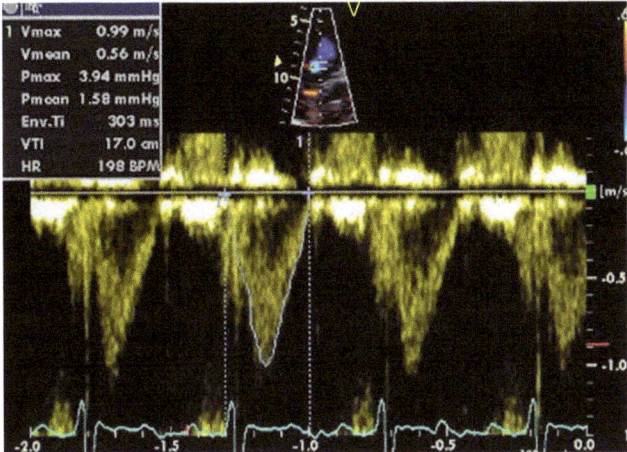

Fig. 13: Spectral Doppler map shows instantaneous velocity (Y-axis) of moving red blood cells (RBCs) over time (X-axis).

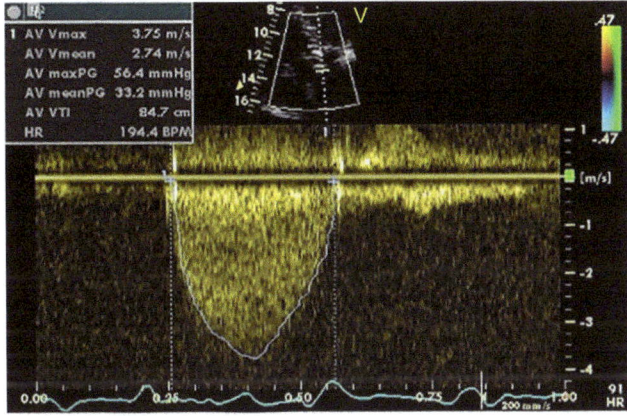

Fig. 14: Continuous wave (CW) spectral Doppler of aortic flow showing peak and mean gradient by applying the modified Bernoulli equation.

Basic Principle of Spectral Doppler Measurement

Spectral Doppler is displayed as a graph, with time depicted along the X- (horizontal) axis and the velocity (of the moving RBCs) depicted along the Y-axis **(Fig. 13)**.

- This spectral Doppler map allows us to measure the peak instantaneous velocity (V). The mean velocity is measured by planimetry of the area circumscribed by the Doppler envelope (the velocity-time integral or VTI) **(Fig. 14)**.
- By applying the modified Bernoulli equation, the peak and mean gradients are then easily calculated.
- Peak gradient (in mm Hg) = $4 \times V^2$ (where V is the velocity in m/s).

- This equation quantifies the peak and mean gradients across either native or prosthetic valves. Stenosis of a valve results in elevated peak and mean gradients, with increasing gradients denoting increasing severity of the stenosis. Doppler formulae can also be used to estimate the orifice area of the mitral or aortic valve.
- In quantifying flow, the flow in mL/beat is calculated across any orifice, e.g., the LV outflow tract (LVOT), RV outflow tract (RVOT), mitral annulus, or tricuspid annulus, by multiplying the cross-sectional area of the orifice and the VTI of the spectral Doppler flow signal **(Fig. 15)**:
  Stroke volume (SV) = [3.14 × (LVOT diameter)^2/4] × (VTI of LVOT Doppler)
  Cardiac output (CO) = SV × Heart rate
- The Doppler quantification of blood flow at the atrioventricular valves and semilunar valves enables us to quantify valvular regurgitation and atrial or ventricular level shunts.

Estimating Right Heart Filling Pressures

The mean RAP or RV end-diastolic pressure (RVEDP) can be roughly estimated by the IVC diameter, the reduction in IVC diameter with inspiration **(Fig. 16)**, and secondary indices (tricuspid flow, tricuspid annular tissue Doppler, and hepatic venous flow). The algorithm followed is as follows:

1. IVC < 20 mm   Inspiratory collapse > 50%   RAP = 3 mm Hg
2. IVC > 20 mm   Inspiratory collapse < 50%   RAP = 15 mm Hg
3. IVC < 20 mm   Inspiratory collapse < 50%   RAP = 8 mm Hg
4. IVC > 20 mm   Inspiratory collapse > 50%   RAP = 8 mm Hg

(In the third and fourth options, if one of the secondary indices is positive (tricuspid valve flow E velocity/A velocity > 2 and/or tricuspid annular E wave

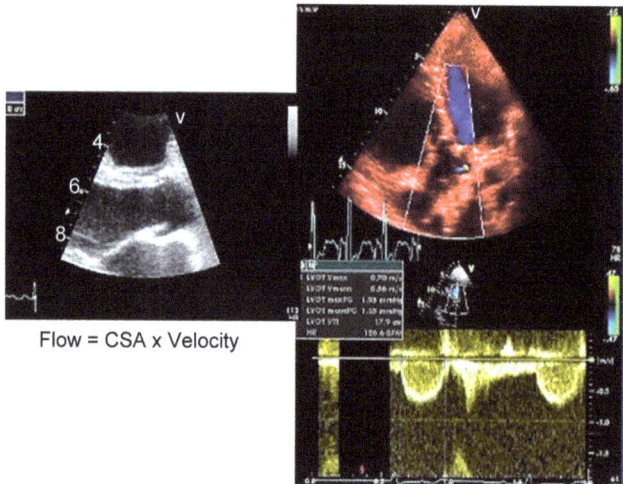

Fig. 15: Calculation of stroke volume by LVOT cross-sectional area (CSA) and LVOT PW Doppler VTI. (LVOT: left ventricular outflow tract; PW: pulse wave; VTI: velocity-time integral)

velocity/e' annular velocity > 6 and/or HV D wave velocity > S wave velocity and A wave flow reversal), the RAP can be upgraded to 15 mm Hg).

Pulmonary Artery Systolic and Diastolic Pressures

By measuring the peak velocity (V) of a TR jet one can calculate the systolic pressure difference (gradient) between the RV and RA chambers. To this difference, if we then add the RAP, we get the RV systolic pressure (RVSP) **(Fig. 17)**.

1. RVSP = PASP = TR jet peak $(4 \times V^2)$ + RAP

   The mean RAP is estimated from the IVC (as described above). The RVSP and the PASP are the same, in the absence of any pulmonary stenosis.

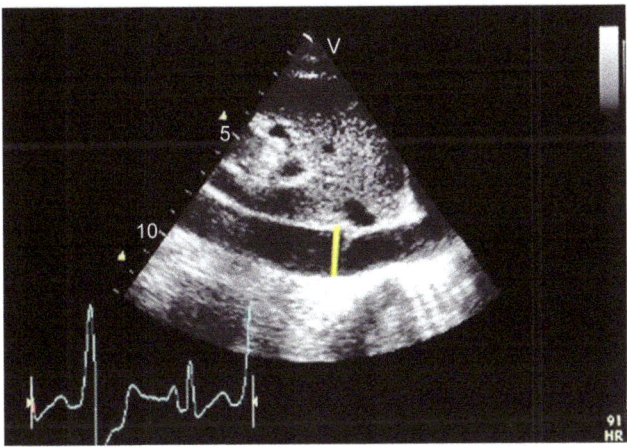

Fig. 16: Inferior vena cava (IVC) diameter (yellow line) before joining of the hepatic vein (HV) tributary.

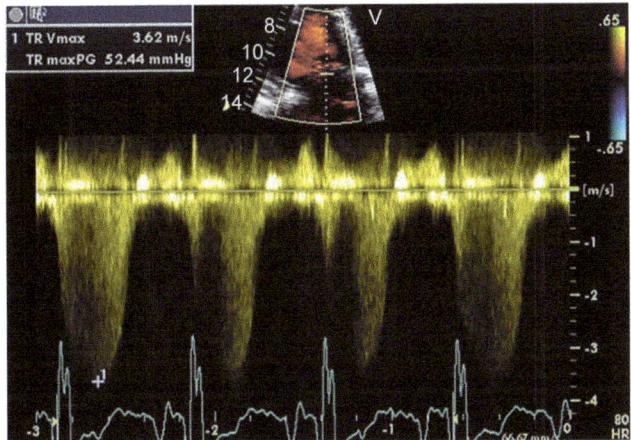

Fig. 17: Calculation of PASP from TR jet by CW Doppler. (CW: continuous wave; PASP: pulmonary arterial systolic pressure; TR: tricuspid regurgitation)

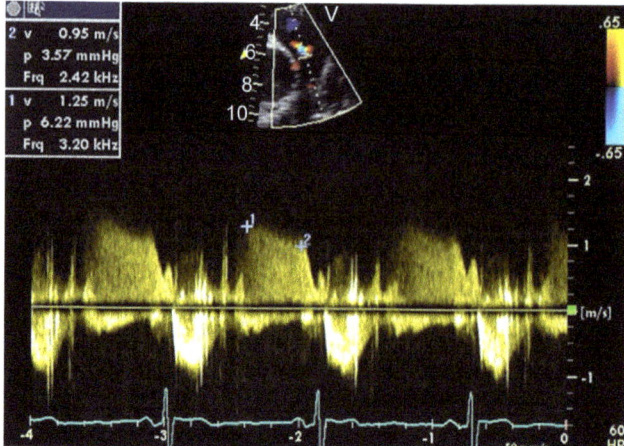

Fig. 18: Calculation of PADP and PA mean pressure from PR jet CW Doppler. (CW: continuous wave; PA: pulmonary artery; PADP: pulmonary artery diastolic pressure; PR: pulmonary regurgitation)

For example, in **Figure 17**, the peak velocity of the TR jet is 3.62 m/s. The peak gradient is therefore $4 \times (3.62)^2 = 4 \times 13.1 = 52.4$ mm Hg.
If the estimated RAP is 8 mm Hg, the RVSP is $52.4 + 8 = 60.4$ mm Hg.
Similarly, by measuring the end-diastolic pulmonary regurgitation (PR) jet velocity, one can calculate the end-diastolic pressure difference between main pulmonary artery (MPA) and RV/RA chambers **(Fig. 18)**.

2. Pulmonary artery diastolic pressure (PADP) = End-diastolic PR jet $(4 \times V^2)$ + RAP

   Mean PA pressure is calculated as PA mean = Early diastolic peak PR jet $(4 \times V^2)$ + RAP

3. In the presence of a ventricular septal defect (VSD), the same principle can be applied for calculating RVSP/PASP as follows:

   RVSP = (LV systolic pressure) − (gradient across the VSD orifice)

   Since the LV systolic pressure is the same as the systolic blood pressure (BP) taken by the sphygmomanometer arm-cuff, in the absence of any aortic stenosis:

   RVSP = Systolic BP − Peak VSD gradient (i.e., $4 \times V^2$)

4. In the presence of a PDA, the same principle can be applied for calculating PASP and PADP as follows:

   PASP = Systolic BP (by arm cuff) − Peak PDA jet $(4 \times V^2)$
   PADP = Diastolic BP (by arm cuff) − Trough PDA jet $(4 \times V^2)$

Estimation of Pulmonary Vascular Resistance (PVR)

By invasive catheterization, PVR is calculated as transpulmonary pressure gradient ÷ transpulmonary flow (normal PVR < 1.5 Wood unit).

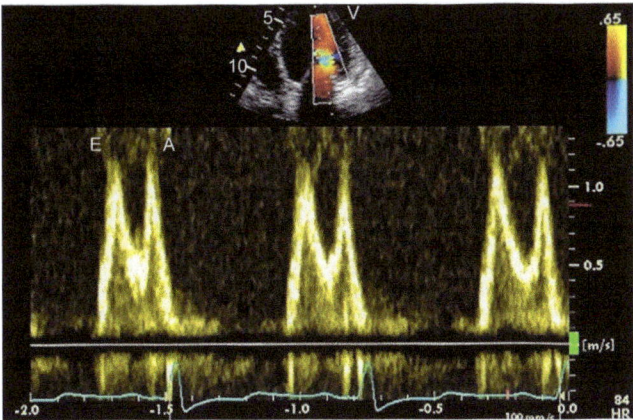

Fig. 19: Mitral flow pulse wave (PW) Doppler showing E and A wave velocities.

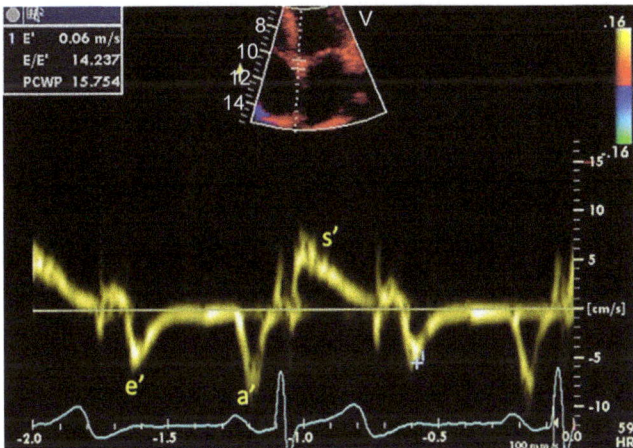

Fig. 20: Mitral annular tissue Doppler showing e′, a′, and s′ waves.

An equivalent Doppler derived equation for PVR has been described as follows:
- PVR = [(TR velocity ÷ RVOT VTI) × 10] + 0.16
- If the TR velocity/RVOT VTI ratio > 0.2 it suggests a PVR > 2 Wood units

Left Heart Filling Pressures (Left Ventricular Mean and Left Ventricular End-diastolic Pressure)

Spectral Doppler of the mitral valve (MV) diastolic (opening) flow shows two peaks: the E wave (first peak) is related to rapid and passive LV filling in early diastole, while the A wave (second peak) corresponds to atrial contraction in late diastole **(Fig. 19)**. Tissue Doppler of the mitral annulus (measured either at its septal or lateral side) shows two negative peaks, the e′ and a′ waves **(Fig. 20)**.

The assessment of LV diastolic function is performed by measuring the mitral flow E and A wave velocities, the mitral annular tissue Doppler e′

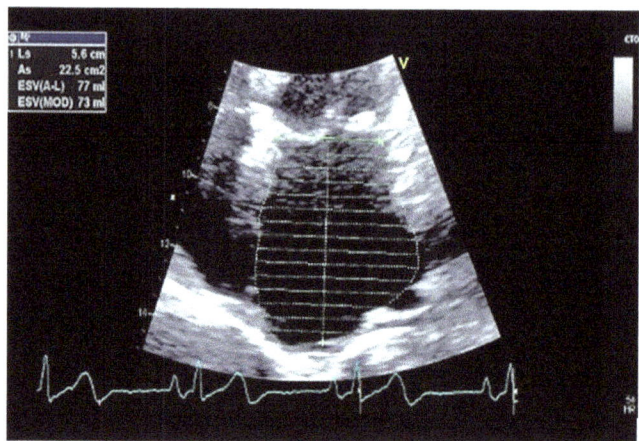

Fig. 21: Calculation of left atrium (LA) volume from planimetering four-chamber and two-chamber views of LA.

velocity, the LA volume **(Fig. 21)** and the TR velocity, and leads to an estimation of left heart filling pressures. The specificity of the algorithm improves in the presence of reduced LVEF or LV hypertrophy/remodeling.

In the presence of reduced LVEF or presence of left ventricular hypertrophy (LVH), evaluate the mitral flow Doppler tracing:
- If E/A ≤ 0.8 and E ≤ 50 cm/s suggests normal mean left atrial pressure (LAP)
- If E/A ≥ 2 suggests raised mean LAP
- If E > 50 cm/s E/A between 0.8 and 2 then evaluate:
  - E/e′ > 14, lateral E/e′ > 13 or septal E/e′ > 15
  - TR velocity > 2.8 m/s, PASP > 36 mm Hg
  - LA volume > 34 mL/m^2

If any two or more are abnormal, it suggests a raised mean LAP.

In the presence of normal LVEF and no LV remodeling, four parameters are evaluated for diastolic dysfunction:
1. e′ velocity (septal e′ < 7 cm/s, lateral e′ < 10 cm/s)
2. Mean E/e′ > 14 or lateral E/e′ > 13 or septal E/e′ > 15
3. TR > 2.8 m/s, PASP > 36 mm Hg
4. LA volume > 34 mL/m^2

If three or more parameters are abnormal, it suggests significant LV diastolic dysfunction. In the presence of clinical signs of pulmonary and/or systemic congestion, and raised N-terminal pro-B-type natriuretic (NT-proBNP) these parameters help in the diagnosis of heart failure with preserved ejection fraction (EF).

Other simpler formulae have also been proposed:

E/e′ < 8 indicates normal filling pressure; E/e′ > 15 indicates raised filling pressure

And

Left ventricular end-diastolic pressure (LVEDP) = 1.24 (E/e′) + 1.9

The parameters of LV filling pressure assessment are not reliable in certain clinical situations such as severe tachycardia or bradycardia, atrial fibrillation (AF), left bundle branch block (LBBB), paced rhythm, MS, MR, MV replacement, LV assist device, and mitral annular calcification.

Left Ventricular and Right Ventricular Systolic Function

The LVEF is estimated qualitatively by an experienced echocardiographer in a portable echocardiography study by a visual estimation; however, quantitative calculation by Simpson's method is recommended when a detailed echocardiography examination is performed **(Fig. 22)**. The

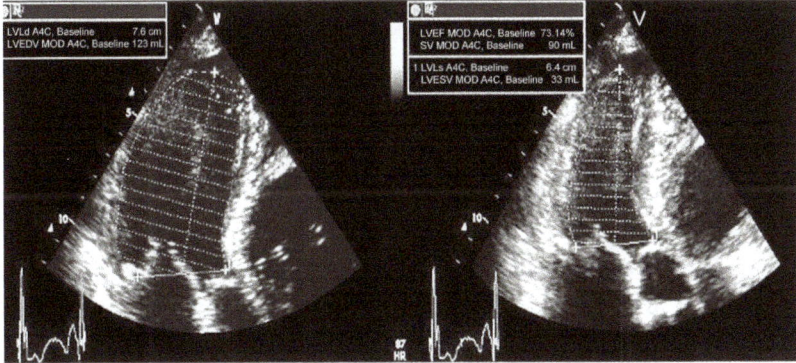

Fig. 22: Left ventricular diastolic and systolic volumes measured by Simpson's method of disks.

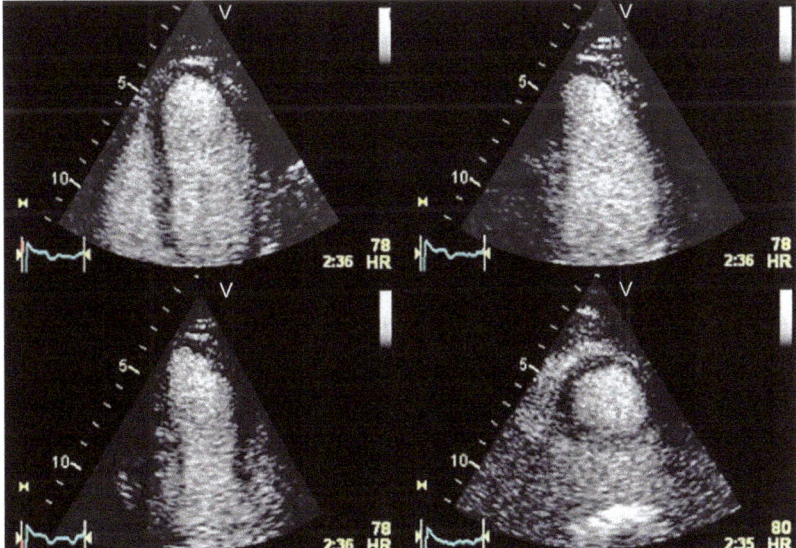

Fig. 23: Left ventricular cavity opacification by intravenous (IV) ultrasound contrast to improve accuracy of left ventricular volume measurement and regional wall motion assessment.

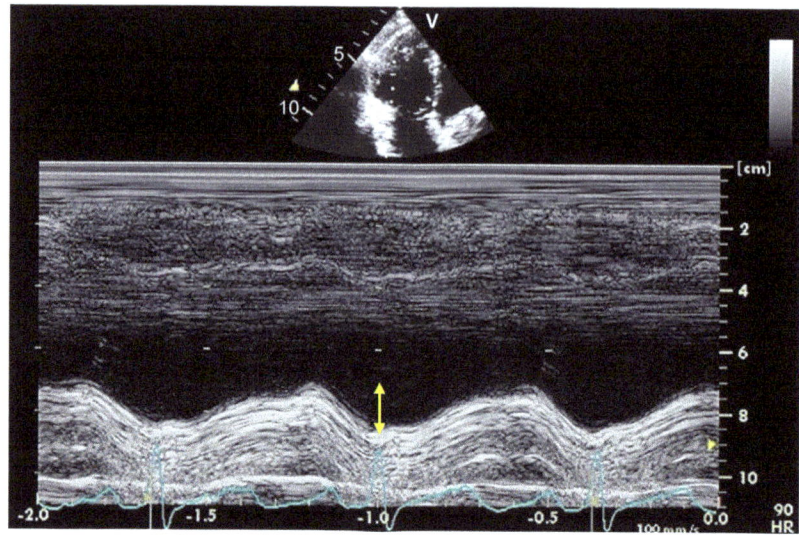

Fig. 24: M-mode derived tricuspid annular plane systolic excursion (TAPSE) shown by yellow arrow.

end-diastolic and end-systolic endocardial contours of the compact myocardium are planimetered in four-chamber and two-chamber views. This accuracy is improved by intravenous (IV) administration of LV cavity opacification ultrasound contrast **(Fig. 23)**. The LV volumes and EF are calculated by summation of the disk volume method. LVEF < 40% is called reduced EF and LVEF in the range of 40–50% is called midrange EF. The LV segmental wall thickness, systolic thickening, and motion are described as per the three coronary arterial distributions in the 16-segment model.

The RV systolic function assessment in the critical care setting is accomplished by M-mode derived tricuspid annular plane systolic excursion (TAPSE) (normal TAPSE $\geq$ 1.7 cm) **(Fig. 24)** or tricuspid annular tissue Doppler S' (normal S' $\geq$9.5 cm/s).

Global RV systolic function can also be assessed by calculating the RV fractional area change FAC (RV fractional area change). This is calculated as:

FAC = (RV end-diastolic area – RV end-systolic area) ÷ RV end-diastolic area.

The normal value, expressed as a percentage, is >35%. The RV is said to be dilated if the RV basal diameter > 40 mm and RVOT proximal diameter in parasternal short axis > 35 mm.

■ GUIDING BEDSIDE INTERVENTION

The point of care echocardiography/vascular ultrasonography can help in guiding bedside interventions:
- For inserting indwelling catheters, the percutaneous vascular access for jugular and femoral veins or radial and femoral arteries can be achieved safely by ultrasound guidance.

- The temporary pacemaker leads can be located and repositioned in the RV cavity by echocardiography guidance
- The distal end of the intra-aortic balloon pump (IABP) catheter can be positioned distal to the left subclavian artery by echocardiographic suprasternal arch view.
- Echocardiographic guidance is vital for safe pericardiocentesis.

SUMMARY

Portable or "point of care" echocardiography in critical care units offers quick and noninvasive imaging of the heart without any radiation or contrast hazards. The data that can be obtained are:
- The size and volume of the cardiac chambers
- The systolic and diastolic function of the ventricles
- The presence of regional wall motion abnormalities of the LV in ischemic heart disease (IHD)
- The presence of any regurgitation or stenosis of the cardiac valves and its quantification
- Evaluation of prosthetic valve function
- The presence of pericardial effusion, its size, and whether there is tamponade
- The presence of intracardiac thrombi, vegetations, or masses
- The possibility of aortic dissection.

Calculation of various parameters enables estimations of:
- The LV filling pressure, the stroke volume, and cardiac output
- The RA, RV, and PA pressures

SUGGESTED READING

1. Baumgartner H, Hung J, Bermejo J, Chambers JB, Evangelista A, Griffin BP, et al. Echocardiographic Assessment of Valve Stenosis: EAE/ASE Recommendations for Clinical Practice. J Am Soc Echocardiogr. 2009;22(1):1-23.
2. Goldstein SA, Evangelista A, Abbara S, Arai A, Asch FM, Badano LP, et al. Multimodality imaging of diseases of the thoracic aorta in adults: From the American Society of Echocardiography and the European Association of Cardiovascular Imaging: Endorsed by the Society of Cardiovascular Computed Tomography and Society for Cardiovascular Magnetic Resonance. J Am Soc Echocardiogr. 2015;28(2):119-82.
3. Harris P, Kuppurao L. Quantitative Doppler Echocardiography. BJA Education. 2016;16(2):46-52.
4. Labovitz AJ, Noble VE, Bierig M, Goldstein SA, Jones R, Kort S, et al. Focused cardiac ultrasound in the emergent setting: A consensus statement of the American Society of Echocardiography and American College of Emergency Physicians. J Am Soc Echocardiogr. 2010;23(12):1225-30.
5. Lang RM, Bierig M, Devereux RB, Flachskampf FA, Foster E, Pellikka PA, et al. Recommendations for chamber quantification: A report from the American Society of Echocardiography's guidelines and standards committee and the Chamber Quantification Writing Group, developed in conjunction with the European Association of Echocardiograph, a branch of the European Society of Cardiology. J Am Soc Echocardiogr. 2005;18(12):1440-63.

6. Mitchell C, Rahko PS, Blauwet LA, Canaday B, Finstuen JA, Foster MC, et al. Guidelines for Performing a Comprehensive Transthoracic Echocardiographic Examination in Adults: Recommendations from the American Society of Echocardiography. J Am Soc Echocardiogr. 2019;32(1):1-64.
7. Mulvagh SL, Rakowski H, Vannan MA, Abdelmoneim SS, Becher H, Bierig SM, et al. American Society of Echocardiography Consensus Statement on the Clinical Applications of Ultrasonic Contrast Agents in Echocardiography. J Am Soc Echocardiogr. 2008;21(11):1179-201.
8. Nagueh SF, Middleton KJ, Kopelen HA, Zoghbi WA, Quiñones MA. Doppler tissue imaging: a noninvasive technique for evaluation of left ventricular relaxation and estimation of filling pressures. J Am Coll Cardiol. 1997;30(6):1527-33.
9. Nagueh SF, Smiseth OA, Appleton CP, et al. Recommendations for the Evaluation of Left Ventricular Diastolic Function by Echocardiography: An Update from the American Society of Echocardiography and the European Association of Cardiovascular Imaging. J Am Soc Echocardiogr. 2016;29(4):277-314.
10. Quiñones MA, Otto CM, Stoddard M, Waggoner A, Zoghbi WA. Recommendations for quantification of Doppler echocardiography: a report from the Doppler Quantification Task Force of the Nomenclature and Standards Committee of the American Society of Echocardiography. J Am Soc Echocardiogr. 2002;15(2):167-84.
11. Rudski LG, Lai WW, Afilalo J, Hua L, Handschumacher MD, Chandrasekaran K, et al. Guidelines for the echocardiographic assessment of the right heart in adults: a report from the American Society of Echocardiography endorsed by the European Association of Echocardiography, a registered branch of the European Society of Cardiology, and the Canadian Society of Echocardiography. J Am Soc Echocardiogr. 2010;23(7):685-713.
12. Silvestry FE, Kerber RE, Brook MM, Carroll JD, Eberman KM, Goldstein SA, et al. Echocardiography-Guided Interventions. J Am Soc Echocardiogr. 2009;22(3):213-31.
13. Troianos CA, Hartman GS, Glas KE, Skubas NJ, Eberhardt RT, Walker JD, et al. Guidelines for performing ultrasound guided vascular cannulation: Recommendations of the American Society of Echocardiography and the Society of Cardiovascular Anesthesiologists. J Am Soc Echocardiogr. 2011;24(12):1291-318.
14. Zoghbi WA, Adams D, Bonow RO, Enriquez-Sarano M, Foster E, Grayburn PA, et al. Recommendations for Noninvasive EvaluatiOn of NativE Valvular ReguRgitation: A Report from the AmericaN Society of Echocardiography Developed in Collaboration with the Society for Cardiovascular Magnetic Resonance. J Am Soc Echocardiogr. 2017;30(4):303-71.
15. Zoghbi WA, Chambers JB, Dumesnil JG, Foster E, Gottdiener JS, Grayburn PA, et al. Recommendations for evaluation of prosthetic valves with echocardiography and Doppler ultrasound: a report from the American Society of Echocardiography's Guidelines and Standards Committee and the Task Force on Prosthetic Valves, Developed in Conjunction With the American ColleGe of CardiOlogy Cardiovascular ImagIng CommittEe, Cardiac ImaGing Committee of the American Heart Association, the European Association of Echocardiography, a registered branch of the European Society of Cardiology, the Japanese Society of Echocardiography and the Canadian Society of Echocardiography, endorsed by the American College of Cardiology Foundation, American Heart Association, European Association of Echocardiography, a registered branch of the European Society of Cardiology, the Japanese Society of Echocardiography, and Canadian Society of Echocardiography. J Am Soc Echocardiogr. 2009;22(9):975-1014.

SECTION 7

Problem Oriented Topics

- **Postoperative Atrial Fibrillation**
  Jamshed Sunavala

- **An Approach to Acute Abdomen**
  Shruti Tandan Pardasani

- **Endocrine Emergencies**
  Nalini S Shah, Kunal Thakkar

- **Management of Exacerbation of Chronic Obstructive Pulmonary Disease**
  Joanne Mascarenhas, Jamshed Sunavala

- **Approach to a Patient with Hyponatremia**
  Bhupendra V Gandhi, Rishit Harbada

- **Intensive Care Unit-acquired Weakness**
  Vibhor Pardasani

- **Seizures in the Intensive Care Unit**
  Vibhor Pardasani

- **Medical Management of Post-traumatic Hemorrhage and Coagulopathy**
  Jamshed Sunavala, Dipsha Kriplani Suvarna

- **Pitfalls in the Diagnosis of Brain Death**
  Sarosh M Katrak

CHAPTER 27

Postoperative Atrial Fibrillation

Jamshed Sunavala

■ INTRODUCTION

Postoperative atrial fibrillation (POAF) is one of the entities in the classification of atrial fibrillation (AF) and typically occurs after cardiothoracic surgery in 30–50% of the patients **(Table 1)**. POAF is more common in the elderly population undergoing cardiac surgery and is associated with a higher incidence of stroke, increased length of stay, and mortality.

Creswell's study, "the hazards of postoperative arrhythmias", was probably one of the first major works published in 1993 in the Annals of Thoracic Surgery. Since then, the underlying triggers, complications and incidence of POAF have practically remained the same. The incidence of POAF is most common after cardiac surgery (50%) and pneumonectomy (30–40%). In contrast, the incidence of any new-onset supraventricular arrhythmias is reported to be very low (<10%) for noncardiac surgery.

■ PERIOPERATIVE RISKS FOR DEVELOPING POSTOPERATIVE ATRIAL FIBRILLATION

The usual perioperative conditions that increase the risk of AF are advanced age and previous history of cardiopulmonary comorbidities. Patients with

TABLE 1 Classification of atrial fibrillation (AF).

Continuous AF	Persists continuously for over a week
Paroxysmal AF	Recurring episodes at variable intervals and terminates spontaneously or after intervention.
Chronic AF	Continuous or repeated episodes of AF for a longstanding period with failure to restore or maintain sinus rhythm. Here no further attempts are made to convert to sinus rhythm and one accepts ventricular rate control as a preferred therapy.
Valvular AF	Could present as any of the above; only difference is that long-term anticoagulation is restricted to vitamin K antagonist, (warfarin), as the use of newer oral anticoagulants are not still validated.
Postoperative atrial fibrillation (POAF)	Occurs during the immediate postoperative period; more common after cardiothoracic surgery and is associated with increased postoperative morbidity and mortality. Usually it is a new-onset AF and attempts should be made to cardiovert after rate control.

history of hypertension, valvular heart diseases, cardiomyopathy, or chronic pulmonary diseases are at a higher risk of getting POAF. It has been shown that patients with hypertension, chronic lung disease, and obstructive sleep apnea may benefit from preoperative optimization, such as weight reduction, controlling hypertension and diabetes mellitus; correcting electrolytes and fluid balance and improving the pulmonary status may help in reducing the incidence of POAF.

▪ PATHOGENESIS

The direct pathology leading to AF is complex and multifactorial, but three important triggers are to be considered: (1) Release of excessive catecholamines following an inflammatory response induced by surgery, plus the administration of vasopressors and inotropes during and after surgery predispose to arrhythmias; (2) type of surgery, especially, where there is undue compression and manipulation of the atria; and (3) new development of ischemic myocardial injury or ventricular dysfunction in the perioperative period can be directly responsible for POAF.

Other factors that can trigger AF, particularly in the postoperative period, include persistent pain, electrolyte and acid-base imbalance, and hemodynamic shifts caused by hypovolemia or hypervolemia. AF is not uncommonly seen in those postcardiac surgery patients who are difficult to wean, possibly because of the respiratory distress with each unsuccessful weaning attempt. In the intraoperative period, AF can be precipitated during induction of anesthesia and during a premature extubation attempt. Studies have also shown that open surgeries are more prone to AF compared to minimally invasive laparoscopic procedures, probably because of less intraoperative inflammatory response.

▪ PROPHYLAXIS FOR POSTOPERATIVE ATRIAL FIBRILLATION

Preexisting modifiable risk factors and correction of possible triggers should be considered before proceeding for surgeries which have a high incidence of POAF. In general, one or more of the following strategies may be employed to decrease the risk of POAF, particularly for patients undergoing cardiothoracic surgeries **(Box 1)**.

- *Empirical use of antiarrhythmic drugs* such as beta-blockers, calcium channel blockers, digoxin, or amiodarone. A meta-analysis published by Crystal et al. in "Circulation 2002" revealed that the use of prophylactic beta-blockers after cardiac surgery, substantially reduced the risk of new-onset of POAF, and this was reconfirmed in a subsequent meta-analysis by the same author in 2004. Soon after this, the "American College of Cardiology Foundation Guidelines" strongly recommended that all patients undergoing coronary artery bypass graft (CABG) should be perioperatively covered with beta-blockers, starting a day prior to surgery. The benefit

> **BOX 1** Strategies for prevention of postoperative atrial fibrillation (POAF) after cardiac surgery.
>
> **Strategies currently recommended**
> - **Antiarrhythmic agents (as perioperative prophylactic agents)**
>   - Beta-blockers and amiodarone
> - **Correctable risk factors**
>   - Maintenance of serum magnesium levels within normal range post cardiac surgery
>   - Maintenance of normal serum electrolytes and acid base balance
>   - Pain management
>   - Monitoring hemodynamic stability and avoiding volume overload
>   - Early weaning, extubation and mobilization
>   - Continue CPAP therapy for obstructive sleep apnea (OSA) patients
>
> **Strategies with inconclusive evidence (not currently recommended)**
>   - Overdrive atrial pacing
>   - Statins, colchicine, and calcium channel blockers
>   - Digoxin (effective for rate control, but no guidelines recommendation for POAF prophylaxis)
>
> **Strategies currently not approved (as side effects outweigh the benefits)**
>   - *Sotalol:* QTc prolongation and torsades de pointes
>   - *Corticosteroids:* Hyperglycemia and infection. Major trials failed to show any benefit
>
> (CPAP: continuous positive airway pressure)

related to the use of empiric beta-blocker therapy in cardiac surgery patients was best observed if started before or immediately after surgery, and was independent of the class of beta-blockers used. However, no such benefit was observed in general surgery patients. On the contrary, in the latter group of patients, the side effects of beta-blockers, such as bradyarrhythmias and hypotension become more prominent, for this reason and the fact that the very incidence of POAF (<10%) is distinctly lower than in postcardiac surgery patients (50%), prophylactic beta-blockers are not recommended for general surgery patients. However, noncardiac, general surgery patients already on longstanding beta-blockers should not discontinue the drug in the perioperative period. In conclusion the current guidelines recommend prophylactic beta-blockers in all patients undergoing CABG surgery.

Sotalol, which is both a beta-blocker and a potassium channel blocking agent, has shown a significant reduction in POAF; however, its use is restricted in clinical practice because of its serious side effects such as prolongation of QTc and torsades de pointes.

Amiodarone has shown a significant reduction in POAF in cardiac surgery patients and it is useful when beta-blockers are contraindicated, particularly in asthmatics. However, amiodarone should not be continued for a prolonged period after the surgery, because it may be associated with pulmonary, thyroid, or hepatic side effects.

- *Magnesium as prophylaxis*: Monitoring and maintaining a normal serum electrolyte balance is mandatory in all postoperative patients; however, magnesium depletion seems to play an important role in inducing AF particularly in patients undergoing CABG. Incidence of supraventricular tachycardias is significantly less with the use of prophylactic magnesium in comparison with controls, and this has been amply demonstrated in two important studies (Shige et al. Am J Med 2004 and Cochrane Database Syst Rev 2013). Current guidelines of ACP strongly recommend maintaining a normal range of magnesium level after cardiac surgery.
- *Inflammatory modulators*: Modulating the inflammatory response to surgery with corticosteroids has not been found to be beneficial and hence it is not recommended as prophylaxis against POAF. Statins by their anti-inflammatory effect have been reported to be beneficial in reducing the incidence of POAF and are hence recommended in the American College of Clinical Pharmacy/American Heart Association (ACCP/AHA) guidelines for prophylactic use in all CABG patients. However, a conflicting view was expressed by the more recent European Society of Cardiology (ESC) guidelines (2016) on the basis of a large randomized controlled trial (RCT) and other current studies, that failed to show a reduction in POAF. None the less, as statins are potentially harmless, many cardiologists continue to use it immediately after surgery in patients undergoing CABG. Other postoperative measures such as pain relief, maintaining hemodynamic stability, earlier weaning plus mobilization, and use of less invasive procedures, should be simultaneously instituted to help in reducing the incidence of POAF in cardiac surgery patients. However, one single "pain management" study has shown a significant reduction in the incidence of AF after cardiac surgery, making pain relief a very important therapeutic measure in the postoperative period.
- *Invasive interventions*: Prophylactic atrial pacing and postoperative drainage of pericardial fluid may be effective in preventing AF after cardiac surgery. Overdrive pacing by setting the pacemaker at 10-20 beats above the intrinsic rate and continuing it for 3-4 postoperative days may help to maintain sinus rhythm. However, there is no clear cut data as there is much ambiguity in literature regards benefit from prophylactic overdrive pacing after cardiac surgery. Two important studies have revealed that postoperative drainage of retained blood from the pericardial space helps in reducing local inflammation and prevents AF after CABG.

■ MANAGEMENT

Chronic AF (in the outpatient community) and POAF are two distinct entities as far as management is concerned. In the former, sinus rhythm is usually not maintained after cardioversion; hence there is no advantage in continuing with repeated attempts at cardioversion. However, it is imperative that ventricular rate is controlled and the underlying causes which increase susceptibility to AF should be treated, as both these strategies improve long-term outcome. On the other hand, in patients with "early-onset of AF" and before chronicity has set in, it is worth attempting cardioversion because these group of patients are likely to maintain sinus rhythm. Similarly, patients with POAF who are mainly cases of "new-onset of AF" are by and large good candidates for cardioversion.

Rate and Rhythm Control in Postoperative Atrial Fibrillation

Approximately 90% of patients who develop AF after CABG are known to revert spontaneously within 2 months and continue to maintain normal rhythm. Hence, there are distinct advantages in reverting these postcardiac surgery patients (with new-onset of AF) back to sinus rhythm as they are more likely to maintain normal rhythm. Further, early cardioversion, rather than delay by waiting for spontaneous reversal to happen, will help improve hemodynamics and decrease the risk of cardiac failure in the crucial postoperative period. Early restoration of rhythm also decreases the risk of thromboembolic episodes.

Initial approach towards patients who are *hemodynamically stable* is to control their ventricular rate below 100/min. Once this is accomplished, cardioversion by either pharmacological or electrical means should be attempted, because in absence of sinus rhythm hemodynamic stability may be compromised. In practice, many of these patients spontaneously convert to sinus rhythm during infusion of medications given to achieve rate control.

Immediate cardioversion is the treatment of choice in all *hemodynamically unstable* patients with POAF and is best performed by a synchronized direct current defibrillator. Unlike stable patients where rate control may suffice, hemodynamically unstable patients can deteriorate rapidly if they are not offered the advantage of atrial kick by converting to sinus rhythm.

Deep sedation is a prerequisite before *cardioversion with electric defibrillator*. Propofol given as a 2 mg/kg stat dose is usually very effective; however, apnea and hypotension are two side effects and one should be prepared to deal with both these complications. Before applying the shock, "R" wave synchronization should be ensured especially for AF where QRS complexes are well defined. Unsuccessful cardioversion may be due to an incorrect positioning of the paddles, chronic AF with a dilated left atrium, tight mitral stenosis, electrolyte imbalance, or uncorrected hyperthyroidism.

Antiarrhythmic Agents

A beta-blocker is usually the drug of choice to control ventricular rate in the postoperative period. Metoprolol or esmolol may be administered intravenously for immediate control of fast ventricular rate and is followed by an oral maintenance dose. Many intensivists prefer intravenous (IV) diltiazem for its efficacy and safety in critically ill patients. IV verapamil should be avoided in patients with left ventricular (LV) dysfunction and no more than a single bolus dose should be repeated, not exceeding 10 mg given over 2–3 minutes. Doses higher than 10 mg given rapidly can precipitate a sharp drop in the blood pressure (BP). Digoxin may be used to control ventricular rate in patients with LV dysfunction, especially if there is no response to other agents. IV amiodarone is more useful for rhythm control and often patients revert abruptly to sinus rhythms during infusion. However, even if it fails to convert the rhythm back to sinus, it is useful for rate control and produces less hypotension than calcium channel blockers or beta-blockers. Dosage of drugs used for rate control is given in **Table 2**.

Present guidelines advocate early conversion to sinus rhythm in all cases of POAF, though for asymptomatic stable patients a deferred cardioversion, after controlling the ventricular rate is acceptable. As mentioned earlier, unstable patients should be cardioverted immediately with a direct current electrical

TABLE 2 Medications for rate control of AF.

Drug	IV stat dose	Oral maintenance dose
Metoprolol tartrate	2.5–5 mg IV bolus over 3–5 minutes. Can be repeated at 5 minutes intervals, not exceeding 10 mg	–
Metoprolol XL	–	50–100 mg OD
Esmolol	500 µg/kg IV bolus over 1 minute followed by 50–200 µg/kg/min IV infusion	–
Carvedilol	–	3.125–25 mg BID
Bisoprolol	–	2.5–10 mg OD
Amiodarone	150–300 mg in 100 mL of 5% glucose IV over 1 hour followed by 600–900 mg in 500 mL 5% glucose over 24 hours (incompatible with 0.9% NaCl). To be given by central vein, not to be given by peripheral vein because of the risk of thrombophlebitis	200 mg TDS for 4 days followed by 100–200 mg OD (monitoring heart rate and QTc)
Diltiazem	0.25 mg/kg IV bolus over 2 minutes	120–360 mg (ER) OD
Verapamil	5–10 mg IV bolus over 2 minutes and repeat 5 mg bolus after 10 minutes, if required	120–240 mg (ER) OD
Digoxin	0.25 mg IV and repeat to a maximum of 1 mg in 24 hours	0.125–0.250 mg OD

(AF: atrial fibrillation; BID: twice a day; ER: extended release; IV: intravenous; OD: once a day; TDS: thrice a day; ER: extended release).
Source: Modified from Am Coll Cardiol 2014:64(21).

shock. In stable patients, amiodarone is the drug of choice for pharmacological conversion and postconversion a maintenance dose should be continued for 6–8 weeks.

Though *amiodarone* is considered the most effective drug for both cardioversion and maintenance of sinus rhythm, it has both short- and long-term side effects. The major side effects on long-term use include thyroid dysfunction in almost one quarter of the patients, and rarely severe hepatotoxicity (though slight elevation of transaminases is common). Pulmonary toxicity is seen more often in the elderly population and with prolonged therapy. It may present with alveolitis, pneumonitis, or in severe form as interstitial pulmonary fibrosis, with CT findings of ground glass opacities and fibrosis and pulmonary function tests reveal a restrictive lung disorder with an impaired diffusion capacity [decreased transfer factor for carbon monoxide (TLCO)]. Frequent monitoring of TLCO is recommended for early detection of this serious complication in all patients on long-term amiodarone therapy. Cardiac side effects include bradyarrhythmias and prolonged QT interval but the incidence of torsades de pointes is rare. Neurological side effects though uncommon, include peripheral neuropathy, and rarely cerebellar dysfunction or cognitive impairment. IV amiodarone should always be administered through the central veins as peripheral infusion of the drug can cause severe thrombophlebitis. Amiodarone should be used with caution when given along with beta-blockers or calcium channel antagonists as it may increase the risk of severe bradycardia, atrioventricular (AV) block, or myocardial depression. It is currently accepted as the first-line antiarrhythmic drug in critically ill patients in the ICU, as it causes minimal myocardial depression. Unlike oral amiodarone, IV administration acts rapidly, hence it is best to overlap the oral maintenance doses along with the IV therapy. The dosage for cardioversion and maintenance remains the same as for the rate reduction (*see* **Table 2**).

Studies have shown that amiodarone is superior to beta-blockers and propafenone for maintenance of sinus rhythms. However, *sotalol*, despite its serious side effects, would be a good alternative to amiodarone as it is very effective in maintaining sinus rhythm. Sotalol is given in a starting dose of 80 mg twice daily, but in patients with a creatinine clearance of <60 mL/min, the dose should be reduced to once daily, and if the creatinine clearance is <40 mL/min, it is contraindicated. During sotalol therapy, frequent ECG monitoring of QT interval is mandatory. Gradual increments by 80 mg/day, but not exceeding 160 mg twice daily, may be given if required, provided the QT interval remains <500 ms and there is no bradycardia. *Propafenone and flecainide* are less effective than amiodarone and sotalol in maintaining sinus rhythm and both these drugs are not recommended in patients suffering from a prior myocardial infarction or decreased LV function. *Dofetilide* is not contraindicated in patients with compromised LV function, but should be used with utmost caution with very close monitoring of QT interval as the danger of precipitating torsade de pointes is more likely with this drug compared to others. *Dronedarone* is another drug structurally similar to amiodarone, but it has serious side effects and is reported to have increased mortality when used in patients with congestive heart failure; in fact, it is not freely available in the market.

In a critical care scenario, one should be aware that drugs administered orally may not be well absorbed, and at times, IV amiodarone may have to be continued for a longer period of 48–72 hours till the overlapping maintenance dose takes effect. Drugs such as digoxin, sotalol, atenolol, and dofetilide are renally excreted and their dosage needs to be carefully adjusted according to the serum creatinine levels, whereas drugs such as amiodarone, metoprolol, and diltiazem are hepatically excreted, and hence can be safely used in patients with renal insufficiency or during dialysis. Verapamil and flecainide are partly excreted both by the liver and the kidneys and will require renal dose adjustment. As for amiodarone, one should try to restrict its use for not >3 months postoperatively. For one, it may not be required as most patients will stabilize to sinus rhythm without the need for further antiarrhythmic medications, and secondly, as prolonged use of amiodarone is associated with serious pulmonary side effects. Amiodarone may be safely replaced by beta-blockers if required for long-term therapy. The usual maintenance dosage of drugs is given in **Table 3**.

Anticoagulation Strategies

In critically ill patients, the use of anticoagulants is a double-edged weapon. On one hand, these patients are at an added risk of developing spontaneous bleeds and on the other hand, they are at high risk of succumbing to thromboembolic complications. Hence, one has to carefully balance the risk versus the benefits of short-term or long-term anticoagulation. In demanding situations, transesophageal echocardiography (TEE) helps in detecting left atrial clots which are missed on transthoracic echo, as it gives a good view of the left atrial appendage. Once the clot is demonstrated, electrical cardioversion can be confidently performed under cover of heparin followed by an oral anticoagulant.

TABLE 3 Commonly used oral antiarrhythmic drugs as maintenance for AF.

Drugs	Dosages
Amiodarone	100–400 mg once a day
Sotalol	80–160 mg (12 hourly)
Flecainide	50–200 mg (12 hourly)
Propafenone	150–300 mg (8 hourly)
Dofetilide	0.125–0.5 (12 hourly)
Quinidine	300–600 mg (6 hourly)

In patients with AF for >48 hours, anticoagulation before cardioversion is a standard recommendation. Normally for most stable patients with long-term AF, 3 weeks of anticoagulation is recommended before cardioversion. However, the scenario is different in hemodynamically unstable surgery patients or in patients with AF after cardiac surgery. Here immediate cardioversion is a pressing issue and hence heparin is given as a bridge to oral anticoagulants, which then follow as maintenance therapy.

In cases of new-onset POAF (<48 hours) where chances of developing left atrial thrombus are less likely, there is limited data regards the need for anticoagulation before electrical cardioversion. However all postsurgical patients have an increased inflammatory response which predisposes to hypercoagulable states, resulting in an imminent risk of a thromboembolic episode. Hence, it would be prudent to selectively anticoagulant patients with <48 hours duration of AF, before cardioversion. However, the risk of potential postsurgical hemorrhage should always be weighed against the benefits of anticoagulation, especially as there is limited data regards the possible benefit in this group of patients.

Usual recommendation regarding long-term anticoagulation after reverting POAF to sinus rhythm is to continue oral anticoagulation for 2–3 months. Postcardioversion risk of thromboembolic events (stroke) in patients with AF > 48 hours is not uncommon, particularly after cardiac surgery, because of the underlying atheromatous disease and poor LV function. There is also a transient decrease in the atrial mechanical function occurring after cardioversion to sinus rhythm, which may last from a few days to a month. Further, studies have shown that incidence of thromboembolism is higher in patients who discontinued therapy after cardioversion or took subtherapeutic doses. However, in selective cases who are at high risk of developing stroke, may require lifelong anticoagulation. Scoring guidelines shown in **(Tables 4 and 5)** give an objective assessment to help in making a decision towards lifelong anticoagulation. Usually a score of 2 or more points favors anticoagulation in either of the scoring systems.

Platelet inhibitors (aspirin or clopidogrel) are less effective than anticoagulants in stroke prevention in patients with AF, and hence are not

TABLE 4 CHADS$_2$ (acronym). European Society of Cardiology (ESC) risk stratification scoring system for AF.

CCF	1
Hypertension	1
Age > 75	1
Diabetes mellitus	1
Stroke/TIA/TE	2
Total	6

(CCF: congestive cardiac failure; TE: thromboembolism; TIA: transient ischemic attack)

TABLE 5 CHA$_2$DS$_2$-VASc (acronym). Scoring and risk stratification for AF (ESC).

Risk factors	Points
CCF	1
Hypertension	1
Age ≥ 75	2
Age 65–75	1
Diabetes mellitus	1
Stroke/TIA/TE	2
Sex—female	1
Vascular disease or prior MI or PAD	1
Total	9

(CCF: congestive cardiac failure; MI: myocardial infarction; PAD: peripheral arterial disease; TE: thromboembolism; TIA: transient ischemic attack)

recommended. The usual anticoagulants used for stroke prophylaxis in AF are (1) vitamin K antagonist—warfarin or (2) the novel oral anticoagulants (NOACs)—rivaroxaban, apixaban, or dabigatran. However, the current guidelines do not recommend NOACs in patients with valvular heart disease and in those with prosthetic valves (mainly metallic valves), and hence the vitamin K antagonist (warfarin) is advised for anticoagulation in such patients. Unlike NOACs which have a standard dose, warfarin needs to be titrated according to the international normalized ratio (INR), as measured by the prothrombin time. According to studies, an INR of 2.5 or more has shown the least incidence of thromboembolic events; hence, it is best to maintain an INR of 2.5–3 which is considered safe and effective.

CONCLUSION

- Major cardiac surgery or pneumonectomy has the maximum impact on the incidence of POAF. Degree of manipulation and compression of the atria is also associated with POAF.
- Prophylactic strategies against POAF include one of the four interventions—antiarrhythmic therapy, maintenance of electrolyte and magnesium balance, postoperative pain and stress management, and overdrive atrial pacing. Corticosteroids and sotalol are currently not approved as their side effects outweigh the benefits.
- All patients with AF after cardiac surgery will benefit from cardioversion.
- Rate reduction followed by attempts at pharmacological cardioversion is acceptable for stable patients.
- Anticoagulation using heparin is mandatory for all patients of POAF undergoing urgent electrical cardioversion, particularly those with AF of >48 hours.

- Anticoagulation should be temporarily continued for 2-3 months after restoration of sinus rhythm.
- It may be prudent to initiate anticoagulation also in patients with AF < 48 hours if the risk of thromboembolism is substantially high, when balanced against the risk of postoperative bleeding.

SUGGESTED READING

1. Aranki SF, Shaw DP, Adams DH, Rizzo RJ, Couper GS, VanderVliet M, et al. Predictors of atrial fibrillation after coronary artery surgery. Current trends and impact on hospital resources. Circulation. 1996;94(3):390-7.
2. Archbold RA, Schilling RJ. Atrial pacing for the prevention of atrial fibrillation after coronary artery bypass graft surgery: a review of the literature. Heart. 2004;90(2):129-33.
3. Arsenault KA, Yusuf AM, Crystal E, Healey JS, Morillo CA, Nair GM, et al. Interventions for preventing post-operative atrial fibrillation in patients undergoing heart surgery. Cochrane Database Syst Rev. 2013;2013(1):CD003611.
4. Brathwaite D, Weissman C. The new onset of atrial arrhythmias following major noncardiothoracic surgery is associated with increased mortality. Chest. 1998;114(2):462-8.
5. Creswell LL, Schuessler RB, Rosenbloom M, Cox JL. Hazards of postoperative atrial arrhythmias. Ann Thorac Surg. 1993;56(3):539-49.
6. Crystal E, Connolly SJ, Sleik K, Ginger TJ, Yusuf S. Interventions on prevention of postoperative atrial fibrillation in patients undergoing heart surgery: a meta-analysis. Circulation. 2002;106(1):75-80.
7. Gillinov AM, Bagiella E, Moskowitz AJ, Raiten JM, Groh MA, Bowdish ME, et al. Rate Control versus Rhythm Control for Atrial Fibrillation after Cardiac Surgery. N Engl J Med. 2016;374(20):1911-21.
8. Kirchhof P, Benussi S, Kotecha D, et al. 2016 ESC Guidelines for the management of atrial fibrillation developed in collaboration with EACTS. Eur Heart J. 2016; 37(38):2893-2962.
9. Kowey PK, Stebbins D, Igidbashian L, Goldman SM, Sutter FP, Rials SJ, et al. Clinical outcome of patients who develop PAF after CABG surgery. Pacing Clin Electrophysiol. 2001;24(2):191-3.
10. Manning WJ, Silverman DI, Katz SE et al. Impaired left atrial mechanical function after cardioversion: relation to the duration of atrial fibrillation. J Am Coll Cardiol. 1994;23(7):1535-40.
11. Shiga T, Wajima Z, Inoue T, Ogawa R. Magnesium prophylaxis for arrhythmias after cardiac surgery: a meta-analysis of randomized controlled trials. Am J Med. 2004;117(5):325-33.
12. Singer DE, Albers GW, Dalen JE, Fang MC, Go AS, Halperin JL, et al. Antithrombotic therapy in atrial fibrillation: American College of Chest Physicians Evidence-Based Clinical Practice Guidelines (8th Edition). Chest. 2008;133(6 Suppl):546S-92S.
13. St-Onge S, Perrault LP, Demers P, Boyle EM, Gillinov AM, Cox J, et al. Pericardial Blood as a Trigger for Postoperative Atrial Fibrillation After Cardiac Surgery. Ann Thorac Surg. 2018;105(1):321-8.
14. Van Gelder IC, Hemels ME. The progressive nature of atrial fibrillation: a rationale for early restoration and maintenance of sinus rhythm. Europace. 2006;8(11):943-9.
15. Whitlock RP, Devereaux PJ, Teoh KH, Lamy A, Vincent J, Pogue J, et al. Methylprednisolone in patients undergoing cardiopulmonary bypass (SIRS): a randomised, double-blind, placebo-controlled trial. Lancet. 2015;386(10000):1243-53.
16. Zheng Z, Jayaram R, Jiang L, Emberson J, Zhao Y, Li Q, et al. Perioperative Rosuvastatin in Cardiac Surgery. N Engl J Med. 2016;374(18):1744-53.

CHAPTER 28

An Approach to Acute Abdomen

Shruti Tandan Pardasani

■ INTRODUCTION

The symptom of a sudden onset, often excruciating pain in the abdomen with accompanying signs of tenderness, guarding, with or without rigidity, often presents itself to the emergency room as acute abdomen.

Acute abdomen encompasses a widespread gamut of conditions that nearly always require immediate attention, for some of these may be life or organ threatening. It has generally an onset within <5 days. Nearly a third of the times, this pain may originate from renal colic, biliary colic, or appendicitis, these being the next most common causes.

The foremost step in approaching a case of acute abdomen is assessment of vital parameters and attention to airway, breathing, and circulation (ABC).

■ DETERMINING THE ORIGIN OF THE PAIN (TABLE 1)

When we encounter acute pain, our prime interest is always in diagnosing its cause, but the foremost step, in fact, should be stabilization of vitals, not localization. No matter how well-versed one is with differentials, it always helps to enlist all the anatomical structures in the area and the pathologies of these, which can produce this type of pain. Pain originating from superficial structures such as skin, subcutaneous tissue, abdominal musculature (injury/hematoma), or nerves (herpes zoster/porphyria), may occasionally be intense, but there is no associated guarding or rigidity. Presence of severe abdominal pain, devoid of signs like guarding/rigidity, but with tachycardia, hypertension or other autonomic disturbances and with neurologic manifestations like seizures or neuropathic pain and with psychiatric features like anxiety or hallucinations, especially if episodic, should raise suspicion of porphyria.

Similar acute moderate-to-severe pain with paucity of signs may be present in young individuals due to sickle cell crisis, which can be life-threatening and thus requires immediate attention. Though analgesia, hydration, blood transfusion, and correction of hypoxemia are the mainstay, many of the other causes of acute abdomen such as cholelithiasis, bowel, or mesenteric ischemia may overlap, and hence these must be excluded.

It is helpful to recollect that the abdomen has dual innervations—visceral and somatic. Visceral nerves arise from the autonomic nervous system and hence the irritation of these nerves by distension, smooth muscle contraction, inflammation, or ischemia of the viscera, causes a dull and poorly localized

TABLE 1	Six major clinical presentations of acute abdomen.
Major clinical presentation	**Examples**
1. Abdominal pain with hemodynamic compromise *Presentation*: Shock	• Acute abdominal aortic dissection • Ectopic pregnancy • Acute mesenteric ischemia • Severe acute pancreatitis • Ruptured spleen • Septic abdomen
2. Generalized peritonitis *Presentation*: Diffuse abdominal pain, toxic look, peritoneal signs—board like rigidity, rebound tenderness and guarding, and very gentle palpation best over the umbilical groove.	• Perforated ulcer • Colonic perforation • Perforated appendix • Severe acute pancreatitis may occasionally present with generalized peritonitis
3. Localized peritonitis *Presentation*: Clinical signs confined to one quadrant of the abdomen.	• Acute appendicitis • Acute cholecystitis • Acute diverticulitis • Acute salpingitis
4. Intestinal obstruction *Presentation:* Vomiting and colicky pain in small bowel obstruction. Constipation and abdominal distension in colonic obstruction. Absence of bowel sounds.	• Adhesions • Strictures • Volvulus • Tumors • Obstructed hernia
5. Abdominal pain of medical disease *Presentation*: Abdominal pain devoid of signs but accompanied by tachycardia, autonomic disturbances, neurological or psychiatric symptoms, hypoxemia, fever, etc.	• Porphyria • Diabetic ketoacidosis • Sickle cell disease • Inferior myocardial infarction • Pneumonia
6. Abdominal wall pain *Presentation*: Pain from superficial structures such as skin, subcutaneous tissue, or abdominal musculature. Burning sensation, pain on contraction of muscles or on movements, rash of herpes zoster, and palpation of a hematoma.	• Herpes zoster • Abdominal wall hematoma • Muscle sprain • Muscle injury

pain in the midline. The parietal peritoneum has somatic innervations; thus, once the serosa or peritoneum is irritated, as in perforation, the pain is sharp and well localized. A classic example is the dull, diffuse ache of acute appendicitis which changes to sharp right iliac fossa pain when an abscess is formed.

Acute pain associated with obstipation, localizes to a bowel pathology and warrants early imaging to distinguish medical from surgical causes. Right iliac fossa pain often originates from the appendix; appendicular pain can be generalized to begin with and may be central or pelvic depending on the position of the appendix. Diverticular pain may be similar in character to that of appendicular origin and though commonly described in the left iliac fossa, it is not restricted to any characteristic location and is almost always accompanied by a history of long-standing constipation. The presence of rigidity, especially with obstipation, is an ominous sign pointing to a perforated viscus—in such a case stabilize vitals, alert the surgeon and obtain urgent imaging, erect and supine X-rays to demonstrate free gas or CT, if feasible. The pain of renal colic is localized to the loin or flanks but may sometimes present in the iliac fossa. Importantly, it is often severe or at best moderate, which slowly builds up to a momentum and then, may swoop down suddenly in intensity.

Gallbladder colic on the other hand is a misnomer, as the characteristic buildup of colicky pain is absent. Instead, there may be a constant upper abdominal/right hypochondriac pain, which may radiate to the shoulder or the back. Likewise, pain in the right hypochondrium may originate from liver injury or abscess and an accompanying pleuritic character or shoulder radiation may be indicative of diaphragmatic irritation.

Pain of pancreatic origin is localized in the upper abdomen, often central, deep seated, and severe, which may radiate to the back. The pain of aortic dissection is a close differential, being similar in location, but is more often excruciating with no guarding. Hemodynamic instability is a late feature. Aortic dissection must be excluded early, as it holds a narrow therapeutic window and carries a high mortality.

Presence of syncope may hint to a ruptured ectopic, aortic dissection, or massive gastrointestinal (GI) blood loss. Assessment of vitals and circulatory reserve will help distinguish this from a neurogenic syncope or a vasovagal episode resulting from severe pain.

Examination of hernial sites must be done in all patients. Rectal examination must be done in cases of obstipation or lower GI bleed.

If the presentation is lower abdominal pain, a pelvic examination should be done in females and in men the testes must be examined to exclude testicular torsion.

Splenic injury or splenic infarction can produce a sharp often pleuritic pain in the upper abdomen, or often in the left hypochondrium. Splenic injury is associated with guarding and free fluid demonstrated on focused assessment with sonography for trauma/ultrasonography (FAST/USG) screening with unstable hemodynamics.

Imaging Modalities

Ultrasonography abdomen is a quick bedside imaging modality of choice, not only for abdominal trauma, but a diagnosis can also be achieved in a few minutes with a focused examination for gallbladder pathologies, pancreatitis, hydronephrosis, and ruptured ectopic pregnancy.

If there is rigidity/obstipation, a CT abdomen or a quick X-ray abdomen, erect and supine, may help localize free air. Alternately, the presence of >3 air-fluid levels is reassuring of an ileus, warranting conservative management.

■ DETERMINING URGENCY

While the name acute abdomen itself warrants emergency care, a few red flags must alert the clinician to act immediately:
- Severe or sudden onset pain, especially one that disturbs sleep
- Pain associated with gross abdominal distension and guarding
- Rigidity or rebound tenderness
- Pain accompanied by hemodynamic instability
- Pain disproportionate to clinical findings
- Patient who is either too still or writhing in pain
- Hematemesis or hematochezia
- Bile in the vomit or in the blood (jaundice)
- Comorbid conditions: Age >50, history of prior abdominal surgery, and ischemic heart disease (IHD)
- Absent bowel sounds.

■ INVESTIGATIONS

A complete blood count and serum electrolytes including magnesium and calcium must be done in all patients. Serum amylase and lipase may be elevated in several conditions including bowel ischemia or perforation, but their elevation over three times is almost diagnostic of acute pancreatitis. Two sets of blood cultures must be sent when sepsis or an infective etiology is suspected *before* an antibiotic is administered. While urine ketones may not always be positive, serum ketones will help to diagnose diabetic ketoacidosis. Arterial blood gas (ABG) will help calculate the anion gap and rule out tissue hypoxemia; in addition arterial lactate is useful when suspecting bowel ischemia or sepsis.

Electrocardiogram (ECG) may warn of atrial fibrillation or hemodynamic instability in conditions such as mesenteric ischemia and bowel perforation and thus preempt better perioperative management.

Urine analysis and a urine culture are helpful when pyelonephritis is a possibility. A urine pregnancy test must be done when a woman in the child-bearing age presents with acute abdomen, especially when suspecting a ruptured ectopic pregnancy.

■ TREATMENT

After immediate resuscitation and a quick assessment, a large number of patients would require surgical intervention. Thus, it becomes important to appreciate and exclude the diagnoses where surgery has no role at all, such as diabetic ketoacidosis, porphyria, sickle cell crisis, peptic ulcer disease, acute pyelonephritis, vis-à-vis those conditions where surgical intervention is best delayed, namely, acute pancreatitis, acute appendicitis, and acute cholecystitis. The role of the acute care physician is to identify and triage the patients with conditions that require immediate surgery—aortic dissection, perforated viscus, mesenteric ischemia of the bowel or mesentery, acute bowel obstruction, and hemoperitoneum with solid organ lacerations. Sieving out this subgroup is paramount and is indeed distinguishing of an astute clinician.

SUGGESTED READING

1. Patterson JW, Kashyap S, Dominique E. Acute abdomen. Treasure Island (FL): StatPearls Publishing; 2020.
2. Solomkin JS, Mazuski JE, Bradley JS, Rodvold KA, Goldstein EJC, Baron EJ, et al. Diagnosis and management of complicated intra-abdominal infection in adults and children: guidelines by the Surgical Infection Society and the Infectious Diseases Society of America. Clin Infect Dis. 2010;50(2):133-64.
3. Silen W. Cope's Early Diagnosis of Acute Abdomen, 20th edition. Oxford: Oxford University Press; 2011.

CHAPTER 29

Endocrine Emergencies

Nalini S Shah, Kunal Thakkar

■ INTRODUCTION

The topic of endocrine emergencies is vast and includes various diabetic and nondiabetic endocrine conditions. Although diabetic emergencies are common, the relative rarity of nondiabetic endocrine emergencies requires a high index of suspicion for diagnosis and management. Treatment of the latter must be started based on suspicion, before diagnostic confirmation, provided the appropriate samples have been taken before the start of the treatment. As the evidence-based assessment of management of endocrine emergencies is limited in literature, we have tried below to outline in brief the clinical features, diagnosis, and management steps for various endocrine emergencies.

■ DIABETES-RELATED EMERGENCIES

Diabetic Ketoacidosis

Diabetic ketoacidosis (DKA) is an acute and life-threatening complication of diabetes requiring prompt recognition and aggressive treatment to improve clinical outcomes. As the name suggests, this condition is characterized by hyperglycemia, ketosis, and acidosis. Hyperglycemia results from absolute or relative insulin deficiency and relative glucagon excess. Insulin deficiency impairs peripheral glucose uptake and promotes fat catabolism, while glucagon excess promotes hepatic gluconeogenesis. Ketosis is caused by fat catabolism of adipose tissue leading to oxidation of excess free fatty acids in the liver, generating ketone bodies acetoacetate and β-hydroxybutyrate. The dissociation of ketone bodies (weak acids) results in metabolic acidosis. There is significant fluid loss to the extent of 5–7 L in critically ill adult patients, leading to severe dehydration. In addition there is also depletion of sodium, potassium, chloride, magnesium, and phosphate. Factors responsible for precipitation of DKA include infection, trauma, cardiovascular emergencies, etc., especially if associated with omission of, or inadequate insulin therapy. Most patients with DKA have pre-existing type 1 diabetes, although patients with advanced and severe type 2 diabetes also can develop DKA during an acute illness. It can be the presenting symptom complex for many children and adolescents leading to diagnosis of type 1 diabetes. DKA is also associated with a severe proinflammatory state characterized by elevation of levels of various cytokines, C-reactive protein, reactive oxygen species, and plasminogen activator inhibitor 1.

Clinical Manifestations

Clinical manifestations of DKA are predictable from its pathophysiology. Most patients give history of polyuria, polydipsia, fatigue, and blurred vision, present for at least few hours to days before the episode as a result of hyperglycemia. Dehydration due to osmotic diuresis results in variable circulatory stress ranging from normal blood pressure and pulse rate to severe circulatory collapse depending on severity. Ketosis leads to fruity odor in breath, as well as variable degrees of abdominal pain, with or without vomiting. Metabolic acidosis leads to tachypnea, regular deep breaths (*Kussmaul breathing*) with compensatory respiratory alkalosis. Patients often have clinical features pertinent to precipitating factors as stated above. Increased levels of stress hormones due to DKA, as well as due to precipitating factors leads to increased insulin resistance, manifesting as nonresponsiveness of hyperglycemia to usual doses of subcutaneous insulin. It should also be kept in mind that errors of insulin administration alone can lead to development of DKA without any other precipitating factor.

Laboratory Findings

The earliest and most urgent tests are determination of blood glucose by fingerprick and urine analysis for ketones by reagent stripes, both of which can be checked by the patient at home. These tests usually lead to detection of, or at least strong suspicion of DKA, if matching with the clinical profile. The list of tests for initial laboratory evaluation of a patient with suspected or confirmed DKA is extensive and is as depicted in **Table 1**.

The diagnostic criteria for DKA include blood glucose above 250 mg/dL, arterial blood pH <7.3, serum bicarbonate <15 mEq/L, and moderate degree

TABLE 1 Initial laboratory tests for patients with DKA and HHS.

Metabolic evaluation	Infectious disease evaluation*	Others*
• Glucose and serum ketones	• CBC with differential counts	• Electrocardiogram (ECG)
• Electrolytes (Na$^+$, K$^+$, Cl$^-$, HCO$_3^-$, Ca^{++}, PO$_4^{3-}$, and Mg^{++})	• Chest X-ray	• Urine toxicology panel
	• Urine culture	• Pregnancy test
	• Blood culture	
• Serum osmolality		
• Blood urea nitrogen, creatinine, and liver function tests		
• Arterial blood gases (ABGs)		
• HbA1c		
• Urine analysis		

*As clinically indicated
(CBC: complete blood count; DKA: diabetic ketoacidosis; HbA1c: hemoglobin A1c; HHS: hyperglycemic hyperosmolar state)

TABLE 2	Diagnostic criteria for diagnosis of DKA and HHS.			
	DKA			
	Mild	Moderate	Severe	HHS
Plasma glucose (mg/dL)	>250	>250	>250	>600
Arterial pH	7.25–7.3	7.00–7.24	<7.00	>7.3
Serum bicarbonate (mEq/L)	15–18	10–15	<10	>18
Serum and urine ketones	Positive	Positive	Positive	None to small
Effective serum osmolality (mOsm/kg water)	Variable	Variable	Variable	>320
Anion gap	>10	>12	>12	Usually normal
Mental status	Alert	Alert/drowsy	Stupor/coma	Stupor/coma

Effective serum osmolality = 2 × [measured sodium (mEq/L)] + glucose (mg/dL)/18.
(DKA: diabetic ketoacidosis; HHS: hyperglycemic hyperosmolar state)
(*Source*: Adapted from Kitabchi AE, Umpierrez GE, Murphy MB, Barrett EJ, Kreisberg RA, Malone JI, et al. Management of hyperglycemic crises in patients with diabetes. Diabetes Care. 2001;24(1):131-53).

of ketonemia and/or ketonuria. Approximately 10% of patients with DKA may have blood glucose levels below 250 mg/dL sometimes due to insulin administration beforehand by self of by primary care physician, advanced liver disease, or if patient had been taking sodium-glucose cotransporter-2 (SGLT2) inhibitor class of drugs. Categorization of DKA to indicate severity is as depicted in **Table 2**.

Accumulation of ketones results in anion gap metabolic acidosis. Anion gap is calculated by subtracting major measured anions (chloride and bicarbonate) from major measured cation (sodium). An anion gap >10–12 mEq/L suggests presence of anion gap acidosis.

The key laboratory feature of DKA is ketonemia or ketonuria. β-hydroxybutyrate is the predominant ketone body in blood in patients with DKA. However, nitroprusside reaction used in urine ketone strips, semiquantitatively detects only acetoacetate and acetone, underestimating the severity of ketoacidosis. Direct measurement of serum β-hydroxybutyrate can be helpful in diagnosis, if available.

At admission many patients have factitiously low serum sodium (pseudohyponatremia) because of hyperglycemia and hyperlipidemia. The corrected sodium can be calculated by adding 1.6 mEq to the reported sodium value for each 100 mg/dL of glucose above 100 mg/dL. As a result, normal or high reported sodium indicates severe state of dehydration. Although total body potassium store is depleted, initial serum potassium level may show hyperkalemia due to acidosis and insulin deficiency. Osmotic diuresis and acidosis-induced shifting of phosphate out of cells lead to negative phosphate balance.

Leukocytosis around 10,000–15,000/mm^3 due to elevation of stress hormones is a common finding in patients with DKA and does not necessarily indicate infection or sepsis. However leukocytosis above 25,000/mm^3 is indicative of septic process and should lead to aggressive evaluation for the same. Elevated serum amylase levels are also common in patients with DKA and do not always indicate pancreatitis, for which serum lipase should be more relied upon. Moderate hypertriglyceridemia is also common in the setting of DKA because of insulin deficiency leading to lipolysis and generation of free fatty acids, which accelerate formation of very low density lipoproteins (VLDL) in the liver.

Differential Diagnosis

Differentiation of DKA from other causes of ketoacidosis is not difficult. Patients with starvation and alcoholic ketoacidosis usually do not have hyperglycemia, and serum bicarbonate is usually >18 mEq/L. Other causes of anion gap metabolic acidosis include lactic acidosis, acute renal failure, ethylene glycol/salicylate/methanol poisoning, etc. Measurement of ketone concentration in plasma or in urine helps identifying origin of anion gap.

Treatment

Patients with DKA should preferably be managed in an intensive care unit (ICU) due to requirements of continuous monitoring, frequent blood testing, and frequent titration of therapy. Therapeutic goals for management of DKA include:
- Restoration of volume status
- Correction of hyperglycemia and ketoacidosis
- Correction of electrolyte abnormalities
- Treatment of precipitating factor
- Prevention of complications of DKA.

Fluid therapy: The average fluid loss in DKA is approximately 5–7 L. Intravenous (IV) normal saline should be started before insulin infusion. Normal saline is generally started at the rate of 15–20 mL/kg or 1–1.5 L in the first hour. After initial stabilization, if corrected serum sodium is normal or elevated, normal saline should be replaced by half-normal saline (0.45% saline), at a rate of 250–500 mL/hour. If corrected sodium is low, normal saline can be continued at a similar rate. Estimated fluid deficit should be corrected in 24 hours, with 50% correction in approximately the initial 8 hours. Once the serum glucose is 200–250 mg/dL, insulin infusion rate should be reduced to 1–2 units/hour and 5% dextrose should be added to IV fluids. This technique prevents hypoglycemia and allows continuation of insulin infusion in sufficient amount to reduce ketoacidosis. The response to fluid therapy is judged by monitoring hemodynamic parameters, clinical examination, urine output, and laboratory parameters. Electrolytes, bicarbonate, and venous pH should be monitored 4 hourly.

TABLE 3: Suggested algorithm for adjusting the IV insulin infusion during treatment of DKA/HHS.

Hourly change in blood glucose	Action
Blood glucose increases	Repeat bolus (0.1 U/kg) and double infusion rate
Blood glucose decreases by 0–49 mg/dL/h	Increase insulin drip rate by 25–50%
Blood glucose decreases by 50–75 mg/dL/h	No change in insulin drip
Blood glucose decreases by >75 mg/dL/h	Hold insulin drip for 30 minutes and then restart at 50% of previous rate

(DKA: diabetic ketoacidosis; HHS: hyperglycemic hyperosmolar state)

Insulin therapy: It is advised not to start insulin infusion if baseline serum potassium is <3.3 mEq/L; waiting till normalization of potassium levels with IV fluids and potassium replacement is justified. Insulin treatment should start with IV bolus dose of 0.1 unit/kg and regular human insulin followed by 0.1 unit/kg/hour infusion. Ideally insulin therapy should decrease blood glucose by 50–75 mg/dL/hour. Overly aggressive reduction of glucose can lead to brain edema. A suggested algorithm for adjusting IV insulin infusion is depicted in **Table 3**. Blood glucose should be monitored using capillary readings hourly initially, and every 2-3 hours once stabilized.

Potassium replacement: Despite total body potassium deficit, serum potassium concentration can be normal or elevated due to acidosis and insulin deficiency. Administration of insulin results in intracellular shift of potassium and consequent fall in serum level. Approximately 10-20 mEq/hour potassium chloride is usually added to IV fluids provided initial serum potassium concentration is <5.5 mEq/L. Potassium deficit in DKA is usually in the range of 300 mEq, but can be as high as 1,000 mEq, and such patients require higher replacement doses. Potassium deficit may persist even after DKA is treated and hence oral replacement should continue.

Phosphate replacement: This is usually required only if serum phosphate concentration at baseline is <1.5 mg/dL, to prevent hypophosphatemic syndrome due to further fall with insulin therapy. Such patients would require 500–1,000 mg elemental phosphate over 12-24 hours.

Bicarbonate therapy: Acidosis generally resolves with adequate fluid and insulin therapy, and usually bicarbonate therapy is not required. Bicarbonate replacement should be initiated only if initial pH <6.9. The replacement is done using the following formula:

$$\text{Bicarbonate (mmol)} = \text{Base deficit} \times \text{weight (kg)} \times 0.3$$

Half of the total dose is given as a bolus and the rest as a slow infusion over the next 8 hours. Hypokalemia, if present, should be corrected before bicarbonate administration.

Search for Treatment of Precipitating Factor

As mentioned earlier, various precipitating factors include infection, cardiovascular, and other acute stresses. Evaluation is required for identifying any such potential precipitating factor (*see* **Table 1**) for its simultaneous appropriate treatment. Errors in insulin administration, if found as a precipitating factor for DKA, should be addressed adequately to prevent future episodes of DKA.

Resolution of Diabetic Ketoacidosis

The criteria for resolution of DKA include plasma glucose <200 mg/dL and at least two of these criteria: bicarbonate ≥ 15 mEq/L, pH > 7.3, and anion gap ≤ 12. Serum bicarbonate can still be low even after resolution of DKA, due nongap acidosis related to aggressive IV crystalloid replacement. Thus the anion gap is the best indicator of DKA resolution.

Transition to Subcutaneous Insulin Therapy

Intravenous insulin infusion can be replaced by subcutaneous insulin injections once DKA has resolved and patient is eating and drinking without vomiting. It is not necessary to wait for the urine to become clear of ketones, as this usually takes a longer time. Shifting to subcutaneous insulin can be more convincingly done with the next planned meal. It is important to overlap with continuation of IV insulin till at least 1-2 hours after subcutaneous insulin injection to prevent recurrence of hyperglycemia and ketosis. If the patient is already a known type 1 diabetic, then the previous insulin regimen can be restarted after addressing the errors, if any. In newly diagnosed patients, multidose insulin (MDI) regimen should be started with total insulin dose ranging from 0.5 to 0.8 units/kg body weight.

Complications

Hypokalemia and hypoglycemia are the most common iatrogenic complications while treating DKA. These can be prevented by appropriate potassium supplements with frequent monitoring and appropriate insulin adjustment along with use of dextrose containing fluids.

Hyperchloremic nonanion gap metabolic acidosis is commonly seen after resolution of DKA, usually due to high amounts of chloride administered as IV fluids. It can be prevented by replacing normal saline with 0.45% saline as maintenance fluid, once patient is stabilized and corrected serum sodium is normal or high.

Cerebral edema is an uncommon but very serious complication of DKA treatment, associated with increased mortality. Overzealous hydration and rapid normalization of hyperglycemia leading to rapid changes in osmolality are associated with increased risk of cerebral edema. It should be suspected based on a change in mental status in a patient who is otherwise recovering from DKA.

Hyperglycemic Hyperosmolar State

Hyperglycemic hyperosmolar state (HHS) is characterized by greater severity of plasma glucose elevation, marked increase in plasma osmolality, absent to mild ketosis, and altered mental status. This condition is predominantly observed in elderly patients with type 2 diabetes, and is typically of gradual onset. There is usually a medical condition that has exacerbated the often undiagnosed type 2 diabetes. Although pathophysiology is somewhat similar to DKA, small residual insulin secretion often prevents development of ketosis and acidosis. Infection is the major precipitating factor for HHS (pneumonia, pyelonephritis, etc.) occurring in about 50% of patients. Other acute illnesses such as myocardial infarction, stroke, and pancreatitis can precipitate HHS due to release of counter-regulatory hormones.

Clinical Manifestations

Contrary to onset of DKA which is relatively acute, HHS usually evolves over days to weeks. The typical osmotic symptoms of unrestrained hyperglycemia are often present for few days to weeks, along with physical findings suggestive of severe dehydration. Mental status is usually altered in patients with HHS, varying from lethargy to stupor or coma. Even though infection is a common precipitating factor, body temperature can be misleadingly normal or low due to peripheral vasodilation.

Laboratory Findings

The initial laboratory evaluation of a patient with suspected HHS is the same as for DKA (*see* **Table 1**). A search for the precipitating factor must be started simultaneously. The criteria for diagnosis and usual laboratory features are listed in **Table 2**. Patients with HHS usually present with profound hyperglycemia (blood glucose > 600 mg/dL), elevated plasma osmolality (>320 mOsm/kg), and severe dehydration/volume contraction. Anion gap is usually normal and bicarbonate levels >18-20 mEq/L in patients with HHS. The dehydration as well as depletion of electrolytes (sodium, potassium, chloride, and phosphate) are more marked in HHS as compared to DKA due to gradual and prolonged duration of osmotic diuresis and decreased fluid intake.

Treatment

The therapeutic goals are almost similar to those for managing DKA as described above. The treatment protocols are also essentially the same as for DKA, with some modifications. The IV fluids should be started before starting insulin. The fall in blood glucose should be approximately 50-100 mg/dL/hour with insulin and IV fluids. The change in serum osmolality should not exceed 3 mOsm/kg/hour. In the majority of patients with HHS, serum osmolality and mental status are normalized by the time hyperglycemia is corrected, when simply lowering insulin infusion rate can be sufficient and addition of 5%

dextrose is often not necessary. However, due to concerns that lowering blood glucose too fast may promote development of cerebral edema, some authorities recommend adding 5% dextrose to IV fluids when blood glucose is in the range of 250-300 mg/dL, until the patient is mentally alert. Otherwise the fluid replacement, insulin therapy, monitoring, and replacement of electrolytes, as well as treatment of precipitating factors remain the same as described for DKA. Resolution of HHS is characterized by normal serum osmolality (<315 mOsm/kg) and normal mental status. The mortality rate in HHS is higher than that in DKA due to advanced age, associated comorbidities, underlying acute illness, thrombotic events, etc.

Hypoglycemia

Hypoglycemia is the limiting factor in the glycemic management of diabetes. Iatrogenic hypoglycemia induced by either insulin, sulfonylureas, and/or glinides causes recurrent morbidity in most people with type 1 diabetes and in many with advanced type 2 diabetes, and it can be fatal. Indeed, while early studies indicated 2-4% mortality due to hypoglycemia in type 1 diabetes, more recent data indicates mortality rates as high as 6-10%. Hypoglycemic deaths occur in patients with type 2 diabetes as well, but the mortality rate is not known. Again hypoglycemia impairs defense against subsequent falling plasma glucose (hypoglycemia unawareness) and thus leads to a vicious cycle of recurrent hypoglycemia. The incidence of iatrogenic hypoglycemia in insulin treated type 2 diabetes is about one-third of that in type 1 diabetes, but the frequency increases with time. However, because the prevalence of type 2 diabetes is about 20-fold more than that of type 1 diabetes, most episodes of hypoglycemia occur in people with type 2 diabetes.

In contrast, hypoglycemia is an uncommon clinical event in individuals without diabetes. Nonetheless there is a list of differential diagnosis of hypoglycemia in nondiabetic individuals **(Table 4)**. The leading causes of hypoglycemia in such individuals are drugs, other than those used to treat diabetes. Clearly, intentional, accidental, surreptitious, and even malicious drug use should be considered when the mechanism of a hypoglycemic episode is obscure.

Clinical Features and Diagnosis

Clinical hypoglycemia is most convincingly documented by Whipple's triad: clinical features consistent with hypoglycemia; a low measured plasma glucose concentration; and resolution of those symptoms and signs, once plasma glucose concentration has been raised.

Neurogenic (or autonomic) symptoms include both adrenergic (palpitations, tremulousness, and anxiety/arousal) and cholinergic (sweating, hunger, and paraesthesia) symptoms. Neuroglycopenic symptoms as a result of brain glucose deprivation include cognitive impairments, behavioral changes,

TABLE 4	Differential diagnosis of hypoglycemia.

Ill or medicated individuals	• Drugs
	  – Insulin and insulin secretagogue
	  – Alcohol
	  – Many other drugs
	• Critical illness
	  – Renal, hepatic, and cardiac failure
	  – Sepsis
	  – Inanition
	• Hormone deficiency
	  – Cortisol deficiency
	  – Glucagon and epinephrine deficiency (in insulin deficient diabetes mellitus)
	• Nonislet cell tumor

Seemingly well individuals	• Endogenous hyperinsulinism
	  – Insulinoma
	  – Functional β-cell disorders (nesidioblastosis)
	  – Autoimmune hypoglycemia (autoantibody to insulin or insulin receptors)
	  – Insulin secretagogue
	  – Others
	• Accidental, surreptitious, and malicious hypoglycemia

(*Source*: Adapted from (1) Cryer PE, Lloyd Axelrod, Ashley B Grossman, Simon R Heller, Victor M Montori, Elizabeth R Seaquist, et al. Evaluation and management of adult hypoglycemic disorders: an Endocrine Society Clinical Practice Guideline. J Clin Endocrinol Metab. 2009;94:709-28. (2) Murad MH, Coto-Yglesias F, Wang AT, Sheidaee N, Mullan RJ, Elamin MB, et al. Clinical review: Drug-induced hypoglycemia: a systematic review. J Clin Endocrinol Metab. 2009;94(3):741-5.)

and psychomotor abnormalities; confusion, seizures, and coma occur at lower plasma glucose concentrations. Awareness of hypoglycemia is largely the result of perception of neurogenic symptoms. Signs of hypoglycemia include pallor and diaphoresis, the result of adrenergic cutaneous vasoconstriction, and cholinergic activation of sweat glands, respectively. Neuroglycopenic signs are often observable.

Treatment

The issue of hypoglycemia should be addressed in every contact with people with diabetes, especially those who are treated with insulin or sulfonylureas, and the target should be its prevention. However obviously when prevention fails, treatment becomes necessary.

Most episodes of asymptomatic hypoglycemia (detected on self-blood glucose testing at home) and mild-to-moderate symptomatic hypoglycemia (patient is conscious with minimal neuroglycopenic symptoms) can effectively be self-treated by ingestion of glucose tablets or carbohydrate containing fruit juice, candy, soft drink, other snack, or a meal. A reasonable dose is 20 g glucose. Clinical improvement should occur in 15–20 minutes; if not, then the same dose should be repeated for up to three times. Parenteral treatment becomes necessary when patient is unable to take carbohydrates orally or is unconscious. Intramuscular or subcutaneous glucagon injection (usual dose 1 mg in adults) by patient's attendant is often used in people with type 1 diabetes. That can be lifesaving, but it often results in side effects such as nausea or even vomiting and transient hyperglycemia. Smaller doses of glucagon (150 µg), repeated if necessary, have also been found to be effective without side effects. Because it acts by stimulating hepatic glycogenolysis, glucagon is ineffective in glycogen-depleted individuals (following a binge of alcohol and repeated hypoglycemia, especially with recent use of glucagon). Although glucagon can be administered intravenously, IV glucose or dextrose is the preferred parenteral therapy for most. A common initial dose is 25 g (100 mL of 25% dextrose or 50 mL of 50% dextrose). The glycemic response to oral or IV glucose is of course transient in the setting of ongoing hyperinsulinemia. Thus, ingestion of a more substantial snack or meal after regaining consciousness and after normal glucose concentration is generally advisable. The duration of iatrogenic hypoglycemia depends on the underlying cause—shorter if caused by rapid-acting insulin and prolonged if caused by long-acting sulfonylurea. The latter can result in recurrent episodes of hypoglycemia over few hours to even days, requiring hospitalization.

■ THYROID-RELATED EMERGENCIES

Myxedema Coma

Myxedema coma is characterized by severe and prolonged depletion of thyroid hormone, leading to altered mental status associated with hypothermia and other organ system disturbances. Although it has become rare nowadays with the widespread availability and measurement of thyroid tests, its early recognition is important due to the high mortality associated with delays in treatment. Myxedema coma can result from usual causes of hypothyroidism such as autoimmune hypothyroidism, postablative or postsurgery hypothyroidism. Precipitating factors such as infection, myocardial infarction, surgery, or use of sedative drugs in a patient with long-standing untreated hypothyroidism may lead to development of myxedema coma.

Clinical Features and Laboratory Findings

The classic presentation of myxedema coma is that of an elderly female with long-standing, improperly/inadequately treated hypothyroidism, who develops any of the precipitating factors, is given sedatives/narcotic drugs or is exposed to cold weather and develops altered mental status and hypothermia. The features of severe untreated hypothyroidism are usually present. The term myxedema coma is however a misnomer, as most patients do not

> **BOX 1** Clinical features and laboratory findings in patients with myxedema coma.
>
> *Hypothermia:*
> - Core body temperature < 35°C or 95°F
> - Infection with absence of fever
>
> *Decreased mental status*
> - Confusion, lethargy, obtundation, or coma
>
> *Cardiovascular abnormalities:*
> - Bradycardia
> - Decreased myocardial contractility
> - Low cardiac output
> - Hypotension or shock
>
> *Respiratory abnormalities:*
> - Central depression of respiratory drive
> - Respiratory muscle weakness
>
> *Laboratory abnormalities:*
> - Respiratory acidosis due to hypoventilation
> - Hypoglycemia directly due to hypothyroidism or due to associated adrenal insufficiency
> - Hyponatremia due to impaired free water excretion
> - Normocytic normochromic anemia due to decreased erythropoiesis
> - Elevation of creatinine phosphokinase due to increased muscular permeability

usually present with frank coma but only with signs of cognitive deterioration such as lethargy or confusion. The common clinical features and laboratory abnormalities are as described in **Box 1**.

Along with described laboratory findings, elevated thyroid-stimulating hormone (TSH) and low free T4 would characterize untreated hypothyroidism in most patients. TSH may not be as elevated as expected for the level of low free T4, usually due to intercurrent illness or because of use of drugs such as dopamine and glucocorticoids. On the other hand, low normal to low TSH coupled, with low free T4, point towards central hypothyroidism as an etiology. However, it is difficult to distinguish central hypothyroidism in such patients from nonthyroidal illness (sick-euthyroid), assessing other pituitary axis provides clue if these are affected.

Management

As myxedema coma is associated with high mortality, management should be aggressive pending laboratory confirmation. Treatment of myxedema coma consists of replacement with thyroid hormones, glucocorticoids, supportive management, and treatment of precipitating factor.

Thyroid hormone replacement: There is no consensus on the optimal mode of thyroid hormone replacement as there are no clinical trials considering the condition's rarity, and recommendations are based mostly on expert opinion.

The preferred route of thyroid hormone replacement is IV replacement with both T4 and T3 and one such approach is given below:
- *Levothyroxine (LT4)*: Loading dose of 200–250 µg IV followed by 100 µg after 24 hours of loading dose. After that maintenance dose of 50–75 µg IV/orally daily.
- *Liothyronine (LT3)*: Loading dose of 10–20 µg IV followed by 10 µg IV every 8–12 hours, until patient can take orally, then switch to LT4 oral regime only (1.5 µg/kg/day)

Although IV route is preferred considering the variable oral absorption due to gastric atony or ileus, the clinical response after oral dose occurs promptly and in one small observational study, the route of administration (oral or IV) did not affect mortality. Hence if IV LT4 and LT3 are not readily available, treatment should be started with 200–500 µg LT4 orally or through nasogastric tube. Heart rhythm should be continuously monitored during early phase of replacement in all patients, especially those with ischemic heart disease.

Intravenous glucocorticoids: About 10–15% of patients with myxedema coma have decreased adrenal function; therefore IV glucocorticoids should be started before starting thyroid hormone replacement. Stress dose of steroids should be started immediately, i.e., hydrocortisone 50 mg IV 6–8 hourly, should be continued for first 48 hours and then tapered over next few days in parallel with clinical improvement, unless the patient proves to be having adrenal insufficiency by further biochemical tests.

Supportive measures: Supportive measures are important components of care for patients with myxedema coma. Early intubation and mechanical ventilation is lifesaving for patients with profoundly altered mental status and hypoventilation. Passive rewarming is indicated such as with space blankets, while active rewarming should be avoided, as it may lead to vasodilatation and hypotension. Vasopressors are to be used if hypotension is present. Free water restriction helps in correcting hyponatremia, while transient hypertonic saline is used for severe hyponatremia (Na <120 mEq/L).

Finally, all the possible precipitating factors should be searched for and treated appropriately. Addressing all these components of care in an aggressive manner led to a significant decrease in mortality from 100% to 30–50%.

Thyroid Storm (Thyrotoxic Crisis)

Thyroid storm is defined as a life-threatening augmentation of manifestations of hyperthyroidism. The pathogenesis of thyroid storm is not fully understood as there is usually no difference in thyroid hormone levels between patients with uncomplicated thyrotoxicosis and those developing thyroid storm. One hypothesis that may explain the pathogenesis is increased catecholamine sensitivity due to increased β-adrenergic receptor density. The most common underlying thyroid condition is Grave's disease (TSH receptor antibody-mediated hyperthyroidism). Rare causes of thyrotoxicosis that can lead to thyroid storm are toxic adenoma, toxic multinodular goiter, TSH secreting pituitary tumor, struma ovary, or human chorionic gonadotropin (hCG)-secreting hydatidiform mole. A precipitating factor usually causes transition from thyrotoxicosis to thyroid storm. Such precipitating factors include any of the systemic stressors such as surgery, severe infection, trauma, myocardial infarction, and parturition. Thyroid storm has also been reported to be precipitated by excessive oral or IV (amiodarone or radiocontrast dye) iodine administration, radioiodine therapy, and even pseudoephedrine and salicylate use, where discontinuation of antithyroid drugs is a common denominator.

Clinical Features and Diagnosis

Thyroid storm is part of a continuum that begins with the development of decompensated thyrotoxicosis. The point at which thyrotoxicosis transforms into thyroid storm is not clear and is relatively subjective. So to standardize and objectify thyroid storm, Burch and Wartofsky have delineated point scale criteria for diagnosis of thyroid storm **(Table 5)**. However, it is prudent to aggressively treat the thyrotoxicosis state of a patient who is suspected of having a thyroid storm, rather than waiting for many investigations to decide whether this case meets the criteria to diagnose thyroid storm or not.

Treatment

The principles of treatment of thyroid storm include: (1) inhibition of thyroid hormone synthesis and release; (2) reducing the peripheral and biologic effects of thyroid hormones; and (3) treatment of systemic complications as well as precipitating factors.

It is important to start antithyroid drug therapy with thionamide at least by 1-2 hours before iodine therapy, to prevent new thyroid hormone synthesis that can occur initially with iodine therapy.

Management of thyroid storm is outlined in **Table 6**.

Once the life-threatening aspects of thyroid storm are treated, decisions should be made for definitive therapy of thyrotoxicosis. Thionamide therapy in gradually decreasing doses is needed for months after thyroid storm. β-adrenergic receptor blockers should be continued till the patient is thyrotoxic, while the other treatment modalities are usually tapered and discontinued coinciding with clinical improvement. Radioactive iodine ablation as definitive therapy cannot be used for weeks to months following treatment with iodine in thyroid storm. Thyroidectomy, if chosen as definitive therapy, should be performed once the patient is euthyroid for several weeks. The goal of definitive therapy is to prevent future recurrence of thyroid storm.

TABLE 5 Point scale criteria for diagnosis of thyroid storm.

Criteria	Points
Thermoregulatory dysfunction *Temperature (°F)*	
99.0–99.9	5
100.0–100.9	10
101.0–101.9	15
102.0–102.9	20
103.0–103.9	25
≥104.0	30
Cardiovascular tachycardia	
100–109	5
110–119	10
120–129	15
130–139	20
≥140	25
Atrial fibrillation	
Absent	0
Present	10
Congestive heart failure	
Absent	0
Mild (pedal edema)	5
Moderate (basilar rales)	10
Severe (pulmonary edema)	20
Gastrointestinal-hepatic dysfunction	
Absent	0
Moderate (diarrhea, abdominal pain, and nausea/vomiting)	10
Severe (unexplained jaundice)	20
Central nervous system disturbance	
Absent	0
Mild (agitation)	10
Moderate (delirium, psychosis, and extreme lethargy)	20
Severe (seizures and coma)	30
Precipitating history	
Absent	0
Present	10

Total score ≥ 45: Thyroid storm; 25–44: impending thyroid storm; <25: unlikely thyroid storm.
(*Source*: Adapted from Burch HB, Wartofsky L. Life-threatening thyrotoxicosis. Thyroid storm. Endocrinol Metab Clin North Am. 1993;22:263-77.)

TABLE 6	Management of thyroid storm.
• Inhibition of thyroid hormone synthesis[a]	
Methimazole	20–30 mg PO q6 h
Propylthiouracil	200–400 mg PO q6–8 h
• Inhibition of thyroid hormone release from thyroid gland[a]	
Saturated solution of potassium iodide (SSKI)	5 drops PO q6 h or 5–10 drops per rectum q6–8 h
Lugol's iodine solution	4–8 drops PO q6 h or 5–10 drops per rectum q6 h
• Counteraction of peripheral effects of thyroid hormones	
β-blockers[a]	
Propranolol	80–120 mg PO q6 h or 0.5–1 mg IV over 10–15 minutes every few hours as needed
Atenolol	50–200 mg PO qd (or divided bid)
Metoprolol	100–200 mg PO qd (or divided bid)
Steroids[a]	
Hydrocortisone	100 mg IV q8 h
Dexamethasone	2 mg IV q6 h
• Supportive therapy	
Acetaminophen	325–650 mg PO/per rectum q4–6 h
Thiamine	IV as clinically indicated (to prevent Wernicke's encephalopathy)
Fluids	D5%NS or D10%NS
• Treatment of systemic complications and precipitant factor	
• Alternative therapies	
Lithium carbonate	300 mg PO q8 h
Cholestyramine	4 g PO qd

[a]Use one agent of group as clinically indicated.
(*Source*: Adapted from (1) Nayak B, Burman K. Thyrotoxicosis and Thyroid Storm. Endocrinol Metab Clin N Am. 2006;35:663-86. (2) Alfandhli E, Gianoukakis A. Management of Severe Thyrotoxicosis When the Gastrointestinal Tract is Compromised. Thyroid. 2011;21(3):215-20.)

■ PARATHYROID-RELATED EMERGENCIES

Acute Hypocalcemia

Calcium is the single most abundant mineral ion in the human body and it serves as a critical ion for many physiological processes such as blood coagulation, platelet adhesion, neuromuscular activity, endocrine and exocrine secretory functions as well as bone metabolism. The adult human body contains approximately 1 kg of calcium, with most of it (99%) incorporated in bones and <1% in serum. Approximately 40–50% calcium in blood is bound to plasma proteins, predominantly albumin, and an equivalent amount being free or ionized calcium, which is physiologically active. The serum calcium level is closely regulated and maintained in normal range (8.5–10.1 mg/dL) by the endocrine system [parathyroid hormone (PTH) and vitamin D]. The regulation of serum calcium concentration is accomplished by coordinated action of PTH and active vitamin D (1, 25-dihydroxyvitamin D) on three predominant organs: intestine, bone, and kidney. In the short term, plasma proteins chiefly albumin, serves as the calcium buffer to maintain normal ionized calcium levels in serum. This calcium-albumin buffer is highly sensitive to pH. Disturbances in any of the axis maintaining calcium balance may lead to development of hypocalcemia **(Table 7)**. The most common cause of acute hypocalcemia is postoperative hypoparathyroidism after thyroid or other neck surgery, during which damage to or unintentional removal of most or all functioning parathyroid glands has taken place.

Clinical Features

The clinical manifestations depend on the degree and rapidity of development of hypocalcemia. An acute decrease in serum calcium concentration increases neuronal excitability, while chronic hypocalcemia, even at relatively lower calcium concentrations, can be asymptomatic. Patients with acute hypocalcemia will present with neurologic symptoms such as perioral tingling, paresthesias, and tingling in distal extremities and even carpopedal spasm (tetany). Trousseau's and Chvostek's signs are signs of

TABLE 7 Causes of hypocalcemia.

Reduced PTH secretion/action	Reduced vitamin D action	Calcium deposition
Hypoparathyroidism • Surgical • Idiopathic • Autoimmune • Postradiation • Genetic • Hypomagnesemia (functional)	Vitamin D deficiency • Limited sunlight exposure • Malabsorption Abnormal vitamin D metabolism • Liver or kidney disease • Abnormal enterohepatic circulation • Anticonvulsants	Hyperphosphatemia • Rhabdomyolysis • Renal failure • Tumor lysis syndrome • Phosphate administration Acute pancreatitis • Blood transfusions
PTH resistance • Pseudohypoparathyroidism • Renal failure	Vitamin D resistance • Vitamin D dependent rickets	Excessive skeletal deposition • Hungry bone syndrome • Osteoblastic metastasis

(PTH: parathyroid hormone)

neuromuscular excitability demonstrated by brachial artery occlusion by sphygmomanometer and facial nerve stimulation by tapping in front of the tragus, respectively. Severe and acute drop in calcium levels can present with severe central nervous system manifestations such as confusion, delirium, seizure, or with laryngospasm and bronchospasm. Cardiac manifestations of acute hypocalcemia include decreased myocardial contractility, congestive heart failure, and arrhythmias due to QT prolongation.

Laboratory Findings

Evaluation in a case of hypocalcemia should include estimations of serum calcium, phosphorus, creatinine, albumin, PTH, and 25-hydroxyvitamin D in all cases. Low levels of PTH associated with hypocalcemia and high normal to high phosphorus indicate hypoparathyroidism. Vitamin D-related hypocalcemia is associated with low calcium and phosphorus with elevated PTH. Serum magnesium concentration should be measured in patients with hypocalcemia in whom PTH is low but the cause is not obvious. Measurement of active form of vitamin D (1,25-dihydroxyvitamin D) is indicated only in few patients where biochemical features of vitamin D-related hypocalcemia is associated with normal 25-hydroxyvitamin D levels and when vitamin D-dependent hypocalcemia is suspected based on clinical features.

Treatment

Acute symptomatic hypocalcemia requires urgent medical attention. Parenteral infusions of either calcium gluconate or calcium chloride are indicated when rapid correction of serum calcium levels is required. Although calcium chloride contains nearly four times more elemental calcium, calcium gluconate is the preferred molecule for peripheral venous administration as calcium chloride can lead to tissue necrosis, if extravasation occurs. The suggested doses for bolus injections are as follows:
- *Calcium chloride*: 10 mL ampoule (272 mg elemental calcium) diluted in 200 mL 5% dextrose, given IV over 30–90 minutes
- *Calcium gluconate*: 10 mL ampoule (92 mg elemental calcium), 1–3 ampoules diluted in 200 mL 5% dextrose, given IV over 30–90 minutes.

However, a single IV bolus injection as above is effective in relieving symptoms only for few hours. A continuous infusion of calcium gluconate [10 ampoules (920 mg elemental calcium) diluted in 1 L of 5% dextrose, IV at a rate of 1–3 mg/kg/hour] is usually required to fully control symptoms and to achieve stable ionized calcium levels above 1.0 mmol/L. Serum calcium levels should be monitored 1–2 hourly initially till symptoms improve, followed by 4–6 hourly. The infusion rate should not exceed 1–2 mg/min because of the risk of potential cardiac arrhythmias associated with rapid calcium infusion. Oral calcium and vitamin D therapy (25-hydroxy or 1,25-dihydroxy depending on etiology) should be started as soon as possible while the IV infusion should be tapered slowly over 24-48 hours.

In patients having low serum magnesium concentration, it is usually difficult to correct hypocalcemia without first correcting magnesium levels. In these cases, 2 g magnesium sulfate in 20 mL D5% should be infused over 10-20 minutes followed by 1 g in 100 mL per hour infusion, as long as serum magnesium concentration is below 1 mg/dL. Continuous supplementation with oral magnesium salts is necessary for extended periods to replete intracellular magnesium which is inadequately mirrored by extracellular serum magnesium levels. Careful monitoring is required in patients with renal impairment.

Severe Hypercalcemia

Hypercalcemia is defined as serum calcium level more than two standards deviation above the laboratory's population mean—commonly total calcium >10.5 mg/dL or ionized calcium 1.3 mmol/L. Under normal conditions, the flux of ionized calcium between the vascular spaces and skeleton, intestine and the kidney is tightly regulated. Consequently, hypercalcemia develops because of disturbances in any of these physiologic processes: (1) increased intestinal absorption, (2) increased bone resorption, or (3) decreased renal calcium excretion. The main action of PTH is to maintain the serum calcium concentration in normal range by promoting bone resorption, enhancing intestinal calcium absorption by stimulating formation of active (1,25-dihydroxy) vitamin D in kidney and renal calcium conservation. The underlying causes of hypercalcemia can be divided into those associated with elevated or inappropriately normal PTH and those associated with appropriately suppressed PTH **(Table 8)**. Patients with severe hypercalcemia (total serum calcium >14 mg/dL) require urgent admission and treatment to prevent complications.

Clinical Features

As in hypocalcemia, clinical features depend on the severity and the rapidity of development of hypercalcemia. However, overt symptoms are rare in patients with total serum calcium <12 mg/dL, while most patients are symptomatic if serum calcium levels are >14 mg/dL. Spectrum of neurological symptoms range from fatigue, lethargy, and depression to even confusion, obtundation, and coma. Gastrointestinal manifestations include anorexia, nausea, vomiting, and abdominal pain with or without development of acute pancreatitis. In a similar fashion, bradyarrhythmias, conduction defects, and digitalis sensitivity manifest with increased ionized calcium levels. Renal manifestations include polyuria and dehydration (nephrogenic diabetes insipidus) with nephrolithiasis or nephrocalcinosis. When fluid intake fails to match the obligatory renal volume losses, prerenal acute kidney injury

| TABLE 8 | Causes of hypercalcemia. |

- Parathyroid hormone (PTH)-dependent hypercalcemia
  - Primary hyperparathyroidism (due to adenoma, hyperplasia, and carcinoma)
  - Familial hypocalciuric hypercalcemia (FHH)
  - Lithium therapy
  - Tertiary (severe secondary) hyperparathyroidism
- PTH-independent hypercalcemia
- Malignancy-associated hypercalcemia (MAH)
  - Humoral hypercalcemia of malignancy (PTH-related protein)
  - Local osteolytic hypercalcemia
- Vitamin D related
  - Vitamin D intoxication
  - Granulomatous disorder (excessive 1,25-dihydroxyvitamin D production)
- Hyperthyroidism
- Immobilization
- Pheochromocytoma
- Vitamin A intoxication

develops. Overall, clinical features of hypercalcemia remain same, irrespective of its etiology.

Laboratory Findings

Laboratory evaluation should be designed to assess the severity of hypercalcemia and to ascertain the underlying etiology. The initial profile should include: serum calcium, phosphorus, alkaline phosphatase, creatinine, and albumin. These initial tests confirm and assess the severity of hypercalcemia, degree of renal impairment, if any, and the levels of serum phosphorus also provide a clue to the probable etiology. Hypercalcemia associated with low serum phosphorus indicates a PTH or PTH-related protein (PTHrP) etiology. On the other hand, high normal to high serum phosphorus levels point toward vitamin D toxicity or granulomatous disorders, as possible causes of hypercalcemia. Next step is measurement of PTH to differentiate between PTH-dependent and PTH-independent hypercalcemia. In patients with PTH-independent hypercalcemia, measurement of serum vitamin D metabolites and search for the undiagnosed malignancy should be initiated. Together, primary hyperparathyroidism (PHPT) and malignancy-associated hypercalcemia (MAH) account for >95% of cases of severe hypercalcemia. However in our country, it is not uncommon to see iatrogenic vitamin D overdoses, leading to vitamin D toxicity presenting with severe hypercalcemia.

Treatment

Severe hypercalcemia is an endocrine emergency that requires prompt action to prevent severe neurologic, cardiac, and renal complications. The emergent treatment should focus on restoring plasma volume and consequent enhancement of renal calcium excretion. In most cases, 500–1,000 mL of normal saline should be infused over the first 1–2 hours followed by 2–5 L over the next 24 hours. Loop diuretics (frusemide) can be added in few cases only after initial volume expansion, especially if the patient develops pulmonary edema or pitting pedal edema. After the volume resuscitation, subsequent treatment should be tailored to the underlying etiology: calcitonin and bisphosphonates (IV zolendronate) for PHPT or MAH to slow the bone resorption, glucocorticoids in granulomatous disorders to slow 1,25-dihydroxyvitamin D synthesis. For patients with congestive heart failure or end-stage renal disease, hemodialysis should be carried out to rapidly reduce serum calcium levels. After the initial management of acute severe hypercalcemia, definitive management should be planned. Cases of PHPT need appropriate localization of pathology followed by parathyroid surgery. However the prognosis of patients with MAH remains relatively bleak, despite adequate management of the severe hypercalcemia episode.

ADRENAL-RELATED EMERGENCIES

Acute Adrenal Insufficiency

Adrenal insufficiency can be either primary or secondary. Primary acute adrenal insufficiency (PAI) is due to destruction of both the adrenal glands. Common causes include autoimmunity, infections, infiltration, hemorrhage, infarction, etc. Both cortisol and aldosterone are deficient in patients with PAI. Secondary acute adrenal insufficiency (SAI) is associated with adrenocorticotropic hormone (ACTH) deficiency due to hypothalamic or pituitary dysfunction and only cortisol is deficient as aldosterone secretion is chiefly regulated by the renin-angiotensin system.

Clinical Features and Laboratory Findings

Clinical features often include weakness, fatigability, weight loss, lethargy, loss of appetite, nausea, vague abdominal pain, and vomiting. Hyperpigmentation of skin and mucus membranes is often present in PAI. Similarly, there may be signs of hypotension varying from postural drop in blood pressure to complete cardiovascular collapse with severe dehydration in patients with PAI. These two signs are not usually observed in patients with SAI due to suppressed ACTH and normal mineralocorticoid secretion, respectively.

The diagnosis of acute adrenal insufficiency is a clinical one: shock, poorly responsive to volume and pressure therapy. Typical laboratory findings in a patient with PAI include hyponatremia, hyperkalemia, and hypoglycemia, especially in children, azotemia, and eosinophilia. As mineralocorticoid secretion is normal, patients with SAI do not develop hyperkalemia. Serum cortisol and ACTH samples should be withdrawn on suspicion of acute adrenal insufficiency. Low cortisol levels confirm adrenal insufficiency, while ACTH levels help differentiate between primary and secondary adrenal insufficiency (high ACTH indicates PAI, whereas low or normal ACTH indicates SAI). Synacthen (ACTH) stimulation test is usually not required to diagnose acute adrenal insufficiency.

Treatment

Management should be initiated based on clinical suspicion while awaiting laboratory results. Hydrocortisone should be injected 100 mg IV or intramuscular stat, followed by 50 mg 6-hourly. At these doses, mineralocorticoid is not needed. Volume expansion is to be undertaken simultaneously with IV normal saline—1 L fluid over the initial 2-4 hours. Further fluid resuscitation is to be guided clinically. Precipitating factors should be addressed properly and broad-spectrum antibiotics may be indicated. Hydrocortisone should be continued at this dose for the initial 24 hours or until the patient is tolerating orally. The dose can then be reduced to 20 mg orally three times a day followed by 10 mg orally three times a day after another 24-48 hours. Once the patient is completely well, the usual dose of hydrocortisone (10 mg at waking, 5 mg at noon, and 5 mg in evening, for most adults) should be started. Oral fludrocortisone replacement should be added at fixed dose of 0.1-0.2 mg/day once IV hydrocortisone therapy is stopped. It is noteworthy that patients with SAI do not require mineralocorticoid replacement and glucocorticoid requirement is also approximately 40-50% lower than that for patients with PAI.

For patients being diagnosed as adrenal insufficiency on first presentation, further assessment should be started to find out the etiology of PAI or SAI, depending on results of plasma ACTH.

Severe Cushing's Syndrome

The most common cause of Cushing's syndrome is exogenous, iatrogenic glucocorticoid overdose, being given through various routes of administration for various clinical conditions. However, Cushing's disease (ACTH-secreting pituitary adenoma) contributes to approximately 70% cases of endogenous Cushing's syndrome. Rest of the cases are due to ACTH-secreting neuroendocrine tumors (NETs) or due to uni/bilateral primary adrenal pathology. Endogenous Cushing's syndrome is rare in incidence and the clinical profile of a patient with Cushing's syndrome is quite variable. The diagnosis is carried out by stepwise carefully selected biochemical tests, followed by imaging tests as indicated to localize the pathology. Description of the whole clinical picture and diagnostic tests is beyond the scope of this chapter. Severe Cushing's syndrome (defined as 24 urine free cortisol levels >1,500 µg) becomes a medical emergency because of the immediate risk of life-threatening complications, hence treatment should be started after withdrawing samples for cortisol and ACTH. If the clinical condition of the patient permits, overnight dexamethasone suppression test (ODST) can be carried out as a single confirmatory test. Ectopic ACTH secretion from NETs or adrenocortical carcinoma (ACC) is responsible for severe Cushing's syndrome in many cases, although Cushing's disease (pituitary adenoma) associated with severe hypercortisolism is not rare. Hypokalemia and metabolic alkalosis are present in most cases of severe Cushing's syndrome and should be treated aggressively with mineralocorticoid antagonist along with potassium replacement. Antihypertensive therapy should be optimized preferably with mineralocorticoid antagonist (spironolactone) and/or angiotensin-converting enzyme (ACE) inhibitors. Insulin should be started and optimized to combat hyperglycemia, if present. Low-molecular-weight heparin (LMWH) should be initiated as a prophylaxis against deep vein thrombosis. Bacterial or fungal infections should be sought actively, as these patients usually do not develop signs of inflammation such fever or cavity in lungs, etc. Starting a broad-spectrum antibiotic after taking appropriate cultures is well justified in these patients. If the clinical condition of the patient permits immediate surgery, and if the culprit lesion is localized, it should be removed surgically. However, if the lesion is not localized for ACTH-dependent Cushing's syndrome, or if the condition of patient prevents prolonged surgery required for removal of such a lesion, bilateral adrenalectomy is a reasonable and lifesaving alternative to immediately lower cortisol load in such cases. Some of the patients are so moribund, that even bilateral adrenalectomy cannot be performed without significant risk. Rapid control of hypercortisolism with the use of nonanesthetic dose of etomidate (0.02–0.08 mg/kg/hour) for few days, helps to improve general condition and bridging with final surgical procedure in some of these patients. Etomidate acts by inhibiting some of the enzymes involved in cortisol synthesis in the adrenals, and this therapy ideally should be carried out in an ICU setting. Patients with ACTH-dependent Cushing's syndrome who underwent emergency bilateral adrenalectomy should later be evaluated for localization of lesion followed by appropriate treatment.

Pheochromocytoma Crisis

Pheochromocytoma is a rare tumor of the adrenal medulla, characterized by pathological excessive secretion of catecholamines and metanephrines. It is estimated that the overall prevalence of pheochromocytoma is between 1:1,700 and 1:4,500, with an annual incidence rate of three to eight cases per million per year. Most of the tumors are in the adrenal glands (pheochromocytoma—80%), while the rest are due to extra-adrenal tumors (paraganglioma). Crisis is caused by unopposed high circulating levels of catecholamines acting at adrenoreceptors: α-receptor activation causes vasoconstriction, increase in blood pressure and decrease in target organ perfusion, while β-receptor activation leads to positive inotropic and chronotropic action on the heart. The classic symptoms of paroxysms of pheochromocytoma include headache, sweating, and palpitations. Hypertension is present in approximately 90% of patients. Other clinical features include tachycardia, anxiety, pallor, and orthostatic hypotension. Sustained hypertension strongly correlates with levels of norepinephrine while paroxysmal hypertension more commonly occurs in epinephrine-secreting tumors. The frequency of hypertensive spells can

> **BOX 2** Precipitating factors for pheochromocytoma crisis.
>
> *Spontaneous:*
> - Hemorrhage into the tumor
>
> *Others:*
> - Exercise
> - Pressure on abdomen
> - Smoking
> - Postural changes
> - Anxiety
> - *Drugs:* Guanethidine, glucagon, naloxone, metoclopramide, cytotoxics, tricyclic antidepressants, and phenothiazines

vary from rare to daily, while the length of each attack varies from minutes to an hour. The longer lasting episodes evolve often into a hypertensive crisis. A hypertensive crisis refers to a markedly increased blood pressure that is resistant to usual antihypertensive medications. Because of the potentially devastating consequences including acute myocardial infarction, cerebrovascular accidents, congestive heart failure, renal failure, and retinal detachment, crises are usually managed in an ICU setup. These spells can be precipitated by a variety of factors as mentioned in **Box 2**.

The diagnosis of pheochromocytoma is based on assessment of either plasma or urine metanephrines. Catecholamines should not be used for diagnosis of pheochromocytoma because these are secreted episodically, hence have poor sensitivity. Metanephrines are released continuously and independently of catecholamine release, therefore measuring metanephrines provides more sensitivity and specificity for diagnosis of pheochromocytoma. For practical purposes we suggest measuring plasma free normetanephrine levels, collected when the patient is relaxed and supine, for the biochemical screening of patients suspected of having pheochromocytoma.

One should not wait for results of biochemical tests to start treatment of a hypertensive crisis. IV infusion of nitroprusside or phentolamine is used to control blood pressure rapidly in patients with suspected pheochromocytoma with accelerated or malignant hypertension. Once the crisis episode is terminated, patients with pheochromocytoma should be treated with α-1 receptor antagonists (prazosin and doxazosin), in gradually increasing doses to achieve complete α-1 receptor blockade. If this therapy is associated with tachycardia, β-1 receptor blockade with atenolol or metoprolol is to be instituted, but β-1 receptor blockers should not be started before at least 2–3 days of α-receptor blockade, to prevent exacerbation of crisis by unopposed action of catecholamines on α-receptors. The presence of postural hypotension indicates intravascular deficit and should be addressed by extra salt and water intake. The definitive treatment includes surgical removal of the tumor after confirming with anatomical and functional imaging techniques, as indicated.

CONCLUSION

Though relatively uncommon, endocrine emergencies are life-threatening and pose a diagnostic challenge for the physician and intensivist. Careful assessment of clinical features along with a high index of suspicion is important to diagnose such conditions. Aggressive management pending the laboratory confirmation of diagnosis is equally important as these conditions are associated with high complication and mortality rates with delays in treatment.

SUGGESTED READING

1. Burch HB, Wartofsky L. Life-threatening thyrotoxicosis. Thyroid storm. Endocrinol Metab Clin North Am. 1993;22(2):263-77.
2. Cryer PE, Axelrod L, Grossman AB, Heller SR, Montori VM, Seaquist ER, et al. Evaluation and management of adult hypoglycemic disorders: an Endocrine Society Clinical Practice Guideline. J Clin Endocrinol Metab. 2009;94(3):709-28.
3. Kitabchi AE, Umpierrez GE, Miles JM, Fisher JN. Hyperglycemic crises in adult patients with diabetes. Diabetes Care. 2009;32(7):1335-43.
4. Kitabchi AE, Umpierrez GE, Murphy MB, Barrett EJ, Kreisberg RA, Malone JI, et al. Management of hyperglycemic crises in patients with diabetes. Diabetes Care. 2001;24(1):131-53.
5. Lenders JW, Duh QY, Eisenhofer G, Gimenez-Roqueplo AP, Grebe SK, Murad MH, et al. Pheochromocytoma and paraganglioma: an endocrine society clinical practice guideline. J Clin Endocrinol Metab. 2014;99(6):1915-42.
6. Lila AR, Sarathi V, Jagtap VS, Bandgar T, Menon P, Shah NS. Cushing's syndrome: Stepwise approach to diagnosis. Indian J Endocrinol Metab. 2011;15(Suppl 4):S317.
7. Marik PE, Pastores SM, Annane D, Meduri GU, Sprung CL, Arlt W, et al. Recommendations for the diagnosis and management of corticosteroid insufficiency in critically ill adult patients: consensus statements from an international task force by the American College of Critical Care Medicine. Crit Care Med. 2008;36(6):1937-49.
8. Murad MH, Coto-Yglesias F, Wang AT, Sheidaee N, Mullan RJ, Elamin MB, et al. Clinical review: Drug-induced hypoglycemia: a systematic review. J Clin Endocrinol Metab. 2009;94(3):741-5.
9. Nieman LK, Biller BMK, Findling JW, Murad MH, Newell-Price J, Savage MO. Treatment of Cushing's Syndrome: An Endocrine Society Clinical Practice Guideline. J Clin Endocrinol Metab. 2015;100:2807-31.
10. Pimentel L, Hansen KN. Thyroid disease in the emergency department: a clinical and laboratory review. J Emerg Med. 2005;28(2):201-9.
11. Sarlis NJ, Gourgiotis L. Thyroid emergencies. Rev Endocr Metab Disord. 2003;4(2):129-36.
12. Shoback D. Clinical practice. Hypoparathyroidism. N Engl J Med. 2008;359(4):391-403.
13. Stewart AF. Clinical practice: hypercalcemia associated with cancer. N Engl J Med. 2005;352:373-9.
14. Wartofsky L. Myxedema coma. Endocrinol Metab Clin North Am. 2006;35(4):687-98.
15. Wolfsdorf JI, Glaser N, Agus M, Fritsch M, Hanas R, Rewers A, et al. ISPAD Clinical Practice Consensus Guidelines 2018: Diabetic ketoacidosis and the hyperglycemic hyperosmolar state. Pediatr Diabetes. 2018;19:155-77.

CHAPTER 30

Management of Exacerbation of Chronic Obstructive Pulmonary Disease

Joanne Mascarenhas, Jamshed Sunavala

■ INTRODUCTION

Exacerbation of chronic obstructive pulmonary disease (COPD) is part of the natural history of the condition. It is an indicator of treatment adequacy and adherence, severity and progression of disease, worsening of lung function, hospitalization rate and length of stay, comorbidity severity, and quality of life; thereby affecting morbidity and mortality.

■ FEATURES OF EXACERBATION

An exacerbation of chronic obstructive lung disease is characterized by a change for the worse from the current symptoms or baseline condition of the patient that warrants treatment. This includes changes in intensity and frequency of breathlessness, decrease in effort tolerance, new onset or change in frequency and intensity of cough, wheezing, change in nature and quantity of expectoration, fever, and desaturation.

This can be caused or precipitated by a change in weather, exposure to allergens or respiratory irritants, respiratory infection (viral or bacterial), nonrespiratory sepsis, heart failure, and a worsening of the underlying comorbid illnesses. Pneumothorax and pulmonary thromboembolism may also precipitate respiratory distress.

■ INITIAL ASSESSMENT

The initial clinical examination includes the assessment of hemodynamic stability, vitals, peripheral oxygen saturation (SpO_2), sensorium, the severity of respiratory distress and the type of respiratory failure and determination of the cardiac status. The patient needs to be further investigated and evaluated, particularly to rule out other conditions that mimic exacerbation. Some of the common mimics include heart failure, infection, pulmonary thromboembolism, and pneumothorax.

Listed below are some of the essential investigations.
- The *routine biochemistry and hematology tests* will determine the presence of infection, electrolyte imbalance, and adequacy of renal and hepatic function.
- An *arterial blood gas* analysis is essential to assess the type, acuity, and severity of the respiratory failure, as well as associated acid—base disturbances.

- A *chest X-ray* on admission will show evidence of changes compared to the previous ones, in the form of infective shadows, pneumonia, pleural effusions, pneumothorax, venous congestion, evolution or resolution of shadows. Subsequent serial imaging will help determine worsening or improvement. Sometimes, these may be misleading and in these instances, a high-resolution computed tomography (HRCT) chest is more informative regarding the severity of disease and establishing the nature and features of cavitating lesions or masses.
- Serial *electrocardiograms* (ECGs) will establish the initial or baseline pattern with respect to ischemia, pulmonary hypertension, arrhythmias, and also help in monitoring ischemic changes and rhythm disturbances.
- The *brain natriuretic peptide (BNP) or N-terminal-pro BNP (NT-pro BNP)* levels will help rule out associated heart failure. The level on discharge serves as a predictive marker for readmission as well as for mortality.
- A *two-dimensional (2D) echocardiogram* will determine the cardiac status, chamber size, biventricular systolic and diastolic functions, degree of pulmonary hypertension, and inferior vena cava (IVC) phasicity. Any changes compared to the previous findings would help in guiding further therapy.
- *Secretions*: Sputum or endotracheal secretions are to be collected for routine examination and culture.
- Other tests [polymerase chain reaction (PCR) or immunoglobulin M (IgM)] may be required to determine respiratory viral or atypical infections to determine the infective cause.

TREATMENT

The main aspects of treatment of COPD exacerbation are enumerated in **Box 1**. However, the initial attention is focused towards three immediate concerns and these include (1) relief from bronchospasm caused by severe airways obstruction, in order to decrease the work of breathing; (2) noninvasive or invasive ventilation support for impending respiratory muscle fatigue and/or hemodynamic instability; and (3) appropriate antimicrobial to treat the underlying infection or sepsis.

BOX 1 Treatment for acute exacerbation of COPD.
- Bronchodilators: Inhaled and/or systemic
- Steroids: Inhaled and/or systemic
- Antimicrobials
- Diuretics
- Oxygen
- Ventilation
- Physiotherapy
- DVT prophylaxis
- Supportive care

(COPD: chronic obstructive pulmonary disease; DVT: deep vein thrombosis)

It is imperative to recognize that patients with COPD exacerbation have severe and unrelenting airways obstruction with marked respiratory distress and may be difficult to manage on invasive ventilation. These patients are also difficult to wean and extubate and remain for a longer time on ventilator. For this reason, it is now universally accepted to initially support with noninvasive ventilation (NIV) thereby avoiding intubation, sedation, and muscle relaxants, which can jeopardize outcome in such patients.

- *Bronchodilators* are the mainstay of treatment along with *corticosteroids*. The inhaled dilators should include short-acting beta-agonists (SABA) for immediate relief, as well as long-acting beta-agonists (LABA) for maintenance along with muscarinic anticholinergic agents.

  Depending on the extent of the respiratory distress and effort, they may be given in the form of nebulization or inhalers with a spacer.

  Systemic bronchodilators are added if the wheezing or bronchospasm does not respond to inhaled bronchodilators and steroids. Along with the theophylline group of drugs, intravenous magnesium also acts as a bronchodilator and is useful during spells of severe bronchospasm.

  While on these agents, there is a risk of tachyarrhythmias and hypokalemia, which need to be monitored and corrected. Therapeutic monitoring of theophylline levels also helps in guiding further doses.

- *Corticosteroids* are usually started both in the inhaled and systemic forms. The choice of systemic corticosteroid depends on the physician or as per the protocol of the unit. The dose though, is a stress dose or higher than the patient's maintenance dose (in case of long-term steroid therapy). Once the exacerbation improves, it is gradually tapered and stopped, or continued in the lowest dose for maintenance.

- The choice of *antimicrobials* is initially empirical, depending on the antimicrobial history of the patient as well as the local antibiogram. Once the PCR or the culture reports are available and depending on the clinical condition of the patient, the regimen can be modified. The cover for atypical pneumonia is a useful addition to the prescription.

- *Diuretics* are essential in the presence of cor pulmonale and heart failure.

- *Oxygen supplementation* is to be administered depending on the type and severity of respiratory failure. The target is the least possible flow to maintain the SpO_2 above 90%, especially in the presence of chronic hypercarbia, where excess of oxygen demolishes the respiratory drive and worsens the failure. Nasal delivery is the first choice. In the presence of hypercapnic failure, face mask is avoided as it may worsen the hypercarbia.

  High-flow nasal cannula (HFNC) ventilation is an alternative to NIV for hypoxic as well as hypercarbic failure with mild-to-moderate respiratory acidosis. In the case of COPD, higher flow rates (>40 L/min) are usually avoided. HFNC helps in improving the distress, inspiratory effort as well as hypercarbia. The fraction of inspired oxygen (FiO_2) delivered is more accurate as compared to the usual flow meters. The advantage it has over NIV is that it does not cause aerophagia or dryness of the upper airway mucosa. However, for acute on chronic hypercapnic failure, NIV still remains the treatment of choice.

- Depending on the type of respiratory failure and the severity of respiratory distress, the mode of ventilation is chosen.
    - NIV is the standard of care and mode of choice for hypercapnic respiratory failure with persistent respiratory acidosis.
    - Mechanical ventilation is opted for when NIV is contraindicated or has failed.
    - *NIV*: The use of this mode has improved survival, reduced the rate of exacerbation, decreased the need for intubation and mechanical ventilation and its associated complications, thereby reducing cost, duration of stay, and the morbidity and mortality associated with it.

        The first step in this process is to choose an appropriate size and fitting mask. Usually a face mask is preferred. Patients of obstructive sleep apnea (OSA) may already be using a nasal mask with continuous positive airway pressure (CPAP), but this may not be useful in the presence of respiratory distress and failure.

        The portable/bedside machines have a single limb tubing. They are ventilated via a *vented mask* or masks with an expiratory port. While using the mechanical ventilators in the NIV mode, a *nonvented mask* is to be used, as these have a double limbed circuit.

        The usual mode on the bedside/portable machines is bilevel positive airway pressure spontaneous/timed (BiPAP S/T). The two levels that need to be set are the expiratory positive airway pressure (EPAP) and the inspiratory positive airway pressure (IPAP). The EPAP helps in keeping the upper airways, and to some extent the alveoli, open during expiration. The level chosen depends on the degree of hypoxia. The IPAP aids in decreasing the respiratory effort. The level of IPAP is added depending on the degree of hypercarbia and the tidal volume generated. The basic points to note are as follows:
        - The minimum settings IPAP/EPAP are 8/4. It takes some minutes for the patient to get accustomed to this; thereafter the pressures are titrated according to the requirement.
        - The difference between the IPAP and EPAP should be >4.
        - Target a tidal volume of 5–7 mL/kg.
        - Increase the IPAP (keep a higher difference between the IPAP and the EPAP) to correct the hypercarbia or to generate a higher tidal volume.
        - Increase the EPAP to improve hypoxia.
        - Set a backup respiratory rate of 12–16 breaths/minute depending on the spontaneous respiratory rate, the tendency for hypoventilation, the central respiratory drive, and the hypercarbia.

- Monitor the leak. Different machines will have different values of compensation.

The higher versions of the machines have a special technology with the option of setting a fixed tidal volume to be delivered. This mode has the additional settings of tidal volume, respiratory rate, EPAP, pressure support (PS) maximum, and PS minimum. This mode can be chosen in the presence of poor respiratory effort or central hypoventilation.

While being ventilated with the mechanical ventilators in the NIV mode, the parameters that have to be set are the positive end-expiratory pressure (PEEP) (in place of EPAP), PS above PEEP (IPAP = Total PS, i.e., PEEP + PS above PEEP), and FiO_2. These have the advantage of delivering a higher FiO_2.

A trial of NIV is given for about an hour. Failure of NIV is considered if there is persistent acidosis, hypercarbia, tachypnea, tachycardia, and worsening respiratory effort. NIV is contraindicated in the presence of hemodynamic instability, altered sensorium with an inability to protect the airway, diaphragmatic palsy, and facial trauma. While on NIV, the following problems may occur, which need to be taken care of:
- *Aerophagia and gastric distension*: This increases the risk of aspiration and worsens respiratory distress. A nasogastric tube is useful here, serving the dual purpose of gastric decompression as well enabling adequate nutrition.
- *Pressure sores* on the face around the site of mask. An appropriate fitting mask as well as suitable padding (gel or cushioning) can help prevent this.
- *Dryness of the mouth and compromised oral hygiene.*

Invasive ventilation: Endotracheal intubation and mechanical ventilation remain the choice in the case of hemodynamic instability, failure of a trial with NIV or where NIV is contraindicated.

Usually the controlled modes are chosen, keeping a watch on the airway pressures, namely inspiratory pressure, plateau pressure, and peak airway pressure. Patients with COPD and bronchospasm have a tendency to develop auto-PEEP **(Fig. 1)**. This will add to the difficulty in ventilation, hypercarbia as well as the hemodynamic instability.

On ventilating the patient with COPD exacerbation, the principal physiological difference encountered would be an increased inspiratory positive pressure due to the high airflow resistance and a substantial prolongation of exhalation time. If an adequately long expiration is not allowed by the ventilator setting, the risk of air trapping and hyperinflation (intrinsic PEEP) can occur, leading to high intrathoracic and intrapulmonary pressures. These adverse effects, of both the high inspiratory peak pressure and the developing intrinsic PEEP, lead to pulmonary and cardiac compromise such

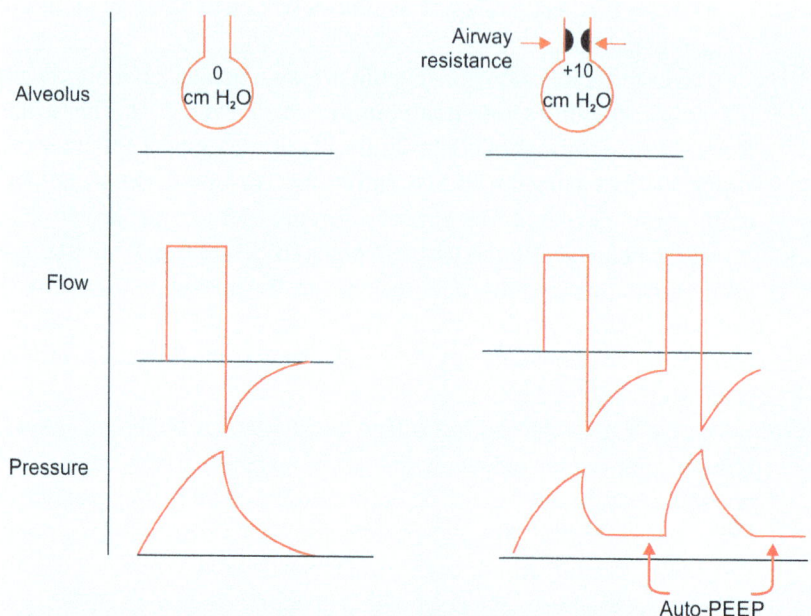

Fig. 1: Auto-positive end-expiratory pressure (PEEP).

as barotrauma and decreased cardiac output, respectively. Further, the marked increased in intrathoracic pressure with chest wall distension and decreased chest wall compliance can cause increased respiratory workload. The workload is further increased because of the patient-ventilator asynchrony due to severe respiratory distress and unchecked spontaneous breathing. To overcome the above-mentioned physiological impairments one may have to use conflicting ventilator strategies as follows:

- Though historically high inspiratory peak pressures were known to increase the risk of barotrauma, in fact it is now accepted that high plateau pressures rather than high inspiratory peak pressures are more harmful in producing barotrauma. Hence, increasing the inspiratory peak pressures to reduce the inspiratory time and better the inspiratory flow rates could be an accepted trade-off under the circumstances.
- Though the pressure limited mode is considered safe, it is best avoided in patients of COPD exacerbation as it will cause small and variable tidal volumes, particularly when higher peak pressures of volume preset modes are believed to be tolerated well. However at all times, high plateau pressures which are known to be harmful should be constantly monitored and kept below 30 cm H_2O.
- Lower tidal volumes of 4–6 mL/kg help to maintain the target plateau pressures under 30 cm H_2O, but the resultant low minute ventilation

could lead to worsening of hypercapnia. Minute ventilation could be improved by increasing the respiratory rate, but it will further decrease the tidal volumes and accelerate air trapping. To minimize air trapping it is best to ventilate at a rate of 12-14 per minute or at a maximum of 18-22 per minute, by decreasing the inspiratory time to 0.5 seconds to achieve an inspiratory:expiratory (I:E) ratio of 1:2.5 or 1:3 thereby increasing the expiratory time. Of course, one could still use smaller tidal volumes, astutely balancing the degree of permissive hypercapnia with the delivered tidal volume.
  - Though PEEP is known to cause hyperinflation of the lungs and is counterproductive in case of COPD exacerbation, it could still be helpful to fix an additional external PEEP in patients with an increasing intrinsic PEEP. The added external PEEP may serve to provide a stenting effect and relieve airflow obstruction. External PEEP should not be > 75% of the internal PEEP.
  - In acute respiratory distress syndrome (ARDS), one accepts partial pressure of arterial oxygen (PaO_2) up to 60-70 mm Hg or arterial oxygen saturation (SaO_2) of 90-92%, so as to provide the lowest optimal level of FiO_2. However, in COPD exacerbation, no optimal level is clearly determined, but higher FiO_2 levels are needed to maintain PaO_2 levels well above those accepted for ARDS, in order to avoid hypoxia induced cardiopulmonary compromise.
  - Most of the predictive values of several criteria to assess the possibility of weaning have their limitations. However, the use of rapid shallow breathing index (RSBI < 100) is one of the better criteria but it is still of uncertain value. Among the side effects and complications associated with invasive ventilation, there is always a risk of difficult weaning and/or dependence.
- *Physiotherapy* is a vital part of management of exacerbation episodes.
  - Chest physiotherapy and postural drainage help in the removal of secretions.
  - Breathing exercises include inspiratory (to improve the chest expansion) and expiratory (assisting in prolonging the expiration and thereby improving the wheeze, bronchospasm and the CO_2 washout).
  - Monitoring the peak flow before and after inhaled bronchodilators gives an indication of the severity of the condition, and the trend indicates the response to treatment.
  - Limb therapy helps in mobilization, improving muscle strength, posture, and balance.
- *Deep vein thrombosis* (DVT) prophylaxis, whether mechanical or chemical, is also essential, as for any sick patient, moreso in the presence of cor pulmonale.
- *Supportive care* includes mucolytics, ensuring glycemic control, adequate nutrition, dietary supplements, maintaining fluid balance, and oral

hygiene. Fluctuations in blood glucose levels are anticipated due to stress, steroids, and also due to fluctuating oral feeds.

Nutrition serves an important role in improving strength, healing, immunity, and overall recovery. It is useful to monitor the caloric and protein intake and adjust the diet and supplements to optimize the nutrition according to the clinical situation.

As the exacerbation comes under control, the intensity of treatment changes and the focus shifts to maintenance therapy and rehabilitation. Eventually, the oxygen and steroids are tapered and discontinued if possible; otherwise, the lowest doses are maintained. The duration of NIV is also gradually decreased. In the presence of OSA, hypoventilation, and chronic hypercapnia, some patients need to continue with NIV support at home as well. A low flow of oxygen may be required continuously for those with severe pulmonary hypertension. If feasible, nebulization is switched to inhaler therapy with a spacer. Breathing exercises and monitoring of the peak flows are continued. Advice on discharge also includes a plan for vaccination (pneumococcal and annual seasonal influenza).

■ SUGGESTED READING

1. Global Initiative for Chronic Obstructive Lung Disease. (2021). 2021 Global Strategy for the diagnosis, management and prevention of COPD. [online] Available from: https://goldcopd.org/2021-gold-reports/. [Last accessed September, 2021].

CHAPTER 31

Approach to a Patient with Hyponatremia

Bhupendra V Gandhi, Rishit Harbada

■ INTRODUCTION

Hyponatremia is one of the most common dyselectrolytemias encountered in clinical settings and is defined as a serum sodium level of <135 mmol/L. It is associated with a wide range of deleterious effects involving various body organs, but mainly the brain. The diverse comorbidities and etiologies associated with hyponatremia pose a great challenge to the treating physician to diagnose and treat patients with this disorder. Hence, an update of the recent consensus statements and guidelines for the diagnosis and management of hyponatremia, with knowledge regarding the newer treatment modalities like vaptans, are essential for all clinicians.

■ PATHOPHYSIOLOGY OF HYPONATREMIA

Hyponatremia has a complex pathophysiology; however, the two main mechanisms of hyponatremia are due to excessive fluid intake or elevated vasopressin, also called as arginine vasopressin [antidiuretic hormone (ADH)] which causes defective water excretion.

The chief regulator of water intake is thirst, which in turn is regulated by increase in serum osmolality. The osmoreceptors located in the hypothalamus sense thirst and stimulate the posterior pituitary to release ADH, which acts on the V2 receptors on the basolateral surface of the collecting duct of the nephrons, and increases water absorption through the shuttle hypothesis. This abolishes thirst and causes water retention.

True volume depletion (hypovolemia) or reduction in tissue perfusion due to either low cardiac output (cardiac failure) or arterial vasodilatation (cirrhosis), cause decrease in effective arterial blood volume (EABV), which is sensed by: (1) baroreceptors at the aortic arch and carotid sinus which regulate the sympathetic activity and release ADH in response to volume depletion; (2) atria and ventricles which release natriuretic peptides and cause water retention; and lastly (3) the afferent arterioles in the glomerular capillary loops which stimulate the renin–angiotensin system. All of these actions result in water retention. Defect in osmoregulation causes inappropriate stimulation of ADH leading to hyponatremia with excretion of concentrated urine.

■ TYPES OF HYPONATREMIA

The total osmolar concentration of solutes in the body is called tonicity. Those solutes that do not cross the cell membrane are called effective solutes, and sodium is the chief effective osmole in the extracellular fluid (ECF). Tonicity affects the movement of water which distributes from areas of higher solute concentration to areas of lower concentration and causes the cells to swell. Hence, most forms of hyponatremia are hypotonic. Osmolality on the other hand includes contributions from not only effective osmoles but also from noneffective osmoles such as urea, ethanol, and glycols which readily move across the cell membrane and do not affect movement of water across the cell membrane. Hence, tonicity is effective osmolality. Normal serum osmolality ranges between 275 and 295 mOsm/kg and is normally calculated by the following equation:

$$\text{Osmolality (mmol/kg)} = [2 \times \text{serum (Na)}] + [\text{serum (glucose)}/18] + (\text{blood urea nitrogen}/2.8)$$

In patients with hyponatremia, serum osmolality is usually low. Hence, this is called true or hypo-osmolal/hypotonic hyponatremia.

Redistributive or translocational hyponatremia is due to osmotically active solutes such as glucose, mannitol, or radiographic contrast that cause translocation of water from intracellular fluid (ICF) to ECF and hence dilutes serum sodium. This type of hyponatremia is associated with hypertonicity, as plasma contains significant amounts of unmeasured solutes. Hence, direct measurement of osmolality is required as calculated osmolality will be high.

Pseudohyponatremia or iso-osmolal hyponatremia is due to hyperlipidemia (triglycerides > 1,500 mg/dL) or hyperproteinemia (>10 g/dL as in myeloma), due to reduction in the water component of plasma, as measured falsely by auto-analyzers due to laboratory artefacts; however, serum sodium levels are normal when measured by ion-selective electrodes or other blood gas analyzers.

ETIOLOGY OF TRUE HYPONATREMIA

Depending upon the ECF volume status of the individual, true hyponatremia is further divided into hypovolemic, hypervolemic, and euvolemic hyponatremia.

Hypovolemic hyponatremia is associated with ECF volume depletion and the reduction in total body sodium exceeds reduction in total body water (TBW). It is associated with decrease in plasma volume which may be either of renal or extrarenal origin. Diarrhea, vomiting, or conditions associated with third space losses such as peritonitis, pancreatitis, muscle trauma, or burns are causes of extrarenal causes of hypovolemic hyponatremia while diuretics (chiefly thiazide diuretics), mineralocorticoid deficiency, salt wasting nephropathy, and cerebral salt wasting (CSW) are a few renal causes.

Hypervolemic hyponatremia is associated with increase in ECF volume and the increase in TBW exceeds the increase in total body sodium. Congestive cardiac failure (CCF), hepatic cirrhosis, and nephrotic syndrome are the most common causes of hypervolemic hypernatremia. These conditions are associated with decreased EABV and cause nonosmotic stimulation of ADH which causes water retention and subsequent hyponatremia. In renal failure, the kidneys cannot maximally excrete excess ingested water thereby causing hyponatremia.

Euvolemic hyponatremia is the most common cause of hypo-osmolal hyponatremia and accounts for 60% of the cases. This type of hyponatremia is associated with normovolemia and an increase in TBW. The most common cause is syndrome of inappropriate secretion of antidiuretic hormone (SIADH). Other causes are hypothyroidism, glucocorticoid deficiency, psychogenic or primary polydipsia, beer potomania, tea and toast hyponatremia, exercise-induced hyponatremia, and drug-induced hyponatremia.

The SIADH is a form of euvolemic hyponatremia due to excessive or inappropriate secretion of ADH. It may occur either due to hypothalamic ADH secretion in conditions such as head injury, stroke, infection or neuropsychiatric disorders, or ectopic ADH production due to small cell cancer of lungs, head neck cancers, thymoma, sarcoma or genitourinary (GU) tract malignancies. It may also occur due to potentiation of the ADH effect as with chlorpropamide or drugs that stimulate ADH release such as selective serotonin reuptake inhibitor (SSRI), carbamazepine, cyclophosphamide, ifosfamide, and nicotine. Other causes of SIADH include postoperative pain, nausea, stress, or respiratory/central nervous system (CNS) infections. ADH secretion is independent of hypertonicity or hypovolemia. This increased ADH causes water retention, dilutional hyponatremia, and expansion of ECF volume. This expanded ECF volume causes stimulation of natriuretic peptides and decreased secretion of aldosterone, which causes natriuresis and isotonic loss of ECF, thereby bringing the ECF volume back to baseline. Hence, SIADH is associated with euvolemia. CSW differs from SIADH only in the context that it is associated with volume depletion and salt wasting.

The SIADH is a diagnosis of exclusion after ruling out other causes of hypo-osmolality. In 1967, Bartter and Schwartz gave the diagnostic criteria for SIADH with essential and supporting criteria **(Box 1)**.

■ CLINICAL FEATURES

The clinical features depend upon the severity of hyponatremia and the rate at which serum sodium is lowered. Hence, acute and severe hyponatremia is symptomatic while chronic and mild hyponatremia is well tolerated.

Development of hyponatremia in <48 hours is called acute hyponatremia and it is associated with cerebral edema because the brain cells do not have sufficient time to adapt to the hypotonic environment. Milder symptoms include nausea, vomiting, lethargy, and headache which can be the first signs of raised intracranial pressure (ICP) due to cerebral edema. Moderate-to-severe symptoms include personality changes, confusion, ataxia, drowsiness, seizures, coma, or rarely death.

> **BOX 1** Bartter and Schwartz diagnostic criteria for syndrome of inappropriate secretion of antidiuretic hormone (SIADH).
>
> *Essential criteria:*
> - Clinical euvolemia
> - Decreased serum osmolality < 270 mOsm/kg
> - Urinary osmolality > 100 mOsm/kg H_2O
> - Urine sodium > 40 mmol/L with normal dietary salt intake
> - Absence of adrenal, thyroid, pituitary, or renal insufficiency or diuretic use
>
> *Supporting criteria:*
> - Failure to improve or worsening of hyponatremia after 0.9% saline infusion and improvement of hyponatremia with fluid restriction
> - Serum uric acid < 4 mg/dL
> - Blood urea nitrogen < 10 mg/dL
> - Fractional sodium excretion > 1% and fractional urea excretion > 55%

Hyponatremia developing over >48 hours is called chronic hyponatremia. In this situation, the brain cells get sufficient time to adapt to the hypotonicity by generation of idiogenic osmoles such as myoinositol, phosphocreatine, and amino acids which act as a protective mechanism and reduce the degree of cerebral edema. Hence, patients with chronic hyponatremia are usually asymptomatic or mildly symptomatic. These patients have more neurocognitive and neuromotor symptoms such as falls, concentration defects, gait disturbances, and fractures. These effects contribute to morbidity and mortality in patient with hyponatremia.

It is very important to identify hyponatremia clinically because this may be an early or first sign of an underlying disease like lung carcinoma. Hyponatremia is associated with increased morbidity and mortality, especially in hospitalized patients causing prolonged hospital stays and increasing expenditure.

■ APPROACH TO A PATIENT WITH HYPONATREMIA

The first step in evaluating a patient with hyponatremia is to confirm the method by which sodium is measured. Ion-specific electrodes (ISE) using direct potentiometry is the ideal way to measure sodium as it is not affected by aqueous phase of plasma or by dilution of plasma and rules out pseudohyponatremia (i.e., low sodium with normal osmolality).

Clinically a thorough history and a comprehensive physical examination should be carried out in all patients, especially to determine whether the hyponatremia is acute (<48 hours) or chronic (>48 hours). Also, an assessment of volume status should be done in all patients, though this does not have a very good sensitivity and specificity, especially in patients with euvolemia or hypovolemia. Volume status is best assessed by clinical observation and the knowledge of the underlying problems, such as CCF and diarrhea, will give a direct clue to volume status. Though measurement of central venous pressure

(CVP) and inferior vena cava (IVC) collapsibility does give a better idea of intravascular volume, it is most often not required.

Serum Osmolality

After serum sodium is confirmed to be low, the next step is to determine whether the hyponatremia is true or is pseudohyponatremia/translocational hyponatremia which can be confirmed with measurement of serum osmolality. The osmolality will be normal in patients with hyperlipidemia and hyperproteinemia and it is high in hyperglycemia. Osmometers should be used to measure serum osmolality, because calculated serum osmolality will be low if other active solutes are present in plasma. For every increase in blood glucose of 100 mg/dL, for every 500 mg/dL rise in serum triglycerides, and for every 1 g/dL rise in serum protein above 8 g/dL, the serum sodium decreases by 1.6 mEq/L, 1.0 mEq/L, and about 4.0 mEq/L, respectively. These calculations should be borne in mind if osmolality is calculated by the equation, rather than being measured by an osmometer.

Urine Sodium and Urine Osmolality

These tests are important to help us understand the pathophysiology involved in hyponatremia. Urine sodium is a measure of the renin-angiotensin-aldosterone system (RAAS), while urine osmolality is a measure of ADH activity. Low urine sodium suggests renal conservation of sodium by aldosterone and angiotensin II. In response to hyponatremia, the body normally causes marked suppression of ADH secretion. ADH suppression causes excretion of very dilute urine with a specific gravity of <1.003 and urine osmolality which is below 100 mOsm/kg. Urinary osmolality values above 100 mOsm/kg indicate persistent secretion of ADH leading to an inability to excrete free water **(Table 1)**.

Serial monitoring of urine sodium concentrations and urine osmolality in response to administration of 1 L 0.9% NaCl can help clarify the diagnosis. After administration of normal saline in a hypovolemic patient the ADH is suppressed promoting the excretion of dilute urine, while in a patient with SIADH, the ADH release is fixed and the osmolality will remain elevated. Hence, improvement of hyponatremia is seen in a hypovolemic patient, while no improvement, or worsening of hyponatremia, is seen in a patient with SIADH.

Acid-base Evaluation

Usually acid-base evaluation is not recommended routinely in patients with hyponatremia, but along with potassium, it can further help in the diagnosis of hyponatremia.

In SIADH, the acid base and potassium levels are normal. Metabolic acidosis and hypokalemia is seen in hyponatremic patients with diarrhea or laxative abuse, while metabolic acidosis and hyperkalemia can be seen

TABLE 1: Urine sodium and osmolality—interpretation.

Urine sodium	Urine osmolality	Interpretation	Clinical setting
Low	High	Both RAAS and ADH acting on the renal tubules	• Hypovolemia • Low effective arterial blood volume (cirrhosis, heart failure, and nephrotic syndrome) • Recent discontinuation of diuretics
High	High	Renal sodium loss with secondary ADH release due to hypovolemia	• SIADH • Active use of diuretics • Adrenal insufficiency and renal or cerebral salt wasting
Low	Low	RAAS activation but no activation of ADH	• Primary polydipsia • Beer potomania • Low solute intake (tea and toast) • Due to low sodium intake or water diuresis

(ADH: antidiuretic hormone; RAAS: renin–angiotensin–aldosterone system; SIADH: syndrome of inappropriate secretion of antidiuretic hormone)

in primary adrenal insufficiency in patients without renal dysfunction. Hyponatremia with metabolic alkalosis and hypokalemia is seen after diuretic use or vomiting, whereas metabolic alkalosis with normokalemia is noted in hypopituitarism.

Since SIADH is a diagnosis of exclusion, tests such as cortisol levels, thyroid profile, CT MRI, and adrenocorticotropic hormone (ACTH) stimulation tests should be done in the evaluation of a patient with euvolemic hyponatremia. Also tests should be done to evaluate the etiology of hyponatremia.

However in cases of emergency when the patient presents with stupor, agitation, coma, seizures, or cardiorespiratory arrest, the patient should be managed urgently in a critical care unit and workup for the diagnosis is carried on simultaneously to establish a cause of hyponatremia. A simplified diagnostic approach is given in **Flowchart 1**.

■ TREATMENT OF HYPONATREMIA

Treatment of hyponatremia should be individualized and tailor made depending upon the etiology, rate of development (acute vs. chronic), severity (mild vs. severe), clinical symptoms and signs (symptomatic vs. asymptomatic), and volume status. A general dictum in treatment is that hyponatremia that develops slowly should be treated slowly, while hyponatremia which develops rapidly should be treated fast. Early diagnosis and prompt and appropriate management of hyponatremia forms the cornerstone to reduce morbidity and mortality in hospitalized patients.

Flowchart 1: Our simplified approach to a patient with hyponatremia.

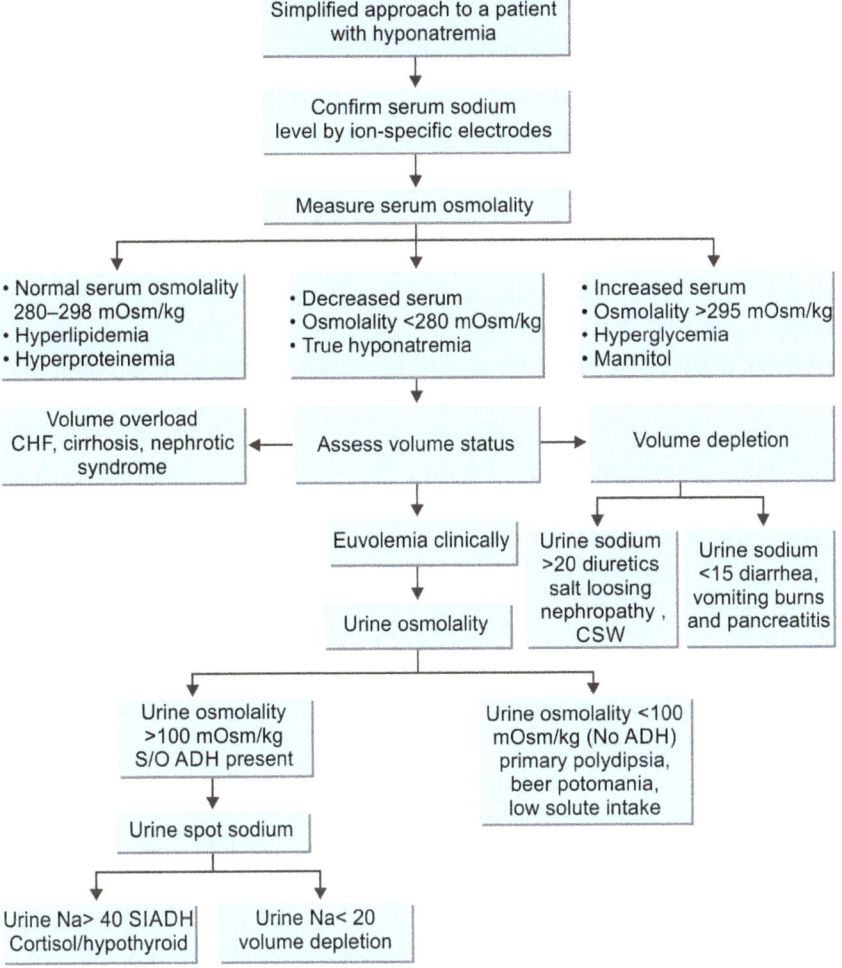

(ADH: antidiuretic hormone; CHF: congestive heart failure; SIADH: syndrome of inappropriate secretion of antidiuretic hormone)

The current recommendations in treatment of hyponatremia are based on consensus and expert opinions rather than on randomized control trials. Over the course of time, the guidelines have become more conservative in terms of rate of correction, due to the increasing incidence of osmotic demyelination syndrome (ODS).

General Guidelines for Treatment of Hyponatremia
- Raise the plasma sodium levels at a safe rate
- Replace sodium deficit or potassium deficit, or both
- Treat the underlying cause of hyponatremia, e.g., discontinuing of thiazide diuretics, restricting intake in patients with psychogenic polydipsia, etc.

- Restrict free water and hypotonic fluids since they aggravate hyponatremia
- Do serial reevaluation of symptoms, signs, volume status, fluid balance, and electrolytes; once symptoms resolve and clinical recovery occurs, step down of treatment should be carried out.

Treatment Based on Acuity of Symptoms

Acute Symptomatic Hyponatremia

Urgent treatment is warranted in patients with acute hyponatremia with moderate-to-severe symptoms. Hypertonic saline infusion is a lifesaving and effective way to increase serum sodium levels rapidly. By giving hypertonic saline into the ECF, water is attracted from the ICF and this helps in reducing cerebral edema. The Adrogué–Madias formula is widely used to predict the rise in serum sodium when hypertonic saline therapy is used. This formula calculates how much serum sodium concentrations will rise when 1 L of various intravenous fluids are given. 1 L of hypertonic saline contains 513 mEq/L of sodium. The TBW is 0.5 times the lean body weight for women and 0.6 for men. It should be always remembered that potassium in the solution should be included in the formula [infusate (Na + K)], as potassium administration raises the serum sodium concentration.

Change in serum sodium = [(Infusate sodium/L – Serum Na) ÷ (Total body water (L) +1]

There is another formula proposed to estimate not only the sodium deficit, but also to help in estimating the direct effect of a given fluid (3% NaCl) on the serum sodium (SNa) concentration.

Sodium deficit = Total body water (TBW) × (desired SNa – actual SNa)

These formulae are good but have their own limitations and cannot be used to precisely predict the magnitude of change in serum sodium; hence frequent measurements are necessary to avoid overcorrection and risk of ODS.

A simple way to calculate the initial volume of infusion of hypertonic saline is based on body weight, i.e., 1.5–2 mL/kg/hour over the first 3–4 hours. This rate is recommended in patients with severe symptoms such as seizures, headache, and decreased mental status. Patients with seizures require anticonvulsants and adequate ventilation. This regimen raises the serum sodium approximately by about 1 mEq/L/hour, which is usually sufficient to improve symptoms and decrease brain edema. In patients with mild-to-moderate symptoms, there is a low risk of herniation; hence hypertonic saline should be infused at a rate of 0.5–1 mL/kg/hour.

Currently a practical approach proposed is that 1 mL/kg of 3% NaCl raises the serum Na by 1 mEq/L approximately. This has the advantage of a simplified and practical approach, as compared to the complexities of difficult calculations in the previously proposed formulae.

The goal is to treat till symptoms improve, sodium is elevated by 5 mEq/L, or sodium levels reach a safe level of around 120 mEq/L, which is usually adequate to improve and help in reversing symptoms of acute hyponatremia. The maximum rate of correction of serum sodium should be around 10-12 mEq/L in 24 hours and around 18 mEq/L in 48 hours. This rate is essential to minimize the rate of ODS. 2-4 hourly monitoring of serum sodium should be done if hypertonic saline is used for treatment of acute hyponatremia.

Autocorrection and Overcorrection of Hyponatremia

Autocorrection occurs when the stimulus for ADH release disappears suddenly, resulting in excretion of a very dilute urine and causing sodium to rise suddenly, thereby precipitating an ODS. Common causes include discontinuation of desmopressin, treatment of hypovolemic hyponatremia, or steroid treatment for adrenal insufficiency. Overcorrection occurs when the actual rise exceeds the predicted rise of serum sodium. These complications should be anticipated during treatment by regularly monitoring serum sodium levels, urine output, and urinary osmolality. If urine output increases with decreased osmolality, it suggests water diuresis with rapid rise in serum sodium levels.

Osmotic demyelination syndrome is also called central pontine myelinolysis (CPM). But CPM has been replaced by ODS because demyelination is more diffuse and does not necessarily involves only the pons. It is a rare but severe and usually irreversible disorder. Osmotic shrinkage of axons occurs, especially in the pons area affecting their connections with the myelin sheaths. Risk factors include elderly females, malnourishment, thiazide diuretics, alcohol abuse, and serum sodium < 105 mEq/L.

Clinical features occur 2-6 days after over- or autocorrection and include paraparesis, quadriparesis, bulbar palsy, dysarthria, locked-in syndrome, and coma, and these are usually irreversible. In high suspicion cases, confirmation may be done by a CT or MRI brain; changes may not be detected immediately, but may take around 4 weeks for radiological signs to appear.

There is no definitive treatment, but discontinuing the treatment of hyponatremia, infusion of hypotonic solutions like dextrose 5% (D5%), and administration of desmopressin (DDAVP). In animal studies, reinduction of hyponatremia in cases with rapid correction has shown to reduce mortality.

Chronic Hyponatremia

In chronic hyponatremia, the brain undergoes adaptation and hence the risk of cerebral edema and brain herniation is low. Thus the aim should be to correct hyponatremia slowly and also to treat the underlying cause. Rapid correction should be avoided since it causes ODS. Current guidelines suggest the rate of correction of sodium by 4-8 mEq/L per 24 hours in patients with low risk of ODS, while it should be only 4-6 mEq/L per 24 hours in patients with high risk of ODS.

Treatment is straightforward in a few cases like stopping the diuretics or treatment of hypothyroidism or hypocortisolism. Hypertonic saline is required in symptomatic hyponatremia, while isotonic saline is required in treatment of hypovolemia. The other treatments are directed towards reducing the intake of electrolyte-free water or promoting water excretion.

Dietary salt and protein intake are recommended in patients with low solute intake. Urea supplementation, loop diuretics, demeclocycline, and fluid restriction are used in treatment of SIADH. Vasopressin receptor antagonists, viz. vaptans, are used in the treatment of SIADH, heart failure, or liver cirrhosis.

The guide to fluid restriction can be determined by a simple formula viz. the sum of urinary sodium and potassium divided by plasma sodium concentration.

$$\frac{\text{Urinary sodium} + \text{Urinary potassium}}{\text{Serum sodium}}$$

If this is >1, recommended fluid intake is <500 mL/day. If it is 1, recommended fluid intake is 500–700 mL/day and if the value is <1, then the recommended fluid intake is 1 L/day. Additional therapy should include salt tablets and a loop diuretic in patients with urine to serum electrolyte ratio >1, if fluid restriction alone does not help to correct the hyponatremia.

Loop diuretics are useful because they abolish the concentration gradient and cause excretion of more water than sodium. Urea causes osmotic diuresis and causes water excretion. Demeclocycline causes nephrogenic diabetes insipidus and water diuresis, but is rarely used. An alternative approach is the initiation of vasopressin antagonist (vaptans), without fluid restriction.

Chronic hyponatremia, even if asymptomatic, is associated with many adverse outcomes such as falls, fractures, neurocognitive decline, and increased morbidity and mortality, and hence should be treated.

Treatment of Hyponatremia Based on Volume Status

It is essential to assess the volume status for patients with hyponatremia as treatment differs in all three groups. However, in cases of severe symptoms, the initial emergency treatment remains the same, irrespective of the volume status.

Hypervolemic Hyponatremia

Fluid restriction (intake should be ideally less than urine output plus insensible losses of water) and use of loop or potassium sparing diuretics, form the mainstay of therapy in hypervolemic hyponatremia. Salt supplementation and 3% saline are contraindicated as they will worsen edema and fluid overload. Specific cause-related treatment is advocated in patients with congestive heart failure (CHF) and cirrhosis.

Hypovolemic Hyponatremia

In hypovolemic hyponatremia, fluid therapy is required to restore intravascular volume. Most cases respond to intravenous infusion of 0.9% sodium chloride (1 L provides 154 mEq of Na^+) and in most cases, 3% normal saline is not indicated. Both potassium and bicarbonate deficits should be corrected along with volume repletion. Normal saline infusion corrects the hyponatremia by restoring the intravascular volume thereby removing the stimulus for ADH, and it also slowly raises the serum sodium by approximately 1 mEq/L for every liter of fluid infused, since 0.9% NaCl has a higher sodium concentration than the hyponatremic plasma.

Thiazides-induced hyponatremia is treated with diuretic discontinuation and sodium and potassium supplementation. These patients should be treated slowly as risk of ODS is high, and as they are at a higher risk for recurrence for hyponatremia, they should not be rechallenged again with a thiazide. Vaptans are not recommended for hypovolemic hyponatremia.

Euvolemic Hyponatremia

Euvolemic hyponatremia is usually, but not always due to SIADH, which is a diagnosis of exclusion after ruling out thyroid, pituitary, adrenal, renal disease, or diuretic use. Fluid restriction is the cornerstone of treatment. If fluid restriction alone is not sufficient then salt tablets, frusemide, urea, increased protein intake, and demeclocycline can be used. It is important to identify and treat the causes of SIADH, such as treatment of pulmonary infections, meningitis, drugs, or postoperative pain. The new kids on the block are vaptans which are safe and effective agents that promote steady and sustained aquauresis with correction of hyponatremia, and treatment with vaptans does not require fluid restriction.

Other causes of hyponatremia should be treated and corrected like water restriction in cases of primary polydipsia. Treatment of adrenal insufficiency and hypothyroidism is a must, because sodium will only correct after treatment of the underlying cause. Increased solute and protein intake should be encouraged in patients with poor intake, e.g., in those with tea and toast hyponatremia.

Vasopressin Receptor Antagonists

Vasopressin receptor antagonists also called as vaptans have revolutionized the treatment of hypervolemic and euvolemic hyponatremia. These drugs act on vasopressin receptors as antagonists. There are total three receptors; the V1A cause vasoconstriction and V1B are associated with release of ACTH while the V2 are associated with antidiuresis. These drugs produce physiological aquauresis without affecting sodium and potassium excretion. These do not stimulate the neurohormonal system.

Classification of Vasopressin Receptor Antagonists

- *Nonselective (mixed V1A/V2):* Conivaptan.
- *V1A selective (V1RA):* Relcovaptan
- *V2 selective (V2RA):* Tolvaptan, lixivaptan, satavaptan, and mozavaptan
- *V1B selective (V3RA):* Nelivaptan

Only conivaptan for intravenous use and tolvaptan for oral use are currently available in India.

Current Uses

These drugs are presently recommended for euvolemic, hypervolemic hyponatremia, and chronic hyponatremia. SALT-1, SALT-2, and SALTWATER trials have demonstrated the efficacy of tolvaptan in patients with hyponatremia due to SIADH. These trials showed that the effect of vaptans on hyponatremia was modest, with improvement of cognitive status; however on stopping tolvaptan, sodium levels reduced.

Therapy is indicated when sodium levels are below 125 mEq/L; above 125 mEq/L it can be given if patient has symptoms. The initial dose is individualized and the starting dose should be between 7.5 and 15 mg/day. The dose of tolvaptan can be increased to 30–60 mg per day if the rise in serum sodium levels is <5 mmol/L in 24 hours. Serum sodium should be monitored every 6 hourly during the initial phase to avoid over- or autocorrection. Fluid restriction is not advocated while using vaptans and the patient's thirst compensates for the aggressive aquaresis.

Vaptans are also useful in treatment of CHF and cirrhosis of liver. Hyponatremia is considered to be a poor prognostic sign and is associated with increased morbidity and mortality. Short-term trials with vaptans, such as EVEREST and ACTIV in CHF showed a rapid increase in serum sodium levels and improvement in hemodynamic parameters; however long-term trials have failed to demonstrate a favorable effect on morbidity and mortality. In cirrhosis, vaptans are used to treat fluid overload and hyponatremia. However due to the hepatotoxicity associated with the use of vaptans, their use is approved by the United States Food and Drug Administration (USFDA) only in patients with end-stage liver disease awaiting liver transplant. Conivaptan causes vasodilatation and is associated with bleeding and hypotension.

Vaptans are contraindicated in hyponatremia due to hypovolemia, vasopressin-independent forms of SIADH, or hyponatremia due to emetic stimuli and adrenal insufficiency. They are also contraindicated in patients with liver injury or hepatic failure not awaiting transplant.

The availability of other vaptans in the course of time will revolutionize the treatment of hyponatremia.

Adverse Effects

Side effects are mainly due to hypernatremia and volume depletion and include dryness of mouth, orthostatic hypotension, increased thirst, encephalopathy, and hyperuricemia. Use of vaptans, especially in higher doses, was associated with almost 2.5 times increase in liver enzymes; hence, regular monitoring of liver enzymes is recommended with the use of vaptans. If liver injury is suspected, tolvaptan should be discontinued. Recently FDA has recommended tolvaptan use but for periods not >4 weeks. Regular monitoring of weight, blood pressure (usually in both supine and standing positions), liver functions, and serum sodium levels should be done.

■ CONCLUSION

Hyponatremia is a frequently encountered but often overlooked problem in clinical practice. Understanding the pathophysiology of hyponatremia with a thorough evaluation helps to establish the cause of hyponatremia. Untreated acute hyponatremia is associated with increased morbidity and mortality due to increased risk of brain herniation, and rapid overcorrection or autocorrection can cause ODS. Treatment of hyponatremia should be individualized and depends upon various factors such as etiology, volume status, duration, and severity of the patient's symptoms. Acute severe hyponatremia requires treatment with hypertonic saline. Treatment of chronic hyponatremia and of hyponatremia depending upon volume status should be individualized. The newer class of drugs viz. the vasopressin receptor antagonists, also called vaptans, are now a preferred and effective treatment option in hypervolemic and euvolemic hyponatremia.

■ SUGGESTED READING

1. Adrogué HJ, Madias NE. The challenge of hyponatremia. J Am Soc Nephrol. 2012;23:1140-8.
2. Berl T, Quittnat-Pelletier F, Verbalis JG, Schrier RW, Bichet DG, Ouyang J, et al. Oral tolvaptan is safe and effective in chronic hyponatremia. J Am Soc Nephrol. 2010;21:705-12.
3. Berl T, Sands JM. Disorders of water metabolism. In: Johnson RJ, Feehally J, Floege J, Tonelli M (Eds). Comprehensive Clinical Nephrology, 6th edition. Amsterdam, Netherlands: Elsevier; 2018.
4. Bondugulapati LR, Kalhan A, Bolusani H, Rees A. Translocational hyponatraemia—an important clue to the diagnosis of hyperosmotic hyponatraemia secondary to hyperglycaemic crisis. Br J Diabetes Vasc Dis. 2012;12(1):54-6.
5. Ellison DH, Berl T. Clinical practice. The syndrome of inappropriate antidiuresis. N Engl J Med. 2007;356:2064-72.
6. Hoorn EJ, Hotho D, Hassing RJ, Zietse R. Unexplained hyponatremia: seek and you will find. Nephron Physiol. 2011;118(3):66-71.
7. Hoorn EJ, Zietse R. Approach to a patient with hyponatremia. In: Turner NN, Lameire N, Goldsmith DJ, Winearls CG, Himmelfarb J, Remuzzi G (Eds). Oxford Textbook of Clinical Nephrology, 4th edition. Oxford: Oxford University Press; 2015.
8. Jovanovich AJ, Berl T. Where vaptans do and do not fit in the treatment of hyponatremia. Kidney Int. 2013;83(4):563-7.
9. Konstam MA, Gheorghiade M, Burnett JC Jr, Grinfeld L, Maggioni AP, Swedberg K, et al. Effects of oral tolvaptan in patients hospitalized for worsening heart failure: The EVEREST Outcome Trial. JAMA. 2007;297:1319-31.

10. McDonald DA. Effects of protein and triglycerides on serum sodium and potassium values obtained by the Kodak dry film potentiometric technique. Can J Med Technol. 1986;48:146.
11. Mohmand HK, Issa D, Ahmad Z, Cappuccio JD, Kouides RW, Sterns RH. Hypertonic saline for hyponatremia: risk of inadvertent overcorrection. Clin J Am Soc Nephrol. 2007;2(6):1110-7.
12. Nguyen MK, Ornekian V, Butch AW, Kurtz I. A new method for determining plasma water content: Application in pseudohyponatremia. Am J Physiol Renal Physiol. 2007;292:F1652-6.
13. Pandya S. Practical Guidelines on Fluid Therapy, 2nd edition. Mumbai: Bhalani Medical Book House; 2015.
14. Reddy P, Mooradian AD. Diagnosis and management of hyponatraemia in hospitalised patients. Int J Clin Pract. 2009;63(10):1494-508.
15. Sahay M, Sahay R. Hyponatremia: A practical approach. Indian J Endocrinol Metab. 2014;18(6):760-71.
16. Schrier RW, Gross P, Gheorghiade M, Berl T, Verbalis JG, Czerwiec FS, et al. Tolvaptan, a selective oral vasopressin V2-receptor antagonist, for hyponatremia. N Engl J Med. 2006;355:2099-112.
17. Schwartz WB, Bennett W, Curelop S, Bartter FC. A syndrome of renal sodium loss and hyponatremia probably resulting from inappropriate secretion of antidiuretic hormone. Am J Med. 1957;23:529-42.
18. Verbalis JG, Goldsmith SR, Greenberg A, Korzelius C, Schrier RW, Sterns RH, et al. Diagnosis, evaluation and treatment of hyponatremia: expert panel recommendations. Am J Med. 2013;126(10 Suppl 1):S1-42.
19. Verbalis JG, Goldsmith SR, Greenberg A, Schrier RW, Sterns RH. Hyponatremia treatment guidelines 2007: Expert panel recommendations. Am J Med. 2007;120: S1-21.
20. Waikar SS, Mount DB, Curhan GC. Mortality after hospitalization with mild, moderate, and severe hyponatremia. Am J Med. 2009;122(9):857-65.

CHAPTER 32

Intensive Care Unit-acquired Weakness

Vibhor Pardasani

■ CASE SCENARIO

A critically ill patient recovering from sepsis wakes up from sedation and is found unable to move his limbs. He has severe weakness of all extremities, more pronounced proximally. Despite resolution of his respiratory illness, the patient continues to need mechanical ventilation and is difficult to wean.

Intensive care unit-acquired weakness, acronymed as ICUAW, is a syndrome of generalized limb weakness that develops while a patient is critically ill and for which there is no alternative explanation other than the critical illness itself.

■ CLINICAL PRESENTATION

It usually involves the extremities but not infrequently the respiratory muscles as well; however, the facial muscles are usually spared. In most patients, the deep tendon reflexes are reduced, but they can sometimes be normal. Sensory modalities are generally spared and the plantar reflexes are flexor. The respiratory muscles, and more specifically the diaphragm, seem to be extremely vulnerable in critically ill patients. This leads to a prolonged need for mechanical ventilation and often a cautious, step-by-step weaning from respiratory support.

Many different terms are used to describe this neurologic syndrome in the sick ICU patient. Some of these include critical illness polyneuropathy (CIP), critical illness myopathy (CIM), acute quadriplegic myopathy, acute necrotizing myopathy of intensive care, and critical illness neuromyopathy. The term ICUAW was adopted in 2009 to denote this syndrome, in order to encompass and include all the previously used terms. ICUAW is most often seen in severely ill patients with multiorgan failure and is considered to be part of the multiorgan failure syndrome, involving nerves and muscles. Nevertheless, severe weakness is also sometimes found in patients who have no other signs of multiorgan failure.

■ WHEN TO SUSPECT INTENSIVE CARE UNIT-ACQUIRED WEAKNESS

The diagnosis of ICUAW is largely dependent on clinical examination and exclusion of other neurologic causes of motor weakness. There is no specific biomarker of ICUAW. The important thing to assess is whether the apparent weakness is true "motor weakness", or just deconditioning of muscles due to prolonged ICU confinement. Through a detailed clinical examination, one can differentiate lower motor neuron type of motor weakness from an upper motor neuron type of involvement.

Presence of hyperreflexia, extensor plantar responses, and a sharp sensory level would support localization in the spinal cord. If the weakness is unilateral or in hemidistribution, one needs to think of a stroke that might have occurred while the patient was critically ill. Severe weakness in some patients, particularly in the presence of severe atrophy, fasciculations, and hyperreflexia, may indicate amyotrophic lateral sclerosis.

■ CHALLENGES IN DIAGNOSIS

Neurologic examination of the critically ill patients is sometimes difficult, especially when the level of consciousness is diminished or altered by sedation. Assessment of strength and sensation is also often unreliable except when limbs are immobile, flaccid, and do not move with nailbed compression. Both proximal and distal muscle groups should be tested whenever possible, including those involved in flexion and extension at the shoulder, elbow, wrist, hip, knee, and ankle joints.

For optimal physical examination and strength assessment, an awake, attentive, and cooperative patient is needed. This can be a limitation in the ICU, as many ICU patients are sedated for variable periods of time. Delirium and lack of cooperation may also jeopardize detailed muscle testing and power assessment.

■ WHY DOES IT OCCUR

In CIP, axonal damage is found in the peripheral as well as in the phrenic nerves. Sepsis induces microvascular changes in the endoneurium, allowing toxic factors to penetrate the nerve ends. In addition, increased vascular permeability may induce endoneural edema, compromising energy delivery to the axon, and resulting in axonal injury. Mitochondrial dysfunction due to stress-induced hyperglycemia may further aggravate this process.

In patients with CIM, loss of muscle mass occurs early and is more pronounced in the presence of multiple organ failure as compared to single organ failure. Atrophy results from increased protein degradation not compensated by protein synthesis. Pathophysiologic factors initiating the catabolic process include inflammation, immobilization, endocrine stress responses, rapidly developing nutritional deficit, impaired microcirculation, and denervation. In addition to structural changes, muscles can be dysfunctional due to other factors including muscle membrane inexcitability due to an acquired sodium channelopathy, mitochondrial dysfunction with resultant bioenergetic failure, and impaired excitation–contraction coupling.

FACTORS INVOLVED IN CAUSATION

Sepsis, the systemic inflammatory response syndrome (SIRS), and multiple organ failure are considered to be central players in the causation of ICUAW. Both severity and duration of SIRS and organ failure are contributing risk factors. Hyperglycemia, frequently present in critically ill patients, is also an independent risk factor for both electrophysiologic and clinical manifestations of ICUAW.

Other patient-related factors that contribute to ICUAW include use of corticosteroids, age, parenteral nutrition, female sex, hyperosmolality, hypoalbuminemia, and renal replacement therapy.

Prolonged confinement to bed, in itself is known to have deleterious effect on the musculoskeletal system and muscle mass disappears quickly. Muscle immobilization rapidly induces loss of muscle mass and strength. Early mobilization is known to effectively reduce ICUAW.

Respiratory weakness and weakness of the diaphragm manifest as difficulty in weaning. 80% of patients with ICUAW demonstrate diaphragmatic weakness of some degree. Mechanical ventilation itself, through immobilization of the diaphragm, may contribute to atrophy of the diaphragm and diaphragmatic muscle weakness in critically ill patients; this is known as ventilator-induced diaphragmatic dysfunction and can confound the assessment of neuromuscular respiratory failure.

Whether the autonomic dysfunction, which is often seen in critically ill patients, is part of CIP it remains to be established. Axonal degeneration of the sympathetic chain and vagal nerves has been noted in selected patients with CIP, and suggests that the autonomic system might be involved in the process.

NEUROELECTROPHYSIOLOGY AND BLOOD MARKERS

Once the clinical diagnosis of ICUAW has been made, the next step is to do a nerve conduction study (NCS). This would contribute by:

- Confirming the involvement of the peripheral nervous system in the neurological weakness;
- Differentiating between CIP and CIM;
- Distinguishing between axonal and demyelinating neuropathies;
- Detecting any preexisting myasthenia gravis.

Due to interference of electric devices in the ICU, NCS can be technologically demanding in the ICU setting. A reduction in the amplitude of the compound muscle action potential (CMAP) is used as a marker of nerve or muscle dysfunction. A normal CMAP on screening electrophysiologic testing, 8 days after ICU admission, practically excludes a neurologic cause for ICUAW. Repetitive stimulation can be used to examine the neuromuscular junction. In ICUAW, the neuromuscular junction is not affected and test results should be normal. Abnormalities in the neuromuscular junction are indicative of ongoing effects of neuromuscular blocking agents or previously undiagnosed myasthenia gravis. Assessment of the morphology and recruitment pattern of motor unit action potentials (MUAPs) on doing a needle electromyography (EMG) can be helpful to diagnose myopathy. Characteristically, with myopathy, MUAPs have a short duration and low amplitude. For optimal EMG, an awake and attentive patient is needed to activate the muscle and to reliably evaluate MUAPs. This is often challenging in sedated, or otherwise unconscious, or delirious critically ill patients.

Muscle Biopsy

This is rarely required in the setting of ICUAW. Muscle tissue can be obtained via open biopsy or needle biopsy techniques. In cases of unclear clinical or electrophysiologic findings, or when a strong suspicion of a myopathy other than CIM exists, muscle biopsy may be helpful.

Blood Markers

Although creatinine kinase (CK) levels in blood are increased in patients with ICUAW, it is not a good biomarker as it can also be elevated with muscle breakdown due to a number of other non-neurologic factors. Plasma neurofilament levels are found to be increased in patients with ICUAW as compared to patients without ICUAW; however, neurofilaments are nonspecific markers of axonal injury and levels can be increased in many other illnesses.

■ HOSPITAL COURSE AND MANAGEMENT

Intensive care unit-acquired weakness is associated with a prolonged need for mechanical ventilation and increased length of stay in the ICU and in the hospital. Mortality rates are higher in these patients during and after the ICU admission. The diagnostic label should be used only if other causes of acute motor weakness, including Guillain–Barré syndrome, myasthenia gravis, etc., have been excluded by clinical examination, electrophysiology, and any additional investigations that might be required. Treatment remains primarily aimed at the primary critical illness, such as sepsis or trauma. There are no specific drugs or agents that are known to reverse or improve ICUAW. As soon as the patient stabilizes, further worsening of the weakness might be prevented by mobilization and muscle exercises through physiotherapy. One should ensure that neuromuscular blockers and sedatives are avoided as far as possible. Serum electrolytes, chiefly potassium, calcium, and magnesium, should be maintained as close to normal as possible.

■ OUTCOME

Different patients recover differently. This heterogeneity represents various clinical phenotypes and results from interaction of ICUAW with other factors such as age, comorbidities, preexisting neuromuscular problems, and ICU length of stay. Recovery from CIM is usually faster, more complete, and less likely to result in severe persisting disability. CIP alone, or coexisting with CIM, usually recovers slowly and at times incompletely. Patients who have not recovered from ICUAW by the end of ICU discharge are more likely to have a higher morbidity and mortality.

■ POINTS TO REMEMBER
- Suspect ICUAW in patients who develop limb weakness after getting admitted to the ICU and inpatients who are difficult to wean off respiratory support.
- A detailed history and clinical examination would suffice for making the diagnosis.
- Nerve conduction studies have a supportive role. At times, investigations may sometimes be required to exclude other causes of motor weakness.
- Treatment is largely supportive and includes early mobilization and avoidance of neuromuscular blocking agents.
- Long-term prognosis depends on the type and severity of ICUAW.

■ SUGGESTED READING
1. Dres M, Goligher EC, Heunks LMA, Brochard LJ. Critical illness-associated diaphragm weakness. Intensive Care Med. 2017;43(10):1441-52.
2. Hermans G, Van den Berghe G. Clinical review: intensive care unit-acquired weakness. Crit Care. 2015;19(1):274.
3. Koch S, Wollersheim T, Bierbrauer J, Haas K, Mörgeli R, Deja M, et al. Long-term recovery in critical illness myopathy is complete, contrary to polyneuropathy. Muscle Nerve. 2014;50(3):431-6.
4. Kramer CL. Intensive care unit-acquired weakness. Neurol Clin. 2017;35(4):723-36.
5. Kress JP, Hall JB. ICU-acquired weakness and recovery from critical illness. N Engl J Med. 2014;370(17):1626-35.
6. Lacomis D. Electrophysiology of neuromuscular disorders in critical illness. Muscle Nerve. 2013;47(3):452-63.
7. Lacomis DJ. Neuromuscular disorders in critically ill patients: review and update. Clin Neuromuscul Dis. 2011;12(4):197-218.
8. Latronico N, Bolton CF. Critical illness polyneuropathy and myopathy: a major cause of muscle weakness and paralysis. Lancet Neurol. 2011;10(10):931-41.
9. Vanhorebeek I, Latronico N, Van den Berghe G. ICU-acquired weakness. Intensive Care Med. 2020;46(4):637-53.

CHAPTER 33

Seizures in the Intensive Care Unit

Vibhor Pardasani

■ INTRODUCTION

Critically ill patients with seizures are either admitted to the intensive care unit (ICU) because of their seizures or are admitted for another systemic illness and then develop seizures.

■ SEIZURE RECOGNITION

Recognizing seizures in the ICU and managing them can be deceptively simple or painstakingly difficult. The first step towards seizure management is recognition of what is a seizure and what is not. The heart of the diagnosis of a seizure lies in it being a transient phenomenon with an onset and an offset, and it largely comprises of positive neurological phenomenon rather than negative. In other words, involuntary limb movements, whether clonic or tonic or dystonic, are likely to be part of seizures rather than transient weakness or loss of power. Similarly, abnormal sensations felt in some part of the body transiently are likely to be part of a seizure rather than a loss or a reduction in sensation(s). Repetitive clonic-like limb movements that occur in specific positions and disappear in others are likely to be signs of upper motor neuron involvement. A truly clonic seizure, partial or generalized, would occur irrespective of limb position. Involuntary movements that involve the entire body would, by rule, impair the consciousness as well, if they are part of a generalized seizure. Consciousness and awareness remain preserved in simple partial seizures, but once generalized, the consciousness is unlikely to remain clear. Violent delirious behavior can be part of a frontal lobe seizure, but only if there is a clear onset and offset to it. The *Gold Standard of diagnosis*, in any patient where a neurologic symptom in the form of an involuntary movement or alteration in behavior is suspected to be a seizure, is an electroencephalogram (EEG) while the patient is having the said symptom.

The initial clinical presentation of patients with seizures depends on the neuroanatomy which is seizing and the underlying cause of the seizure. Clinical findings in patients with ongoing seizures will further depend on the effects of medications and complications. There are positive clinical signs, including twitching, tonic or dystonic movements, automatisms, and rhythmic jerking, and negative signs such as confusion and aphasia. After a seizure has ended, some patients may have motor weakness for several minutes (known as Todd's paralysis), confusion, lethargy, drowsiness, or even sleep. If the level of consciousness does not improve by 20 minutes after the movements/

clinical phenomena have stopped, nonconvulsive seizures (NCSz) should be considered. In the critically ill, it can be especially difficult to distinguish if a patient is having a seizure. These patients often have altered consciousness secondary to systemic disease or medication effect. Among ICU patients who are receiving any form of sedation or neuromuscular blockade, it is especially difficult to recognize seizures.

STATUS EPILEPTICUS

Status epilepticus (SE) is defined as clinical and/or electrographic seizure activity lasting >5 minutes or recurrent seizures in a 5-minute interval without return to neurologic baseline. Early texts had defined SE with a 30-minute duration. However, it is amply clear with animal experiments and clinical experience that 30-minute cutoff is the time when seizures become pharmacoresistant and when significant neurologic damage has already occurred. In adults, generalized convulsive seizures, on an average, are found to last approximately 60 seconds for both behavioral and EEG changes. Thus, if a seizure has lasted 5 minutes or more, it is unlikely to abort spontaneously.

Status epilepticus can be generalized convulsive [generalized convulsive SE (GCSE)] with overt jerking/tonic activity or nonconvulsive [nonconvulsive SE (NCSE)] with seizure activity seen only on EEG without obvious clinical signs. It can also be classified as partial status, which is manifested as focal motor convulsions, focal sensory symptoms, or focal impairments in function, such as aphasia without alternations of consciousness. Focal motor status, also termed epilepsia partialis continua, involves repetitive movements or neurologic symptoms confined to restricted body regions. These seizures are frequently caused by a structural brain lesion and sometimes by nonketotic hyperglycemia.

Diagnostic Workup

Status epilepticus is a neurologic emergency, particularly a GCSE; treatment is started prior to initiating a diagnostic workup. When the clinical diagnosis of GCSE is made or there is concern for NCSE, patients should be assessed first for their airway, breathing, and circulation (ABC). Stabilization of vital sign parameters should be initiated in parallel to terminating clinical and electrographic seizures. One of the first steps in seizure management is checking the blood glucose to eliminate or manage hypoglycemic seizures. A hypoxic seizure would be easily recognized by peripheral oxygen saturation (SpO_2) monitoring in the ICU.

All patients with SE should also be investigated for complete blood count, basic metabolic panel, ionized and total calcium, magnesium, serum levels of the antiseizure medication (ASM) if being already used, and computed tomography (CT) scan of the head. Additional investigations may be required based on the clinical scenario. If one suspects central nervous system (CNS) infection (fever, headache, and nuchal rigidity), then empiric antibiotics and antivirals should be started immediately, and a lumbar puncture should be planned after a CT scan of the head. Empiric antibiotics should be continued until the cerebrospinal fluid profile comes back negative. Those with possible exposure or ingestion as the potential cause for SE should have a comprehensive toxicology panel to include substances that frequently cause seizures.

Patients who are already admitted in the ICU due to a neurologic or non-neurologic cause may have multifactorial causes for seizures. These may include neurologic complications (i.e., brain hemorrhages), multiorgan failure (i.e., development of sepsis or renal failure), metabolic derangements (i.e., hyponatremia or hypocalcemia), and medications (i.e., administration of drugs that may lower seizure threshold such as certain antibiotics or antipsychotics).

Magnetic resonance imaging (MRI) can be used on a case-by-case basis to diagnose stroke, posterior reversible encephalopathy syndrome, abscesses, or metastases. Ongoing seizures may cause restricted diffusion in the hippocampus, thalamus, especially the pulvinar, and the cerebral cortex. Such altered signals should not be misdiagnosed as acute stroke.

Continuous Electroencephalogram Monitoring

Continuous EEG (cEEG) monitoring is required to detect NCSz/NCSE and to direct treatment in SE, particularly if refractory to initial interventions. Specific indications for cEEG include patients who (1) do not attain their preseizure neurologic baseline state; (2) are suspected to have NCSz (coma and altered mental status); and (3) have epileptiform activity or periodic discharges on initial 30 minutes of EEG. Almost 50% of patients with GCSE continue to have electrographic seizures after control of clinical seizures; those who do not show improvement in their mental status by within 20 minutes need evaluation with cEEG for their further management. The diagnosis of NCSE may not always be easy and requires significant improvement in the clinical state, or appearance of previously absent normal EEG patterns following acute administration of a rapidly acting ASM.

Management

Seizure duration, time to first treatment, and time to seizure control are major determinants of morbidity and mortality in patients with SE. The initial approach involves stabilization of vital signs (ABCs of life support) and identifying the underlying cause of SE while trying to terminate the seizures. If the patient's airway is not secure from seizures, at postictal state, or escalation of seizure treatment to intravenous (IV) ASMs, then early intubation should be considered. Strict vitals monitoring (blood pressure, body temperature, and oxygenation) and IV access should be continued throughout ASM administration, as both ASMs and ongoing seizure activity may be associated with life-threatening hypotension and arrhythmias.

The most critical step in stopping clinical (and electrographic) seizure activity involves prompt administration of adequate ASMs. A benzodiazepine (BZD) is given as emergent rescue therapy and later, unless the precipitating cause of seizures is corrected (i.e., hypoglycemia or hypocalcemia) and the patient has stopped seizing, a second ASM, called the control therapy, is invariably required.

Lorazepam is currently considered the most efficacious initial agent in immediate seizure control. Compared to other BZDs such as diazepam and midazolam, lorazepam has a longer duration of antiseizure effect as other BZDs are more lipophilic and get quickly redistributed to other fatty tissues, causing both brain and serum concentrations to decrease quickly.

After lorazepam has been given, patients should receive a second ASM unless the cause of seizures, such as hypoglycemia, is definitively corrected. BZDs are fast acting, but are not a good maintenance therapy to prevent the recurrence of seizures or SE. For those patients whose seizures responded to lorazepam, a loading dose of a second ASM causes a quick rise to therapeutic blood levels and then this ASM is continued for maintenance dosing. If the seizure did not respond to a BZD, then the second ASM needs to be administered without any time lapse. This second agent can be IV fosphenytoin/phenytoin or valproate sodium or levetiracetam. There is not enough data to support any superiority of one over the other. When choosing the second ASM, each clinical scenario, including comorbidities, should be assessed, but the most important goal is to administer an ASM promptly to attain therapeutic serum levels. In patients with known epilepsy who had been taking an ASM, it is reasonable to give an IV bolus of that ASM before moving on to a new agent **(Table 1)**.

Refractory Status Epilepticus

A patient who continues to have seizures clinically or electrographically after two ASMs is considered to be in refractory status epilepticus (RSE) regardless of the elapsed time. After two standard ASMs have been given, only 2% and 5% of GCSE and NCSE, respectively, will respond to a third ASM. Because of this poor response, it is recommended that at this stage, continuous-infusion ASMs should be considered without further delay. These include midazolam, propofol, thiopentone, and ketamine. Respiratory depression and hypotension are expected when using these anesthetic infusions. Patients should be intubated by this time, with central lines in place. The intensivist should be ready to initiate vasopressors and there should be hypotension following the initiation of these infusions. One should not desist from using IV ASMs for fear of hypotension, as it is the rapidity of seizure control that determines the final outcome in these patients. Midazolam and propofol infusions are preferred over thiopentone, as they are shorter acting and cause fewer hemodynamic disturbances.

Once IV ASMs in the form of the above anesthetic agents are started, absence of clinical seizures alone is no longer the target. Many patients

TABLE 1 Antiseizure medications dosing in status epilepticus.

Drug	Loading dose	Onset of action (minutes)	Duration of effect (hours)	Repeat dose	Maintenance dose
Lorazepam	0.1 mg/kg intravenous (IV) up to 4 mg per dose	3–10	12–24	May repeat once in 5 minutes	
Phenytoin	20 mg/kg IV, maximal infusion rate of 50 mg/min	10–25	24	10 mg/kg	5–7 mg/kg/day in two to three divided doses
Fosphenytoin	30 mg/kg IV, maximal infusion rate of 150 mg/min	10–25	24	15 mg/kg	5–7 mg/kg/day in two to three divided doses
Valproic acid	20–40 mg/kg IV at rate of 3–6 mg/kg/min	20–30	8–12	20 mg/kg IV	40 mg/kg/day in three to four divided doses
Levetiracetam	20 mg/kg IV or 1–3 g IV over 15 minutes	15–20	12–18	No recommendation	40 mg/kg/day in two divided doses
Lacosamide	200–400 mg IV over 15 minutes	20–30	12–18	No recommendation	100–200 mg q12 hours
Phenobarbital	20 mg/kg IV, infusion rate of 50–100 mg/min	20–30	>48	5–10 mg/kg	1–3 mg/kg/day in two to three divided doses

continue to have electrographic seizures at this stage while there are no clinical manifestations (NCSz or nonconvulsive status). It is therefore important to put all patients on cEEG monitoring so as to control electrographic seizures. Some experts prefer to achieve burst suppression pattern on the EEG as the target for electrographic status control. Studies suggest that mortality and return to functional baseline is independent of which IV anesthetic agent is used and the extent of electrographic burst suppression. Once the electrographic goal has been reached, the IV infusion is continued for 24-48 hours and then a very gradual weaning of the medication should be done, while conventional maintenance ASMs are optimized. Dosing should be individualized to seizure control with monitoring for toxicity. The withdrawal of these infusions should always be initiated while under cEEG to monitor for recurrent electrographic seizures. If patients have withdrawal seizures, they should be restarted on the same infusion at the rate prior to initiating the weaning and maintained for at least another 24 hours. Prior to tapering the anesthetic drip again, at least one of the nonanesthetic antiepileptic drugs (AEDs) that the patient is already receiving should be optimized (preferably achieve therapeutic levels), or a new nonanesthetic AED should be started **(Table 2)**.

TABLE 2 Antiepileptic drug dosing for refractory and super-refractory status epilepticus.

Drug	Loading dose	Maintenance dosing	Dose range
Midazolam	0.2 mg/kg with 0.2–0.4 mg/kg boluses every 5 minutes until seizures stop, up to maximum 2 mg/kg	Initial rate 0.05 mg/kg/h. If recurrent seizures, give 0.1–0.2 mg/kg bolus, then increase maintenance rate by 0.05–0.1 mg/kg/h	0.05–3 mg/kg/h
Propofol	1–2 mg/kg with 1–2 mg/kg boluses every 3–5 minutes until seizures stop, up to maximum of 10 mg/kg	Initial rate 20 mg/kg/min. If recurrent seizures, increase maintenance rate 5–10 mg/kg/min every 5 minutes or 1 mg/kg bolus plus increasing maintenance rate	20–200 mg/kg/min. Do not exceed a dosage of 5 mg/kg/h for >48 hours (increased risk of propofol infusion syndrome)
Pentobarbital	5 mg/kg, infusion rate 25–50 mg/min with repeated 5 mg/kg boluses until seizures stop	Initial rate 1 mg/kg/h. If recurrent seizures, 5 mg/kg bolus followed by increase in the maintenance rate	0.5–10 mg/kg/h
Ketamine	1–2 mg/kg intravenous (IV) over 1 minute with 1.5 mg/kg bolus every 3–5 minutes until seizures stop, up to a maximum of 4.5 mg/kg	Initial infusion rate is 20 mg/kg/min. If recurrent seizures, a bolus should be followed by increase of maintenance rate by 10–20 mg/kg/min until seizure control	5–125 mg/kg/min

Super Refractory Status Epilepticus

Seizures that are refractory to third-line (anesthetic) agents are rare and are termed as super refractory status epilepticus (SRSE). This is defined as SE that continues for 24 hours or more after the initiation of an IV infusion and includes patients who had attained seizure control with the infusion, but had recurrence on weaning. In these patients one must add an additional continuous IV infusion and optimize all ASMs.

Immunomodulators, steroids (methylprednisolone 1 g/day IV for 5 days, followed by prednisone 1 mg/kg/day for 1 week), IV immunoglobulins (0.4 g/kg/1 day IV for 5 days), plasmapheresis (five sessions), and adrenocorticotropic hormone are recommended in SRSE on a case-by-case basis. These interventions have been reported in select cases to help control seizures in syndromes with underlying immune mechanisms, such as Rasmussen's encephalitis, limbic encephalitis, acute disseminated encephalomyelitis, and paraneoplastic disorders.

Other medications used include topiramate (300-1,600 mg/day by nasogastric tube), gabapentin (in acute intermittent porphyria), magnesium 4 g bolus IV and 2-6 g/h infusion (likely to be helpful only in eclampsia), and pyridoxine 100-600 mg/day IV or via nasogastric tube. Other nonpharmacologic therapies include hypothermia, ketogenic diet, neurosurgical resection of an epileptogenic focus, if any, electroconvulsive therapy, vagal nerve stimulation, deep brain stimulation, and transcranial magnetic stimulation.

Patients in SE can have systemic complications either from ongoing seizure activity or from the ASMs themselves. Life-threatening arrhythmias and stress cardiomyopathy can sometimes occur due to the sympathetic surge. Pulmonary arterial pressures increase with every seizure, resulting in pulmonary edema. Patients with SE typically are not able to protect their airways and are at risk of developing hypoxia and aspiration. Fever can occur due to sustained muscle activity; metabolic acidosis (secondary to excessive anaerobic activity) and an elevated lactate may also be seen, but infection should always be ruled out first. Renal failure can result from increased creatine kinase levels causing rhabdomyolysis. Electrolyte abnormalities such as hyperkalemia can occur from muscle necrosis and metabolic acidosis. These complications can aggravate the underlying etiology, may cause further seizures, and complicate treatment.

Outcome

Status epilepticus is a disease that carries a high morbidity and mortality rate. The neurotoxicity of prolonged or repetitive seizures will cause neuronal death and is associated with a higher mortality and worse clinical outcomes. For SE, at hospital discharge, mortality ranges between 9 and 21% in various studies. The 30-day mortality ranges between 19 and 27%. RSE has a mortality rate between 23 and 61% while SRSE also has been seen to have a very high mortality rate of near 50%. Determinants of outcome include seizure etiology, older age, medical comorbidities, high initial Acute Physiologic Assessment and Chronic Health Evaluation (APACHE) score, and acute symptomatic seizures.

■ SUGGESTED READING

1. Ch'ang J, Claassen J. Seizures in the critically ill. Handb Clin Neurol. 2017;141:507-29.
2. Glauser T, Shinnar D, Gloss D, Alldredge B, Arya R, Bainbridge J, et al. Evidence-Based Guideline: Treatment of Convulsive Status Epilepticus in Children and Adults: Report of the Guideline Committee of the American Epilepsy Society. Epilepsy Curr. 2016;16(1):48-61.
3. Meierkord H, Boon P, Engelsen B, Göcke K, Shorvon S, Tinuper P, et al. EFNS guideline on the management of status epilepticus in adults. Eur J Neurol. 2010;17(3):348-55.
4. Pichler M, Hocker S. Management of status epilepticus. Handb Clin Neurol. 2017;140:131-51.
5. Vossler DG, Bainbridge JL, Boggs JG, Novotny EJ, Loddenkemper T, Faught E, et al. Treatment of refractory convulsive status epilepticus: a comprehensive review by the American Epilepsy Society Treatments Committee. Epilepsy Curr. 2020;20(5):245-64.

CHAPTER 34

Medical Management of Post-traumatic Hemorrhage and Coagulopathy

Jamshed Sunavala, Dipsha Kriplani Suvarna

■ INTRODUCTION

Road traffic accidents and homicidal injuries are the common violence-related emergencies encountered by casualty physicians and intensivists in most general public hospitals. However, unsuspected attacks with mass casualties can expose most hospital's unpreparedness to deal with such a crisis. In recent years such mass casualties are not uncommon, following assaults, bombing, mob violence during riots, and terrorist attacks posing horrendous challenges to most hospitals (particularly private institutions). To deal with extensive injuries with serious bleeding disorders brought en masse and all at once to a private hospital could prove disastrous as these are not specialized trauma centers. There are relatively few hospitals even in most major cities in our country that are well-equipped to handle such emergencies. Hospitals close to the scene of accidents are the ones to experience the first wave of the catastrophe. Hence, all major health centers should be decently equipped and well-prepared to organize a triage and be ready to perform timely surgical interventions to stop the hemorrhage and have a backing of good intensive care unit (ICU) and intensivists knowledgeable in resuscitating patients with continuous bleeding in extremes.

At least one-third of the patients with uncontrolled hemorrhage following trauma will manifest signs of coagulopathy. The very fact that such patients continue to bleed, indicates that they have significant coagulopathy. This group of patients develops organ failure and have a higher mortality than those with similar injuries and blood volume loss but in absence of coagulopathy. Coagulopathy can begin before admission to the hospital as a result of tissue injury, hypoperfusion, and loss of platelets plus clotting factors through hemorrhage. This initial coagulopathy is further accentuated by the combination of hypothermia and acidosis. Hypothermia is caused by infusion of cold saline and packed red blood cell (PRBC) transfusions given in an emergency without warming. In addition the patient has heat loss due to getting exposed to the markedly low temperature of the operation theatres (OTs), very often with exposed chest and abdomen during resuscitation. Hypothermia is known to actively delay the process of coagulation which leads to prolonged bleeding. Patients also continue to be acidotic during the process of hemodynamic resuscitation which worsens the coagulopathic state and infusion of large volumes of normal saline (a common crystalloid of choice) during fluid resuscitation will cause hyperchloremic acidosis plus dilutional coagulopathy.

> **BOX 1** Management of post-traumatic hemorrhage.
>
> *Initial resuscitation (at or near the site of accident):*
> - Bleeding control with compression or tourniquets
> - Cervical collar
> - Clearing and securing airways
> - Oxygen by mask
>
> *Advanced resuscitation (commenced on transfer to major hospital):*
> - Intubation, oxygenation, and ventilation
> - Hemodynamic support
>
> *Rapid assessment of blood loss:*
> - Clinical assessment
> - ATLS classification of blood loss
> - Shock index
> - CVP
> - IVC collapsibility index
>
> *Detecting the source of bleeding (mainly for blunt trauma):*
> - Imaging
> - FAST
> - MSCT
> - X-rays
>
> *Laboratory workup:*
> - CBC, serum creatinine, serum electrolytes, blood sugar, LFT, ABG, PT (INR), aPTT, serum lactate, and early detection of platelet dysfunction
>
> *Antidotes to reverse the effect of prior anticoagulant and anti-platelet therapy (see Table 1):*
> - Prior anticoagulants and platelet therapy
>
> *Damage control surgery (DCS) (for patients with suspected internal bleeding after blunt trauma):*
> - Open abdomen and chest
> - Pressure packs
> - External fixation devices
> - Venous thromboembolism (VTE)
> - Intensivist role post-DCS
>
> *Management of coagulopathy:*
> - Packed red blood cell (PRBC)
> - Fresh frozen plasma (FFP)
> - Platelet transfusions
> - Cryoprecipitate
> - Tranexamic acid
> - Factor VIIa as salvage therapy
>
> (ABG: arterial blood gas; aPTT: activated partial thromboplastin time; ATLS: Advanced Trauma Life Support; CBC: complete blood count; CVP: central venous pressure; FAST: focused assessment with sonography for trauma; INR: international normalized ratio; IVC: inferior vena cava; LFT: liver function test; MSCT: multislice CT; PT: prothrombin time)

■ MANAGEMENT (BOX 1)

Initial Resuscitation

Systemized trauma care should be given at the earliest possible time, at an appropriate facility. This has been accepted in principle to decrease overall mortality significantly, provided there is minimum delay between the time of injury and bleeding control. However, this concept is unlikely as much as it is ludicrous to be put to test by any "randomized controlled trial (RCT)".

Initial resuscitation begins at the healthcare facility closest to the site of the accident, where serious attempt should be made to limit the source of bleeding by applying extra local compression. Alternatively, tourniquet may be applied around the limb proximal to the site of hemorrhage as this has been found to be effective for uncontrollable bleeding, though it is not recommended for close injuries. Application of cervical collar for head and neck injuries, clearing, and securing the airways with oropharyngeal tube and oxygen by mask are essential components of initial resuscitation. These should be immediately extended to the patient at the nearest healthcare center or by a trained paramedic at the site of the accident. If no such facility is available at the nearest site of the accident, the patient is best rushed to the nearest hospital. Most lethal injuries occur, following a severe impact, to the head, cervical vertebrae, chest, and pelvis. Pelvic ring fractures have a high mortality because of resultant multifocal hemorrhage including a severe retroperitoneal bleed, which is not easily compressible nor manageable. These groups of patients require immediate admission to a major hospital which can deal with severe polytrauma needing complex surgeries.

Advanced Resuscitation

Basic resuscitation would have been already offered at the initial facility but once the patient is transferred to a major hospital or a specialized center, necessary advanced resuscitation begins with maintenance of airways, correction of hypoxemia, and stabilizing the deranged hemodynamics. Most likely the patient would be transferred directly to the OT as immediate surgical procedures may be required to contain the source of bleeding.

Intubation, Oxygenation, and Ventilation

Maintaining a patent airway by tracheal intubation is strongly indicated in the presence of either poor sensorium, obstructed airways, severe hemoptysis, lung injury, shock or respiratory failure. However, intubation should be best handled by a skilled operator as it involves considerable risk particularly for patients with cervical spine instability or those with facial, lung, and burn injuries. Sudden hypotension is known to occur by introducing positive pressure during intubation, more so in trauma patients who are already hypovolemic and this can lead to a potentially life-threatening situation.

The main objective of immediate intubation, besides maintaining an adequate airway and ventilation, is to generate optimal oxygenation on a mechanical ventilator. Simultaneously, one needs to ensure "lung protective" ventilation by delivering low tidal volume (6 mL/kg) with a mild-to-moderate positive end-expiratory pressure (PEEP) as most of these patients are at risk of developing acute respiratory distress syndrome (ARDS). The partial pressure of arterial oxygen (PaO$_2$) levels should be ideally maintained between 90 and 95 mm Hg. Very high PaO$_2$ level should be avoided in patients with traumatic brain injury (TBI), as studies have shown that ventilated patients with extreme or moderate hyperoxia have poor chances of survival. This is perhaps related to the altered microcirculation associated with hyperoxia and increased production of oxygen free radicals, particularly in patients with brain injury. Similarly, hyperventilation and hypocapnia in this group of patients may also result in increased mortality compared to nonhyperventilated patients. This is due to the marked vasoconstriction, secondary to hypocapnia resulting in decreased cerebral blood flow.

Life-threatening hypotension is managed with fluid challenge and vasopressors till such time as adequate blood transfusions are able to maintain a target arterial pressure. If trauma is associated with sepsis or septic shock, immediate empirical broad-spectrum antibiotics, fluid challenge with crystalloids, and further management using the septic bundle protocol should be initiated. A few studies showed increased survival with restricted volume replacement and permissive hypotension in patients with trauma-induced injuries. This was based on certain retrospective studies which showed that aggressive volume administration with crystalloids increased the incidence of third spacing, abdominal compartment syndrome, and possibility of further dilutional coagulopathy leading to multiple organ failure and decreased likelihood of survival. In contrast to these studies, existing data shows that permissive hypotension should be carefully considered as they may adversely affect the elderly patients and those with preexisting chronic hypertension and in patients with TBI.

In conclusion, the latest recommendation as per the European guidelines (Critical Care, 2019) is to target the systolic blood pressure at 80-90 mm Hg, mean arterial pressure at 50-60 mm Hg until major bleeding has ceased following trauma. However, in patients with severe TBI [Glasgow Coma Scale (GCS) ≤ 8], the mean arterial pressure should be maintained at 80 mm Hg. It also recommends vasopressors to be used transiently to sustain blood pressure and maintain tissue perfusion for patients with severe hypotension till such time the volume replacement is effective in stabilizing the hemodynamics. Restricted use of crystalloids but avoidance of saline solutions is recommended during resuscitation.

Rapid Assessment of Bleeding

Massive blood loss though obvious is difficult to quantitate, because often a visual observation or even the appraisal of vitals or the measurement of hemodynamic parameters may fail to estimate the extent of bleeding. The anatomical site, mechanism, and type of injury could provide a rough guide in predicting the magnitude of hemorrhage in the initial stages.

The Advanced Trauma Life Support (ATLS) classification for blood loss by the American College of Surgeons was based on certain clinical parameters. It is useful as a rough guide in estimating blood loss during the initial presentation of the patient. In this classification, a clinical spectrum of tachycardia, tachypnea, hypotension, decreased pulse pressure, oliguria, and a decreased GCS was suggestive of moderate-to-severe blood loss (class III to IV). An additional inclusion of base deficit value if less than −10 mEq/L was highly indicative of severe blood loss.

Though, several studies have highlighted discrepancies in this classification, it is still a practical and very useful guideline to be used at the bedside in the initial stages of blood loss following trauma. One simple calculation to assess the magnitude of blood loss is the "shock index (SI)". This index is defined as the ratio of heart rate to systolic blood pressure and is supposed to give a reasonably accurate indication of the size of bleeding and blood transfusion requirement. According to some studies an increment in SI paralleled an increase in volume resuscitation and vasopressor requirement. Interestingly, retrospective data base analysis of 10,234 patients confirmed that the detection of high SI on arrival to the emergency department was a sign of poor outcome. However, in practice, one should not entirely rely on SI but take into consideration other parameters of ATLS. A combination of clinical variables and base deficit may give a better prediction of the need for massive blood transfusion.

After the patient has stabilized following the initial resuscitation, further investigations are mandatory to detect any unidentified source of bleeding caused by the traumatic injury. *Imaging studies* offer immediate and useful information regards the source of blood loss. Focused Assessment with Sonography for Trauma (FAST) uses an ultrasonography to assess free fluid in the thoracoabdominal and pelvic cavities and this technique is now accepted as an essential first line of imaging in the emergency department. It is a rapid noninvasive technique which can be performed by a trained intensivist or emergency room physician at the bed side. One can detect hemorrhage in the pleural, peritoneal, and pericardial cavities by using a few standard cross-sectional planes, which does not necessarily require a specialized sonologist to operate.

Ultrasound can also readily asses the injuries in the abdominal, pelvic, thoracic, and pericardial cavities. Further, ultrasound can also assess volume status noninvasively by evaluating the inferior vena cava collapsibility index. Respective studies have shown good specificity and accuracy of FAST for identifying intra-abdominal injuries in hemodynamically unstable patients but a low sensitivity in hemodynamically stable patients. A negative ultrasound finding may miss intra-abdominal injuries; hence further assessment with multislice computed tomography (MSCT) should be done. However, hemodynamically unstable patients with blunt trauma who have clear physical findings suggesting intra-abdominal injury should not be denied exploratory laparotomy despite a negative FAST. New "contrast-enhanced ultrasound (CEUS)" has been developed with increased capacity to detect parenchymal injuries and may be available to us to enable better diagnostic yield at the bed side.

Multislice computed tomography with its superiority in diagnostic accuracy and a higher sensitivity than FAST allows better delineation of various intra-abdominal injuries and a more specific localization of the source of bleeding. Therapeutically it is superior in planning for better bleeding control, accurate detection of both the major and associated injuries and differentiation between various types of major vascular trauma. MSCT has also been found useful in detecting pelvic fractures with a probable underlying bleed and thoracic stab wound injuries which were undetected on plain X-rays. MSCT is now considered the "gold standard" particularly for intra-abdominal blunt trauma injuries and for identification of retroperitoneal hemorrhage. Modern scanners with its advanced technology can enable fast scanning of the whole torso with good image quality. MSCT facility in the immediate vicinity of the emergency department may result in early diagnosis of patients with polytrauma and significantly increase the probability of survival.

Delay phase CT is often used to detect an active bleed within solid organs which could be missed otherwise. Pooling of contrast in peritoneal cavity in *blunt liver injury* indicates massive bleeding due to a serious trauma and can be responsible for rapid hemodynamic collapse and requires urgent surgery, whereas intraparenchymal pooling of contrast in an unruptured liver capsule mainly indicates limited hemorrhage and these patients may respond to nonoperative treatment.

Standard laboratory tests such as complete blood count, renal functions, serum electrolytes, serum lactate, arterial blood gas estimation, and coagulation profile should be a part of the basic diagnostic workup of all trauma patients. A *low initial hemoglobin (Hb)* or hematocrit (Hct) level is traditionally considered an indicator for serious bleeding and associated coagulopathy, especially in patients with internal or occult bleeding. However, its main limitation in diagnosing internal bleeds is the influence of fluid and blood products during initial resuscitation. None the less, an initial Hb level of <8 g% is an indication for substantial and rapid transfusion. Anemia may also play an adverse role in clotting as the low Hct level has a negative impact on platelet activation.

Measurement of serum lactate and base deficit is useful as a diagnostic parameter and a prognostic marker of hemodynamic shock. Lactate clearing time provides an early and objective sign of patient's positive response to therapy, hence repeated determination of lactate levels is a reliable prognostic index for all patients in shock. Studies have shown that in patients where lactate levels returned to normal range (≤2 mmol/L) within 24 hours had very good chances of survival and in patients where the levels remained abnormal for >24 hours had increase probability of developing organ failure. Mortality was considerably high in those patients where the lactate levels remained abnormal for >48 hours. Lactate determination may not be reliable after alcohol consumption as ethanol metabolism is known to convert pyruvate to lactate via lactate dehydrogenase resulting in an increased level of lactate in the blood. Thus, in patients with traumatic injury associated with alcohol consumption the lactate levels may be spuriously high and unreliable. Monitoring of base deficit may be a better predictor of prognosis in such cases.

Prothrombin time (PT) and activated partial thromboplastin time (aPTT), platelet counts and fibrinogen levels are the standard coagulation parameters monitored in all patients with significant bleeding after a traumatic injury. PT measures the activity of the extrinsic pathway and can be seriously prolonged when any one of the factors II, VII, and X are low. Prolonged PT with an international normalized ratio (INR) of >1.5 may adversely alter the prognosis in patients with traumatic hemorrhage and is an indication for transfusion. Assessment of these standard tests has a prolonged turnover time over 1 hour. Further the coagulation assays such as PT, aPTT, and thrombin have been shown as insufficient to correlate with bleed in acute trauma settings. *Viscoelastic methods (VEM)* such as the thromboelastography (TEG) and the newer rotational thromboelastometry (ROTEM) devices have a faster turnover time of around 10 minutes which becomes a major asset when dealing with life-threatening hemorrhage from severe traumatic injuries. In addition to the rapid assessment of hemostasis which helps in early clinical decision making, VEM also has the ability to detect the most important coagulation deficiencies. Although the use of *TEG* and ROTEM devices are rapidly increasing one has to understand that there are a few limitations associated with the use of these devices and some controversies still remains regarding the use of VEM for detection of post-traumatic coagulopathy. The variance between the standard coagulation tests and VEM has also created doubt and disagreement as to the validity of the results between the two techniques.

Early detection of platelet dysfunction which is associated with traumatic injury is an important parameter in trauma and bleeding induced coagulopathy. Unfortunately, neither the standard coagulation tests nor VEM gives a reliable status of platelet function, hence the present recommendation is to use platelet function analyzer (PFA-1000) or "platelet aggregometry", the former is not readily available in India. Many more devices to check platelet function are available though not in India but some of them have specific application such as the "VerifyNow"—platelet reactivity test for aspirin (VN-ASA) which successfully identifies TBI patients who are on aspirin but in whom the prior intake of the medication was unknown, as in unconscious patients. While patients on vitamin K antagonist (VKA) therapy can be assessed by using INR or platelet function assay by aggregometry, to date there is no validated rapid test for any newer anticoagulants [direct oral anticoagulants (DOACs)].

The immediate intervention to reverse the effect of VKA is intravenous administration of vitamin K and the INR will begin to decrease within 2 hours and normalized by 12–16 hours. However, in case of life-threatening bleed where urgent correction of INR is mandatory, prothrombin complex concentrate (PCC) may be administered in an attempt to achieve satisfactory hemostasis. PCC till late was known to transmit blood-borne infectious diseases but the recent techniques such as pasteurization and nanofiltration have added to its safety. If PCC is not available, fresh frozen plasma (FFP) should be used.

Novel oral anticoagulants (NOACs) do pose a problem as not many antidotes are available. Factor Xa inhibitors (rivaroxaban and apixaban) has no validated reversing agent so far for immediate reversal of the anticoagulant effect. For monitoring the anticoagulant effect of factor Xa inhibitor, the anti-factor Xa assay is available. Recently an antidote (idarucizumab) to reverse the anticoagulant effect of thrombin inhibitor dabigatran has been made available though it is not clear if it is effective for immediate reversal during life threatening bleed. Monitoring of the anticoagulant effect of dabigatran is best done by assessing the thrombin time.

Fondaparinux is a pentasaccharide and effectively inhibits factor Xa. The only agent which so far has been found to effectively reverse the anticoagulant effect of fondaparinux is recombinant factor VIIa (rVIIa)

In case of severe hemorrhage and if there is dire need to reverse the effect of antiplatelet agents (aspirin, clopidogrel, prasugrel, or ticagrelor), platelet concentrate should be the first choice. Another option would be the administration of de-amino d-arginine vasopressin (DDAVA) or desmopressin, if available. It is given in a standard dose of 0.3–0.4 µg/kg in 100 mL saline over 30 minutes as it has an immediate effect **(Table 1)**.

Damage Control Surgery and the Role of the Intensivist

Damage control surgery (DCS) is a part of resuscitation for serious trauma patients with life-threatening hemorrhage and has to be performed immediately on admission to major hospitals. This is mainly essential for patients with suspected internal bleeding, especially in blunt trauma cases. Usually it involves opening up the chest or abdomen to control the bleeds, followed by pressure packs to prevent further bleeding and most patients are transferred from the OT back to the ICU with open body cavities. It is not unusual for patients to remain with open chest and abdomen for days before it is closed, resulting in deranged mechanical and physiological functions due to the altered anatomy and heavy pressure packings. The intensivist would have to adopt advanced modes of ventilation and innovative strategies for respiratory support. Similarly, skilled nursing for wound care, management of pressure dressings and supplemental nutritional strategies would be required in case of open abdomen. Further complication such as severe infection, prolonged ventilator support, and secondary bleeds following coagulopathy from massive transfusions will constantly require expert management.

TABLE 1: Antidotes for reversing the effects of anticoagulants and antiplatelets agents.

Anticoagulant agents	Reversing agents	Monitoring the anticoagulant effect
VKA (warfarin)	• Vitamin K I/V • PCC for immediate reverse	Prothrombin time
New oral factor Xa inhibitors (rivaroxaban and apixaban)	No validated antidote available	Anti-factor Xa assay
Dabigatran	• Idarucizumab	Thrombin time
Fondaparinux (factor Xa inhibitor)	• rVIIa*	—
LMWH	• Protamine sulfate (25–50 mg stat)	—
Anti-platelets (aspirin, clopidogrel, prasugrel, or ticagrelor)	• Platelet concentrate • DDAVP (0.3–0.4 µg/kg in 100 mL normal saline over 30 minutes)*	Platelet aggregation test

(DDAVP: de-amino d-arginine vasopressin; LMWH: low molecular weight heparin; VKA: vitamin K antagonist; PCC: prothrombin complex concentrate)
*From—Levi M. Annual update in intensive care and emergency medicine, 2016.

Patient with polytrauma are most likely to receive definitive treatment with early external fixation as part of damage control orthopedic surgery. In addition to large external fixation devices, there may be binders for pelvic stabilization, cervical collars, and spinal braces which often limit the mobility and restrict the access to proper nursing care of the patient in the ICU.

Patients with major trauma are at risk of developing venous thromboembolism (VTE). Immobility, hypercoagulable state, postsurgery, bone fracture, and damage-related inflammatory response are the common risk factors for VTE in patients with serious traumatic injuries. As the use of prophylactic anticoagulants is not possible in actively bleeding patients various other strategies such as sequential compression devices may be useful. Evidence-based guidelines which help to reduce the incidence of VTE in trauma patients should be a part of a set protocol of every ICU.

Lastly, the failure to recognize missed injuries could seriously affect the outcome, particularly in trauma patients where physical examination is often restricted. Hence, a tertiary survey protocol should be followed, by using faster and newer imaging facilities.

Transfusion Management

Management of acute coagulopathy associated with trauma often involves massive transfusion. The historic approach to transfusion was in the form of a fixed ratio of 1:1:1 of red blood cell units to plasma to platelets. With the availability of VEM, more accurate assessment of transfusion requirements can be made.

Fresh frozen plasma is plasma prepared from single units of whole blood or by apheresis. It contains all the coagulation factors present in blood and thus is an ideal replacement for factors lost in major bleeding. FFP can be frozen up to a year and thus need to be thawed for an hour before being made available for transfusion. ABO compatible units are transfused as plasma contains antibodies to RBC antigens. The European guidelines for management of bleeding following major trauma recommend treatment with FFP at a dose of 10–15 mL/kg. Further doses will depend on coagulation monitoring and the amount of other blood products administered. Each unit of FFP has a volume of 200–250 mL. Massive transfusion can put the patient at risk for circulatory overload.

Packed red blood cell transfusions are given over 4 hours to achieve a respectable Hb level of 7–9 g/dL. Extracellular potassium levels increase in the RBC units towards the end of the maximal storage time. This can add on to the trauma-related hyperkalemia. Administration of calcium in the form of calcium gluconate 1,000 mg over 2–3 minutes rapidly averts the membrane actions of hyperkalemia. Calcium chloride is avoided as it causes local irritation at the injection site.

A platelet count of at least 50×10^9/L should be maintained following injury as bleeding does not occur at this count. However, if disseminated intravascular coagulation and/or hyperfibrinolysis are suspected, the target platelet count should be above 75×10^9/L and in case of massive hemorrhage with TBI, the platelet count should be maintained above 100×10^9/L. ABO compatible platelets should be given (approximately one random donor unit per 10 kg of body weight). Five to six random donor platelets or one single donor platelet provide about 3 to 4×10^{11} platelets. This raises the platelet count by about 30,000/µL within 10 minutes of infusion.

Cryoprecipitate is derived from FFP and contains a major fraction of fibrinogen, factor VIII, factor XIII, and von Willebrand factor. Plasma fibrinogen levels are routinely used for assessment of cryoprecipitate transfusion requirements. However, if available, thromboelastometry is considered more apt for evaluation of transfusion requirements as it provides information on clot formation in real time. Cryoprecipitate administration at a dose of 50 mg/kg is recommended if patient with massive hemorrhage has a plasma fibrinogen level < 1.5–2.0 g/L or if thromboelastometric shows signs of a functional fibrinogen deficit. Massive transfusions have well-known risks such as transfusion-related acute lung injury (TRALI), multiple organ failure, and increased risks of infections. A proactive transfusion strategy should be adopted.

To stabilize coagulopathy in bleeding trauma patients, transfusion of blood products can be supplemented by pharmacological agents. Antifibrinolytic agents like *tranexamic acid* are used when hyperfibrinolysis is an established concern. Antifibrinolytic therapy is best guided by thromboelastometric assessment, if available. An empirical bolus of 10–15 mg/kg followed by an infusion of 1–5 mg/kg per hour is the standard recommended dose.

Recombinant factor VIIa is a salvage therapy option reserved for off label use in cases where major bleeding persists despite standard attempts to control bleeding. This is especially applicable in cases where antidote to patient's ongoing anticoagulant therapy is not available. There are no established doses for these off label uses; however, a dose of about 15 µg/kg has been effective.

■ SUGGESTED READING

1. American College of Surgeons. ATLS® Student Course Manual, 10th edition. Chicago: American College of Surgeons; 2018.
2. Briggs A, Gates JD, Kaufman RM, Calahan C, Gormley WB, Havens JM. Platelet dysfunction and platelet transfusion in traumatic brain injury. J Surg Res. 2015;193(2):802-6.
3. Cap A, Hunt BJ. The pathogenesis of traumatic coagulopathy. Anaesthesia. 2015;70(Suppl 1):96-101, e32-4.
4. Carter JW, Falco MH, Chopko MS, Flynn WJ Jr, Wiles Iii CE, Guo WA. Do we really rely on fast for decision-making in the management of blunt abdominal trauma? Injury. 2015;46(5):817-21.
5. Caspers M, Maegele M, Frohlich M. Current strategies for hemostatic control in acute trauma hemorrhage and trauma-induced coagulopathy. Expert Rev Hematol. 2018;11(12):987-95.
6. Eddy VA, Morris JA Jr, Cullinane DC. Hypothermia, coagulopathy, and acidosis. Surg Clin North Am. 2000;80(3):845-54.
7. Fligor SC, Hamill ME, Love KM, Collier BR, Lollar D, Bradburn EH. Vital signs strongly predict massive transfusion need in geriatric trauma patients. Am Surg. 2016;82(7):632-6.
8. Foster JC, Sappenfield JW, Smith RS, Kiley SP. Initiation and termination of massive transfusion protocols: current strategies and future prospects. Anesth Analg. 2017;125(6):2045-55.
9. Gonzalez E, Moore EE, Moore HB, Chapman MP, Chin TL, Ghasabyan A, et al. Goal-directed hemostatic resuscitation of trauma-induced coagulopathy: a pragmatic randomized clinical trial comparing a viscoelastic assay to conventional coagulation assays. Ann Surg. 2016;263(6):1051-9.
10. Gunn ML, Kool DR, Lehnert BE. Improving outcomes in the patient with polytrauma: A review of the role of whole-body computed tomography. Radiol Clin N Am. 2015;53(4):639-56.
11. Hagemo JS, Christiaans SC, Stanworth SJ, Brohi K, Johansson PI, Goslings JC, et al. Detection of acute traumatic coagulopathy and massive transfusion requirements by means of rotational thromboelastometry: an international prospective validation study. Crit Care. 2015;19:97.
12. Harada MY, Ko A, Barmparas G, Smith EJ, Patel BK, Dhillon NK, et al. 10-year trend in crystalloid resuscitation: reduced volume and lower mortality. Int J Surg. 2017;38:78-82.
13. Harvin JA, Peirce CA, Mims MM, Hudson JA, Podbielski JM, Wade CE, et al. The impact of tranexamic acid on mortality in injured patients with hyperfibrinolysis. J Trauma Acute Care Surg. 2015;78(5):905-11.
14. Holcomb JB, Tilley BC, Baraniuk S, Fox EE, Wade CE, Podbielski JM, et al. Transfusion of plasma, platelets, and red blood cells in a 1:1:1 vs a 1:1:2 ratio and mortality in patients with severe trauma: the PROPPR randomized clinical trial. JAMA. 2015;313(5):471-82.
15. Huber-Wagner S, Biberthaler P, Haberle S, Wierer M, Dobritz M, Rummeny E, et al. Whole-body CT in haemodynamically unstable severely injured patients—a retrospective, multicentre study. PLoS One. 2013;8(7):e68880.
16. Lawton LD, Roncal S, Leonard E, Stack A, Dinh MM, Byrne CM, et al. The utility of Advanced Trauma Life Support (ATLS) clinical shock grading in assessment of trauma. Emerg Med J. 2014;31(5):384-9.

17. Lewi M. Emergency reversal strategies for anticoagulant and anti-platelet agents. In: Vincent JL (Ed). Annual Update on Intensive Care and Emergency Medicine. Berlin/Heidelberg: Springer; 2016.
18. Maegele M, Schöchl H, Menovsky T, Marechal H, Marklund N, Buki A, et al. Coagulopathy and haemorrhagic progression in traumatic brain injury: advances in mechanisms, diagnosis, and management. Lancet Neurol. 2017;16(8):630-47.
19. Miele V, Piccolo CL, Galluzzo M, Ianniello S, Sessa B, Trinci M. Contrast-enhanced ultrasound (CEUS) in blunt abdominal trauma. Br J Radiol. 2016;89(1061):20150823.
20. Mutschler M, Nienaber U, Brockamp T, Wafaisade A, Fabian T, Paffrath T, et al. Renaissance of base deficit for the initial assessment of trauma patients: a base deficit-based classification for hypovolemic shock developed on data from 16,305 patients derived from the TraumaRegister DGU®. Crit Care. 2013;17(2):R42.
21. Nguyen BM, Plurad D, Abrishami S, Neville A, Putnam B, Kim DY. Utility of chest computed tomography after a "normal" chest radiograph in patients with thoracic stab wounds. Am Surg. 2015;81(10):965-8.
22. Olaussen A, Blackburn T, Mitra B, Fitzgerald M. Review article: shock index for prediction of critical bleeding post-trauma: a systematic review. Emerg Med Australas. 2014;26(3):223-8.
23. Podda G, Scavone M, Femia EA, Cattaneo M. Aggregometry in the settings of thrombocytopenia, thrombocytosis and antiplatelet therapy. Platelets. 2018;29(7):644-9.
24. Savage SA, Zarzaur BL, Croce MA, Fabian TC. Redefining massive transfusion when every second counts. J Trauma Acute Care Surg. 2013;74(2):396-400.
25. Schieb E, Greim CA. Emergency sonography. Anaesthesist. 2015;64(4):329-42.
26. Schöchl H, Nienaber U, Maegele M, Hochleitner G, Primavesi F, Steitz B, et al. Transfusion in trauma: thromboelastometry-guided coagulation factor concentrate-based therapy versus standard fresh frozen plasma-based therapy. Crit Care. 2011;15(2):R83.
27. Skitch S, Engels PT. Acute management of the traumatically injured pelvis. Emerg Med Clin North Am. 2018;36(1):161-79.
28. Spahn DR, Bouillon B, Cerny V, Duranteau J, Filipescu D, Hunt BJ, et al. The European guideline on management of major bleeding and coagulopathy following trauma: fifth edition. Crit Care. 2019;23(1):98.
29. Stensballe J, Henriksen HH, Johansson PI. Early haemorrhage control and management of trauma-induced coagulopathy: the importance of goal-directed therapy. Curr Opin Crit Care. 2017;23(6):503-10.
30. Swan KG Jr, Wright DS, Barbagiovanni SS, Swan BC, Swan KG. Tourniquets revisited. J Trauma. 2009;66(3):672-5.
31. Vincent JL, Taccone FS, He X. Harmful effects of hyperoxia in postcardiac arrest, sepsis, traumatic brain injury, or stroke: the importance of individualized oxygen therapy in critically ill patients. Can Respir J. 2017;2017:2834956.

CHAPTER 35

Pitfalls in the Diagnosis of Brain Death

Sarosh M Katrak

■ INTRODUCTION

The criteria for the diagnosis of brain death are well established under the Indian law since 1994. India follows the British system of equating brain death with brainstem death. Before considering the diagnosis of brain death, there are strict prerequisites to be met. The coma should be irreversible and the etiology should be unequivocally established. Complicating medical conditions like drug intoxication or poisoning and hypothermia should be excluded. The systolic blood pressure (BP) should be >100 mm Hg, even if vasopressor drugs are used.

A detailed neurological examination should establish the following:
- The coma is catastrophic and irreversible.
- All brainstem originating motor responses are absent.
- All brainstem reflex activity is absent—absence of the pupillary and corneal reflexes, the oculocephalic maneuver (OCM), the oculovestibular reflex to ice-cold caloric stimulation, and the cough, sucking, and rooting reflexes.
- Lastly, the apnea test, repeated by another physician after 6 hours, is positive.

Most mistakes occur when the above clinical setting and neurological protocols are not followed—the cause of the coma is *not unequivocally established*, a complete neurological examination protocol is *not followed*, and discrepancies from a full neurological examination are *not recognized*. This is avoided by *strict adherence to clinical setting and examination protocol*.

The cause of coma is not unequivocally established. When neuroimaging does not establish the diagnosis, one tends to label that coma as "encephalitis" without establishing the exact etiology. There are many examples of inadvertent transmission of central nervous system (CNS) infection from the host to the solid-organ transplant recipient.

The most common cause of coma of unknown origin is drug poisoning. A collaborative study by the National Institute of Health, USA, in 1978 stated "many more cases of drug intoxication contributed to the clinical picture of deep coma than suspected clinically by experienced physicians". The drugs mainly involved are organophosphorus (OP) compounds, baclofen, lidocaine toxicity, and delayed clearance of vecuronium. OP compounds inhibit cholinesterase, thereby producing cholinergic overstimulation of the central and peripheral nervous systems. Phorate, a diethyl OP compound is lipid

TABLE 1	Pitfalls in clinical examination.
Pupils fixed	• Anticholinergic drugs • NM blocking drugs • Preexisting disease
No OVR	• Ototoxic drugs • Vestibular suppressants • AEDs • Preexisting disease
No respiration	• Post HV apnea • NM blocking drugs • TBI with high Cx cord trauma
No motor activity	• NM blocking drugs • Sedative drugs • Locked-in syndrome

(AEDs: antiepileptic drugs; HV: hyperventilation; NM: neuromuscular; OVR: oculovestibular reflex; TBI: traumatic brain injury)

soluble and is stored in fatty tissues for a prolonged period with slow release. This "coasting" phenomenon may produce high levels of OP compounds in the blood, long after the drug is stopped, giving a false impression of irreversible coma. Vecuronium, a neuromuscular blocking agent is predominantly excreted by the liver but also by the renal route. The causes of impaired excretion of vecuronium are liver and renal dysfunction, metabolic acidosis, hypermagnesemia, and drugs such as fosphenytoin and corticosteroids. All these factors are likely to be prevalent in the intensive care unit (ICU).

Case reports have documented many *mimics of brain death*. These case reports involve the "locked-in" syndrome, traumatic brain together with high cervical cord injury, and fulminant Guillain–Barré syndrome with bilateral facial and total oculomotor nerves palsy. In all these conditions, an electroencephalogram (EEG) may be essential to establish cerebral activity.

The pitfalls in the neurological examination are outlined in **Table 1**.

Deterrents during clinical examination involve certain involuntary movements in a brain dead body. These may be in the cranial nerve distribution or involve the limbs or torso. Involuntary movements in the cranial nerve distribution are facial myokymia, transient eye opening, ocular microtremors and cyclical pupillary dilation and contraction in light-fixed pupils. Facial myokymia may be due to denervation hypersensitivity of the facial nerve nucleus in the damaged pons. Transient eye opening may be due to transient contraction of the Müller's muscle. The exact etiology of the latter two is not known. The cyclical dilation and contraction of the pupil may arise either in the ciliary ganglion or the pupillary muscles which respond cyclically to neurotransmitters in the setting of denervation hypersensitivity.

Spontaneous or stimulus-induced limb or torso movements are spinally mediated. They occur in about 13–79% of cases, usually within the first

24 hours. The spinally mediated deep tendon reflexes and extensor plantar responses may be elicited. Triple flexion at the ankle, knee, and hip, with or without head turning is also described, only to raise false hope of a response to pain. Similarly, spontaneous arm, leg, or respiration-like movements have been described. The movements can be very subtle, such as fine finger tremors, or dramatic, like the Lazarus sign. In the Lazarus sign, there is bilateral arm flexion to the chest, shoulder adduction, and the hands crossing or even touching each other for about 10–30 seconds before returning to the normal posture. As mentioned before, these movements are mediated at the spinal cord level and have no bearing on the diagnosis of brain death. They only serve to "panic" an uninitiated examiner.

In conclusion, all the pitfalls in the diagnosis of brain death can be avoided, if one strictly adheres to the clinical setting criteria and neurological examination protocol. It must be reiterated that the etiology of the coma must be unequivocally established, drug intoxication should be ruled out, particularly in patients with normal neuroimaging, and awareness of the deterrents during examination are the necessary steps. A certain degree of competence to perform a complete CNS examination for brain death is also necessary.

SUGGESTED READING

1. Busl KM, Greer DM. Pitfalls in the diagnosis of brain death. Neurocrit Care. 2009;11:276-2.

Appendices

- Antibiotic Formulary Used in Critically-ill Patients
- Important Scorings Used in Critical Care Patients
- Inotropes Used in ICU
- Mnemonics

APPENDIX

Antibiotic Formulary Used in Critically-ill Patients

Cephalosporins

Drug	Dosage (IV)	Remarks
1st generation Cefazolin	1 g q6h IV 2 g q8h for deep seated/bone infections*	• Drug of choice for MSSA infections and preoperative surgical prophylaxis • Affected by inoculum effect in deep seated Staphylococcal infections in which case cloxacillin/flucloxacillin are preferred. • Most effective for aerobic gram-positive cocci and also effective against *Haemophilus influenzae*. No activity against MRSA, MR CoNS
2nd generation Cefuroxime axetil	• 1.5 g q6–8h IV*	• Drug of choice for preoperative surgical prophylaxis • Effective against both GPC and to some susceptible GNBs • No activity against *P. aeruginosa*
3rd generation Ceftazidime 3rd generation Ceftriaxone	2 g q6–8h IV for CNS/severe infections* 2 g q12h IV (No renal dose adjustment except in patients on HD)	• Most effective against GNB but only ceftazidime has activity against *P. aeruginosa*; however all in this group are inactivated by ESBL producing organisms. 3rd generation cephalosporins are effective against ESBL producers when combined with beta-lactamase inhibitors like sulbactam or avibactam • Ceftazidime has limited activity against *Staphylococcus aureus*. Ceftriaxone is a drug of choice for *Salmonella*. Good activity against *H. influenzae*. • Useful in meningitis, intracranial abscesses as they penetrate inflamed meninges and achieve adequate concentrations in the CNS.

Contd...

Contd...

Drug	Dosage (IV)	Remarks
		• Ceftazidime and ceftriaxone both may elevate INR • Neonates <28 days do not give any Ca containing IV drugs within 48 hours of ceftriaxone • >28 days—Ca can be given after flushing the line but not simultaneously (chemically incompatible)
4th generation Cefepime	1–2 g q8h IV*	• Has excellent activity against *P. aeruginosa* and other susceptible GNB but practically no staphylococcal activity • Use with caution in patients with a history of seizure disorder • May elevate INR
5th generation Ceftaroline	600 mg q12h*	It has excellent activity against GP organisms including MRSA; its activity against GNB is as good as 3rd generation cephalosporins. Its main advantage may be targeting both GNB + MRSA in empirical therapy especially for community acquired pneumonia and skin and soft tissue infections
Cefoperazone + sulbactam (see BLBLI table)	1.5–3 g TDS 1 g Cefoperazone + 0.5 sulbactam	• Good activity against all GNB including *P. aeruginosa* • Good safety profile. Not inactivated by ESBL producing organisms.
Ceftazidime + Avibactam (see BLBLI table)	2.5 g TDS 1.25 g TDS or BID (RF) 0.94 g OD (CrCl< 15 mL)	• It is effective against GNBs and *P. aeruginosa* and is stable against most ESBLs (unlike ceftazidime used alone) and Amp C beta-lactamases but unstable in the presence of Metallo-beta-lactamases • Administer over 2 hours

*Renal dose adjustment required
(HD: hemodialysis; GPC: gram-positive cocci; OD: once a day; BID: twice a day; TIDL thrice a day; RF: renal failure)

Appendix I | Antibiotic Formulary Used in Critically-ill Patients

Beta-lactam beta-lactamase inhibitors (BLBLIs)

Piperacillin tazobactam	4.5 g q6–8h IV*	• Broad spectrum activity against ESBL producing GN organisms including *P. aeruginosa*, anaerobes, and GP organisms except MRSA and penicillin resistant enterococci • *Stenotrophomonas maltophilia* is highly resistant • There is divergent clinical evidence as to whether piperacillin–tazobactam should be used to treat bacteremia or other high inoculum infections due to ESBL producing GNOs • Carbapenems may be considered in the above setting especially if piperacillin tazobactam MICs are > 16 mg/L • CSF penetration is poor
Cefoperazone + sulbactam	1.5 – 3 gm q12h IV 1 g Cefoperazone + 0.5 sulbactam*	• Good activity against all GNB including susceptible strains of *P. aeruginosa* and *Acinetobacter baumannii* • Intrinsically resistant to all enterococci • Good safety profile • Not inactivated by ESBL producing organisms
Ceftazidime/ avibactam (CAZ AVI)	2.5 g TDS*	• This combination is active against carbapenemase-producing (KPC, AmpC and OXA-48-like) GN enterobacteriaceae and *Pseudomonas*. It has no activity against NDM producers. However, combination of CAZ AVI + aztreonam may be used for NDM producing isolates. (This drug should be used only as a *reserve* drug for patients with proven CR infections) • Poor activity against *Acinetobacter spp.* and anaerobes. Additional anaerobic cover advised in patients with intra-abdominal/other anaerobic infections

*Renal dose adjustment required
(CR: carbapenems resistance; GP: gram positive)

Carbapenems

Drugs	Dosage (IV)
Meropenem	1–2 g q8h*
Imipenem	0.5 g q6h*
Doripenem	0.5 g q8h*
Ertapenem	1 g q24h*

Usage
- *All carbapenems require renal dose adjustment
- Excellent broad spectrum activity against GNBs and provides adequate cover against MSSA, MS CoNS and anaerobes including *Bacteroides fragilis*
- They are not hydrolyzed by ESBLs
- Not active against MRSA, MR CoNS, penicillin-resistant enterococci
- Except for Ertapenem they have good activity against *P. aeruginosa*
- Meropenem and Imipenem are drugs of first choice for empiric use in septic shock for their broad spectrum activity and also useful for pelvic infections because of their effective mixed aerobic–anaerobic activity
- Imipenem is rapidly destroyed in the kidney by an enzyme hydropeptidase hence it is combined with cilastatin
- Carbapenems rely on time-dependent killing hence PKPD may be optimized by extended infusions over 3 hours (data exists supporting stability of extended and continuous infusion when admixed with NS at a concentration of 14.3 mg/mL at room temperature) or using a long-acting agent like Ertapenem
- Carbapenems can develop resistance to GNB following hydrolysis by carbapenemases. Combination of carbapenems with polymyxins, tigecycline, Fosfomycin, aminoglycosides may be used for CR infections if the carbapenem MIC <16 mg/L
- They have good CNS penetration. Meropenem is the drug of choice for GN meningitis
- Carbapenams, especially imipenem, have seizurogenic potential especially in elderly patients. They may decrease the serum concentration of divalproex sodium/valproic acid increasing the risk of breakthrough seizures. Doripenem: Not approved for VAP, increased mortality when compared with imipenem and the clinical response rates is lower.

Note: Faropenem (penem-class oral beta-lactamase agent), has a different structure from carbapenems and should not be considered an oral carbapenem. Although active against most GP and ESBL-producing GN Enterobacteriaceae, it has a lower potential for development of resistance. It has no activity against *Pseudomonas*, *Acinetobacter*, MRSA and *Enterococcus faecium*.

Aminoglycosides

Drug: Amikacin

Dose: 15 mg/kg q24h (dosing interval extended for reduced renal clearance)
- Ideal body weight and adjusted body weight formulas should be used for determining dosage in obese and morbidly obese patients, respectively
- Once daily, extended interval dosing as compared to traditional thrice daily dosing offers the potential advantages of reduced nephrotoxicity, ease of administration and serum concentration monitoring. This administration rationale is based on the pharmacodynamics properties of aminoglycosides—concentration dependent killing and postantibiotic effect
- Aminoglycoside infusion should be given over 60 minutes
- Avoid coadministration of beta-lactams in the same solution as they may inactivate the aminoglycoside (based on in vitro data)
- Therapeutic drug monitoring is not routinely recommended. Consider through monitoring in patients at higher risk of nephrotoxicity, e.g., ICU, elderly, concomitant use of nephrotoxic agents

Usage in ICU
- Most active of the aminoglycosides
- Good activity against GNB including *P. aeruginosa* and *Acinetobacter baumannii*, may show susceptibility to some carbapenem-resistant strains
- Aminoglycosides have no anaerobic activity
- Traditionally used for neutropenic patients and those in septic shock combined with a beta-lactam drug. However, superiority of combination therapy has not been established and should be weighed against potential for drug toxicity and selection of drug resistance
- Higher loading dose up to 25–30 mg/kg are advised to achieve adequate concentrations in critically ill patients due to increased volume of distribution and unpredictable clearance
- Nephrotoxic, hence dose adjustment required as per creatinine clearance
- *Adverse reactions:* Neurotoxicity, ototoxicity
- Avoid concomitant use with other nephrotoxic agents (colistin, vancomycin, amphotericin B, mannitol). Avoid loop diuretics as concomitant use may enhance cochlear toxicity
- Use with caution in patients with neuromuscular disorders (myasthenia gravis/Parkinsonism). Neuromuscular blockade and respiratory paralysis have been reported following use soon after anesthesia or muscle relaxants
- Avoid use of man nitol with amikacin as it enhances its nephrotoxic effect.

Gentamicin: The place of gentamicin in the ICU is now restricted to select indications like part of a combination regimen for prosthetic valve endocarditis due to enterococci or *S. aureus* and for neonatal sepsis and meningitis.

Antibiotics against MRSA

Drugs	*Dosage (IV)*
Vancomycin	*Loading dose:* 20–35 mg/kg in critically ill/meningitis (not to exceed 3 g) *Maintenance dose:* 15 mg/kg q8–12h (as per therapeutic drug monitoring) Target trough concentrations (before 4th dose): *Mild-mod infections:* 10–15 mcg/mL *Severe/CNS/deep-seated infections:* 15–20 mcg/mL

- Most effective if used in the highest possible dose recommended as per the creatinine clearance
- Other than nephrotoxicity, flushing due to vasodilation (red man's syndrome) and thrombocytopenia may occur occasionally. Vancomycin infusion over 2 hours to avoid red man's syndrome. IV vancomycin is an irritant, extravasation and thrombophlebitis may occur (slow infusion rates, dilute solution 5 mg/mL and rotate injection site)
- Broad aerobic and anaerobic gram-positive coverage. Should be reserved for MR *S. aureus*/CoNS and resistant enterococcal species
- Inferior option for methicillin sensitive staphylococcal isolates (cloxacillin, 1st G cephalosporins are preferred options)

Teicoplanin	• Loading dose 12 mg/kg (400 mg q12h) × 3 doses • Maintenance dose – 6 mg/kg (400 mg q24h) • Higher maintenance doses of 12 mg/kg/d (400 mg q12h) have been recommended for serious/deep-seated infections.

- Spectrum of activity similar to vancomycin. Inferior option for methicillin sensitive staphylococcal isolates.

Linezolid	600 mg BID (no renal/hepatic dose adjustment recommended)
Daptomycin	• 4–6 mg/kg OD for soft tissue infections • 8–10 mg/kg/d for deep-seated/complicated infections

Usage

- Linezolid and daptomycin are alternatives to vancomycin and may be useful in strains with reduced vancomycin susceptibility
- Linezolid has good lung penetration unlike daptomycin which is inactivated by surfactants in the lungs. However, daptomycin may be used in infections with lung involvement due to a hematogenous source of infection, for example, IE with pulmonary emboli
- Drug reaction with eosinophilia and systemic symptoms (DRESS) has been reported with daptomycin use. Myopathy/rhabdomyolysis has also been reported
- Statins may enhance the adverse effects of daptomycin. It is advisable to temporarily stop statins prior to initiating daptomycin. If continued, monitor CPK levels
- Linezolid–lactic acidosis, cytopenias, peripheral neuropathy, and optic neuritis are among the important adverse effects reported
- Avoid coadministration of Linezolid with serotonergic psychiatric drugs (SSRI, SNRI, TCA, MAOI) unless indicated due to increased risk of serotonin syndrome. May increase serotonin CNS levels by MAO-A inhibition

Antibiotics for multidrug-resistant GNBS (polymyxin B and E)

Drugs	Dosage	Usage
Colistin (Polymyxin-E) Colistin is available as the prodrug colistimethate sodium (CMS)	CMS 9 MIU stat followed by 4.5 MIU twice a day after 12–24 hours of the stat dose as maintenance dose. Renal dose adjustment is necessary and recommended dosing in patients on renal replacement therapy must be adhered to See International Consensus Guidelines for the Optimal Use of the Polymyxins. [*Tsuji et al. Pharmacotherapy. 2019;39(1):10-39.*]	• The Polymyxins (Colistin/ Polymyxin E and Polymyxin B) have the identical spectrum of activity and should be used as reserve antibiotics for carbapenem resistant gram-negative organisms particularly CR *Pseudomonas* and *Acinetobacter* spp • Polymyxins are intrinsically resistant to gram-positive organisms, anaerobes, and many gram-negative agents such as *Burkholderia* spp., *Proteus* spp., *Morganella* spp. *Serratia* spp., *Brucella* spp., etc • MIC using the broth microdilution technique is the only recommended method for drug susceptibility testing • Polymyxins have a narrow therapeutic index with major dose limiting nephrotoxicity and neurotoxicity. They should be avoided in cases with myasthenia, and in patients on neuromuscular blocking agents • Combination therapy with other susceptible agents (carbapenems/ tigecycline/fosfomycin, etc.) is encouraged in critically ill patients especially in infections where polymyxins achieve suboptimal drug concentrations, for example, lung, CNS, bones • Unlike Polymyxin B, colistin achieves levels in the urine and is preferred in treatment of urinary tract infections.
Polymyxin B	*Loading:* 20,000–25,000 units/kg *Maintenance:* 12,500–15,000 units/kg every 12 h (No renal dose adjustment is recommended)	• Polymyxin B is not a prodrug, hence achieves rapid steady-state concentration in the blood unlike colistin which can take up to 36 hours. It is, hence, a preferred option in critically ill ICU patients • It does not achieve levels in urine and hence to be avoided in urosepsis.

Contd...

Contd...

Drugs	Dosage	Usage
Fosfomycin	12–24 g/day IV (higher doses in critically ill patients) Oral 3 g sachets for uncomplicated carbapenem-resistant GN UTI	• Reserve antibiotic for carbapenem-resistant GN infections. Must be used in combination with another effective drug for complicated/deep-seated infections due to early development of resistance when used as monotherapy • Monotherapy may be considered in uncomplicated UTI due to resistant organisms • Achieves good concentrations in the lung and CSF and has excellent biofilm activity making it an attractive option for implant associated infections • Broad spectrum GN and GP activity including MRSA and VRE • Higher MICs for *Klebsiella oxytoca, Enterobacter* spp., *Pseudomonas aeruginosa, Morganella morganii, Providencia rettgeri* • No activity against *Acinetobacter* spp., *Stenotrophomonas* spp., *Bacteroides* spp., *Burkholderia cepacia, Bordetella, Brucella, Borrelia, Legionella, Moraxella* spp.

Tetracyclines for ICU use

Drugs	Dosage (IV)
Doxycycline	100 mg BID
Minocycline	200 mg stat then 100 mg BID

Usage
- No dose adjustment for renal or hepatic failure (Doxycycline may be preferred in patients with renal insufficiency)
- Contraindicated in pregnancy, children
- Usual indication—community-acquired infections such as atypical pneumonia (*Chlamydia, Mycoplasma*), scrub typhus, rickettsial infections, Lyme disease, brucellosis, leptospirosis, cholera, nocardia, STIs and pelvic inflammatory diseases
- Useful agents in GN sepsis due to *Acinetobacter, E. coli, Enterobacter* spp. when susceptible
- For SSTIs due to *S. aureus* if susceptible on culture
- Minocycline should be infused over 60 minutes to avoid reaction
- *Retinoids:* Administration of isotretinoin should be avoided shortly before, during and shortly after minocycline therapy. Each drug alone has been associated with pseudotumor cerebri (benign intracranial hypertension)
- Absorption impaired with concomitant administration with Fe, Ca, Mg bismuth, AL and Zn

Appendix I | Antibiotic Formulary Used in Critically-ill Patients

	Glycylcycline
Drugs	***Dosage (IV)***
Tigecycline	Loading dose (LD) 100 mg stat; maintenance dose—50 mg BID

Usage
- Has a reduced potential for resistance, as it is not affected by the ribosomal protection proteins and many efflux pumps. Thus, tigecycline may have activity against tetracycline-resistant organisms
- *Broader spectrum of activity compared to other tetracyclines including DR GN and GP organisms including MRSA and VRE.* Not active against *P. aeruginosa* but activity against *Acinetobacter* species has been reported in studies
- No dose adjustment for patients in renal failure
- In patients with hepatic failure (Child-Pugh C), loading dose 100 mg stat, maintenance 25 mg BID
- Best used for skin and soft tissue infections, complicated intra-abdominal infection
- FDA black box warning stating that tigecycline should be reserved for use in situations when alternative agents are not suitable, based on a 2013 meta-analysis showing greater mortality with Tigecycline use in CAP, complicated intra-abdominal, skin and soft tissue infections. However, higher doses of tigecycline (200 mg LD, followed by 100 mg 12 hourly), to achieve optimum concentrations, have been safely and successfully used for the above indications in multiple clinical studies

APPENDIX II

Important Scorings Used in Critical Care Patients

1. Acute Physiology and Chronic Health Evaluation (APACHE) II Score

It is used as a clinical scoring system to classify the severity of illness. It uses the worst values in the last 24 hours.

APACHE II = Acute Physiological score + Age points + Chronic health points

A. Acute Physiological Points

	4	3	2	1	0	1	2	3	4
Temperature (°C)	≥ 41	39–40.9		38.5–38.9	36–38.4	34–35.9	32–33.9	30–31.9	≤ 29.9
MAP	≥ 160	130–159	110–129		70–109		50–69		≤ 49
HR (bpm)	≥ 180	140–179	110–139		70–109		55–69	40–54	≤ 39
RR	≥ 50	35–49		25–34	12–24	10–11	6–9		≤ 5
(A-a)D FiO$_2$ ≥ 0.5	≥ 500	350–499	200–349		< 200				
(A-a)D FiO$_2$ < 0.5					> 70	61–70		55–60	< 55
Arterial pH	≥ 7.7	7.6–7.69		7.5–7.59	7.33–7.49		7.25–7.32	7.15–7.24	< 7.15
HCO$_3$	≥ 52	41–51.9		32–40.9	22–31.9		18–21.9	15–17.9	< 15
Sodium (mmol/L)	≥ 180	160–179	155–159	150–154	130–149		120–129	111–119	< 110
Potassium (mmol/L)	≥ 7	6–6.9		5.5–5.9	3.5–5.4	3–3.4	2.5–2.9		< 2.5
Creatinine (mg/dL)	≥ 3.5	2–3.4	1.5–1.9		0.6–1.4		< 0.6		
Hct (%)	≥ 60		50–59.9	46–49.9	30–45.9		20–29.9		< 20
WBC/mm³	≥ 40		20–39.9	15–19.9	3–14.9		1–2.9		< 1
GCS	Score = 15 minus actual GCS								

[(A-a)D: alveolar–arterial gradient; HR: heart rate; HCO$_3$: serum bicarbonate, use only if no ABG; Hct: hematocrit; GCS: Glasgow Coma Scale; MAP: mean arterial pressure; RR: respiratory rate]

B. Age Points

Age	≤ 44	45–54	55–64	65–74	≥ 75
Points	0	2	3	5	6

C. Chronic Health Points

- 2 points for elective postoperative admissions, or
- 5 points if emergency operation or nonoperative admission, if patient has significant chronic liver, cardiovascular, respiratory, or renal disease or is immunocompromised

Source: Knaus WA, Draper EA, Wagner DP, Zimmerman JE. APACHE II: a severity of disease classification system. Critical Care Medicine. 1985; 13 (10): 818–29.

2. Glasgow Coma Scale

	Response	*Points*
Eye opening	Spontaneous	4
	To voice	3
	To pain	2
	None	1
Verbal response	Oriented	5
	Confused	4
	Inappropriate words	3
	Incomprehensive words	2
	None	1
Motor response	Obeys commands	6
	Localizes	5
	Withdraws	4
	Flexion (decorticate)	3
	Extension (decerebrate)	2
	None	1

Source: Teasdate GM, Jennet B. Assessment of coma and impaired consciousness. A practical scale. Lancet. 1978;304:81-4

3. Sequential Organ Failure Assessment (SOFA) Score

	0	1	2	3	4
Respiratory					
PaO_2/FiO_2 mm Hg	> 400	< 400	< 300	< 200	< 100
SaO_2/FiO_2		221–301	142–220	67–141	< 67
Coagulation					
Platelets $10^3/mm^3$	> 150	< 150	< 100	< 50	< 20
Liver					
Bilirubin (mg/dL)	< 1.2	1.2–1.9	2.0–5.9	6.0–11.9	> 12.0
Cardiovascular					
Hypotension	No hypotension	MAP < 70	Dopamine ≤ 5 or dobutamine any dose	Dopamine > 5 or Norepinephrine/ Epinephrine ≤ 0.1	Dopamine > 15 or Norepinephrine / Epinephrine > 0.1
CNS					
Glasgow coma score	15	13–14	10–12	6–9	< 6
Renal					
Creatinine (mg/dL)	< 1.2	1.2–1.9	2.0–3.4	3.5–4.9 or UO < 500 mL/day	> 5.0 or UO < 200 mL/day

(MAP: mean arterial pressure; SaO_2: peripheral arterial oxygen saturation; UO: urine output)

PaO_2/FiO_2 ratio used preferentially. If not available SaO_2/FiO_2 ratio used. Vasoactive medication administered for at least 1 hour (dopamine and norepinephrine doses in μg/kg/min)

Source: Vincent JL, Moreno R, Takala J, Willatts S, Mendonca A, Bruining H. The SOFA (Sepsis-related Organ Failure Assessment) score to describe organ dysfunction/failure. On behalf of the Working Group on Sepsis-Related Problems of the European Society of Intensive Care Medicine. Intensive Care Med. 1996;22(7):707-10.

Inotropes Used in ICU

Agent	Standard infusion
Noradrenaline	4 or 8 mg/50 mL (mL/hour → μg/min OR μg/kg/min) Dose: 0.01–1 μg/kg/min
Adrenaline	3 or 4 mg/50 mL (mL/hour → μg/min OR μg/kg/min) Dose: 0.01–0.5 μg/kg/min
Dobutamine	500 mg/50 mL (mL/hour → μg/kg/min) Dose: 2–10 μg/kg/min
Dopamine	200 or 400 mg/50 mL (mL/hour → μg/kg/min) Dose: 2–20 μg/kg/min
Isoprenaline	4 mg/50 mL (mL/hour → μg/min) Dose: 0.01–1 μg/kg/min
Levosimendan	12.5 mg/250 mL 5% dextrose Loading dose: 6-12 μg/kg over 10 minutes followed by Infusion: 0.05–0.2 μg/kg/min for 24 hours only NB: Loading dose may cause marked hypotension, therefore may be omitted or reduced
Milrinone	10 mg/50 mL Loading dose: 50 μg kg/20 minutes Infusion: 0.375–0.75 μg/kg/min
Vasopressin	40 units/ 40 mL (mL/hour = units/minute) Dose: 0.01–0.04 units/minute
Phenylephrine	10 mg/50 mL (mL/hour = μg/min OR μg/kg/min) Dose: 10–100 μg/min 0.1–1 μg/kg/min

Note:
- All inotropes are to be administered in a syringe pump via a central venous catheter
- All dilutions are upto 50 mL. The amount of diluent will vary depending on the amount of drug.
- For example: 3 mg adrenaline = 3 mL of drug
  Add 47 mL of 5% dextrose to make a total of 50 mL
- All dilutions are preferred to be in 5% dextrose (isotonic) but 0.9% normal saline may also be used.
- May vary as per individualized institutional protocols.

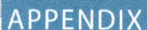

Mnemonics

1. Mnemonic **SEPSIS** as guide to selection of empirical antibiotics in patients with sepsis

S	Site of infection—meningitis, Subacute bacterial endocarditis, hepatobiliary infection, etc.
E	Epidemiology—community acquired, healthcare facility acquired, ICU acquired, ventilator associated pneumonia
P	Previously used—avoid if possible using antibiotic used in the last 3 months
S	Severity of infection—In severe sepsis, start with a broad spectrum cover
I	Immunocompromised or neutropenic—broad spectrum cover
S	Side effects—nephrotoxicity (aminoglycosides)

2. Mnemonic **CATHETER** to avoid catheter related blood stream infection (CRBSI)

C	Catheter site—subclavian most aseptic; femoral least aseptic
A	Aseptic procedure –strict aseptic precautions during the procedure and routine handling
T	Transparent dressing—always use a transparent dressing over puncture site
H	Hand hygiene—always wash hands or wear gloves during any manipulations of the lines or bivalves etc.
E	Exchange—avoid exchanging catheters over guidewire
T	Triple lumen catheter for Total parenteral nutrition —never use same lumen for drugs, parenteral nutrition and blood collection
E	Education and training to all health care providers who maintain central lines and is of almost importance
R	Removal—prompt and early (remove central line at the earliest) and removed all unnecessary central lines

3. Mnemonic **SPECIFIC** for specific causes of ICU related fevers.

S	Sites which are usually missed—surgical wounds, sinuses, sinusitis, bed sores, skin rash, lymph nodes, oral cavity
P	Pulmonary embolism/Deep vein thrombosis/Thrombophlebitis
E	Endocarditis
C	CRBSI
I	Inflammation (pancreatitis, burns) and Iatrogenic (drugs, blood products, Total parenteral nutrition)
F	Foleys catheter (catheter related urinary tract infection)
I	Ischemic bowel disease
C	C. difficile infection

4. Mnemonic **A to H** as a check list for weaning failure

A	Is the patient conscious enough to be **Aware** of attempting to breathe
B	**Breathing**—use of accessory muscles of respiration or paradoxical breathing will cause failure to wean. Also, rule out critical care neuropathy
C	Underlying **Cardiac failure** and fluid overload
D	**D**rugs—recent use of sedative or use of prolonged steroids during the illness
E	**E**lectrolytes and fluid imbalance
F	**F**ever—mild fever due to underlying or smouldering infection
G	**G**as—any significant ABG abnormality (persistent acid base imbalance /$PaCO_2$-$P_{ET}CO_2$ gap suggestive of dead space effect)
H	**H**indrance—Any external hindrance–pain, full bladder, anxiety, abdomen distension

5. Mnemonic **'S'** as check list for extubation (especially for patients who have been on prolonged ventilator support)

S	**S**ensorium—patient should be fully conscious
S	**S**ecretions—excessive secretions and inability to maintain trachea-bronchial toilet
S	**S**trength—Forced vital capacity ≥ 10 mL/kg BW
S	**S**tamina—should be able to tolerate > 3 hours without ventilator support and RSBI <100
S	**S**eepage—cuff leak test

6. Mnemonic **BURNS** for medical management of severe burns comprise of the following

B	BSA—initial assessment is as per the BSA rule of 9
U	Urine output—The most important monitoring parameter in severe extensive burn. Urine output < 0.5 mL/kg/hr × 3 consecutive hours left uncorrected by fluid resuscitation can be fatal due to hypovolemic shock
R	Resuscitation—Fluid resuscitation according to Parkland formula, most essential in the first 8 hours
N	Nutrition—Patents with extensive burns are severely hypercatabolic with increased energy expenditure and have negative protein balance
S	Sepsis—after successful resuscitation–sepsis is the commonest cause of mortality requiring appropriate antibiotic cover

7. Mnemonic **BIPAP** to check for absolute contraindications for Non-invasive ventilation

B	Brain—poor sensorium, seizures
I	Injury to head, face, mouth, neck or thoracic cage
P	Pressure—external laryngeal pressure or laryngeal edema
A	Aspiration risk from copious secretions, vomiting, hematemesis
P	Pulmonary—life-threatening cardiopulmonary problems

8. Mnemonic **COUGH** for causes of unexplained coughing in ICU patient- having ruled out the usual causes like - upper or lower respiratory infections, allergy or drugs

C	**Cardiac**—early left ventricular failure
O	Small airways **Obstruction**—mucus plugging, inflammation and infection
U	**Upper** airways secretions and micro aspirations
G	**Ga**stro esophageal reflux disease
H	**Hoarseness** with cough following post extubation after a prolonged ET intubation

9. **Mnemonic CHAMP**

After early stabilization of cardiac failure, the CHAMP mnemonic suggested by the European Society of Cardiology gives a comprehensive list of acute reversible conditions that could provide benefit at this stage (see Chapter 6, Management of acute heart failure and cardiogenic shock)

C	**C**oronary syndromes
H	**H**ypertension
A	**A**rrhythmia
M	**M**echanical complications of acute coronary syndrome
P	**P**ulmonary embolism

10. Mnemonic **DIARRHOEA** as a check list to rule out causes of diarrhea in patients on enteral nutrition (EN)

D	Drugs to be avoided	Inappropriate use of antibiotics, laxatives & prokinetics
I	Infection	Contamination of feeds
A	Allergy	Intolerance to certain foods
R	Rectal examination	For impaction and overflow diarrhea
R	Rate of feeding	Increased rate of feeding. This may have to be reduced.
H	Hypoalbuminemia	Seen mainly in patients on tube feeding who have albumin < 2 g/dL due to chronic malnutrition
O	Osmolality	Shift to iso-osmolar feeds
E	Excess	Fluid intake, glucose polymer or medium chain triglycerides
A	Assess further	? Colonoscopy

11. Mnemonic **GOLDMARK** is an useful to memorize the important causes of high anion gap metabolic acidosis (see Chapter 25, Arterial blood gases)

	Causes of high anion gap metabolic acidosis
G	Ethylene **g**lycol ingestion
O	**O**xoproline
L	**L**actic acidosis
D	**D** lactic acid
M	**M**ethanol
A	**A**spirin (salicylate toxicity)
R	End stage **R**enal failure
K	**K**etoacidosis

12. Mnemonics **COMAH** to rule out the common unexplained causes of coma in ICU

C	**C**entral—trauma, tumor, stroke, viral encephalitis, absent seizures, and meningitis
O	**O**xygen deficiency—hypoxic encephalitis following sever hypotension, respiratory arrest or failure
M	**M**etabolic—severe metabolic acidosis of any cause
A	**A**buse—drugs, alcohol
H	**H**ypo/Hyper—Glucose, Na, Ca and hypophosphatemia

"H" is added at the end as an etymology. In Latin Coma is derived from a word meaning Hair of the Head (from which the word 'comb is derived). From ancient Greek - Kómē or Hair. Hence interesting to remember the letter "H"

Index

Page numbers followed by *b* refer to box, *f* refer to figure, *fc* refer to flowchart, and *t* refer to table.

A

Abdomen, acute 374, 375*t*
Abdominal compartment syndrome 440
Abdominal pain 375, 392
   severe 374
Abdominal wall pain 375
Abscess 432
   drainage of 155
   ruptured 217*f*
Acetaminophen 393
   cases 131
Acid-base
   abnormalities 322
   evaluation 415
   imbalance 322, 325, 337
Acid-base disorder 325, 326*t*, 327
   assessing mixed 329
   mixed 326
   primary 325, 325*t*, 326*t*, 328, 329
   triple 331
   type of 328
Acid-fast
   organisms 181
   stain 181
Acidosis 334, 379, 381, 383
   development of 385
Acinetobacter baumannii 172, 215, 223
Acinetobacter spp 172, 173, 177
   drug-resistant 177
Acremonium 204
Activated immune cells 127
Activated partial thromboplastin time 438
Acute confusional state 104-106
Acute coronary syndrome 72, 117, 345
Acute exacerbation, treatment for 404*b*
Acute kidney injury
   etiology of 85, 86*b*
   pathophysiology of 87
   staging systems for 84
   systemic effects of 87
   treatment of 93
Acute liver failure 126, 128, 129, 129*b*, 130, 132, 135
   causes of 127*b*
   clinical features 128
   epidemiology 126
   etiology 126
   extracorporeal treatments in 135
   management 132
   pathogenesis 127
Acute lung injury, transfusion-related 58
Acute respiratory
   distress syndrome 35, 36, 39, 56, 58, 62, 64, 100, 208, 232, 235, 246, 253, 409, 440
   distress, physical signs of 231*b*
   failure 35, 37, 37*f*, 56, 232
Acute stroke
   clinical approach to 113
   complications of 117
Adenoma 397
Adequate organ perfusion 83
Adjuvant treatment 204
Administer oxygen 74
Adrenal insufficiency
   acute 398
   diagnosis of acute 398
   primary 416
      acute 398
   treatment of 421
Adrenaline 467
Adrenal-related emergencies 398
Advanced renal failure 333
Advanced resuscitation 439
Advanced trauma life support 438, 441
Aerophagia 407
Agar dilution susceptibility testing 183
Air
   fluid levels 217*f*
   trapping, risk of 407
Airflow resistance, increased 252
Airway
   anatomy of 19
   assessing adequacy of 19
   breathing, and circulation 431
   difficult 21
   function of 19
   management 20, 24*t*

manoeuvre, triple 20
obstruction 237
pressure 236
  release ventilation 247, 248, 248f
  waveform 240
resistance 237, 238
Akinetic mutism 106
Albumin 101, 204, 394
Alcoholic ketoacidosis 332
Aldosterone 398
Aldosteronism, primary 324
Alimentary tract, nonfunctioning 286
Alkalosis 101, 334
Alternaria 204
Alveolar pressure 314f
Alveolar ventilation 46, 48
Alveolar-arterial gradient 44
Ambler classification 175
Amikacin 173, 216
Amino acid 286
  losses 101
Aminoglycoside 162, 223, 459
Amiodarone 365, 368-370
Amphotericin B 162, 203
Amrinone 303
Analgesia 374
Aneurysm, ruptured 122
Angiographic vasospasm 122
Angiotensin receptor blockers 86
Angiotensin-converting enzyme 86
  inhibitors 400
Anion gap 331
Annual seasonal influenza 410
Antacids 324
Antiarrhythmic drugs 364, 365, 367
Antibiotic 150, 151, 215, 226, 460
  broad-spectrum 440
  de-escalation of 152
  incorrect spectrum of 190
  inhaled 209
  resistance 8
    collection of 167
  stewardship 186
  susceptibility test 173
  tissue penetration 191
Antibodies 9
Anti-Candida therapy 196, 197fc
Anticoagulant 119
  agents 445
  effects of 445t
Anticoagulation strategies 370
Antidiuretic hormone 411, 413, 416, 417
Antiepileptic drug 435t, 450
Antifibrinolytic agents 446

Antifungal therapy 205
Antihypertensive 226
  therapy 117, 400
Antimicrobial agents 190
Antimicrobial combinations 161
Antimicrobial resistance 171
  mechanisms 171
  types of 171
Antimicrobial sensitivity testing, caveats of 190
Antimicrobial synergism 161
Antimicrobial therapy 155, 170t, 211
  characteristics of 162t
  targeted 164
Antineutrophil cytoplasmic antibody 89, 227
Antioxidants supplements 295
Antiplatelet
  agents 444, 445t
  role of 116
Antipseudomonal activity 177
Antiretroviral agents 304
Antiretroviral therapy 200
  highly active 201
Antiseizure medication 431, 434t
Antithyroid drugs 226
Aorta 343, 344
  arch of 348f
Aortic dissection 117, 347, 376, 378
  acute 345
Aortic pressure waveform 266f
Aortic regurgitation 344f, 346
Aortic stenosis 346
  severe 348
Aortic valve leaflets 343f
Apixaban 372
Apneusis 108
Appendicular pain 375
Arachidonic acid 294
Arginine 284, 292, 295
Arousal 104
Arrhythmia 81, 123, 231, 312, 364, 404, 432
Arterial blood
  gas 26, 72, 74, 287, 322, 327, 337, 403, 438
  volume 411
Arterial carbon dioxide, partial pressure of 256
Arterial oxygen
  partial pressure of 36, 39, 56, 256, 304
  saturation 304
    peripheral 466
Arterial pressure monitoring 307
Arterial pulse pressure 319
  variation 319

Arteriovenous 346
Arthropod envenomation 86
Aspergillosis 202
Aspergillus 196, 202, 226
    species 198
Aspiration pneumonia 234
Aspirin 371, 444
Asthmatic patients 253
Asymptomatic candiduria 188
Asymptomatic hypoglycemia 387
Ataxia 413
Ataxic breathing 108
Atelectrauma 62
Atenolol 393, 401
Atrial fibrillation 392
    classification of 363t
    postoperative 363, 367
    prevention of postoperative 365b
    prophylaxis for postoperative 364
Atrial mechanical function 371
Atrial pressure
    left 300
    right 300
Attacks, unsuspected 437
Autoimmunity 398
Automated instrument methods 184
Autonomic dysfunction 289
Autophagia 290
Auto-positive end-expiratory pressure 239f, 408f
Avibactam 172, 218, 456, 457
Azathioprine 9
Azoles, dinteractions with 205t
Azotemia 398
Aztreonam 162, 172, 177, 218

B

Baclofen 449
Bacterial infections 128
Bacterial latex agglutination 189
Bacterial pneumonias 128
Balloon assistance 267
Balloon inflation 309
Balloon rupture 312
Barotrauma 61, 251
Basal ganglia 118
Bedside echocardiography
    advantages of 341
    limitations of 341
Bedside intervention, guiding 358
Bernoulli equation, modified 351f
Beta-agonists, long-acting 405
Beta-human chorionic gonadotropin 130
Beta-hydroxybutyrate 332

Beta-lactama 162, 175
    ambler classification of 176t
    extended-spectrum 168, 175, 218
Bicarbonate 89, 382
    therapy 383
Bilateral pulmonary infiltrates 52
Bilevel ventilation 248
Bioenergetic failure 426
Biomarkers 204
Biotrauma 62, 251
Bisoprolol 368
Bisphosphonates 398
Biventricular failure 263
Biventricular systolic 404
Bleeding 30
    rapid assessment of 440
Blood
    glucose 380
    loss 348
    markers 428
    products, transfusion of 134
    transfusion 374
    urea nitrogen 89
Blood culture 181, 208
    sensitivity of 173t
Blood flow 318
    velocity 318
Blood pressure 27, 116, 305
    management of 116
    systolic 70, 449
Blood sugar 153
    low 339
Bloodstream infection, catheter-related 181, 288
Body fluids, cultures of 155
Body mass index 277, 293
Body surface area 281
Bone resorption 396
Bradyarrhythmias 396
Bradycardia 30
    severe 369
Brain 124, 202
    death, diagnosis of 449
    hemorrhages 432
    herniation, risk of 423
    injury, secondary 28
    natriuretic peptide 404
Brainstem 124
    depression 107
    function 108
    reflexes 108
Breath pattern 243
Breathing 4
    index 255

Bronchoalveolar lavage 58, 187, 208
  galactomannan 197
Bronchodilators 405
Bronchospasm 405
  severe 234, 405
Broth dilution susceptibility
    testing 183
Brucella 181
Budd-Chiari syndrome 127
Bugs, battle of 8
Bullae formation 214
Burkholderia 173
Burkholderia
  cepacia 221
  pseudomallei 172
Burn injury 439

C

Calcium
  albumin buffer 394
  chloride 395
  concentrations, lower 394
  gluconate 395
    infusion of 395
Calcofluor stain 198f
Caloric requirements 280
Calorimetry, indirect 277
Candida 129, 194, 218
  auris 171
  chorioretinitis 194f
  isolation of 195
  species 289
Capillary perfusion 44
Capnocytophaga spp 190, 226
Capnometry 51
Carbamazepine 413
Carbapenem 110
  resistance 178
Carbapenemase 175, 177
Carbon dioxide 241, 322
  arterial partial pressure of 327
  partial pressure of 27, 36
  role of 27
Carbon monoxide, transfer factor for 369
Carbonic acid 323
Carcinoma 397
Cardiac arrest 27, 28b
  out-of-hospital 28
Cardiac chambers 343
Cardiac complication 397
Cardiac consequences 241
Cardiac failure 13, 411
Cardiac function 251
  estimation of 341

Cardiac output 39, 145, 268, 303, 4
  measurement 315
  pulse-induced contour 317
Cardiac performance 299
  determinants of 299, 300fc
Cardiac power output 269
Cardiac precipitants 72
Cardiac remodeling, chronicity of 349
Cardiac surgery 363
  after 365b
Cardiogenic edema 57
Cardiogenic shock 50, 69, 145, 268, 269
  severe 262
Cardiomyopathy 348, 364
Cardiopulmonary complications 123
Cardiopulmonary failure, severe 263
Cardiopulmonary resuscitation 27, 28
Cardiorespiratory compromise 72
Cardiovascular abnormalities 389
Cardiovascular emergency 379
Cardiovascular tachycardia 392
Carvedilol 368
Caspofungin 204
Catecholamine 400
  release 401
Catheter 289
  and cannula placement 270
  design 309
  large-bore 266
  shaft 270
  types of 309
  with tubes 291
Causative organism diagnosis 207
Cefazolin 455
Cefepime 110, 173, 456
Cefmetazole 175
Cefoperazone 134, 173, 456, 457
Cefotetan 175
Cefoxitin 175
Ceftaroline 456
Ceftazidime 172, 173, 218, 455-457
Cefuroxime axetil 455
Cellulitis 214
Central herniation, signs of 107
Central nervous system 9, 104, 191, 431
  disturbance 392
  infections 189
Central pontine myelinolysis 419
Central venous
  catheter 288
  pressure 145, 300, 438
    monitoring 307
Cephalosporins 110, 172, 455
Cerebellar artery, posterior inferior 107
Cerebellar hematomas 120

Cerebellar hemorrhage 120
Cerebellar strokes, large 117
Cerebral arteries 202
　right middle 203*f*
　right posterior inferior 203*f*
Cerebral blood flow 440
Cerebral edema 384, 414
Cerebral hemispheres 107
Cerebral infarction 122
Cerebral ischemia 122
　delayed 122
Cerebral performance category scale 31
Cerebrospinal fluid 121, 189, 199, 200*f*
Cerebrovascular accident 36
Chemotherapy 194*f*
Chest
　cuirass 235
　pain, acute 345
Cheyne-Stokes respiration 108
Chikungunya 180
Chlamydia 185
Chloramphenicol 177
Chloride 379
　resistant 324, 336
　　metabolic alkalosis, causes of 336
　responsive 324
Cholestyramine 393
Chronic care, inadequate 72
Chvostek's signs 394
Ciliospinal reflex, preserved 107
Circulatory failure 136
Citrobacter 217
Clindamycin 162, 222
Clopidogrel 116, 371, 444
Clostridium difficile 185, 189
　antigen 189
Coagulation abnormalities 119, 143
Coagulation pathways, activation of 59
Coagulopathy 134
Cognitive and motor function 105*f*
Cognitive impairments 386
Cold-dry profiles 78
Cold-wet profiles 78
Colistin 216, 223
Colloid, type of 148
Colonization 164, 166*fc*, 191
Coma 104, 106, 110*t*, 413
　clinical classification of 109
　deep 449
　etiologies of 106
　nontraumatic 111
　of unknown origin, cause of 449
　outcome of 110
　with focal signs 109
　without focal signs 109

Commercial feeding formulae 283
Community-acquired pneumonia,
　treatment of 164
Complete blood count 89, 169, 291, 377,
　380, 438
Concentration dependent drugs 162
Concomitant fungal infection 146
Conduction defects 396
Confusion 430
Congestive cardiac failure 371, 372, 412
Congestive heart failure 392, 417
Consciousness
　deteriorates, level of 104
　pathophysiology of 104
Constipation, long-standing 376
Continuous cardiac output
　monitoring 316
Continuous electroencephalogram
　monitoring 432
Continuous positive airway pressure 74,
　248*f*, 249, 365, 406
Continuous renal replacement therapy 95,
　159
Continuous venovenous
　hemodiafiltration 98
　hemodialysis 98
　hemofiltration 95
Contraction alkalosis 324, 337
Convulsive seizures 431
Copenhagen 5
Copper 295
Corneal reflex 108, 111
Coronary artery bypass graft 364
Coronary perfusion 269
　pressure 305
Coronary syndromes 81
Coronavirus disease-2019 pandemic 11
Correct wedging procedure 311
Corrective stress factors 281
Corticosteroid 153, 405
　systemic 405
Co-trimoxazole 173
Cough 403
　reflex 207
C-reactive protein 145, 169, 187, 214, 379
Creatinine 214
　kinase 428
Cricothyrotomy, surgical 23
Critical care
　echocardiography in 341
　medicine 3
　neuropathy 253
　patients 464
Critical illness 158
　myopathy 425

Index

Critically ill
　obese 293*t*
　patients 277*b*, 292, 294, 322, 430
　　malnutrition in 274
Cryoprecipitate 446
Cryptococcal antigen 190
Cryptococcal meningitis 199*f*
Cryptococcal meningoencephalitis 200
Cryptococcus 173, 199, 204
　infection 199
Crystalloid, type of 148
Cuff leak test 259
Cushing's disease 399
Cushing's syndrome 324, 399
　severe 399
Cyclical pupillary dilation 450
Cyclophosphamide 413
Cyclosporine 9, 204
Cytokines 143, 379
Cytomegalovirus 130

D

Dabigatran 372, 445
Damage control surgery 444
Daptomycin 162, 167, 222
Dead space ventilation 47
Deep vein thrombosis 263, 404, 409
Dehydration, severe 379
Delirium 106
Dengue 88, 180
Deoxyribonucleic acid 130, 180
Device components 269
Dexamethasone 393
Dexmedetomidine 65
Diabetes 108, 109
　mellitus 199, 213
　related emergencies 379
　type 1 386
Diabetic ketoacidosis 332, 375, 379-381, 383
　resolution of 384
Dialysis machine 98
Dialytic therapy 93
Diaphragm crura 250
Diaphragmatic irritation 376
Diaphragmatic muscle weakness 427
Diarrhea 331, 392
　checklist 283*t*
　infectious 189
Diastolic functions 404
Digoxin 80, 368
Dilated right ventricle 349*f*
Diltiazem 368, 370
Dilution methods 183
Dilutional hyponatremia 413

Diminished cardiac contractility 123
Disease etiology 37
Disk diffusion susceptibility tests 182
Dissection flap 348*f*
Disseminated intravascular coagulation 13, 144
Diuretic 405
　therapy 324
D-lactic acidosis 332
Dobutamine 79, 303, 467
Docosahexaenoic acid 294
Dofetilide 369, 370
Dopamine 79, 149, 303, 467
Dopaminergic effect 150
Doppler shift 342
Doripenem 175, 458
Doxazosin 401
Doxycycline 222, 462
Dronedarone 370
Drowsiness 413, 430
Drug
　interactions 204
　poisoning 449
Drug-resistant pathogens, risk factors for 157
Dysfunctional right ventricle 347*f*
Dyslipidemias 109
Dysphagia, severe 281
Dyspnea 42
　acute 350

E

Early intubation 74
Echinocandins 196
Echocardiogram 72
Echocardiography 76
　Doppler modalities 346*t*
　information 345
　modalities of 342
　window 341
Eclampsia 117
Edema 88
Eicosapentaenoic acid 294
Ejection fraction 76
Electric defibrillator 367
Electrocardiogram 26, 72, 404
　postrecovery 30
Electrolyte 89, 382
　balance 134
　imbalance 133
　replacement of 386
Elemental feeds 284
Elevated natriuretic peptides
　cardiac causes of 75*t*
　noncardiac causes of 75*t*

Emergency
  medical services 40
  room 113
Emergent therapy 111
  principles of 111
Empiric antituberculosis treatment 204
Empiric treatment 209
Empirical antimicrobial
  selection 155
  therapy 155
Empirical therapy 155
Encephalitis 158
Encephalomyelitis, acute disseminated 435
Encephalopathy 133, 134
  syndrome 432
End-diastolic
  pressure 300
  volume 299
End-inspiration pressure 238
Endocarditis, infective 181, 318
Endocrine
  conditions, nondiabetic 379
  emergencies 379
  topic of 379
Endoneural edema 426
Endophthalmitis 194
End-organ
  dysfunction 73
  perfusion 269
Endotracheal aspirate 188
Endotracheal intubation 21, 63, 118
Endotracheal secretions 208
Endotracheal tube 130, 207, 210, 252
Endovascular coiling 122
Endovascular infections 194
End-tidal carbon dioxide 27
Enteral feeds, mechanical obstruction to 273, 274
Enteral nutrition 281, 286b, 287, 291, 293
  related complications 285t
Enterobacter 217
Enterobacteriaceae 172, 175
Enterococcus
  faecalis 174
  faecium 172, 174
  spp 173
Entirely noninvasive methods 319
Enzyme 200
  immunoassay 180
  modification 172
Eosinophilia 398
Epilepsy 433
Epinephrine 149, 150
Episodes, acute 70

Epstein-Barr virus 130
Equipment and procedure 266
Ertapenem 172, 175, 177, 458
Escherichia coli 217
Eskape pathogens 172
Esmolol 368
Essential interventions 28b
Estimated glomerular filtration rate 85
E-test 182
Ethyl alcohol 333
Ethylene glycol 333
Euvolemic hyponatremia 413, 421
Evidence-based medicine 10
Exacerbation 403
  episodes, management of 409
Extensor plantar responses 426
Extracellular fluid 412
Extracorporeal albumin dialysis 135
Extracorporeal blood purification 100
Extracorporeal life support organization 67
Extracorporeal membrane oxygenation 67, 97, 261, 264
Extracorporeal therapies 159
Extubation 258
  prerequisites before 259b
Eye
  living 105
  movements 108

F

Facial injury 439
Facial myokymia 450
Fasciotomy 216f
Fatigue 231
Fecal samples 189
Fentanyl 65
Fever 432
  acute undifferentiated 179
Fibrin-platelet clot 144
Fibrotic phase 59
Filling pressure, function of 306
Flecainide 369, 370
Fluconazole 196
Fluid
  overload, avoid 148
  responsiveness 299, 306t
    determinants of 305
  restriction 420
  resuscitation 92, 148
  therapy 382
    phases of 92b
  type of 148
Fluoroscopic equipment 310
Focal motor convulsions 431

Focal sensory symptoms 431
Fondaparinux 444
Forced vital capacity 259
Fosfomycin 216, 223, 462
Fosphenytoin 434
Fraction of inspired oxygen 27, 38, 56, 58, 64, 232, 256
Frank-Starling
 curve 305*f*
 relationship 299
Fresh frozen plasma 446
Functional disorder 113
Functional residual capacity 6
Fungal infection 128
Fungal pathogens 193*t*
 clinical manifestations 193*t*
 risk factors 193*t*
 treatment 193*t*
Fusarium 204, 226

G

Gabapentin 436
Gag reflex 108
Galactomannan 187, 204
Gallbladder colic 376
Gamma-aminobutyric acid 333
Ganz thermodilution catheter 267
Gas exchange 37*f*
 alterations 240
Gastric aspirates 189
Gastric distension 407
Gastric secretions, regurgitated 117
Gastric stasis 273
Gastrointestinal blood loss, massive 376
Gastrointestinal cause 334
Gastrointestinal infections 189
Gastrointestinal-hepatic dysfunction 392
Gastrostomy 282
Genitourinary tract malignancies 413
Gentamicin 173, 216, 459
Glasgow coma scale 108, 465
Glomerular filtration rate 84
Glucocorticoid deficiency 413
Glucose
 concentration, normal 388
 control 153
Glutamine 292, 294
Gradient diffusion method 183
Graft-versus-host disease 187
Gram stain 181
Gram-negative resistance 175
Gram-positive infections 204
Granulomatous disease, chronic 197
Granulomatous disorders 397

Grave's disease 391
Guiding therapy 146*f*
Guillain-Barré syndrome 231, 428
Gut inflammation 204

H

Haemophilus influenzae 190
Half life procalcitonin 187
Hand hygiene 210
Hantavirus 88
Harris-Benedict equation 281
Headache 107, 432
Health
 evaluation, chronic 464
 points, chronic 465
Healthy granulation tissue 216*f*
Heart 299
 filling pressures, left 355
 rate 303
Heart failure 117, 233, 348
 acute 69, 70*t*, 71, 71*f*, 72, 72*t*, 75
 chronic 69
 signs of 69
 symptoms of 69
Helicobacter pylori 189
Hematology tests 403
Hematoma 118, 374
 large superficial 119
Hemato-oncology 156
Hematopoietic stem cell
 transplant 193
Hematuria 188
Hemispheric stroke, large 117
Hemodialysis therapies 93
Hemodialyzer 98
Hemodynamic
 compromise 69
 deterioration 347
 devices 307
 instability 71
 monitoring 299
  physiological basis of 299
 parameters 303
 stability, assessment of 403
 support 6
 values, normal 302*t*
Hemofiltration 93
Hemoglobin 46, 214, 256, 304
Hemolytic anemia 295
Hemoperfusion therapy 100
Hemophagocytic lymphohistiocytosis 127
Hemorrhage 398, 437
 acute 114
 intracerebral 118, 119

management of
  intraventricular 120
  post-traumatic 438*b*
medical management of post-traumatic 437
putaminal 120
severe 444
simultaneous 144
subarachnoid 75, 121, 122
traumatic 443
Hemorrhagic changes 114
Hemorrhagic fevers 158
Hemorrhagic shock 145
Henderson-Hasselbalch equation 323, 327
Heparin anticoagulation 119
Heparin-induced thrombocytopenia 144
Hepatic cirrhosis 412
Hepatic dysfunction, serious 290
Hepatic encephalopathy 128
Hepatic gluconeogenesis 379
Hepatic vein 346
  tributary 353*f*
Hepatitis 180
  A 227
    virus 130
  autoimmune 127, 129
  B 227
    core antigen 130
    surface antigen 130
  C virus 130
  E virus 130
  ischemic 127
Hepatocellular failure 339
Hepatocytes 129
Hepatorenal syndrome 128
Herpes simplex virus 130
Herpes zoster 374
Hip joint effusion, right 219*f*
Hippocrates 3
  after 4
Histoplasma 204
  capsulatum 173, 188
Hormone, adrenocorticotropic 416
Human chorionic gonadotropin 391
Human immunodeficiency virus 180, 193, 197, 227
Hydatidiform mole 391
Hydration 374
Hydrocephalus 123
Hydrocortisone 393, 399
  dose of 399
Hydrogen ion 322
Hydrophilic drugs 161
Hyperammonemia 133
Hypercalcemia 396
  causes of 396, 397, 397*t*
  dependent 397
  episode, severe 398
  malignancy-associated 397
  severe 396, 397
Hypercapnia 47, 49
  chronic 410
  physiological basis of 47
Hypercapnic failure
  acute 406
  chronic 406
Hypercapnic respiratory failure 35, 36, 231, 406
Hypercarbia, degree of 406
Hypercatabolic phase 273
Hypercatabolic state, level of 279
Hyperchloremic acidosis 437
Hyperfibrinolysis 446
Hyperglycemia 287, 289, 379, 381, 384, 385, 426, 427
Hyperglycemic hyperosmolar state 380, 381, 383, 385
Hyperinflation 407
Hyperinsulinemia 388
Hyperkalemia 30, 133, 398
  membrane actions of 446
Hyperlactatemia, causes of 304
Hyperlipidemia 381
Hypermagnesemia 133, 450
Hyperoxia 54, 440
  moderate 440
Hyperplasia 397
Hyperreflexia 426
Hypersomnia 104, 105
Hypertension 81, 109, 118, 219, 231, 337
  control of 118
  evidence of 108
  history of 364
  renovascular 324
Hypertensive crisis, treatment of 401
Hypertensive effect, acute 116
Hypertensive encephalopathy 117
Hypertriglyceridemia 287
  moderate 382
Hyperventilation 49, 323, 329, 450
Hypervolemia 133
  mild 123
Hypervolemic hypernatremia, causes of 412
Hypervolemic hyponatremia 412, 420, 422
Hypervolemic therapy, mild 123
Hypoalbuminemia 159
Hypoalbuminemic malnutrition 275
Hypocalcemia 101, 395, 396, 432
  acute 393, 394

acute symptomatic 395, 418
causes of 394*t*
D-related 395
Hypocapnia 440
Hypoglycemia 114, 129, 134, 289, 384, 386, 387, 389, 398
  clinical 386
  diagnosis of 387*t*
  elative 289
  mild-to-moderate symptomatic 387
  signs of 387
Hypokalemia 30, 336, 337, 384, 399
Hypomagnesemia, severe 324
Hyponatremia 124, 133, 389, 390, 398, 411-415, 417*fc*, 422, 423, 432
  autocorrection of 419
  causes of 421, 423
  chronic 413, 414, 419, 420, 422
  correction of 421
  development of 413
  diagnosis of 411
  etiology of true 412
  management of 411
  mild 413
  overcorrection of 419
  pathophysiology of 411, 423
  redistributive 412
  severe 390
  translocational 412, 415
  treatment of 416, 417, 420
    chronic 423
  types of 411
Hyponatremic plasma 421
Hypoperfusion 437
  cold 70
  symptomatic 80
  warm 70
Hypotension 30, 86, 144, 149, 348, 432
  symptomatic 80
Hypothermia 101, 436, 437
Hypothyroidism, severe untreated 388
Hypotonic hyponatremia 412
Hypoventilation 323, 390, 410
Hypovolemia 92, 101, 324, 411, 422
  severe 308
Hypovolemic hyponatremia 412, 421
Hypoxemia 38, 44, 57
  approach to 38
  causes of 39*f*
  correcting 51
  correction of 374
  nonrespiratory causes of 38*t*
  respiratory causes of 38*t*
Hypoxemic respiratory failure 35, 231
Hypoxia, refractory 64

Hypoxic brain injury 27
Hypoxic respiratory failure 233

I

Iatrogenic causes 334
Iatrogenic complications 54
Iatrogenic hypoglycemia 386
Idarucizumab 444
Ideal body weight 293
Ifosfamide 413
IIntra-abdominal infection, treatment of serious 191
Iliopsoas bursitis 219*f*
Imipenem 175, 458
Immobilization 426
Immune
  function 190
  nutrition 296
Immunochromatographic test 188
Immunoglobulin M 130
Immunonutrients 292
Impaired renal perfusion 87
Impella controller 271
  system 270
Impella device 267, 270*f*
  physiological effect of 269*fc*
Improved respiratory function 83
Infarction 398
Infection 101, 134, 139, 156, 164, 165*t*, 166*fc*, 191, 312, 379, 398, 404
  c-induced 313
  healthcare-associated 206
  hospital-associated 206
  secondary 13
  serious 86
  severe 391
  site of 153
  specific organ-related 187
  wide spectrum of 213
Infectious disease evaluation 380
Infiltration 398
Inflammation 426
  local 366
  signs of 400
Inflammatory modulators 366
Infratentorial lesion 107
In-hospital cardiac arrest 29
Initial ventilatory settings 63
Inotropes 73
Insertion technique 310
Inspiratory positive airway pressure 406
Insulin 386
  administration of 383
  deficiency 379, 381, 382

infusion 382
therapy 383
    inadequate 379
Intact oculocephalic maneuver 107
Intensive care management 69
Intensive care unit 21, 44, 102, 132b, 155, 193, 254, 273, 293, 341, 346, 425, 428, 437
    acquired weakness 425
    seizures in 430
Interatrial septum 346
Interferon γ 204
Intermittent hemodialysis 93
Intermittent mandatory ventilation 241, 242, 256, 257
Interstitial lung disease 36, 38, 39
Intestinal absorption 396
Intestinal obstruction 375
Intoxication 107, 109
Intra-abdominal
    infection 191, 217, 219
    injuries 441
Intra-aortic balloon pump 73, 265, 271, 359
Intracellular fluid 412
Intracranial pressure 117
Intraoperative tissue 215
Intrapulmonary pressures 407
Intravenous
    drugs 201
    glucocorticoids 390
    insulin infusion 384
    thrombolysis 114, 115
Invasive arterial pressures 73
Invasive aspergillosis 187
Invasive candidiasis, risk factors for developing 194
Invasive fungal infections 193
Invasive mechanical ventilation 232
Invasive pulmonary aspergillosis 197
Invasive samples 208
Invasive ventilation 74, 407
Ireton-Jones equation 281
Iron lung 235
Isavuconazole 198, 203
Ischemia 86
    pulmonary hypertension 404
Ischemic stroke 116, 118
    role of thrombectomy in 115
Isoniazid 333
Isoprenaline 467
Isotonic saline 420

J

Jejunostomy 282
Joint aspiration 220f
Jugular venous pressure 88

K

Ketamine 435
Ketoacid, primary 332
Ketoacidosis 332
Ketogenic diet 436
Ketone
    accumulation of 381
    bodies, accumulation of 332
Ketonemia 381
Ketonuria 381
    test for 332
Ketosis 379
    development of 385
Kidney
    biopsy 89
    disease 85, 97
        chronic 88, 110, 187, 193, 197
    failure 84
    function 101
    hypoperfusion 101
    injury
        acute 13, 84-88, 90, 91, 97, 101, 102, 128, 149
        management of acute 91, 102fc
Klebsiella 163, 217, 221, 226, 227
    penumoniae 163, 172, 223, 227
        carbapenemase 218
    spp 171
Kussmaul breathing 380

L

Labored breathing 313
Lacosamide 135, 434
Lactate clearance 304
Lactic acid acidosis 332
Lactic acidosis 331
Laryngeal edema 259, 260
Laryngeal mask airway 21f
Laryngeal reflexes 21
Laryngospasm 259
Lazarus sign 451
Left atrium 342-344
    calculation of 356f
Left bundle branch block 357
Left ventricular
    cavity opacification 357f
    diastolic and systolic volumes 357f
    dysfunction 368
    ejection fraction 348
    end-diastolic pressure 267, 355
    failure 253
    hypertrophy 75, 76
    outflow tract 346, 352
    stroke volume 317

systolic
  dysfunction 350
  function 357
Legionella 181
  pneumophila 188
Leptomeningeal enhancement 199*f*
Leptospira 180
Leptospirosis 88
Lethargy 430
Leukocytoclastic vasculitis 227*f*
Leukocytosis 382
Levetiracetam 135, 434
Levofloxacin 173
Levosimendan 79, 467
Levothyroxine 390
Lidocaine toxicity 449
Life-threatening
  hypotension 440
  organ failure 143
Limb, stimulus-induced 450
Limbic encephalitis 435
Linezolid 110, 162, 222
Liothyronine 390
Lithium carbonate 393
Liver
  disease, chronic 197
  dysfunction 450
  failure 293, 333
  function test 438
  injury
    acute 13, 128, 313
    drug-induced 127
    malignant infiltration of 127
    transplantation 131*b*, 135
      contraindications for 136*b*
Lmipenem 173
Lobar, surgery for 120
Locked-in syndrome 450
Long chain triglycerides 284
Loop diuretics 324
Lorazepam 65, 433, 434
Low initial hemoglobin 442
Low molecular weight heparin 445
Low serum
  osmolality 124
  sodium 124
Lower limb 225*f*
  right 213*f*
Lower respiratory
  pathogens 189
  tract infection 223
Lugol's iodine solution 393
Lung
  compliance 237
  damage 62
  disease, structural 209

  hyperinflation of 409
  injury 439
    acute 56
    severity of 60
    ventilator-induced 59, 60
  parenchyma 224
  pathology, unresolved 254
  protection ventilation 62
  protective strategy 61, 251
  small cell cancer of 413
  ultrasonography 77*f*
  ultrasound 76
  units 44
Lymphocytic pleocytosis 199

M

Macrolides 162
Maculopapular skin lesions 194*f*
Magnesium 379
Malaria 88
Malicious drug 386
Malnutrition 273
  acute disease-related 273, 274
  assessment of 276
  chronic disease-related 274
  classification of 273
Mask
  nonvented 406
  vented 406
Mean airway pressure 240
Mean arterial pressure 466
Mechanical circulatory supports 265
Mechanical thrombectomy 114, 115
Mechanical ventilation 19, 62, 64*b*, 64*t*, 132, 152, 240, 245, 315, 427
  advanced modes of 245, 245*b*, 247
  basics of 235
  effects of 315
  indications of 231, 232*t*
  strategies in 245
  weaning from 252
Membranoproliferative
  glomerulonephritis 89
Meningeal signs 109
Meningoencephalitis, chronic 157
Mental obtundation 214
Mental status 384
  decreased 389
  normal 386
Meropenem 173, 175, 458
Mesenteric ischemia 378
Metabolic abnormalities 145
Metabolic acidosis 252, 325, 322, 330, 332, 335*b*, 336, 450

causes of 331, 331t
development of 134
severe 133
Metabolic alkalosis 323-325, 330, 331, 336, 399
analysis of 336
causes of 324t, 336, 337
secondary 340
type of 336
Metabolic complication 289
Metabolic derangements 291, 432
Metabolic disorder 322, 328, 333
Metabolic encephalopathies 110
Metabolic evaluation 380
Metanephrines 401
Metastases 432
Metastatic infections 196
Metformin 304
Methanol 333
Methicillin-resistant *Staphylococcus aureus* 168, 174
Methimazole 393
Methylprednisolone 435
Metoprolol 393, 401
tartrate 368
XL 368
Metronidazole 110, 162
Midazolam 65, 435
Midbrain involvement 108
Milrinone 79, 123, 467
Minimal bactericidal concentration 160
Minimally conscious state 104, 105, 111
Minocycline 462
Minute ventilation 46, 409
Mitochondrial damage, severe 304
Mitral annular tissue 355f
Mitral flow pulse wave 355f
Mitral leaflet 343f
flail anterior 350f
Mitral regurgitation 345f, 346, 350f
Mitral stenosis 346
severe 348
Mixed venous oxygen 303, 309, 317t
Mnemonics 468
Molecular adsorbent recirculating system 135
Monitoring 297
devices 299
Monobactam aztreonam 175
Monoclonal antibodies 199
Morganella 173
Morphine 80
Motion, equation of 237
Motor weakness 426

Mucor 201, 202
Multidrug-resistant
bacteria 208
enterococcus spp 172
Multifocal myoclonus 108
Multiorgan failure 128, 432
Multiple organ dysfunction syndrome 88
Multislice computed tomography 441
Muscle biopsy 428
Musculoskeletal system 427
Myasthenia gravis 428
Mycobacteria 185
Mycobacterium tuberculosis 181
Mycophenolate 9
Mycoplasma 185, 226
Myeloid leukemia, acute 194f
Myocardial depression 369
Myocardial infarction 76, 372, 391
acute 265
inferior 375
Myocardial perfusion 269
gradient 269
Myxedema coma 388, 389, 389b

N

Nasal cannula ventilation, high-flow 405
Nasal delivery 405
Nasal mucosa 19
Nasal oxygen
device, humidified high-flow 53
high-flow 12, 233
Nasogastric aspiration 324
Nasogastric tube 282, 436
Nasojejunal tube 282
Natriuretic peptide 72
B-type 72
Nausea 392
Nebulization 410
Nebulized prostaglandins 66
Neck cancers 413
Necrotizing fasciitis 201, 213f, 214
Necrotizing infective pancreatitis, severe 293
Needle cricothyrotomy 23
Neoplasms 109
Nephrocalcinosis 396
Nephrogenic diabetes insipidus 396
Nephrolithiasis 396
Nephrotic syndrome 412
Nephrotoxic drugs 86, 101
Nephrotoxic injury 87
Nervous system, peripheral 202
Nesiritide 79
Neuroglycopenic symptoms 386, 387

Neurohormonal system 421
Neuroimaging 114
Neurologic complication 432
  severe 397
Neurologic damage 431
Neurologic deficit 114, 115, 123
Neurologic examination 426
  rapid 113
Neurologic syndrome 425
Neurological examination 108
Neurological injury 27, 28
Neurological phenomenon, positive 430
Neuromuscular blockade 431
Neuromuscular junction 427
Neuromuscular problems, preexisting 428
Neuromuscular respiratory failure 427
Neurosurgical intervention 119
Neutropenia 194
Neutropenic patients 157
Nicardipine 123
Nicotine 413
Nimodipine 123
Nitrofurantoin 223
Nitrogen balance 275, 280, 291
  calculation 279b
Nitroglycerin 79, 303
Nitroprusside 79, 303, 401
Nocardia spp 181
Nonabsorbable 324
Nonacetaminophen cases 131
Nonanesthetic antiepileptic drugs 434
Nonaneurysmal perimesencephalic subarachnoid hemorrhage 124
Nonanion gap acidosis, causes of 333
Nonconvulsive status 434
Nonculture-based tests 195
Non-Hodgkin's lymphoma 226
Noninvasive positive pressure ventilation, contraindications of 52f
Noninvasive ventilation 12, 21, 52, 57, 63, 71, 72, 231, 232, 253
Nonrebreathing masks 52
Nonsteroidal anti-inflammatory drug 72, 86
Noradrenaline 79, 80, 149, 467
Norepinephrine 123, 133, 150, 303
Normocapnia 132
North-south syndrome 264
Nuchal rigidity 432
Nutrition 134
  inadequate 339
Nutritional planning 275

Nutritional support 274, 276t, 291, 293
  approach to 273
  disease modified 292
  indications of 275, 277b
  monitoring of 290
Nutritional syndrome 274fc

O

Obstructive pulmonary disease, chronic 36, 72, 75, 197, 233, 232, 237, 249, 253, 313, 403, 404
Obstructive sleep apnea 406
Ocular movements, external 107
Oculocephalic maneuver 449
Oculovestibular reflex 107, 450
Ofloxacin 173
Oliguria 89
Omega-3 fatty acids 294
Omega-6 fatty acids 292
Opioids 226
Opportunistic bacterial illnesses 156
Oral antiarrhythmic drugs 370t
Oral anticoagulants, direct 119, 443
Oral nimodipine 123
Orbital cellulitis with palate 201f
Organ dysfunction 33, 72, 141, 142
  sepsis-induced 145
Organ failure 136
Organ perfusion 304
Organ support system 100
Organ transplant 8
Organophosphorus compounds 449
Oropharyngeal seal 20
Orthostatic hypotension 422
Osmolality 416t
Osmotic demyelination syndrome 419
Osmotic diuresis 381
Osteomyelitis 194
Oxacillins 172
Oxins 127
Oxygen
  consumption index 302
  delivery 303
    devices 51
  index 302
  dissociation curve 41
  high flow 57
  partial pressure of 27
  saturation 27, 206, 312
    peripheral 132
  supplementation 405
Oxygenation 304b
  support of 74
Oxyhemoglobin 303

P

Pacemaker, temporary 359
Packed red blood cell 446
Pain
   acute 375
   origin of 374
Pancreatic origin, pain of 376
Pancreatitis 146, 293
Papillary muscle rupture 347
Paraganglioma 400
Paraneoplastic disorders 435
Parasite lactate dehydrogenas 179
Parathyroid
   glands 394
   hormone 394, 397
   related emergencies 393
Parenteral nutrition 286, 287, 291, 293, 427
   complications of 288, 288t
   peripheral 290
   total 287
Paresthesias 394
Paroxysmal hypertension 400
Paroxysmal nocturnal dyspnea 70
Parsimony, rule of 157
Partial parenteral nutrition 287
Particularly imipenem 178
Parturition 391
Passive leg raising 319
Patent foramen ovale 346
Pathogen activated molecular pattern 143
Pelvic stabilization 445
Penicillin plus, combination of 161
Penicillium 204
Percutaneous coronary
        intervention 267
   triage for 30
Percutaneous tracheostomy 23
Percutaneous transluminal coronary
        angioplasty 265
Pericardial effusion 318, 347f
Pericardial tamponade 350
Pericarditis 345
Peripheral arterial disease 372
Peritoneal dialysis 93
Peritonitis, localized 375
Permissible hypercapnia 62, 251
Persistent respiratory acidosis 406
Persistent vegetative state 105, 111
Pharmacodynamics 158
Pharyngeal reflexes 21
Phentolamine 401
Phenylephrine 123, 467
Phenytoin 434
Pheochromocytoma 400, 401
   crisis 400, 401b
   diagnosis of 401
Phosphate 379
   replacement 383
Phosphodiesterase 73
Physical examination 279
Physiological abnormality 35
Physiology health evaluation,
        acute 464
Piperacillin 110, 134, 173, 457
Pitting pedal edema 398
Pituitary adenoma 399
Pituitary tumor 391
Plasma
   concentrations 97
   exchange, high volume 135
   natriuretic peptide levels 75
   separation 100
   triglyceride 287
Plasmalyte 133
Plasmodium
   falciparum 180
   species 180
Plateau pressures 238
Platelet
   count 446
   dysfunction, early detection of 443
   inhibitors 371
Pneumomediastinum 13
Pneumonectomy 363
Pneumonia 117, 206, 375
   bundle, ventilator-associated 210b
   causes of ventilator-associated 207
   community-acquired 157
   hospital-acquired 206
   prevention of ventilator-associated
        210, 211b
   ventilator-associated 206, 207, 208, 224
Pneumothorax 235
Point of care echocardiography 341
Poisoning 109
Polio epidemic 5
Polyclonal antibody 9
Polydipsia, primary 413, 421
Polyethersulfone 99
Polymerase chain reaction 179, 197, 208,
        404
Polymicrobial culture 215
Polymicrobial infections 161
Polymyxin 172, 177, 218
   B 173, 223, 461
   E 461
Polytrauma 275, 445
Polyurethane balloon 266
Polyvinyl chloride 309

Population, increasing 8
Porphyria 374, 375
Posaconazole 198, 203
Positive end-expiratory pressure 5, 53, 56, 64, 238, 239, 245, 301, 315, 439
Postcardiac arrest care 26
Postcardiac surgery 365
Potassium 379
  depletion, severe 324
  iodide, saturated solution of 393
  replacement 383
Potential adverse events 271
Potential cardiac arrhythmias 395
Prasugrel 444
Prazosin 401
Precipitating causes 70
Precipitating factor, treatment of 384
Predisposing conditions 57
Preeclampsia 117
Pregnancy 127
Prerenal causes 86
Pressure control ventilation 236, 236*f*
Pressure sores 407
Pressure waveform configuration 311*f*
Pressure-regulated volume control 247
Preweaning tests 255
Primary disorders, severe 326
Procalcitonin 145, 146
  concentration, interpretation of 146*f*
  test 169
Propafenone 369, 370
Prophylactic agents, perioperative 365
Propofol 435
  infusions 433
Propranolol 393
Prostate 191
Protein
  C 128
  S 128
Prothrombin complex concentrate 119, 444, 445
Providencia 173
Pseudohyponatremia 381, 412, 414, 415
Pseudomonas 173, 178, 215, 221, 226, 227
  aeruginosa 172, 177, 209
    drug-resistant 177
  infection 170
Public health systems, deficient 86
Pulmonary arterial systolic ressure 353
Pulmonary artery 312, 354
  catheter 312
    complications of 312
    diastolic pressure 311, 312, 353, 354

main 346
pressure 313, 314*f*, 344
pressure monitoring 308
  indications for 310*b*
  systolic pressures 353
Pulmonary capillary wedge pressure 56, 145, 300, 303, 312
Pulmonary catheter, triple-lumen 311*f*
Pulmonary circulation 38
Pulmonary complications, postoperative 234
Pulmonary diseases, chronic 364
Pulmonary edema 233, 350
  high-altitude 40
  noncardiogenic 56
Pulmonary emboli 81
Pulmonary embolism 39, 40, 241, 263, 345, 348, 350
  subacute 347*f*
Pulmonary hypertension 240, 308
  degree of 404
Pulmonary infarction 313
Pulmonary regurgitation 346, 354
Pulmonary vascular resistance 346, 350
  estimation of 354
Pulmonary vasoconstriction 251
Pulmonary venous pressure 314, 314*f*
Pulmonary wedge position 310
Pulse
  oximetry 50
  wave 346, 352
Pupillary reflex 111
Purpuric rash 225*f*
Pyelonephritis 377
  acute 378

Q

Quinidine 370
Quinolones 110

R

Radial artery 307
Randomized controlled trials 10
Rankin scale, modified 31
Rapid diagnostic tests 179
Rapid shallow breathing index 256, 259
Rash 158
Rasmussen's encephalitis 435
Reactive oxygen species 379
Rebreathing, partial 52
Recognizing seizures 430
Red blood cell 121, 351*f*, 437
Red impella plug 270

Refractory hypoxemic failure, severe 36
Remifentanil 65
Renal causes 334, 335
   intrinsic 86
Renal clearance, augmented 159
Renal complication 397
Renal dysfunction 133, 293, 450
Renal failure 134
   development of 432
   early 334
Renal replacement therapy 84, 86, 94, 95, 102, 133, 278, 293
   acute 93
   complications of 101
   discontinuation of 100
   dose of 99
   modality of 95
   prolonged intermittent 98
Renin-angiotensin-aldosterone system 415, 416
Residual insulin secretion 385
Respiration 108
   types of 108
Respiratory abnormalities 389
Respiratory acid-base disorders, chronic 323
Respiratory acidosis 322, 330, 336, 389
   acute 36, 325
   chronic 325, 340
   mild-to-moderate 405
   severe 326
Respiratory alkalosis 330
   acute 325
   chronic 325
Respiratory arrest 231
Respiratory compensation 323
Respiratory disorder 322, 328
Respiratory distress
   severe 69
   severity of 403, 406
   signs of 231
   syndrome, severe acute 261
Respiratory drive, decreased 253
Respiratory failure 38, 231
   chronic 35
   classification of 35, 36t
   combined 35
   gas exchange in 37
   of acute 42
   type of 403, 406
Respiratory illness 425
Respiratory infection 82, 403
Respiratory irritants 403
Respiratory muscle
   disuse 253
   fatigue 253

Respiratory quotient, higher 252
Respiratory support 5
Respiratory tract infections 188
Resting energy expenditure 277
Resuscitation 17
   early 147
   initial 438
Reye syndrome 127
Rickettsiae 180
Right atrium 312
   vegetation in 220f
Right heart filling pressures 352
Ringer's acetate 148
Ringer's lactate 133, 148
Rivaroxaban 372
Road traffic accidents 437
Rotadynamic centrifugal pump 261

S

Salicylate overdose 333
Saline infusion, normal 421
Saliva 117
Salmonella spp 173, 189
Sarcoma 413
Sedation 63
Seizure 413
   drug-induced 110t
   duration 432
   management 119
   nonconvulsive 431
   recognition 430
   treatment 432
Self-calibrated devices 317
Sensorium 259
Separate arterial pressure 267
Sepsis 86, 100, 141, 144, 159fc, 180, 404, 428
   biomarkers for 186
   catheter-induced 320
   failure, development of 432
   features of 142
   pathogenesis of 143
   syndrome 194
Septic arthritis 221
Septic shock 141, 146, 148, 153, 157
Sequential compression devices 124
Sequential organ failure assessment 142, 197
   score 466
Serotonin reuptake inhibitor 413
Serratia 173
Serum
   calcium concentration 394
   electrolyte balance 366

glutamic
  oxaloacetic transaminase 130
  pyruvic transaminase 130
lactate 304
  measurement of 442
osmolality 415
sodium 411
Session length 99
Shigella 189
Shock 231, 241, 348, 375, 442
  hemodynamic profile in 145*t*
Shoulder adduction 451
Shunt 342
  fraction, degree of 45
  physiological 44
  quantifying 44
Sickle cell disease 375
Sinus of Valsalva 347
  ruptured 345
Sinus rhythm 367, 371
Sirolimus 9
Skin 374
  biopsy 227*f*
  hyperpigmentation of 398
  turgor 88
Slow continuous ultrafiltration 98
Smooth muscle contraction 374
Sodium 214
  depletion of 379
Solid organ
  lacerations 378
  transplant 193, 197
Solid tumors 226
Sotalol 365, 370
Spectral Doppler measurement 351
Spectrum of disease 194, 197, 199, 201
Spinal cord 124
Spontaneous breathing 235, 253, 306
  trial 65, 256
    procedure 257*b*
Spontaneous circulation, return of 26, 29
ST elevation myocardial infarction 347
ST segment elevation myocardial infarction 30
Standard polymeric formula 284
Staphylococcus 227, 289
  aureus 129, 161, 165, 172, 183, 209, 221, 289
Starvation ketoacidosis 332
Static drugs 196
Statins, role of 116
Status epilepticus 431, 434*t*, 436
  refractory 433
  super refractory 435, 435*t*

Stenotrophomonas 221
Steroid 13, 66, 199, 324, 393, 435
  treatment 66
Straightforward syndromes 158
Streptococcus
  agalactiae 224
  pneumoniae 181, 188
Stress 276*t*
  cardiomyopathy 123
  levels 281*t*
  starvation 275
Stroke 113
  acute 117
  onset 114, 115
  volume variation 306, 318
Stupor 106
Subcutaneous insulin therapy 384
Subcutaneous tissue 374
Sublingual nifedipine 117
Sulbactam 134, 173, 456, 457
Sulfamethoxazole 216, 222
Sulfonylureas 386
Superior vena cava 308, 346
Support 229
Supratentorial compartment 106
Surviving sepsis campaign 147
Synacthen stimulation test 398
Synchronized intermittent mandatory ventilation 242*f*
Syndrome of inappropriate secretion of antidiuretic hormone 414*b*, 416, 417
Systemic complications 436
  treatment of 391
Systemic inflammatory response syndrome 141, 187, 294, 427
Systemic vascular resistance 145, 302, 304
Systems requiring calibration 317
Systolic function, right ventricular 357
Systolic pressure variations 307

T

Tachycardia, severe 357
Tachypnea 231
Tacrolimus 204
Tazobactum 110, 134, 173, 457
Technical complications 289
Teicoplanin 167, 222, 460
Temporal lobe, part of 107
Terminally ill, end-of-life care for 10
Tetracycline 162, 173
Therapeutic drug monitoring 205
Therapeutic hypothermia 28, 29*b*
  management 29*b*

Thermodilution technique 315, 316
Thiazide 324
   diuretics 412, 417
   induced hyponatremia 421
Thionamide therapy 391
Thrombocytopenia 144
Thromboelastography 30
Thromboembolic events 371
Thromboembolism 371, 372
Thrombolytic treatment 117
Thrombotic microangiopathy 89
Thymoma 413
Thyroid hormone
   release, inhibition of 393
   replacement 389
   synthesis 393
Thyroid related emergencies 388
Thyroid storm 390
   diagnosis of 392t
   management of 391, 393t
   treatment of 391
Thyrotoxic crisis 390
Ticagrelor 444
Tigecycline 177, 216, 218, 223, 463
Tissue
   hypoperfusion 141
   hypoxia, causes of 46b
   oxygenation 299, 303
   perfusion
      determinants of 304b
      organ-specific 304
Today's intensive care units, genesis of 7
Todd's paralysis 430
Torso movements 450
Total body water 412
Toxic alcohols 333
Toxic encephalopathies 110
Toxicity, severe 333
Toxins 333
Tracheostomy 23
   complications of 24t
   tube 257
Tranexamic acid 446
Transducer monitoring
      technique 307
Transesophageal Doppler monitoring
      devices 318
Transesophageal echocardiography 318, 341, 370
Transfalcine herniation 106
Transfusion management 445
Transient ischemic attack 371, 372
Transplant medicine 156
Transpulmonary thermodilution 317
Transthoracic echocardiography 220

Trauma 146, 379, 391, 428
   sonography for 438
   systemized 438
Traumatic brain 450
   injury 440, 450
Trichosporon 173
   beigelii 190
Tricuspid annular plane systolic excursion 358f
Tricuspid regurgitation 346, 353
Triglycerides, medium chain 284
Trimethoprim 216, 222
Trophic feeds 290
Tropical fever 179
Trousseau's signs 394
Truma ovary 391
Tube feeding 286b, 287fc
Tubular necrosis
   acute 90
      ischemic 128

U

Ularitide 79
Ulcer, nonhealing 226f
Uncal herniation 107
Unit-acquired weakness 425
Upper gastrointestinal dysfunction 281
Upper lobe, left 203f
Upper respiratory
   pathogens 188
   tract infections 188
Uremia 133, 331
Uric acid, excretion of 90
Urinalysis 89
Urinary anion gap 335
Urinary chloride 324, 337
Urinary tract 191
   infection 128, 157, 223
Urine 89
   analysis 89
   osmolality 415, 416
   output 382, 466
   sodium 415, 416, 416t
      high 124
Urosepsis 187

V

Valproic acid 434
Valvar regurgitation 342
Valvular heart diseases 364
Vancomycin 167, 221, 222, 460
   detection of 183
Varicella zoster virus 130

Vascular access 99
Vascular territory implies 113
Vascular trauma, types of major 442
Vasculitis
   causes for 226
   types for 226
Vasodilator 79
   inhaled 66
   therapy 303
Vasopressin 133, 149, 150, 467
   receptor antagonists 421
      classification of 422
Vasopressor
   doses of 150*b*
   effects of 150, 150*b*
   support 148
Vena cava
   inferior 133, 262*f*, 346, 353*f*
   junction of superior 220*f*
Venoarterial extracorporeal membrane oxygenator 264
Venous admixture, treating 45
Ventilation 44, 46, 132, 303, 444
   adaptive support 241, 250
   advanced modes of 245
   assist control 64, 241, 248
   basic modes of 244*b*
   controlled 247
   discontinuation of 74
   inverse ratio 247
   modes of 243
      classification of 243*b*
   positive pressure 236, 240
   pressure support 249, 249*f*, 258
   pressure-controlled 236
   prone position 246
   proportional assist 250
   volume-controlled 236
Ventilator
   interventions 210
   support 51
Ventilator-associated conditions 206*b*
Ventilatory assist, neurally adjusted 250
Ventricular arrhythmias, refractory 263
Ventricular compliance 300
Ventricular contraction 301
Ventricular fibrillation 28
Ventricular septal rupture, acute 265
Ventricular tachycardia 28

Verapamil 123, 368
Very low density lipoproteins 382
Vibrio cholerae 189
Viral hepatitis 127
Viral illnesses 156
Viruses 185
Visceral protein levels 280
Viscoelastic methods 443
Vital interventions 5
Vitamin 295
   C 284
   D 395
      toxicity 397
   E 284
   K 444
      antagonist 443, 445
Vocal cords 259
Volutrauma 61, 251
Vomiting 324, 392
Voriconazole 198, 204

W

Warfarin 363
Warm-dry profiles 77
Warm-wet profiles 77
Weaning 65
   difficult 260
   failure
      causes of 252
      indicators of 254
   procedure 254
   stages of 255*b*
   trials 260
Wheezing 403, 405
Whipple's triad 386
White blood cell 187, 214
Wilson's disease 127
Witzel technique 282
Worsening hypotension 134

X

Xenotransplantation 9

Z

Zinc 295
Zolendronate 398

EU GSPR Authorised Reprsentative
Logos Europe, 9 rue Nicolas Poussin
1700, La Rochelle, France
Phone: +33 (0) 6 67 93 73 78
E-mail: contact@logoseurope.eu

www.ingramcontent.com/pod-product-compliance
Ingram Content Group UK Ltd.
Pitfield, Milton Keynes, MK11 3LW, UK
UKHW050427150426
5217IPUK00019B/1278